THERE IS NO RIGHT OR WRONG WAY TO HAVE A BODY.

— PATRICIA BERNE
    DISABILITY JUSTICE ORGANIZER AND ARTIST

CONTENTS

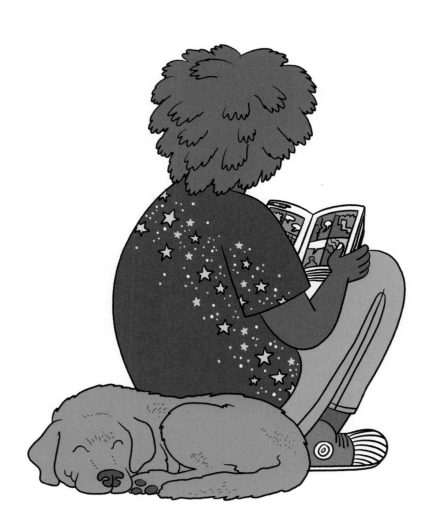

LETTER TO THE READER

THANK YOU FOR PICKING UP OUR BOOK!

LEARNING ABOUT BODIES, GENDER, SEX, AND PUBERTY IS DIFFERENT THAN LEARNING ABOUT OTHER THINGS. IT'S NOT BECAUSE THOSE TOPICS ARE BAD, WEIRD, STRANGE, OR UNCOMFORTABLE—WE JUST DON'T TALK ABOUT THEM NEARLY AS MUCH AS WE TALK ABOUT THINGS LIKE MOVIES, VIDEO GAMES, MUSIC, OR SPORTS.

SO, I WANT TO POINT OUT A FEW THINGS BEFORE YOU START READING THIS BOOK.

1. SOME PEOPLE THINK SEX EDUCATION IS A SCIENCE LESSON, LIKE THERE'S ONLY ONE RIGHT ANSWER TO EACH QUESTION. THAT'S NOT HOW WE WROTE THIS BOOK. WE'RE GUIDED BY SOMETHING DISABILITY JUSTICE ORGANIZER AND ARTIST PATTY BERNE SAYS: THERE'S NO RIGHT OR WRONG WAY TO HAVE A BODY.

   IF SOMETHING IN THIS BOOK DOESN'T FIT FOR YOU, IT ISN'T YOUR FAULT OR YOUR PROBLEM. YOU MAY HAVE WAYS OF THINKING AND FEELING THAT WE LEFT OUT. YOU MAY BE LEFT WITH MORE QUESTIONS THAN ANSWERS; I KNOW I FEEL THAT WAY A LOT OF THE TIME.

2. THIS BOOK IS A LOT! THERE'S FUNNY STUFF AND FASCINATING STUFF—BUT ALSO A LOT OF HARD STUFF, LIKE TALKING ABOUT DISCRIMINATION AND VIOLENCE. IF SOMETHING YOU'RE READING FEELS LIKE TOO MUCH, TAKE A BREAK (FOR AN HOUR, A WEEK, A MONTH, OR A YEAR). LEARNING DOESN'T HAPPEN QUICKLY. YOU KNOW BEST WHAT YOU CAN HANDLE AND WHEN, AND TRUSTING YOUR INSTINCTS IS WHAT THIS BOOK IS ALL ABOUT. SO, IF YOU COME ACROSS A QUESTION OR ACTIVITY IN THE BOOK AND IT DOESN'T FEEL RIGHT, SKIP IT. OR COME UP WITH YOUR OWN QUESTION OR ACTIVITY.

3. THIS BOOK IS FOR ADULTS TOO! MOST ADULTS DIDN'T HAVE THE OPPORTUNITY TO THINK AND TALK ABOUT SEX AND GENDER WHEN THEY WERE YOUNGER. THERE WILL BE THINGS IN THIS BOOK THAT ARE NEW FOR ADULTS. THERE WILL BE OTHER THINGS THEY DON'T EXPECT TO FIND IN A BOOK FOR YOUNG PEOPLE (LIKE PREGNANCY LOSS AND TRAUMA). IF YOU KNOW AN ADULT WHO IS OPEN TO READING THIS BOOK WITH YOU, REMIND THEM THAT THEY MAY NEED TIME BEFORE THEY ARE READY TO TALK ABOUT SOME OF WHAT THEY LEARN HERE.

   IT TOOK FIONA AND ME SEVEN YEARS TO MAKE THIS BOOK. I HOPE YOU FIND SOME THINGS IN IT THAT ARE HELPFUL, FUNNY, INTERESTING, CHALLENGING, AND USEFUL. OUR BOOKS GET BETTER WHEN READERS LET US KNOW BOTH WHAT WORKED FOR THEM AND ALSO WHAT DIDN'T. IF YOU HAVE THOUGHTS OR QUESTIONS ABOUT ANYTHING IN THIS BOOK, PLEASE BE IN TOUCH! YOU CAN FIND ME THROUGH MY WEBSITE, WWW.CORYSILVERBERG.COM.

   —CORY SILVERBERG, TORONTO

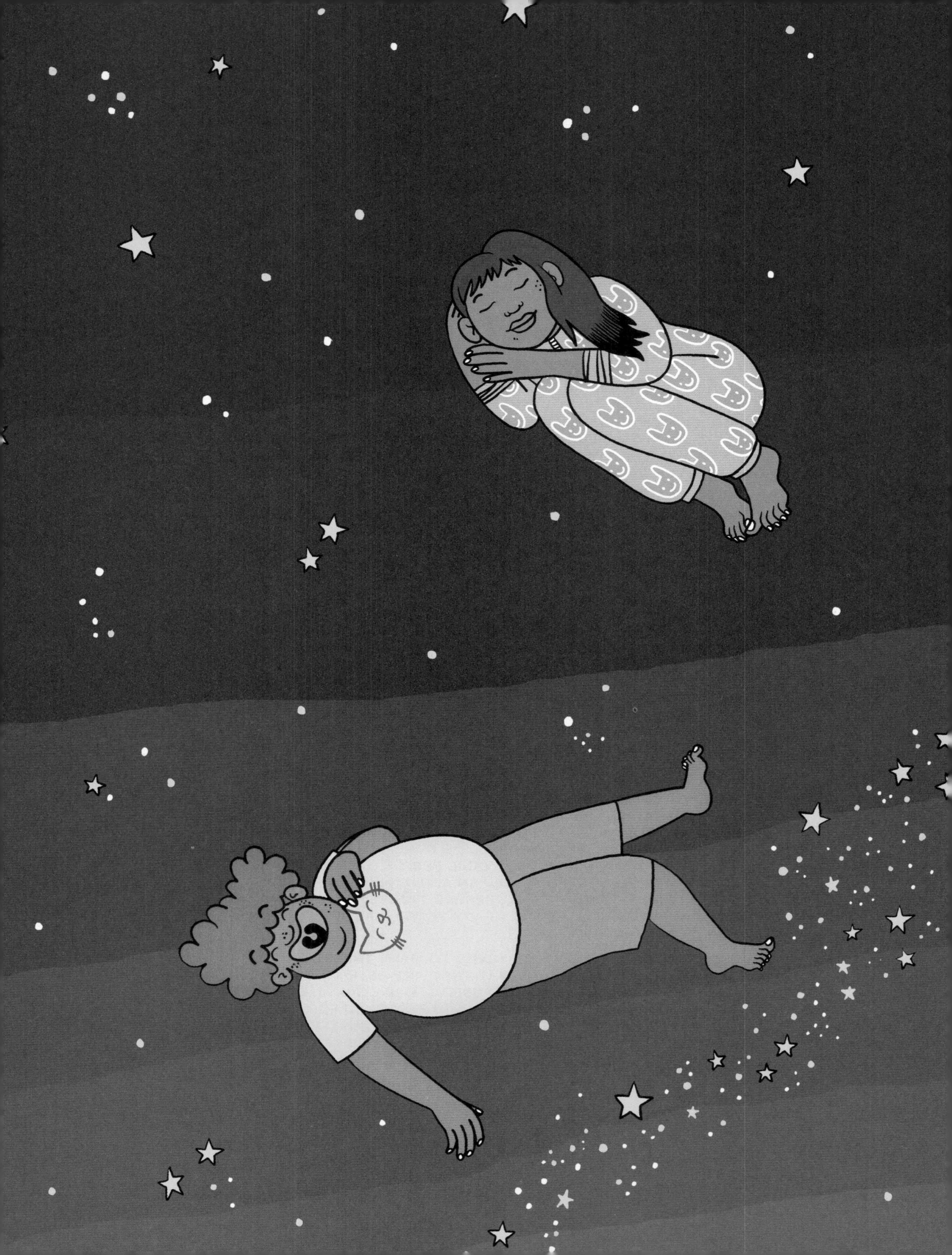

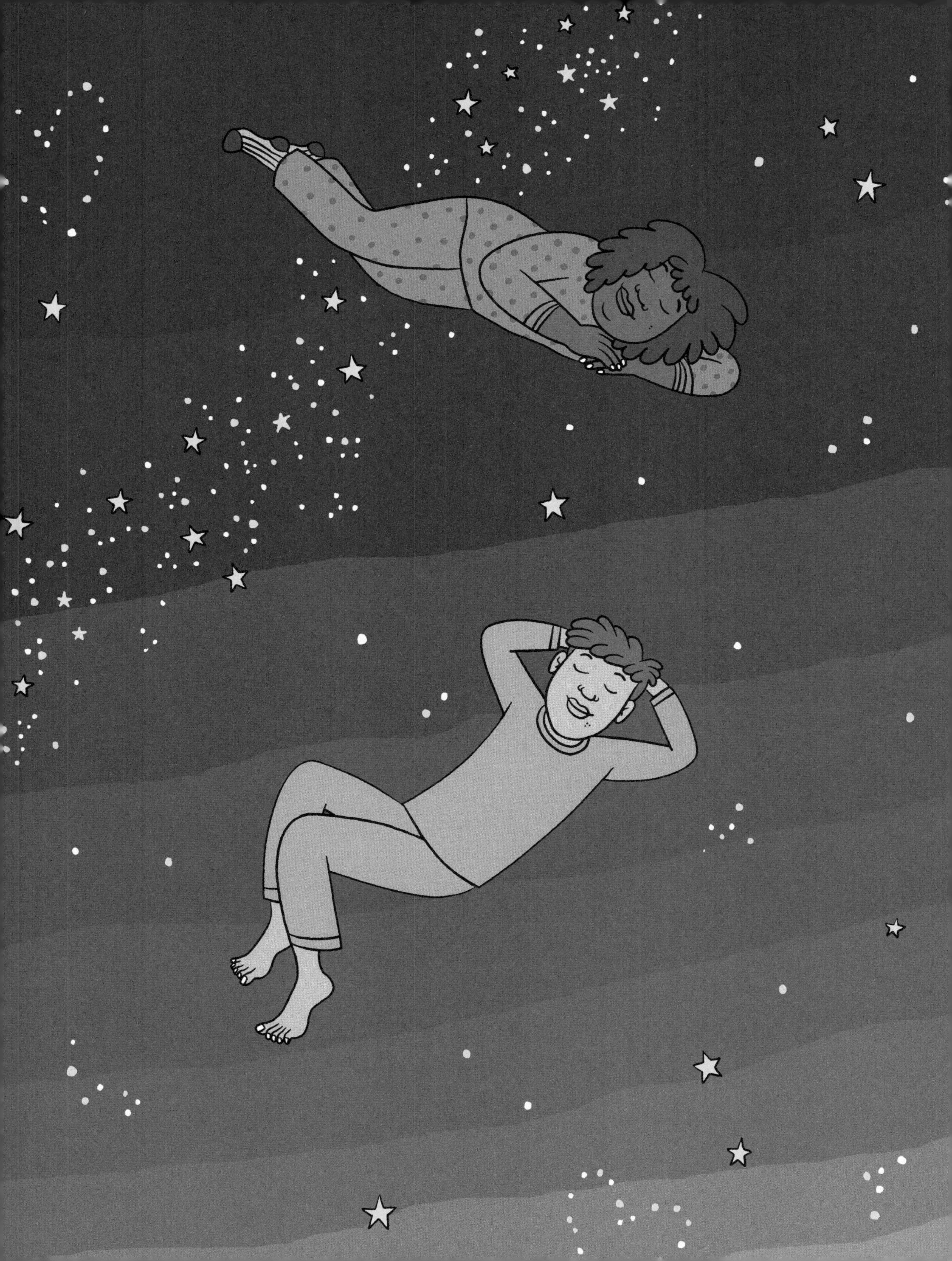

YOU KNOW, SEX

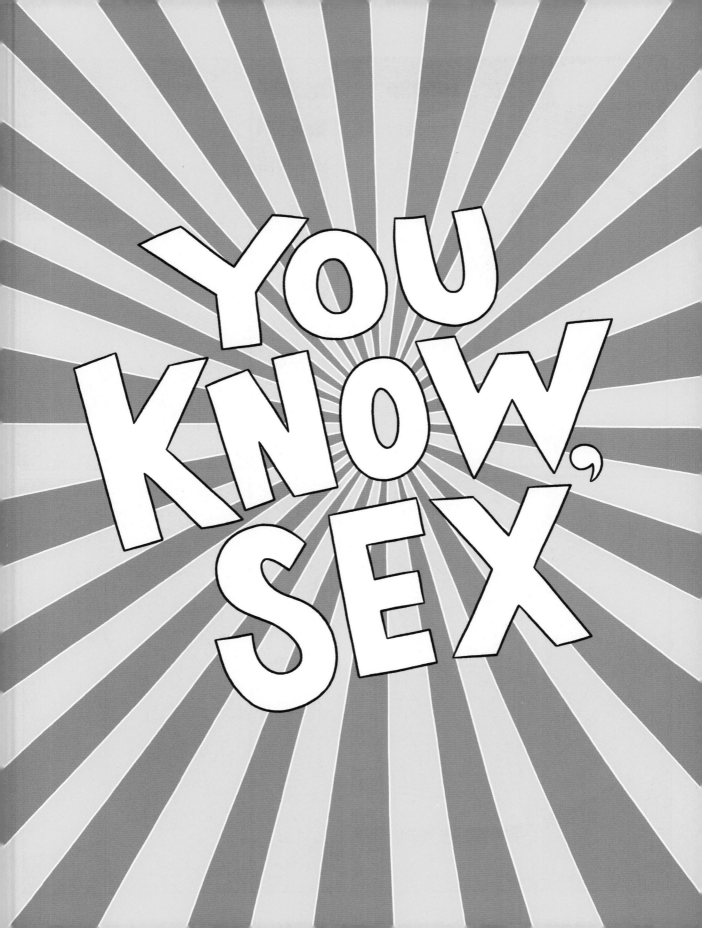

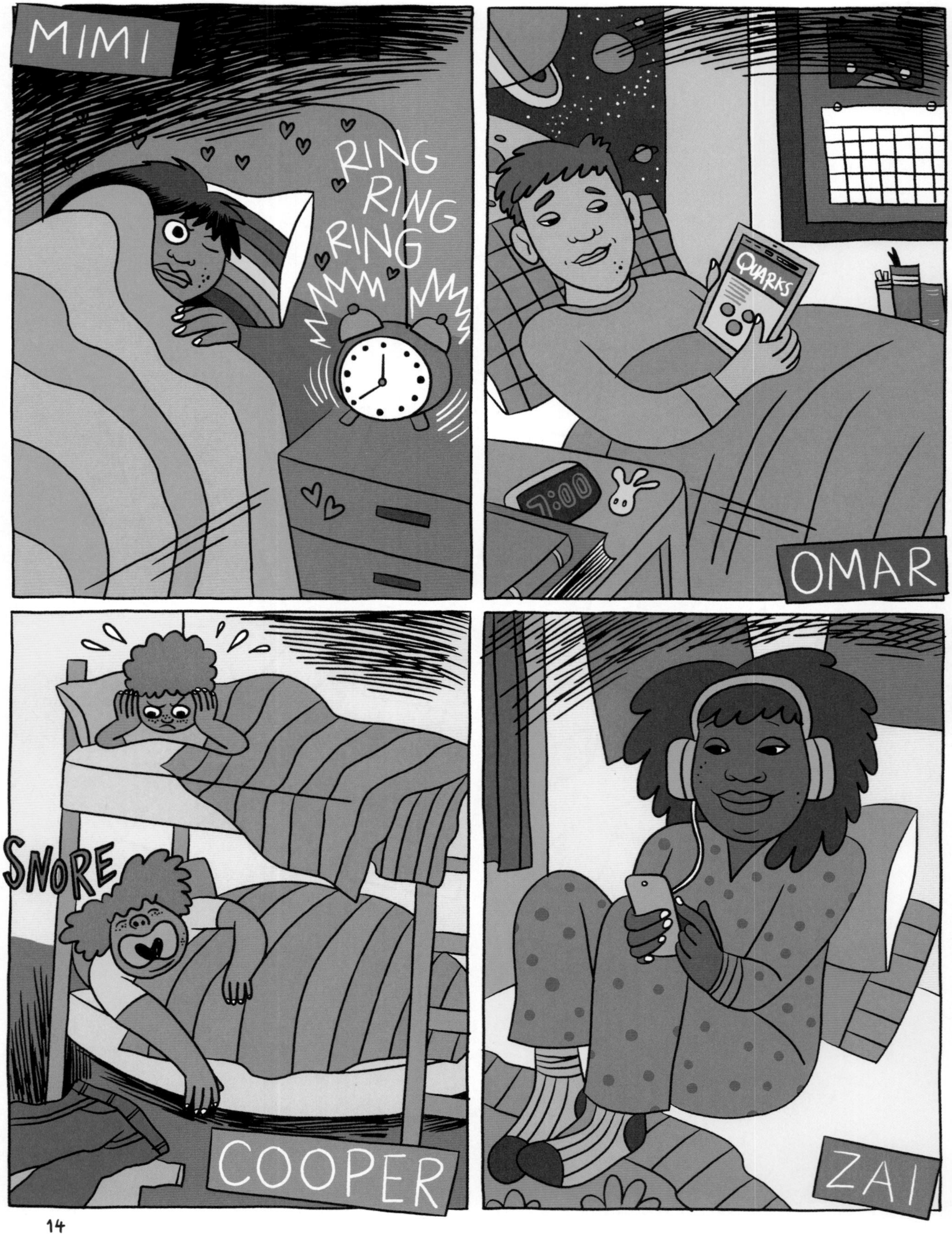
MIMI
RING
RING
RING
OMAR
QUARKS
7:00
SNORE
COOPER
ZAI

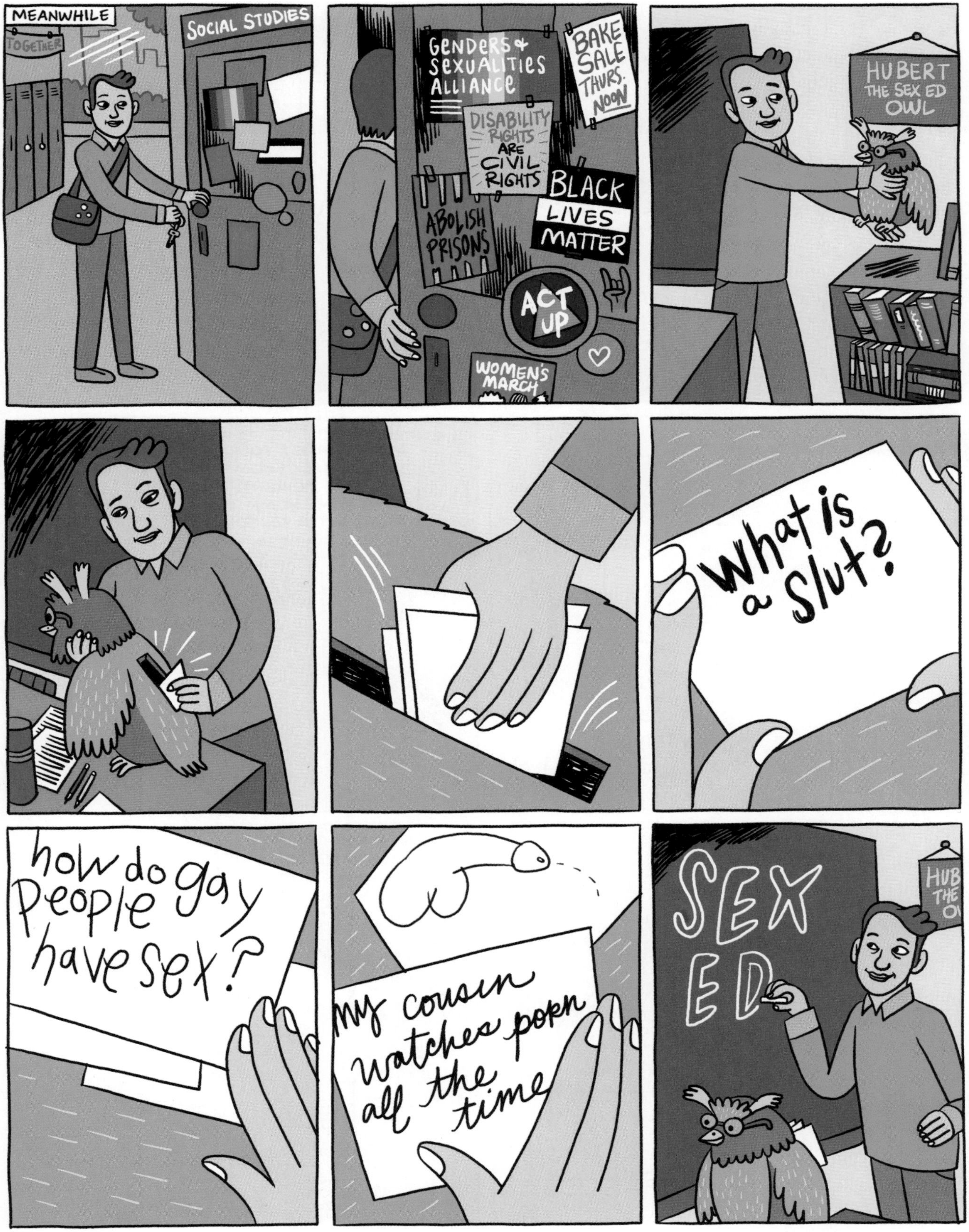
MEANWHILE
TOGETHER
SOCIAL STUDIES
GENDERS & SEXUALITIES ALLIANCE
BAKE SALE THURS. NOON
DISABILITY RIGHTS ARE CIVIL RIGHTS
ABOLISH PRISONS
BLACK LIVES MATTER
ACT UP
WOMEN'S MARCH
HUBERT THE SEX ED OWL
what is a slut?
how do gay people have sex?
my cousin watches porn all the time
SEX ED

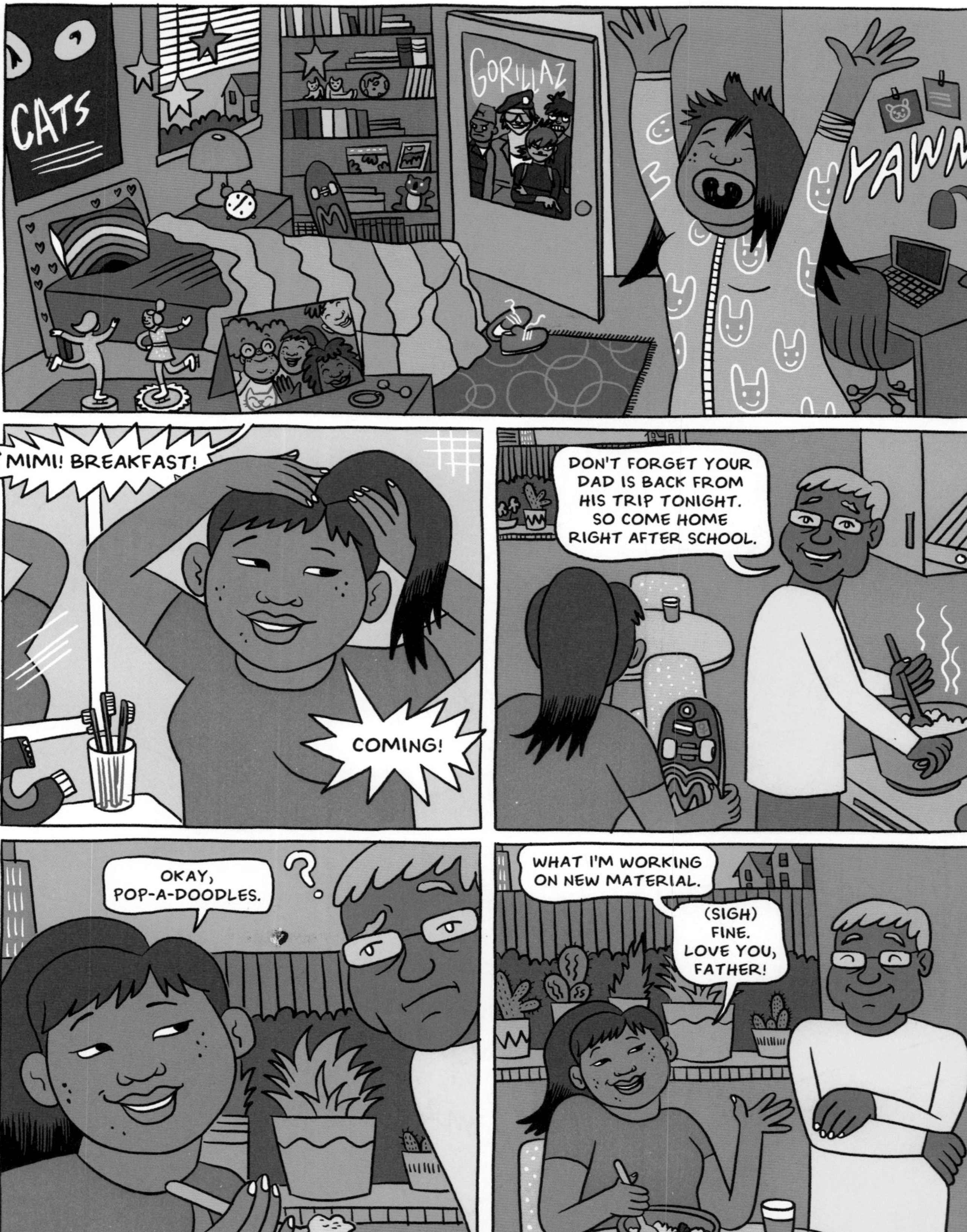
CATS
GORILLAZ
YAWN
MIMI! BREAKFAST!
COMING!
DON'T FORGET YOUR DAD IS BACK FROM HIS TRIP TONIGHT. SO COME HOME RIGHT AFTER SCHOOL.
OKAY, POP-A-DOODLES.
?
WHAT I'M WORKING ON NEW MATERIAL.
(SIGH) FINE. LOVE YOU, FATHER!

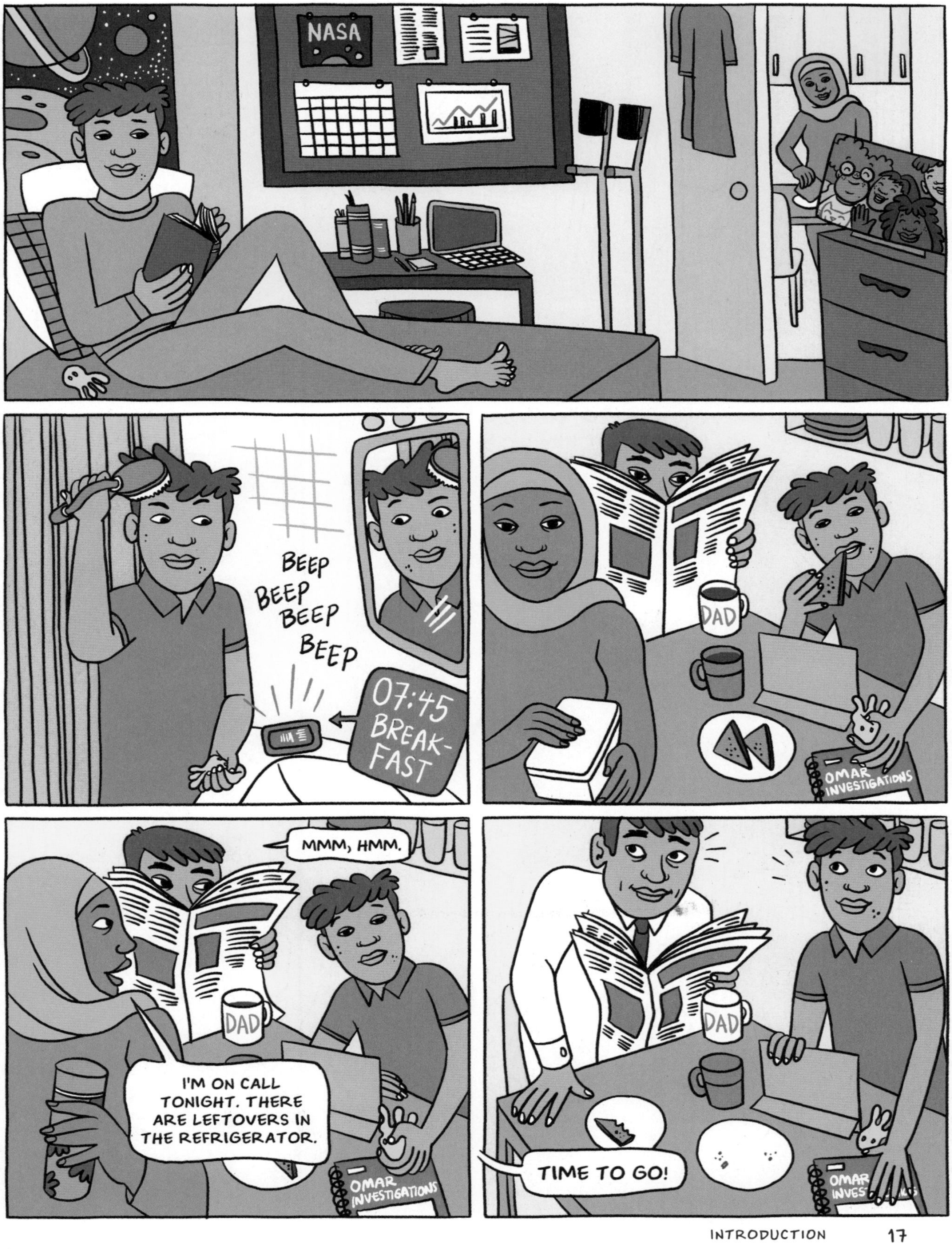
NASA
BEEP
BEEP
BEEP
BEEP
07:45 BREAK-FAST
DAD
OMAR INVESTIGATIONS
MMM, HMM.
DAD
I'M ON CALL TONIGHT. THERE ARE LEFTOVERS IN THE REFRIGERATOR.
OMAR INVESTIGATIONS
DAD
TIME TO GO!

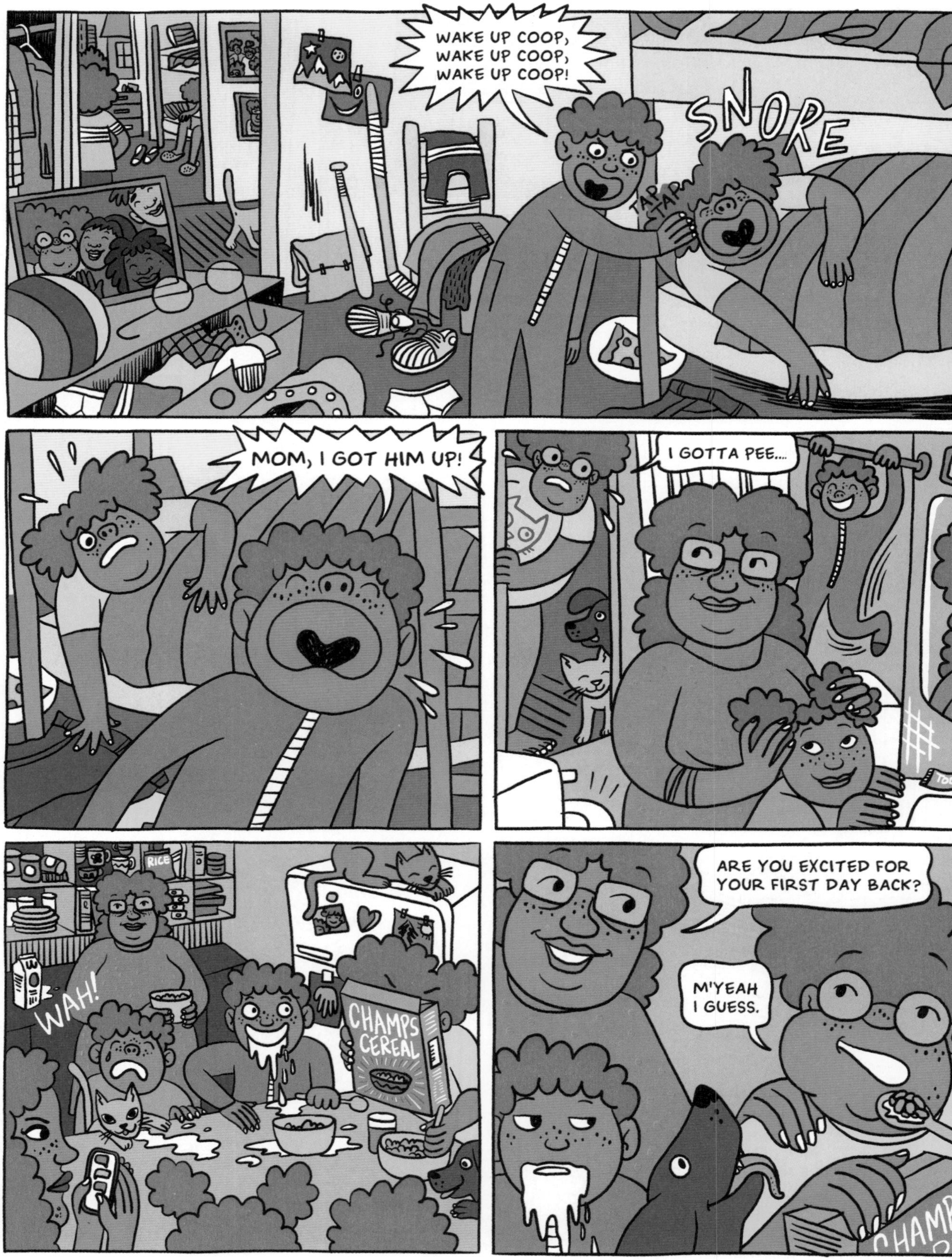
WAKE UP COOP,
WAKE UP COOP,
WAKE UP COOP!
SNORE
TAP TAP
MOM, I GOT HIM UP!
I GOTTA PEE....
RICE
WAH!
CHAMPS CEREAL
ARE YOU EXCITED FOR YOUR FIRST DAY BACK?
M'YEAH I GUESS.

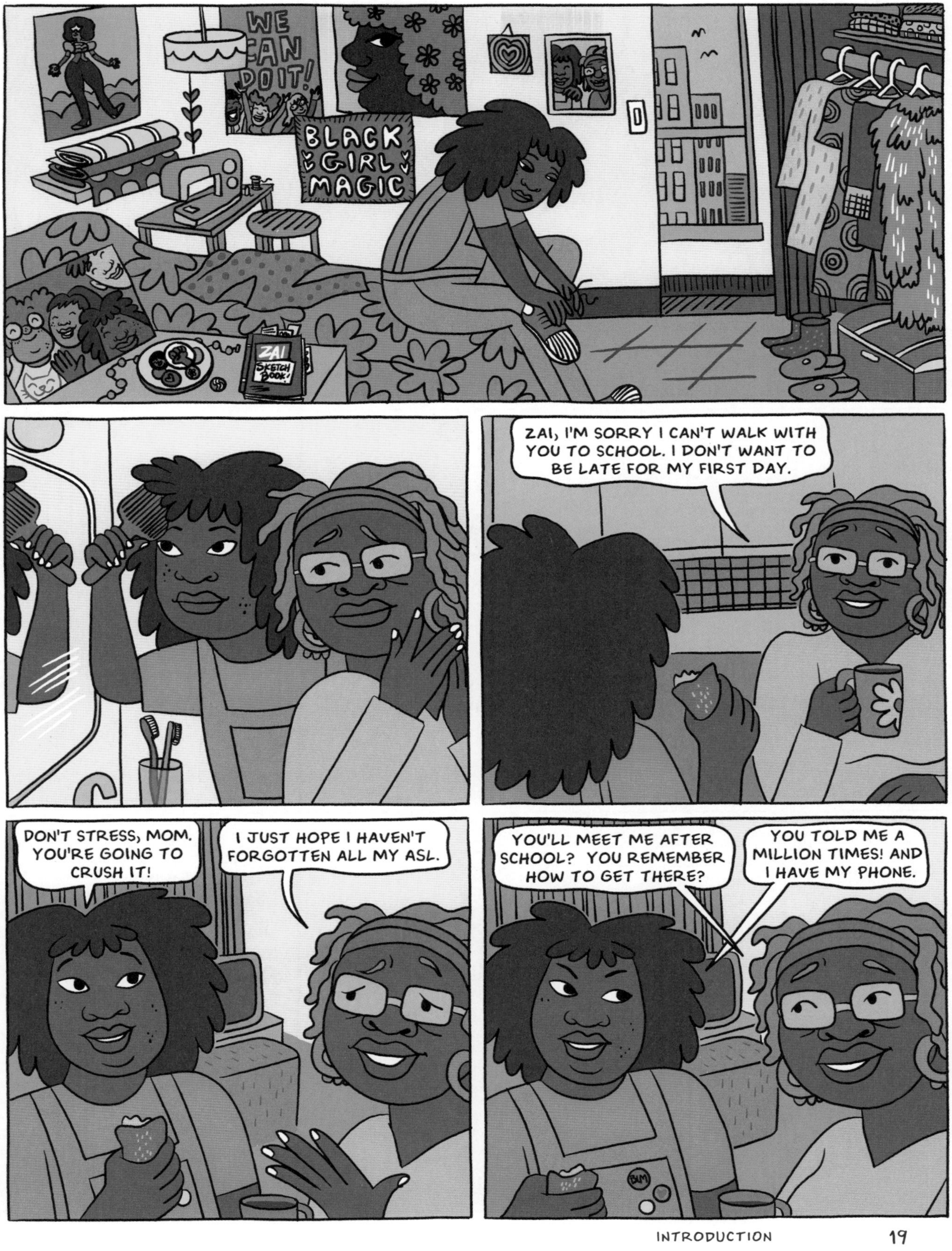
WE CAN DO IT!
BLACK GIRL MAGIC
ZAI SKETCH BOOK!
ZAI, I'M SORRY I CAN'T WALK WITH YOU TO SCHOOL. I DON'T WANT TO BE LATE FOR MY FIRST DAY.
DON'T STRESS, MOM. YOU'RE GOING TO CRUSH IT!
I JUST HOPE I HAVEN'T FORGOTTEN ALL MY ASL.
YOU'LL MEET ME AFTER SCHOOL? YOU REMEMBER HOW TO GET THERE?
YOU TOLD ME A MILLION TIMES! AND I HAVE MY PHONE.

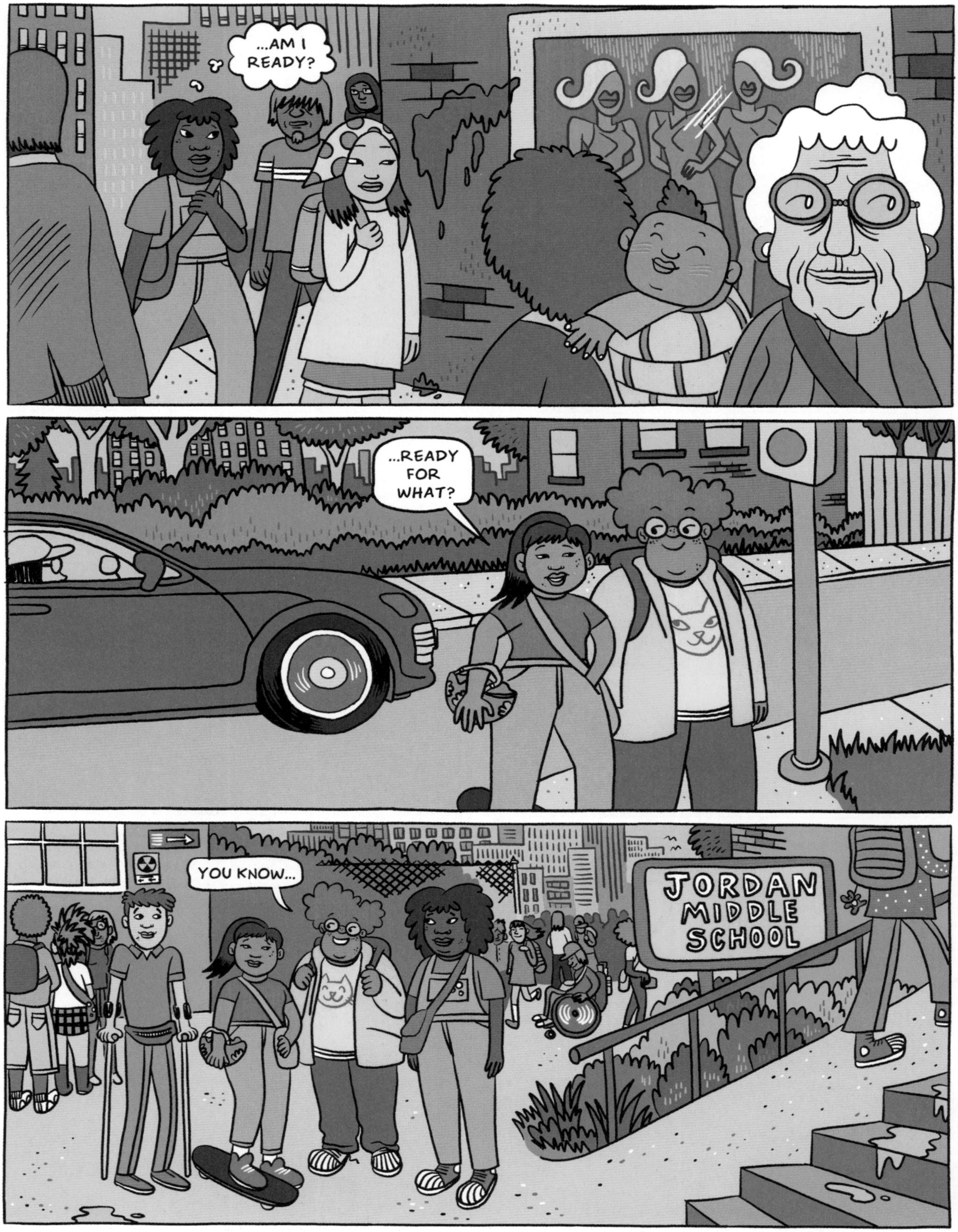
...AM I READY?
...READY FOR WHAT?
YOU KNOW...
JORDAN MIDDLE SCHOOL

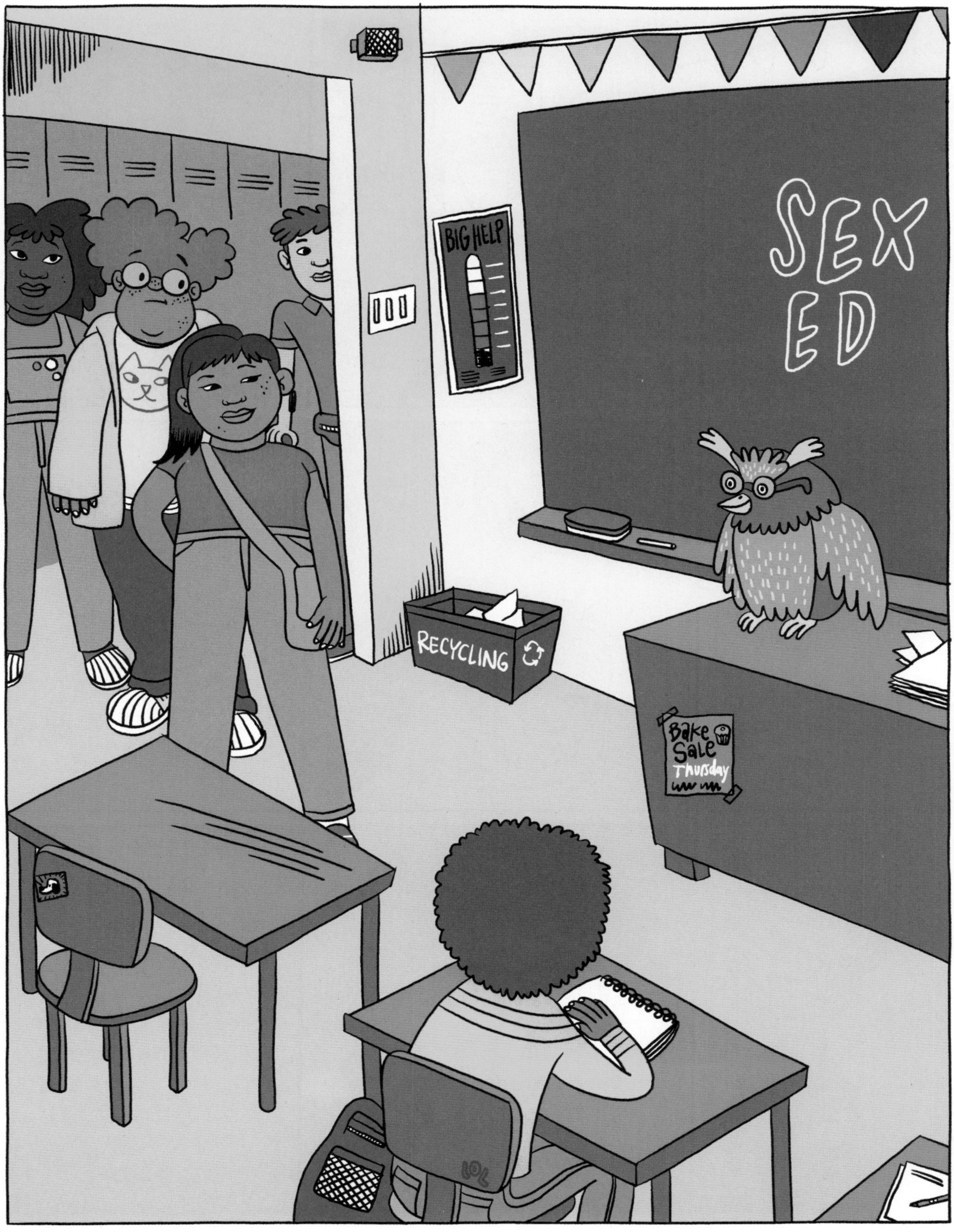
BIG HELP
SEX
ED
RECYCLING
Bake Sale
Thursday

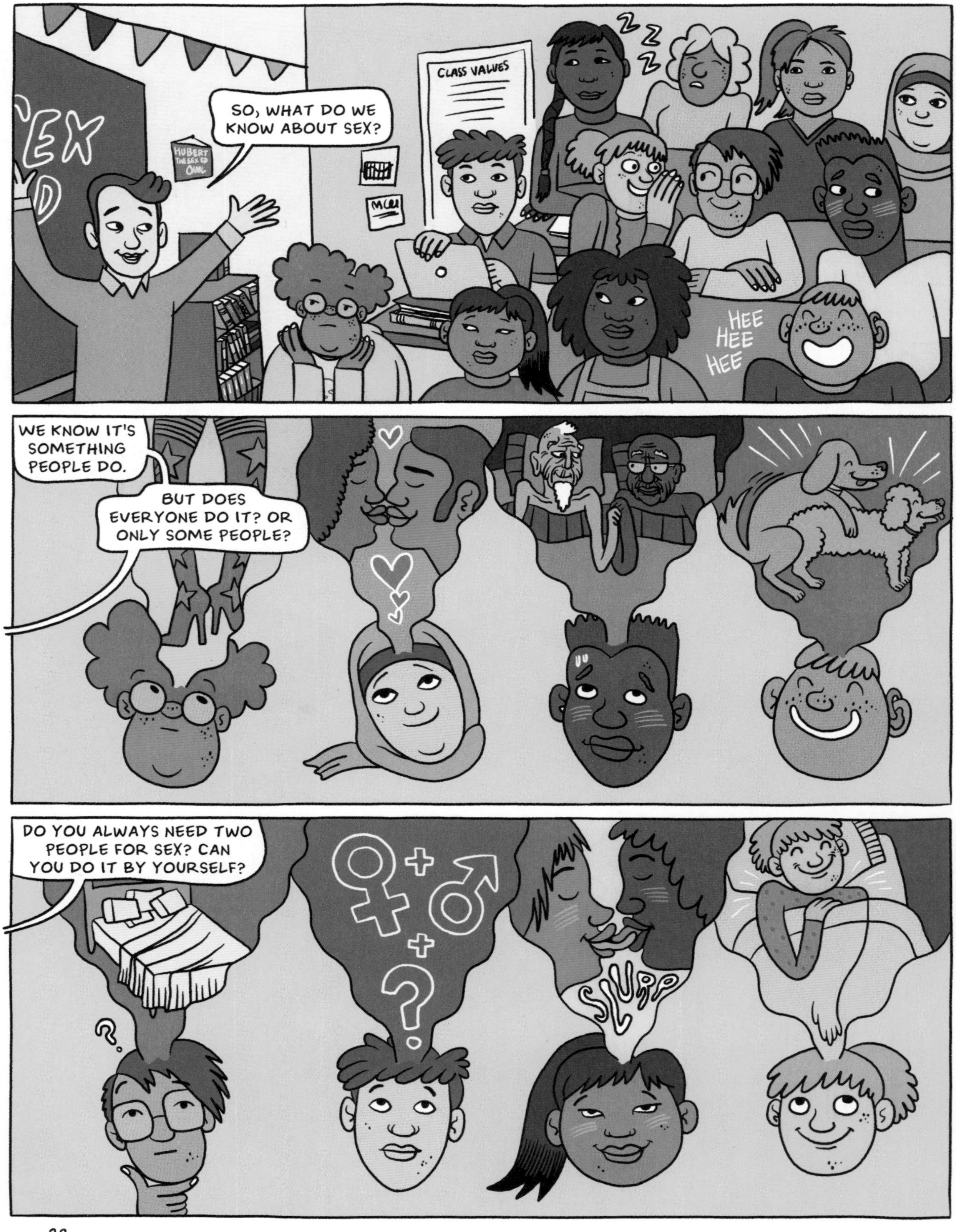
SO, WHAT DO WE KNOW ABOUT SEX?
CLASS VALUES
HUBERT THE SEX ED OWL
SEX ED
HEE HEE HEE
WE KNOW IT'S SOMETHING PEOPLE DO.
BUT DOES EVERYONE DO IT? OR ONLY SOME PEOPLE?
DO YOU ALWAYS NEED TWO PEOPLE FOR SEX? CAN YOU DO IT BY YOURSELF?
SLURP

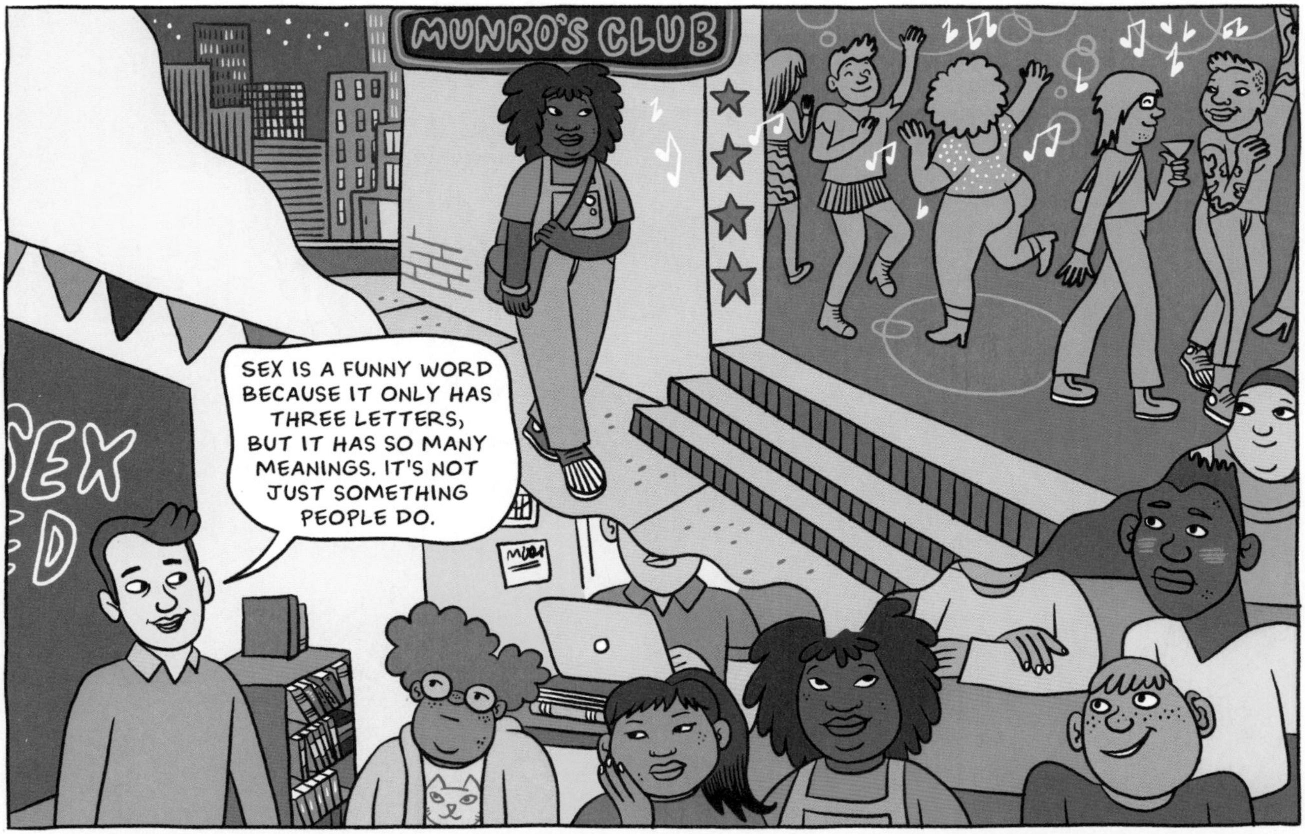
MUNRO'S CLUB
SEX ED
SEX IS A FUNNY WORD BECAUSE IT ONLY HAS THREE LETTERS, BUT IT HAS SO MANY MEANINGS. IT'S NOT JUST SOMETHING PEOPLE DO.

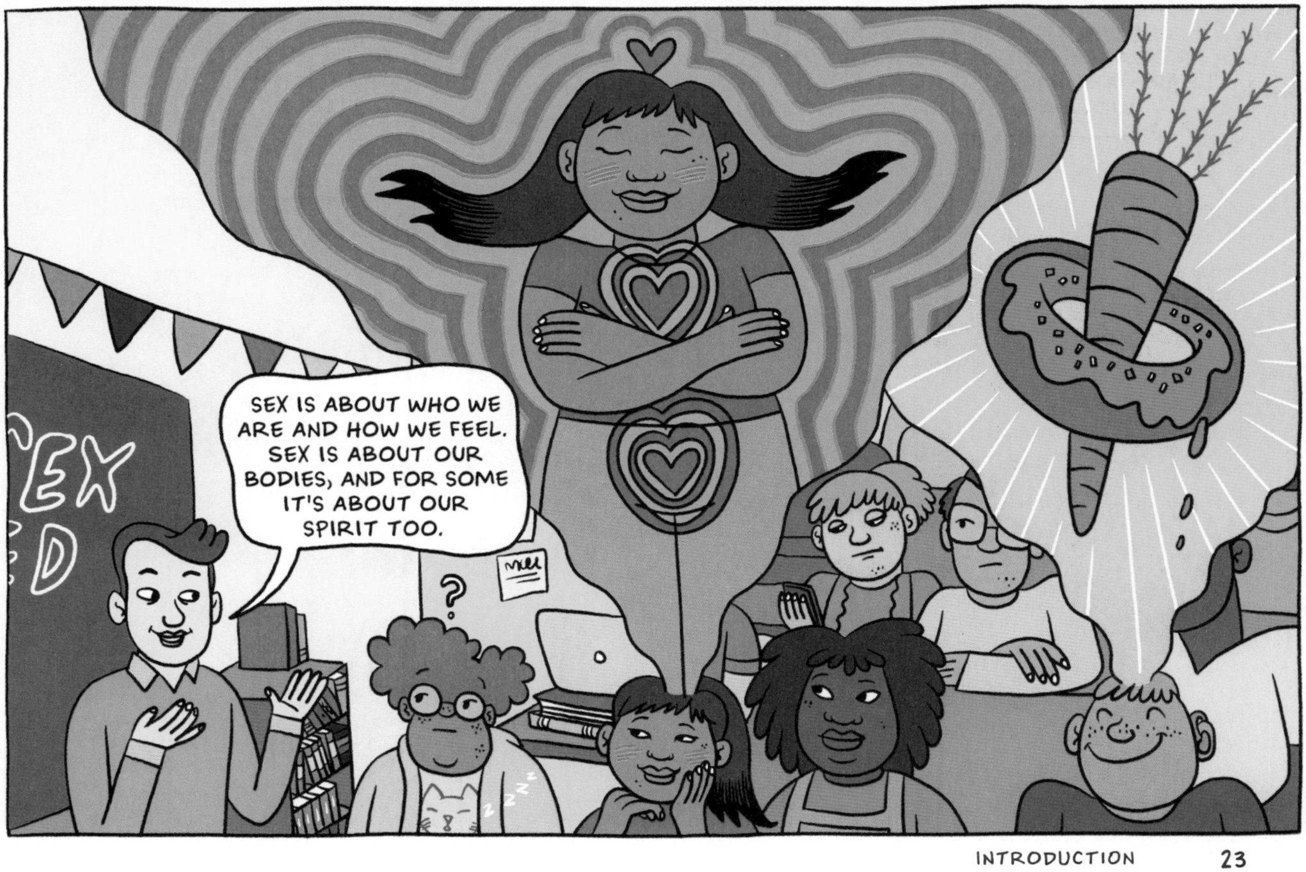
SEX ED
SEX IS ABOUT WHO WE ARE AND HOW WE FEEL. SEX IS ABOUT OUR BODIES, AND FOR SOME IT'S ABOUT OUR SPIRIT TOO.

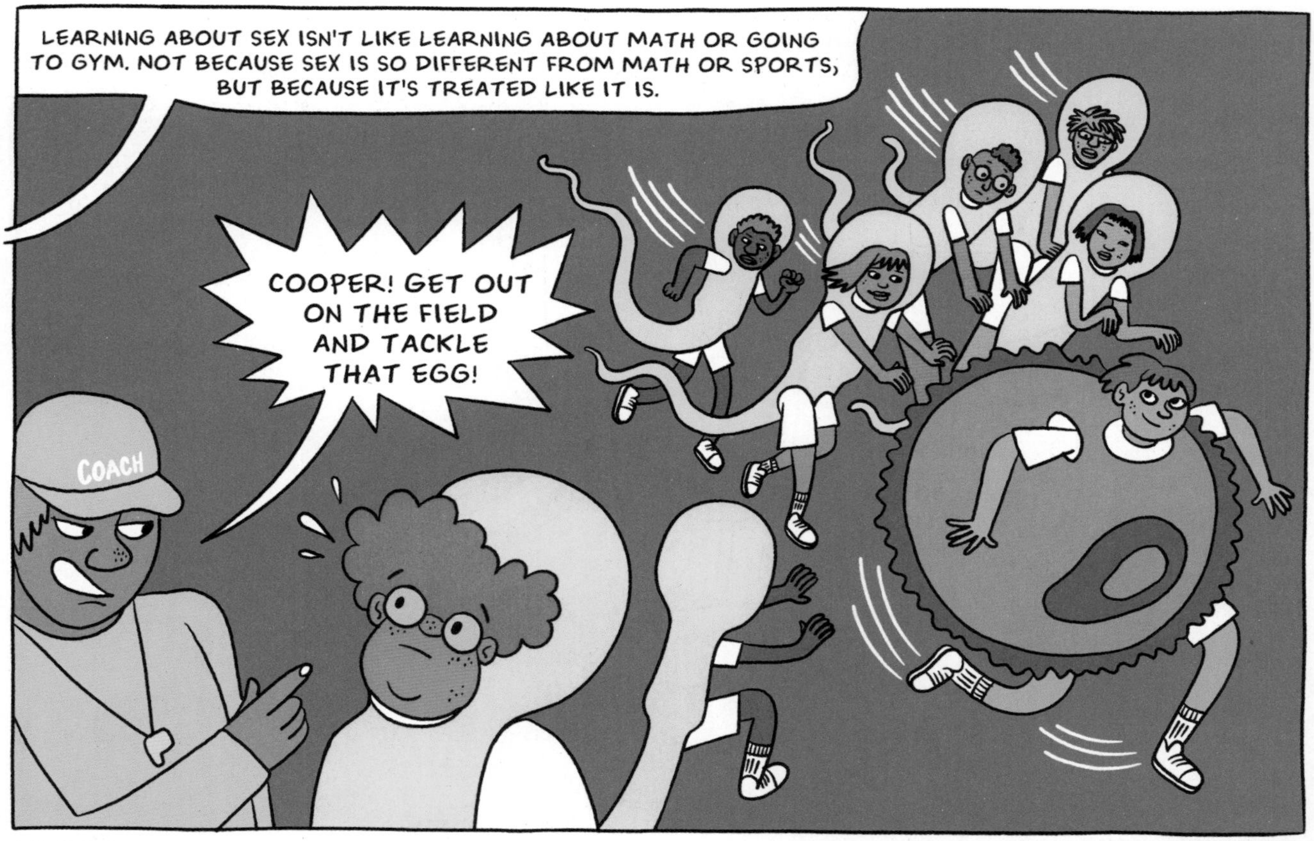
LEARNING ABOUT SEX ISN'T LIKE LEARNING ABOUT MATH OR GOING TO GYM. NOT BECAUSE SEX IS SO DIFFERENT FROM MATH OR SPORTS, BUT BECAUSE IT'S TREATED LIKE IT IS.
COOPER! GET OUT ON THE FIELD AND TACKLE THAT EGG!
COACH

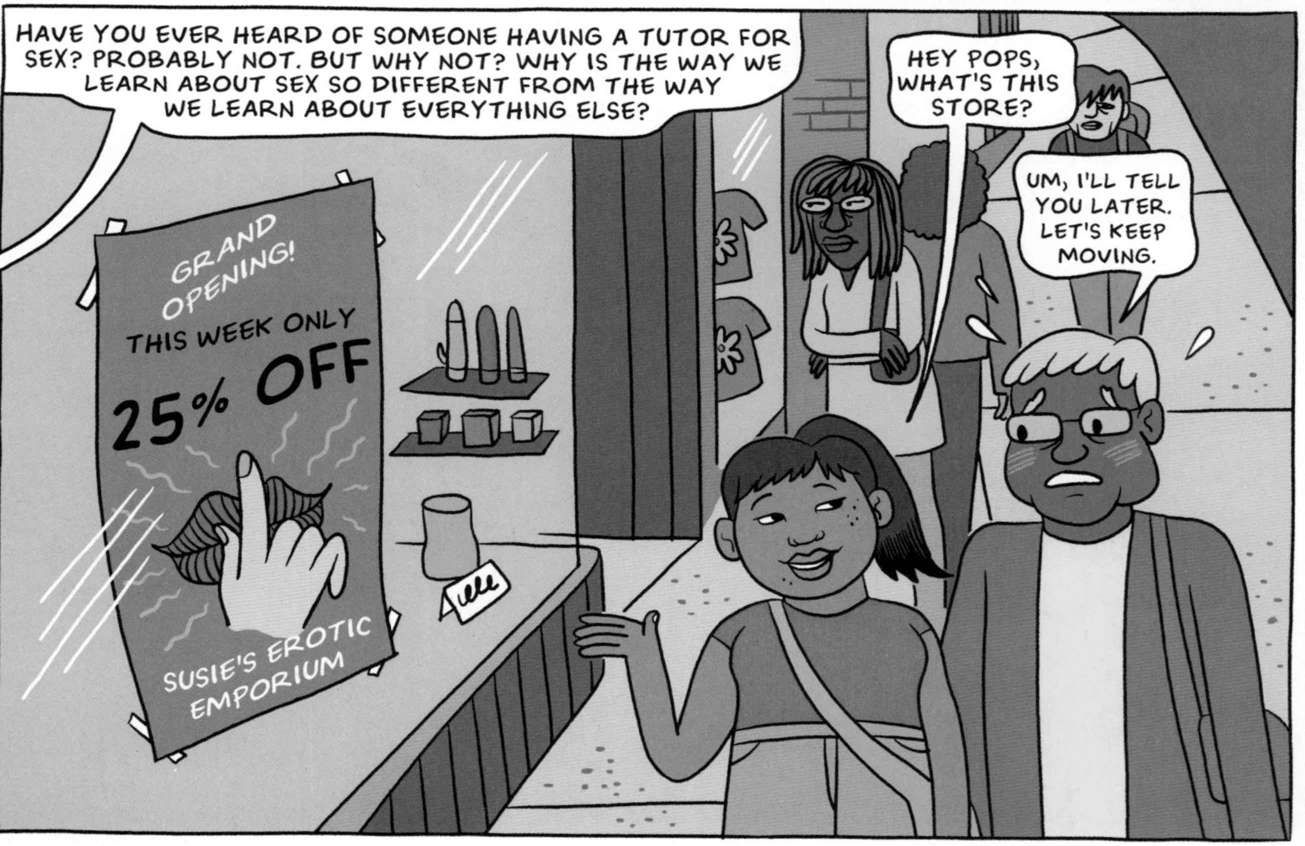
HAVE YOU EVER HEARD OF SOMEONE HAVING A TUTOR FOR SEX? PROBABLY NOT. BUT WHY NOT? WHY IS THE WAY WE LEARN ABOUT SEX SO DIFFERENT FROM THE WAY WE LEARN ABOUT EVERYTHING ELSE?
GRAND OPENING!
THIS WEEK ONLY
25% OFF
SUSIE'S EROTIC EMPORIUM
HEY POPS, WHAT'S THIS STORE?
UM, I'LL TELL YOU LATER. LET'S KEEP MOVING.

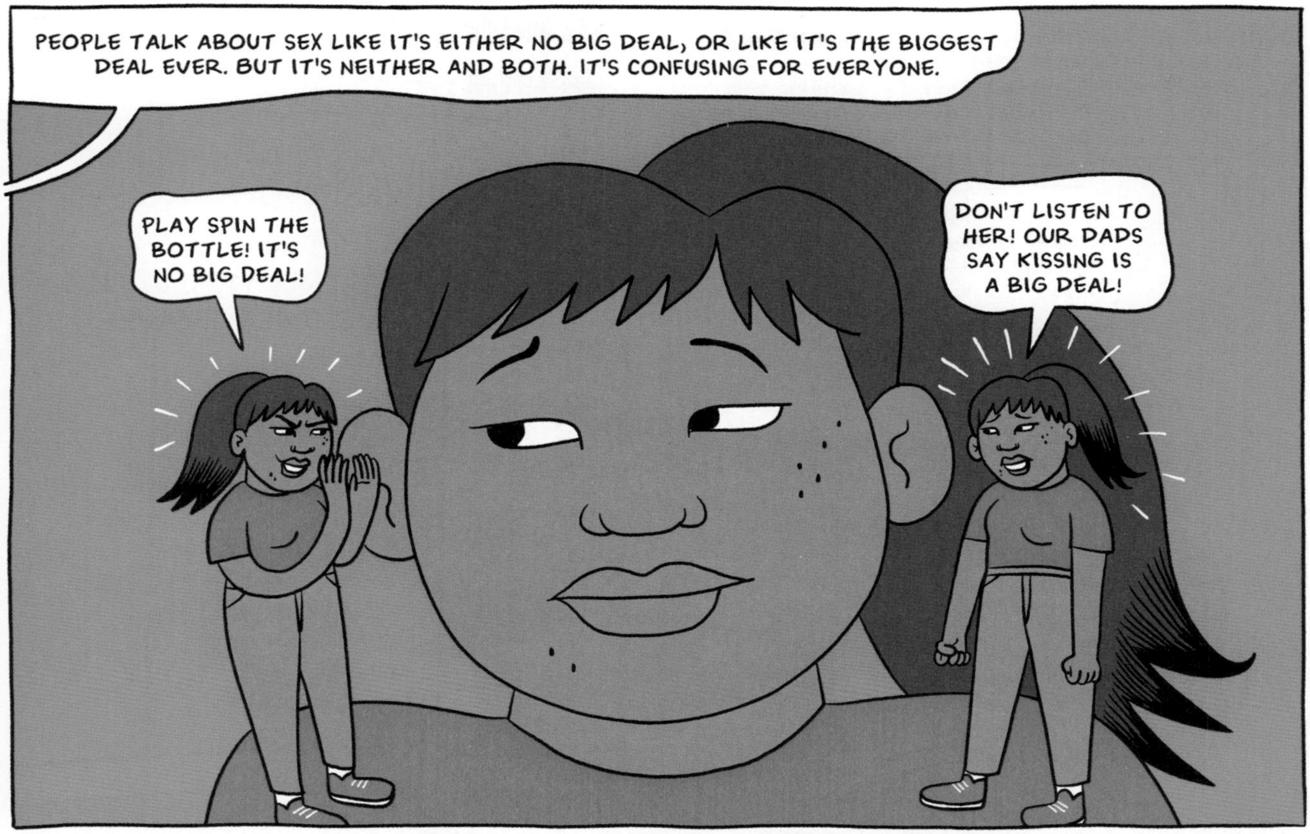
PEOPLE TALK ABOUT SEX LIKE IT'S EITHER NO BIG DEAL, OR LIKE IT'S THE BIGGEST DEAL EVER. BUT IT'S NEITHER AND BOTH. IT'S CONFUSING FOR EVERYONE.
PLAY SPIN THE BOTTLE! IT'S NO BIG DEAL!
DON'T LISTEN TO HER! OUR DADS SAY KISSING IS A BIG DEAL!

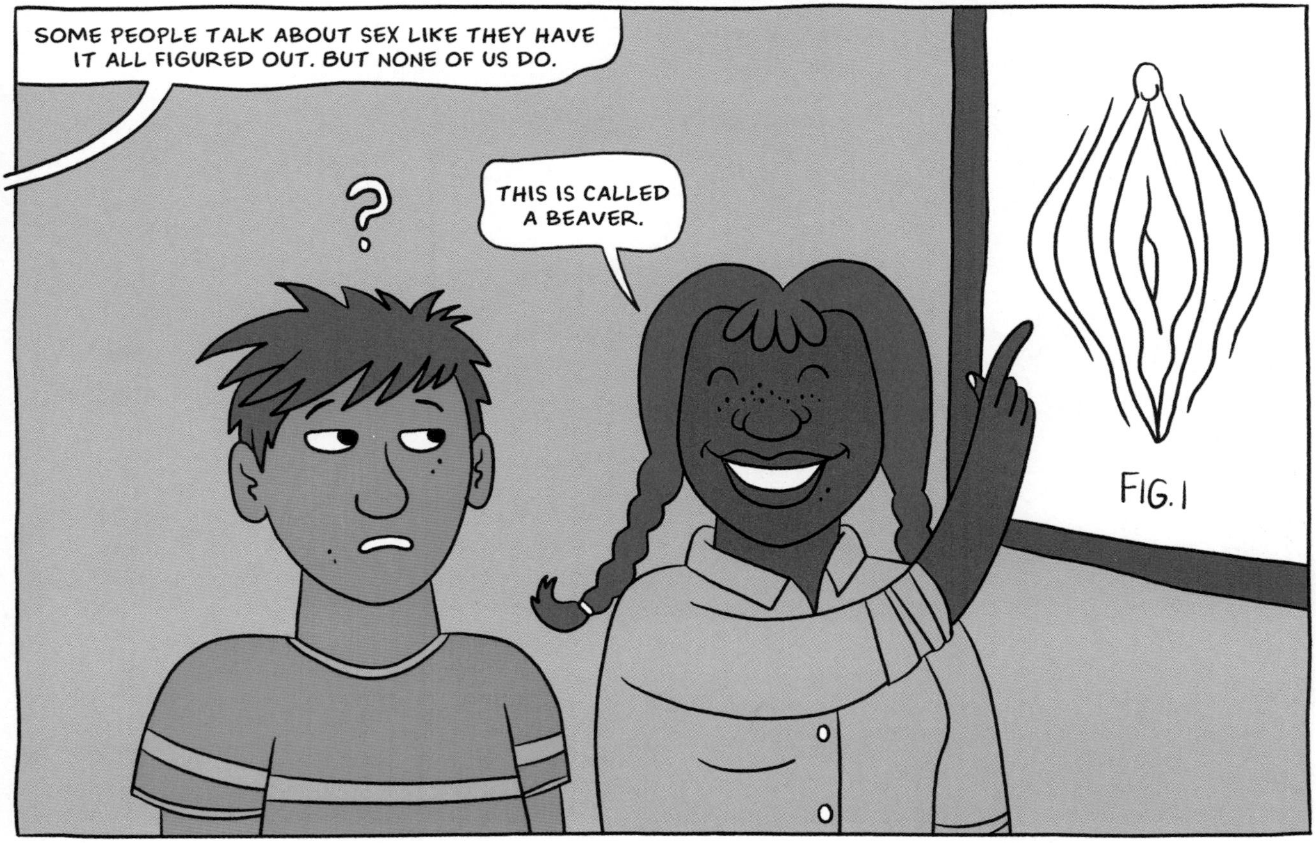
SOME PEOPLE TALK ABOUT SEX LIKE THEY HAVE IT ALL FIGURED OUT. BUT NONE OF US DO.
?
THIS IS CALLED A BEAVER.
FIG. 1

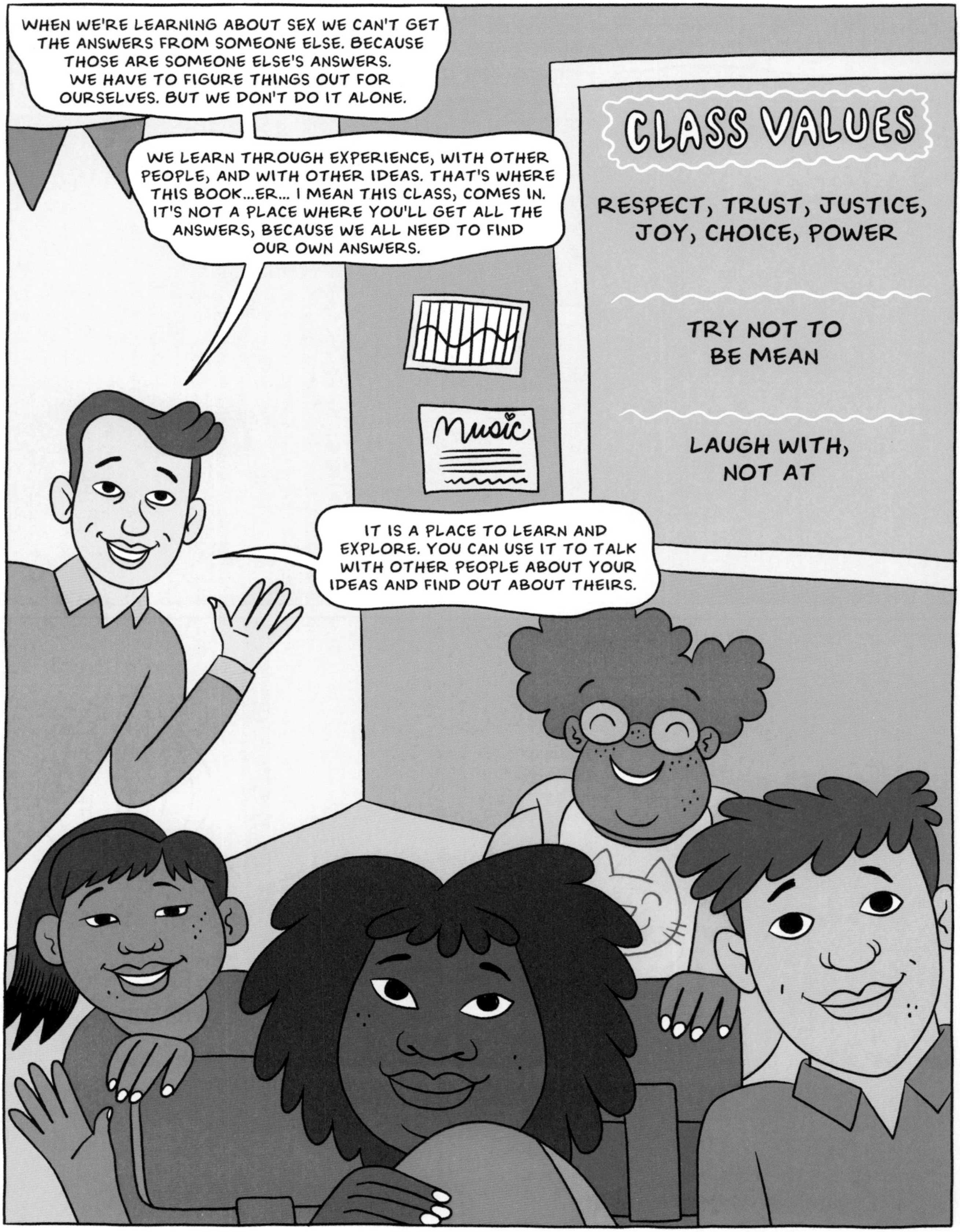
WHEN WE'RE LEARNING ABOUT SEX WE CAN'T GET THE ANSWERS FROM SOMEONE ELSE. BECAUSE THOSE ARE SOMEONE ELSE'S ANSWERS. WE HAVE TO FIGURE THINGS OUT FOR OURSELVES. BUT WE DON'T DO IT ALONE.
WE LEARN THROUGH EXPERIENCE, WITH OTHER PEOPLE, AND WITH OTHER IDEAS. THAT'S WHERE THIS BOOK...ER... I MEAN THIS CLASS, COMES IN. IT'S NOT A PLACE WHERE YOU'LL GET ALL THE ANSWERS, BECAUSE WE ALL NEED TO FIND OUR OWN ANSWERS.
CLASS VALUES
RESPECT, TRUST, JUSTICE, JOY, CHOICE, POWER
TRY NOT TO BE MEAN
LAUGH WITH, NOT AT
Music
IT IS A PLACE TO LEARN AND EXPLORE. YOU CAN USE IT TO TALK WITH OTHER PEOPLE ABOUT YOUR IDEAS AND FIND OUT ABOUT THEIRS.

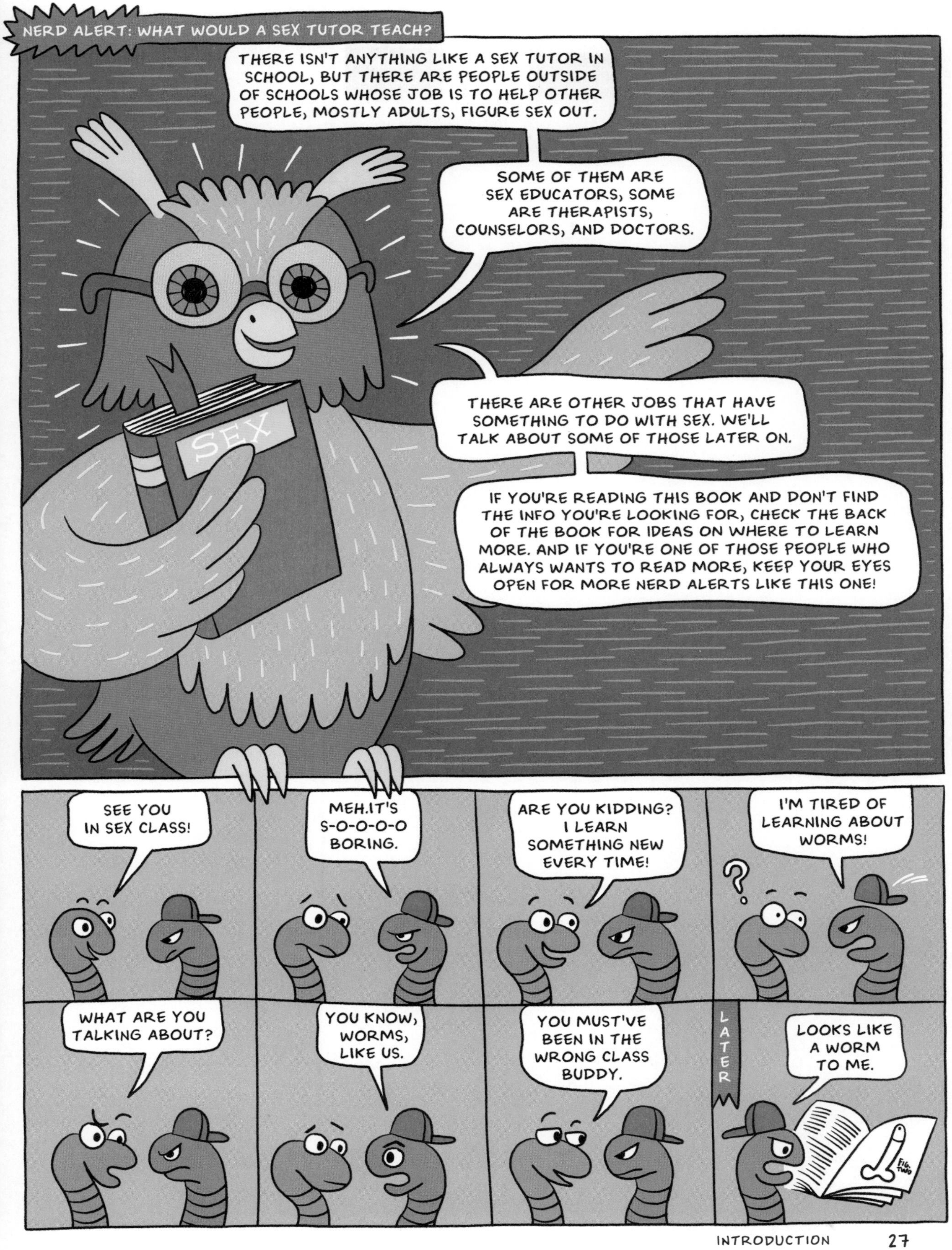
NERD ALERT: WHAT WOULD A SEX TUTOR TEACH?
THERE ISN'T ANYTHING LIKE A SEX TUTOR IN SCHOOL, BUT THERE ARE PEOPLE OUTSIDE OF SCHOOLS WHOSE JOB IS TO HELP OTHER PEOPLE, MOSTLY ADULTS, FIGURE SEX OUT.
SOME OF THEM ARE SEX EDUCATORS, SOME ARE THERAPISTS, COUNSELORS, AND DOCTORS.
SEX
THERE ARE OTHER JOBS THAT HAVE SOMETHING TO DO WITH SEX. WE'LL TALK ABOUT SOME OF THOSE LATER ON.
IF YOU'RE READING THIS BOOK AND DON'T FIND THE INFO YOU'RE LOOKING FOR, CHECK THE BACK OF THE BOOK FOR IDEAS ON WHERE TO LEARN MORE. AND IF YOU'RE ONE OF THOSE PEOPLE WHO ALWAYS WANTS TO READ MORE, KEEP YOUR EYES OPEN FOR MORE NERD ALERTS LIKE THIS ONE!
SEE YOU IN SEX CLASS!
MEH. IT'S S-O-O-O-O BORING.
ARE YOU KIDDING? I LEARN SOMETHING NEW EVERY TIME!
I'M TIRED OF LEARNING ABOUT WORMS!
?
WHAT ARE YOU TALKING ABOUT?
YOU KNOW, WORMS, LIKE US.
YOU MUST'VE BEEN IN THE WRONG CLASS BUDDY.
LATER
LOOKS LIKE A WORM TO ME.
FIG. TWO

SEE YOU TOMORROW!
LATER, GATOR!

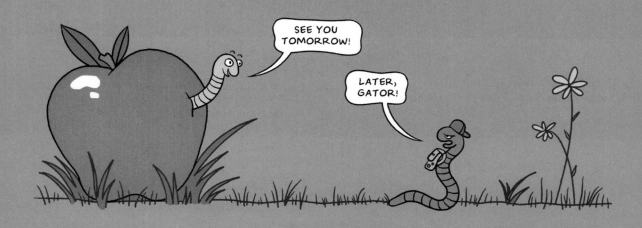

1

WHAT IS SEX?

THE TITLE OF THIS SCULPTURE IS "PORNICATION."
?
I DON'T GET IT.

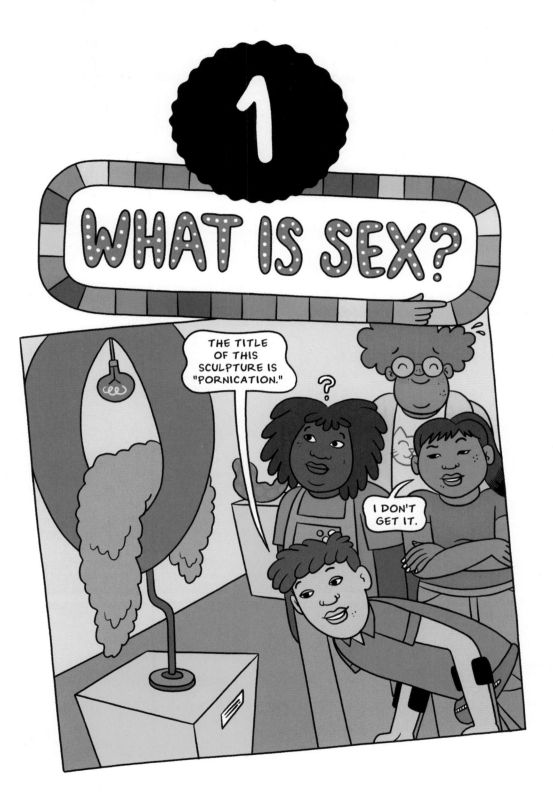

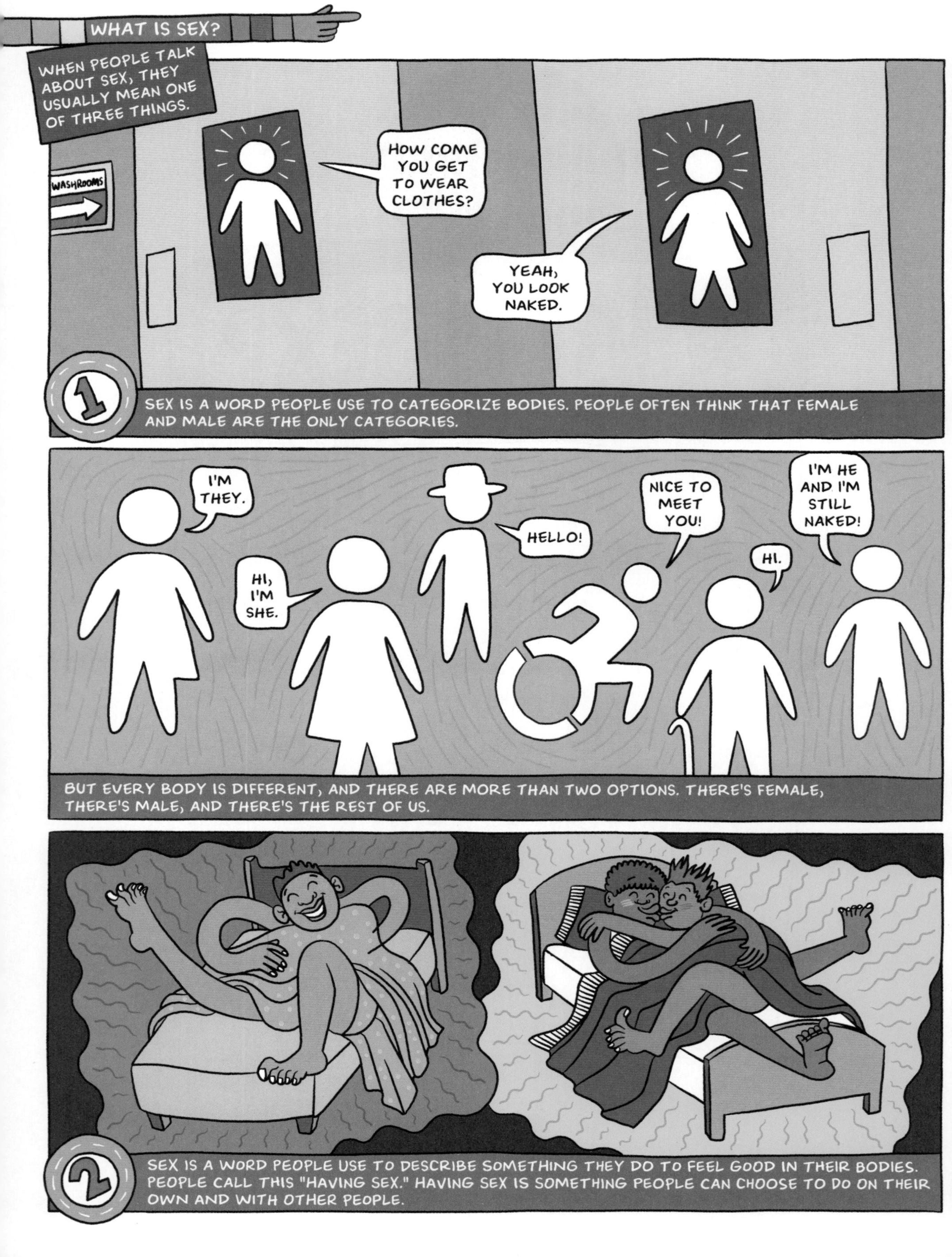
WHAT IS SEX?
WHEN PEOPLE TALK ABOUT SEX, THEY USUALLY MEAN ONE OF THREE THINGS.
WASHROOMS
HOW COME YOU GET TO WEAR CLOTHES?
YEAH, YOU LOOK NAKED.
1
SEX IS A WORD PEOPLE USE TO CATEGORIZE BODIES. PEOPLE OFTEN THINK THAT FEMALE AND MALE ARE THE ONLY CATEGORIES.
I'M THEY.
HI, I'M SHE.
HELLO!
NICE TO MEET YOU!
HI.
I'M HE AND I'M STILL NAKED!
BUT EVERY BODY IS DIFFERENT, AND THERE ARE MORE THAN TWO OPTIONS. THERE'S FEMALE, THERE'S MALE, AND THERE'S THE REST OF US.
2
SEX IS A WORD PEOPLE USE TO DESCRIBE SOMETHING THEY DO TO FEEL GOOD IN THEIR BODIES. PEOPLE CALL THIS "HAVING SEX." HAVING SEX IS SOMETHING PEOPLE CAN CHOOSE TO DO ON THEIR OWN AND WITH OTHER PEOPLE.

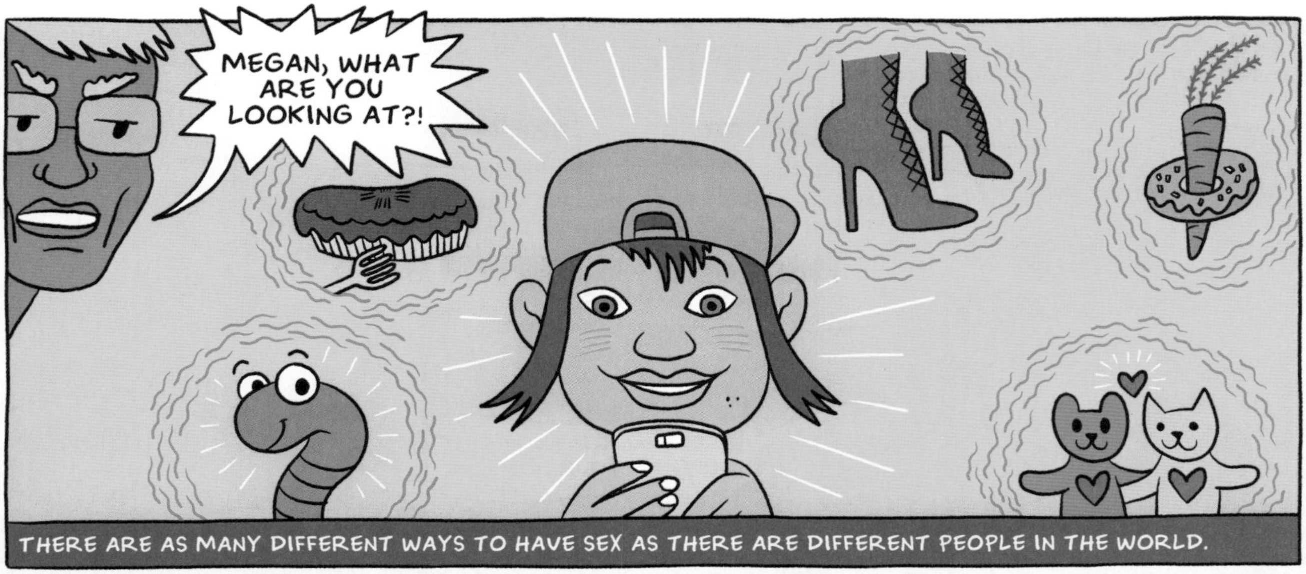
MEGAN, WHAT ARE YOU LOOKING AT?!
THERE ARE AS MANY DIFFERENT WAYS TO HAVE SEX AS THERE ARE DIFFERENT PEOPLE IN THE WORLD.

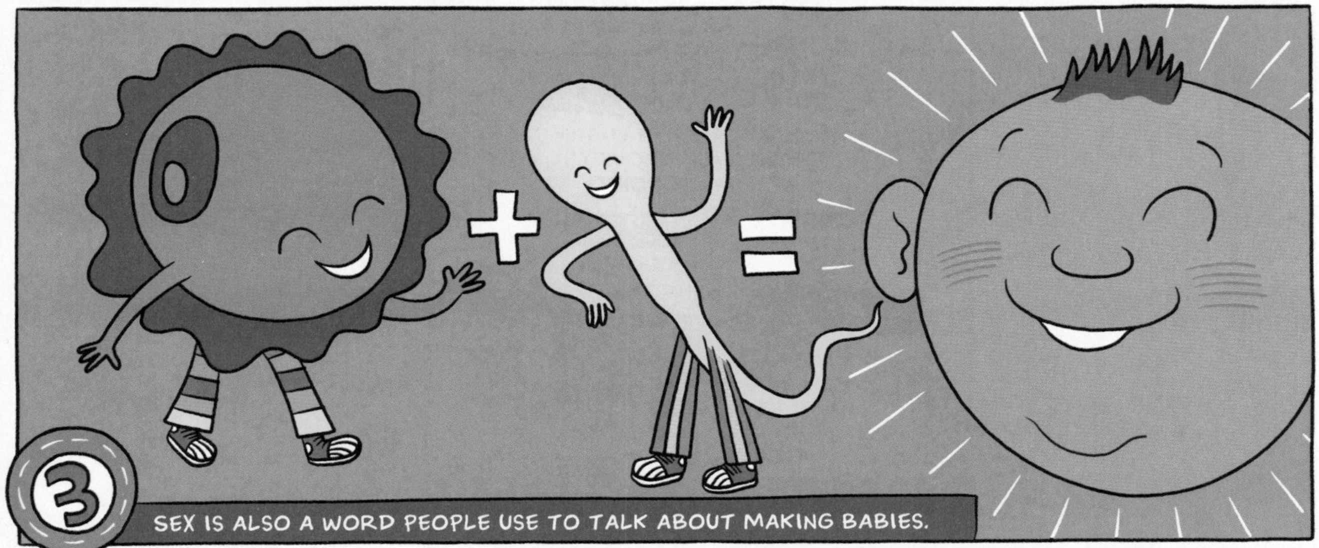
+
=
3
SEX IS ALSO A WORD PEOPLE USE TO TALK ABOUT MAKING BABIES.

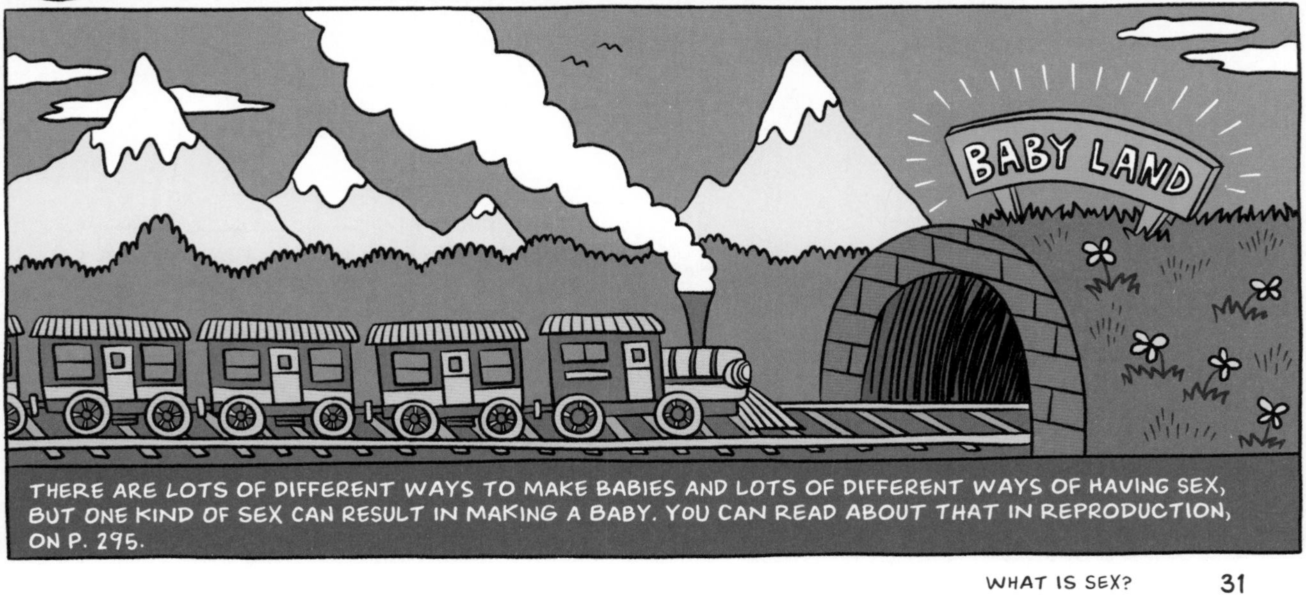
BABY LAND
THERE ARE LOTS OF DIFFERENT WAYS TO MAKE BABIES AND LOTS OF DIFFERENT WAYS OF HAVING SEX, BUT ONE KIND OF SEX CAN RESULT IN MAKING A BABY. YOU CAN READ ABOUT THAT IN REPRODUCTION, ON P. 295.

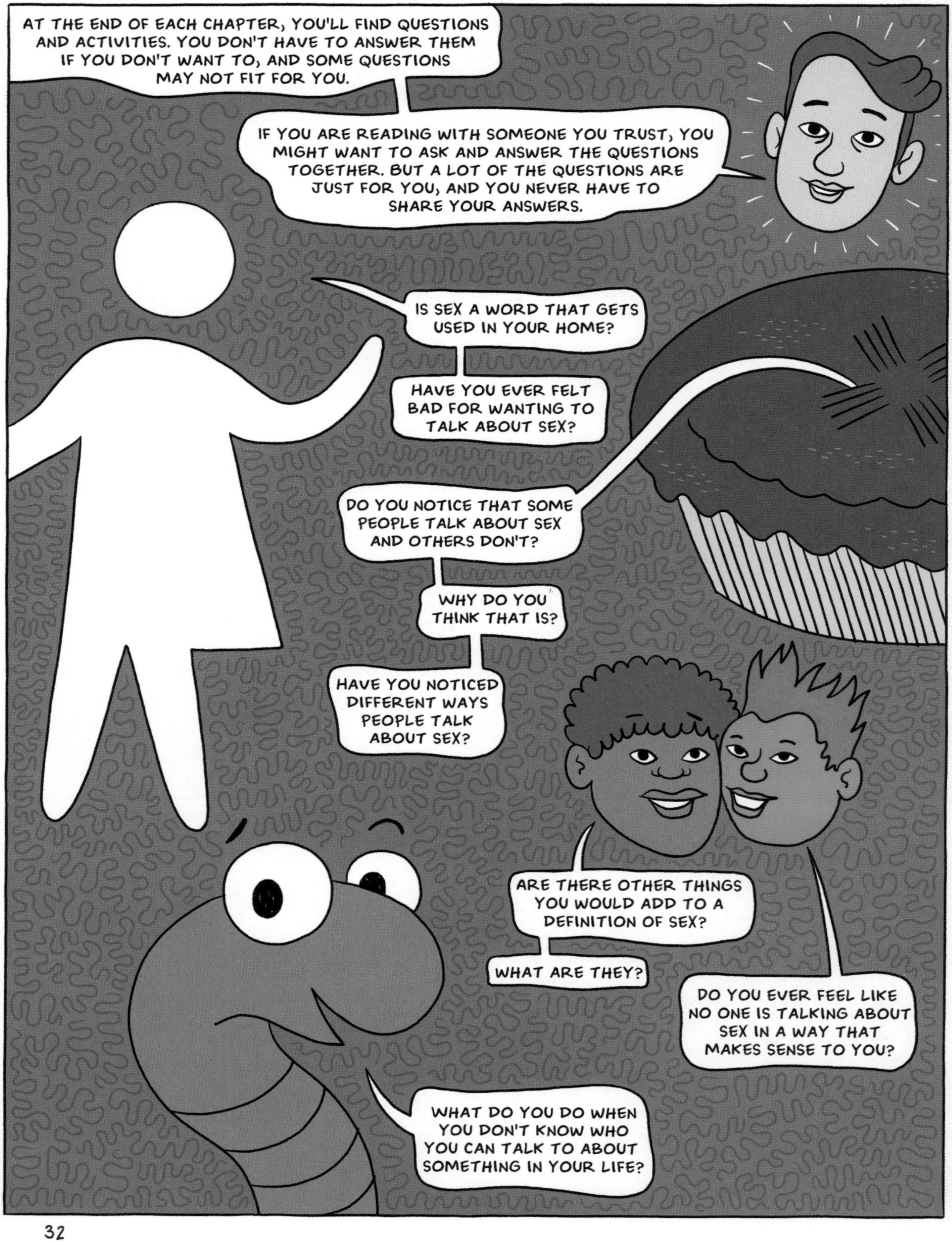
AT THE END OF EACH CHAPTER, YOU'LL FIND QUESTIONS AND ACTIVITIES. YOU DON'T HAVE TO ANSWER THEM IF YOU DON'T WANT TO, AND SOME QUESTIONS MAY NOT FIT FOR YOU.
IF YOU ARE READING WITH SOMEONE YOU TRUST, YOU MIGHT WANT TO ASK AND ANSWER THE QUESTIONS TOGETHER. BUT A LOT OF THE QUESTIONS ARE JUST FOR YOU, AND YOU NEVER HAVE TO SHARE YOUR ANSWERS.
IS SEX A WORD THAT GETS USED IN YOUR HOME?
HAVE YOU EVER FELT BAD FOR WANTING TO TALK ABOUT SEX?
DO YOU NOTICE THAT SOME PEOPLE TALK ABOUT SEX AND OTHERS DON'T?
WHY DO YOU THINK THAT IS?
HAVE YOU NOTICED DIFFERENT WAYS PEOPLE TALK ABOUT SEX?
ARE THERE OTHER THINGS YOU WOULD ADD TO A DEFINITION OF SEX?
WHAT ARE THEY?
DO YOU EVER FEEL LIKE NO ONE IS TALKING ABOUT SEX IN A WAY THAT MAKES SENSE TO YOU?
WHAT DO YOU DO WHEN YOU DON'T KNOW WHO YOU CAN TALK TO ABOUT SOMETHING IN YOUR LIFE?

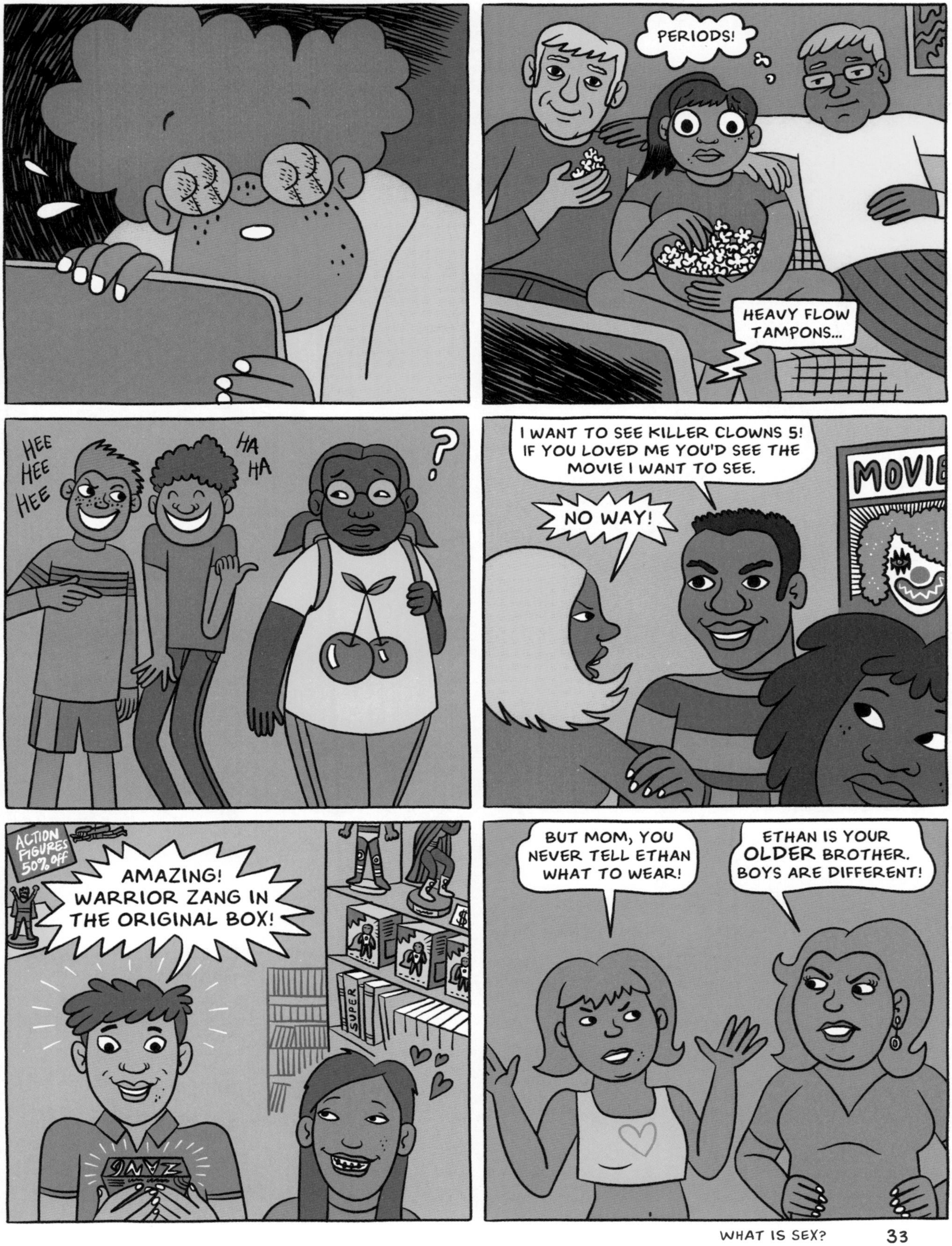
PERIODS!
HEAVY FLOW TAMPONS...
HEE HEE HEE
HA HA
?
I WANT TO SEE KILLER CLOWNS 5! IF YOU LOVED ME YOU'D SEE THE MOVIE I WANT TO SEE.
NO WAY!
MOVIE
ACTION FIGURES 50% OFF
AMAZING! WARRIOR ZANG IN THE ORIGINAL BOX!
SUPER
ZANG
BUT MOM, YOU NEVER TELL ETHAN WHAT TO WEAR!
ETHAN IS YOUR OLDER BROTHER. BOYS ARE DIFFERENT!

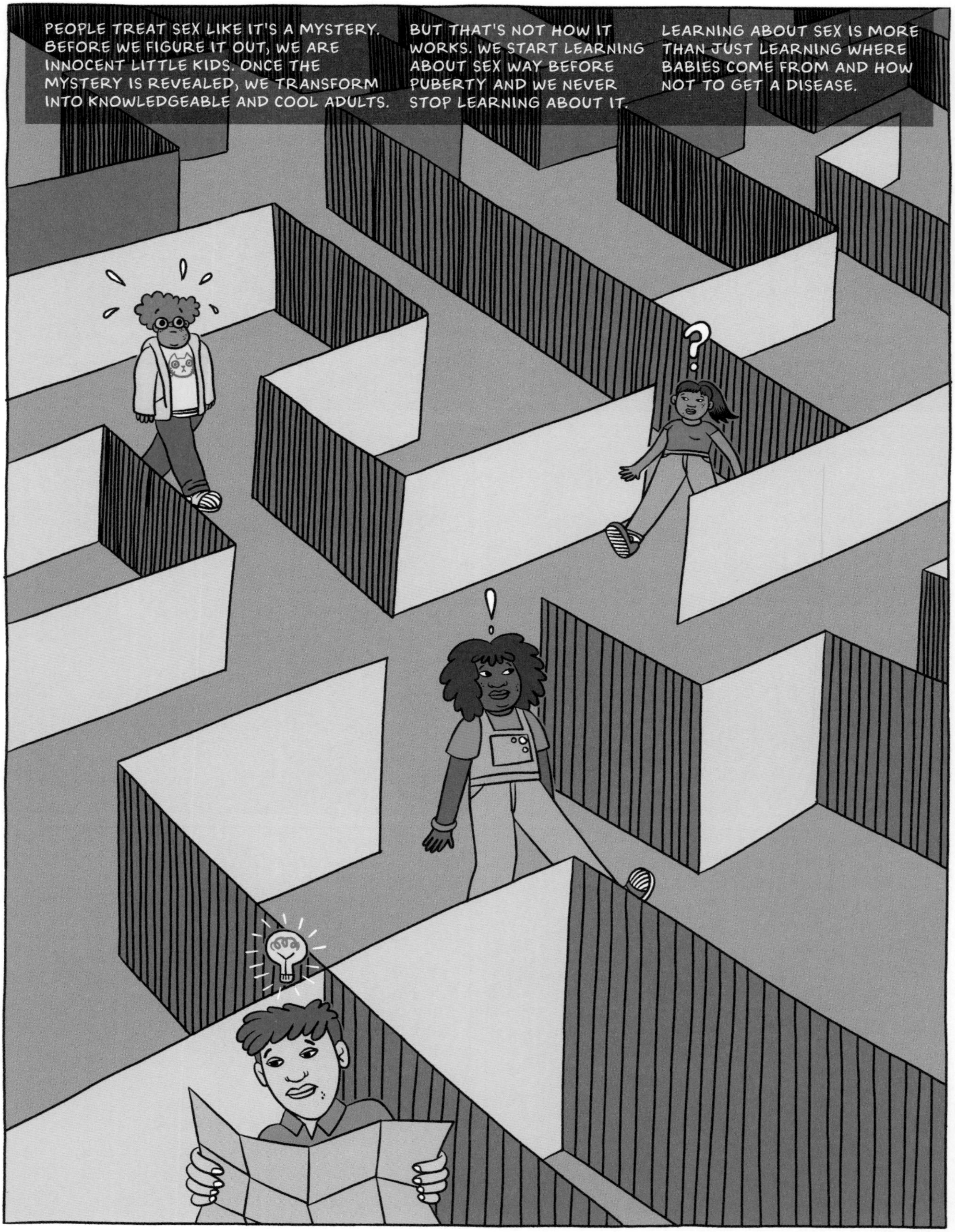
PEOPLE TREAT SEX LIKE IT'S A MYSTERY. BEFORE WE FIGURE IT OUT, WE ARE INNOCENT LITTLE KIDS. ONCE THE MYSTERY IS REVEALED, WE TRANSFORM INTO KNOWLEDGEABLE AND COOL ADULTS.
BUT THAT'S NOT HOW IT WORKS. WE START LEARNING ABOUT SEX WAY BEFORE PUBERTY AND WE NEVER STOP LEARNING ABOUT IT.
LEARNING ABOUT SEX IS MORE THAN JUST LEARNING WHERE BABIES COME FROM AND HOW NOT TO GET A DISEASE.

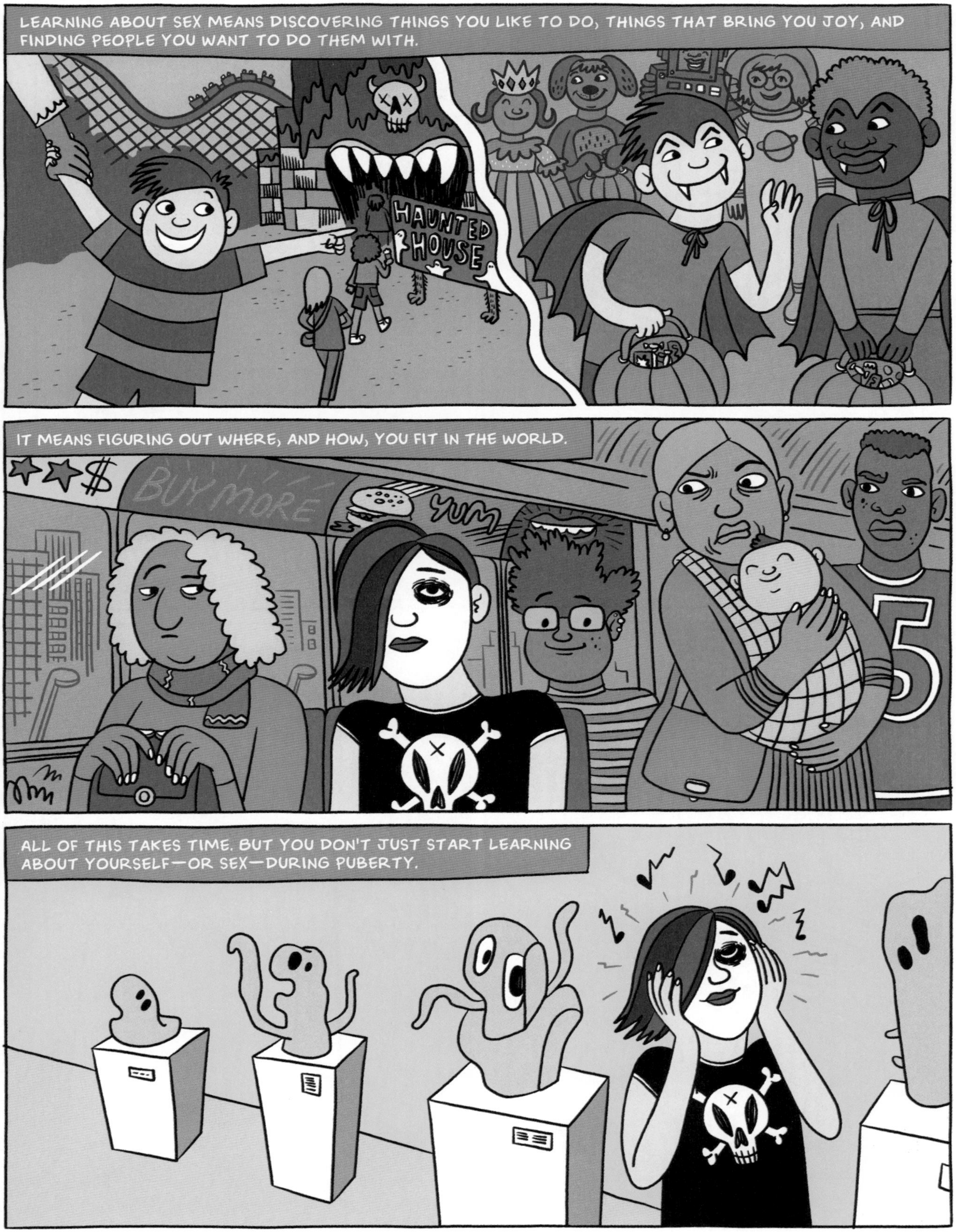
LEARNING ABOUT SEX MEANS DISCOVERING THINGS YOU LIKE TO DO, THINGS THAT BRING YOU JOY, AND FINDING PEOPLE YOU WANT TO DO THEM WITH.
HAUNTED HOUSE
IT MEANS FIGURING OUT WHERE, AND HOW, YOU FIT IN THE WORLD.
BUY MORE
YUM
ALL OF THIS TAKES TIME. BUT YOU DON'T JUST START LEARNING ABOUT YOURSELF—OR SEX—DURING PUBERTY.

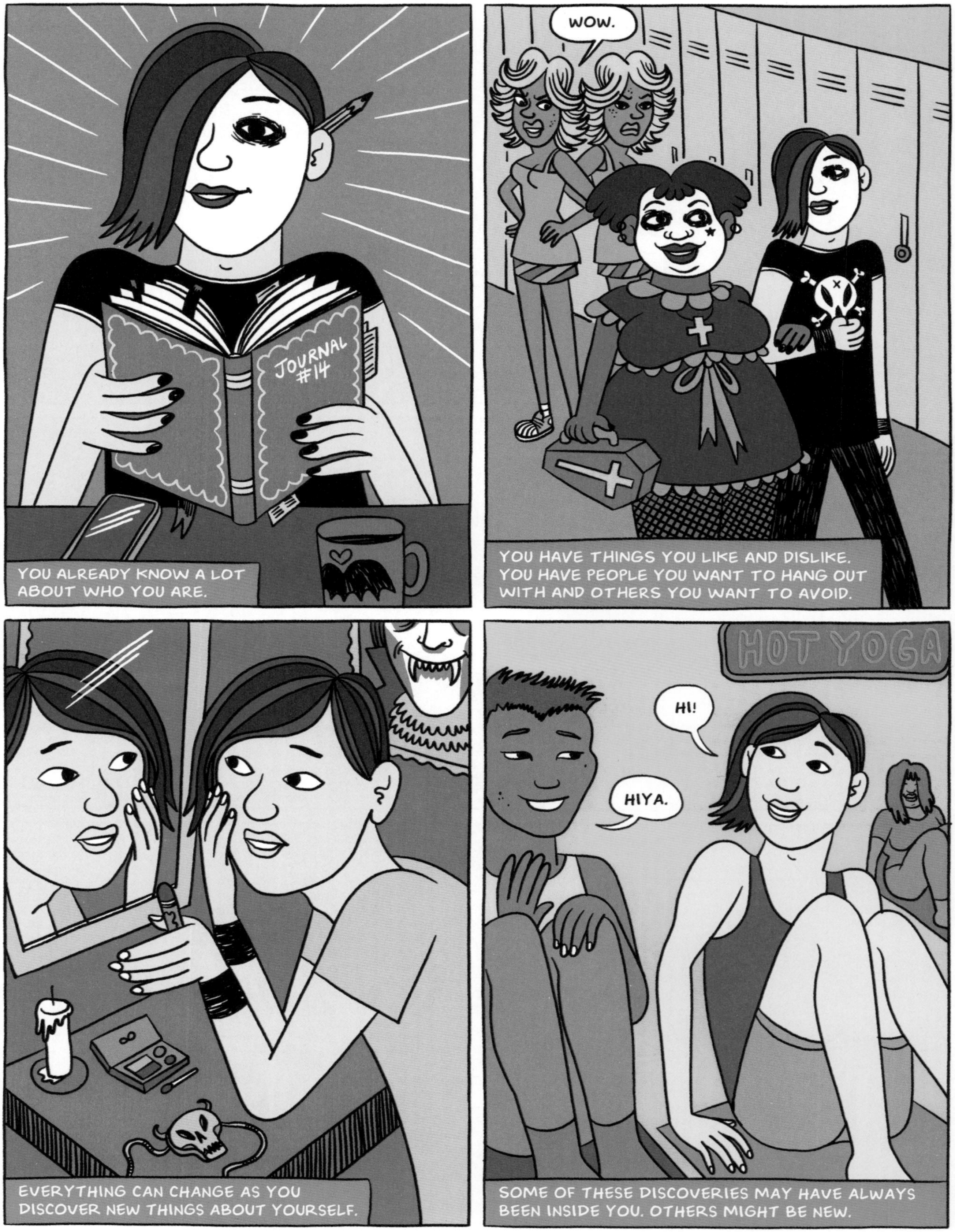
JOURNAL #14
YOU ALREADY KNOW A LOT ABOUT WHO YOU ARE.
WOW.
YOU HAVE THINGS YOU LIKE AND DISLIKE. YOU HAVE PEOPLE YOU WANT TO HANG OUT WITH AND OTHERS YOU WANT TO AVOID.
EVERYTHING CAN CHANGE AS YOU DISCOVER NEW THINGS ABOUT YOURSELF.
HOT YOGA
HI!
HIYA.
SOME OF THESE DISCOVERIES MAY HAVE ALWAYS BEEN INSIDE YOU. OTHERS MIGHT BE NEW.

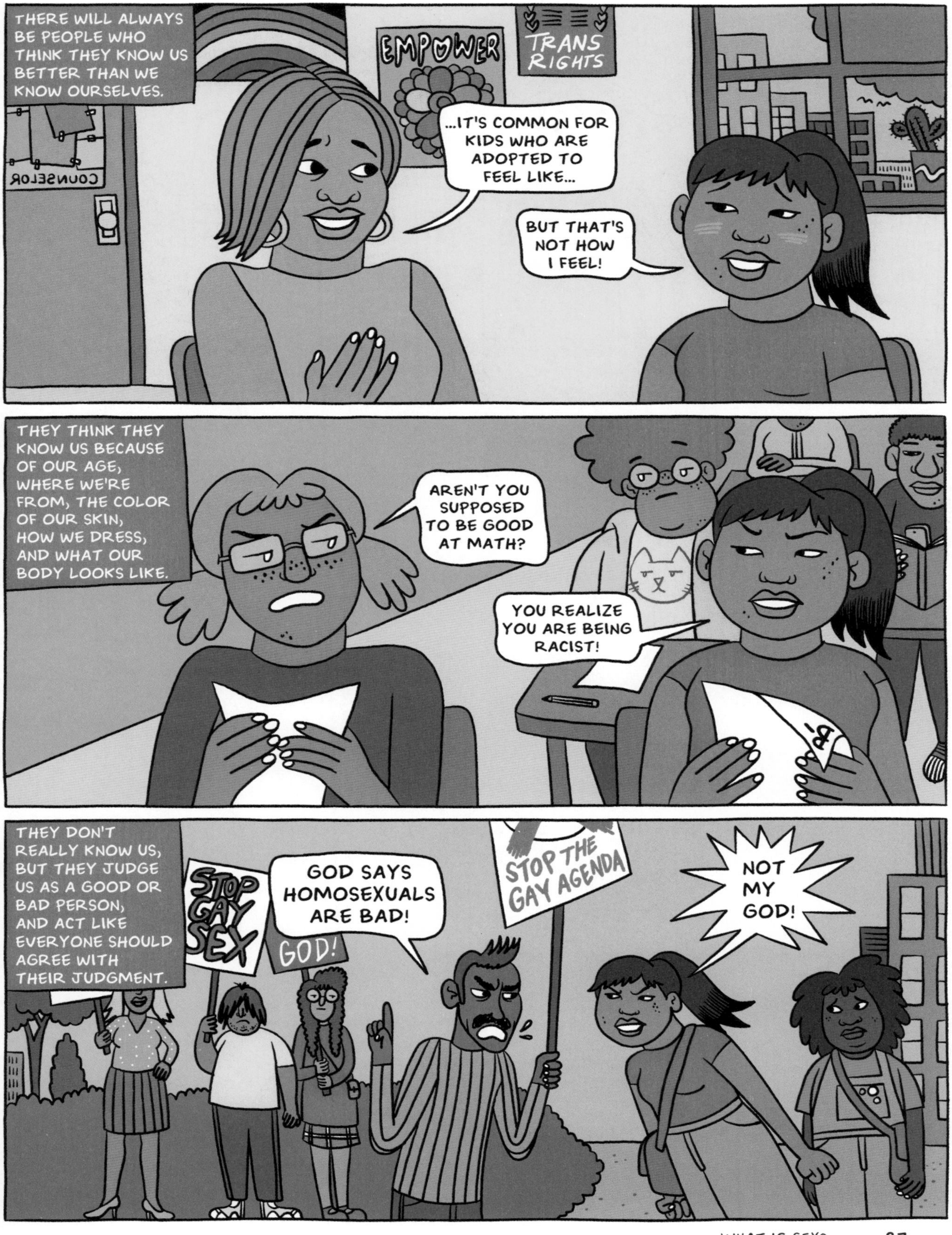
THERE WILL ALWAYS BE PEOPLE WHO THINK THEY KNOW US BETTER THAN WE KNOW OURSELVES.
EMPOWER
TRANS RIGHTS
COUNSELOR
...IT'S COMMON FOR KIDS WHO ARE ADOPTED TO FEEL LIKE...
BUT THAT'S NOT HOW I FEEL!
THEY THINK THEY KNOW US BECAUSE OF OUR AGE, WHERE WE'RE FROM, THE COLOR OF OUR SKIN, HOW WE DRESS, AND WHAT OUR BODY LOOKS LIKE.
AREN'T YOU SUPPOSED TO BE GOOD AT MATH?
YOU REALIZE YOU ARE BEING RACIST!
B-
THEY DON'T REALLY KNOW US, BUT THEY JUDGE US AS A GOOD OR BAD PERSON, AND ACT LIKE EVERYONE SHOULD AGREE WITH THEIR JUDGMENT.
STOP GAY SEX
GOD!
GOD SAYS HOMOSEXUALS ARE BAD!
STOP THE GAY AGENDA
NOT MY GOD!

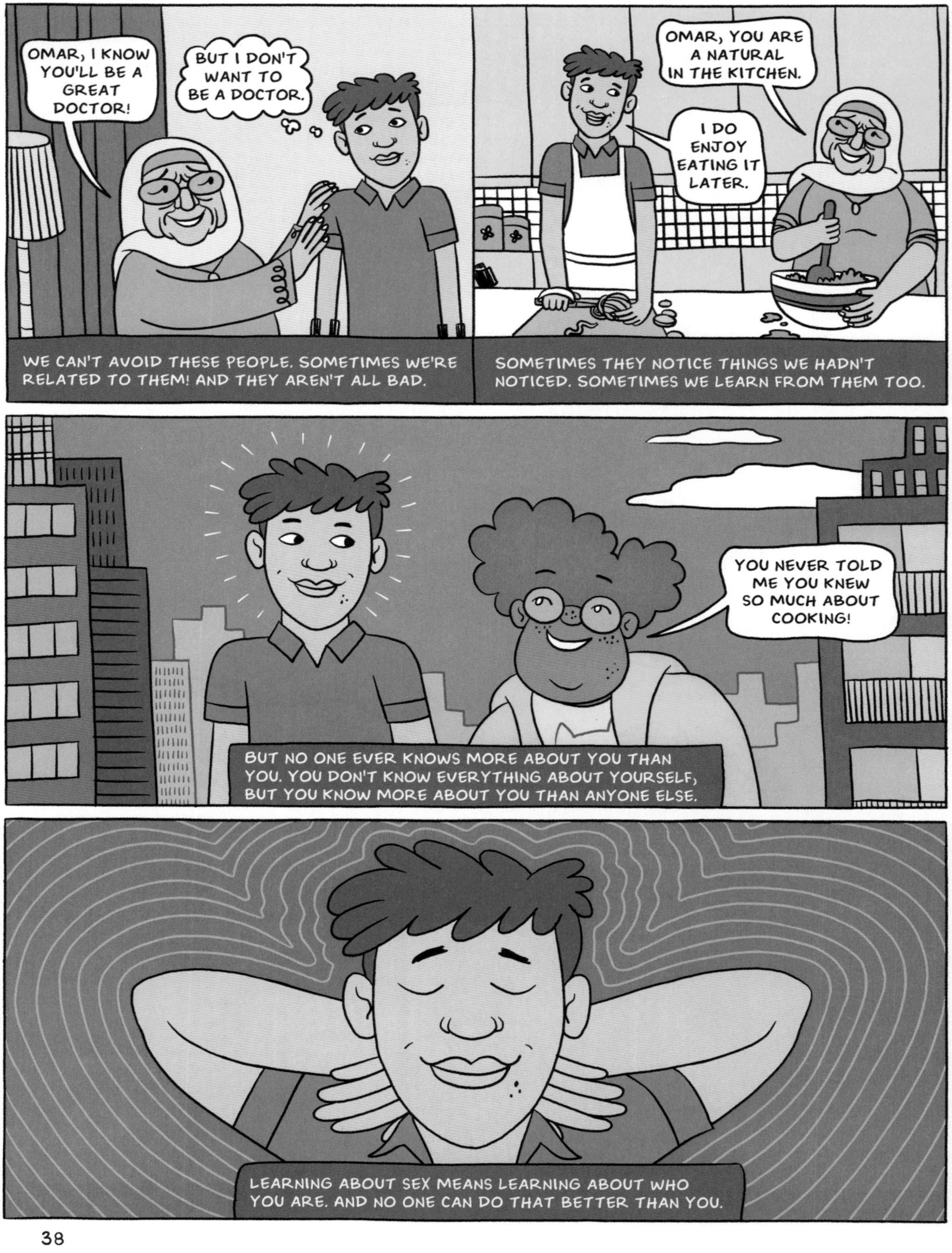
OMAR, I KNOW YOU'LL BE A GREAT DOCTOR!
BUT I DON'T WANT TO BE A DOCTOR.
WE CAN'T AVOID THESE PEOPLE. SOMETIMES WE'RE RELATED TO THEM! AND THEY AREN'T ALL BAD.
OMAR, YOU ARE A NATURAL IN THE KITCHEN.
I DO ENJOY EATING IT LATER.
SOMETIMES THEY NOTICE THINGS WE HADN'T NOTICED. SOMETIMES WE LEARN FROM THEM TOO.
YOU NEVER TOLD ME YOU KNEW SO MUCH ABOUT COOKING!
BUT NO ONE EVER KNOWS MORE ABOUT YOU THAN YOU. YOU DON'T KNOW EVERYTHING ABOUT YOURSELF, BUT YOU KNOW MORE ABOUT YOU THAN ANYONE ELSE.
LEARNING ABOUT SEX MEANS LEARNING ABOUT WHO YOU ARE. AND NO ONE CAN DO THAT BETTER THAN YOU.

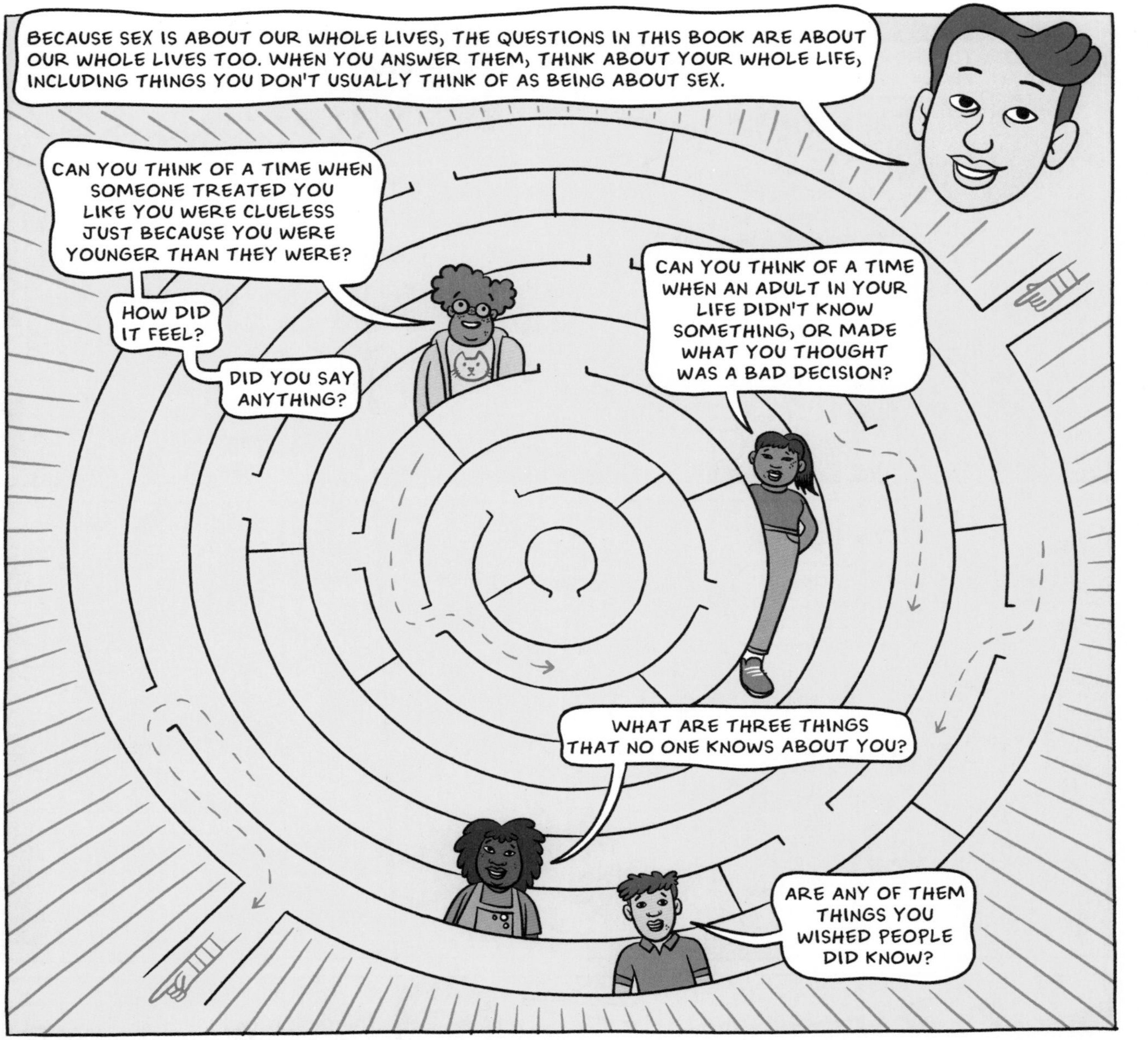
BECAUSE SEX IS ABOUT OUR WHOLE LIVES, THE QUESTIONS IN THIS BOOK ARE ABOUT OUR WHOLE LIVES TOO. WHEN YOU ANSWER THEM, THINK ABOUT YOUR WHOLE LIFE, INCLUDING THINGS YOU DON'T USUALLY THINK OF AS BEING ABOUT SEX.
CAN YOU THINK OF A TIME WHEN SOMEONE TREATED YOU LIKE YOU WERE CLUELESS JUST BECAUSE YOU WERE YOUNGER THAN THEY WERE?
HOW DID IT FEEL?
DID YOU SAY ANYTHING?
CAN YOU THINK OF A TIME WHEN AN ADULT IN YOUR LIFE DIDN'T KNOW SOMETHING, OR MADE WHAT YOU THOUGHT WAS A BAD DECISION?
WHAT ARE THREE THINGS THAT NO ONE KNOWS ABOUT YOU?
ARE ANY OF THEM THINGS YOU WISHED PEOPLE DID KNOW?

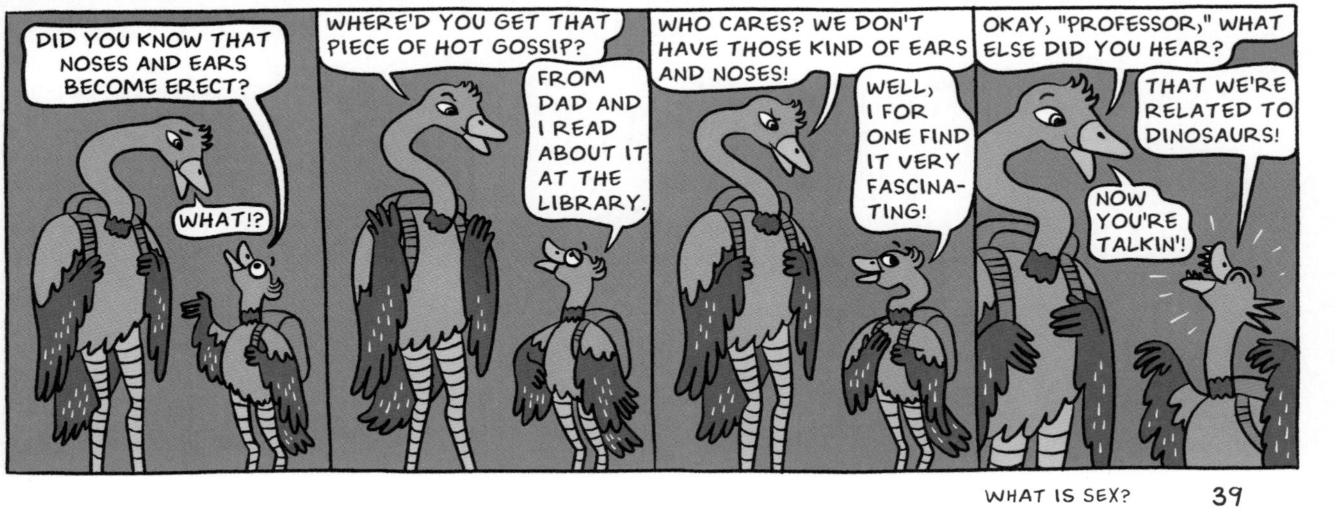
DID YOU KNOW THAT NOSES AND EARS BECOME ERECT?
WHAT!?
WHERE'D YOU GET THAT PIECE OF HOT GOSSIP?
FROM DAD AND I READ ABOUT IT AT THE LIBRARY.
WHO CARES? WE DON'T HAVE THOSE KIND OF EARS AND NOSES!
WELL, I FOR ONE FIND IT VERY FASCINATING!
OKAY, "PROFESSOR," WHAT ELSE DID YOU HEAR?
THAT WE'RE RELATED TO DINOSAURS!
NOW YOU'RE TALKIN'!

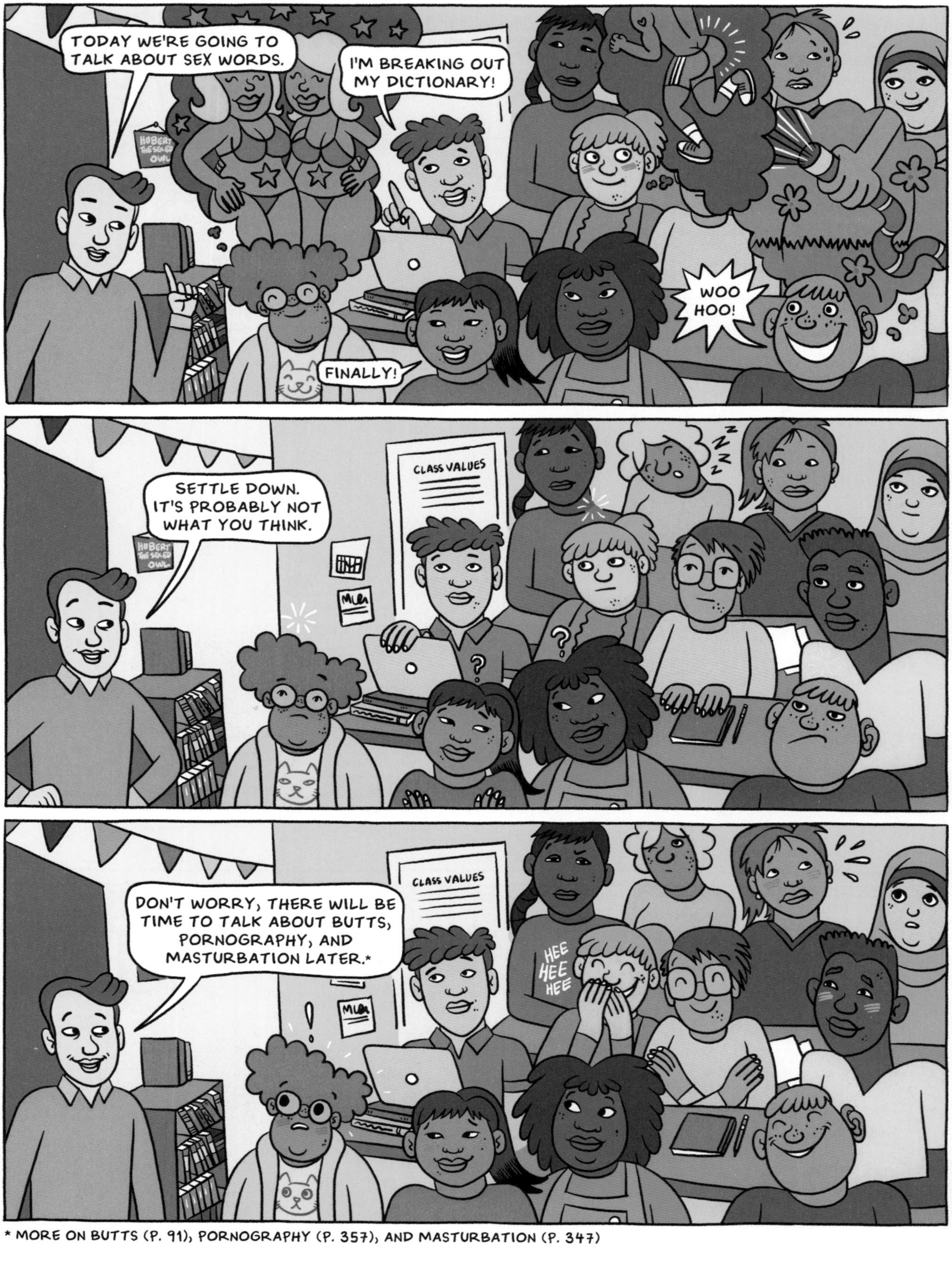
TODAY WE'RE GOING TO TALK ABOUT SEX WORDS.
I'M BREAKING OUT MY DICTIONARY!
HUBERT THE SEX ED OWL
WOO HOO!
FINALLY!
SETTLE DOWN. IT'S PROBABLY NOT WHAT YOU THINK.
CLASS VALUES
DON'T WORRY, THERE WILL BE TIME TO TALK ABOUT BUTTS, PORNOGRAPHY, AND MASTURBATION LATER.*
HEE HEE HEE

* MORE ON BUTTS (P. 91), PORNOGRAPHY (P. 357), AND MASTURBATION (P. 347)

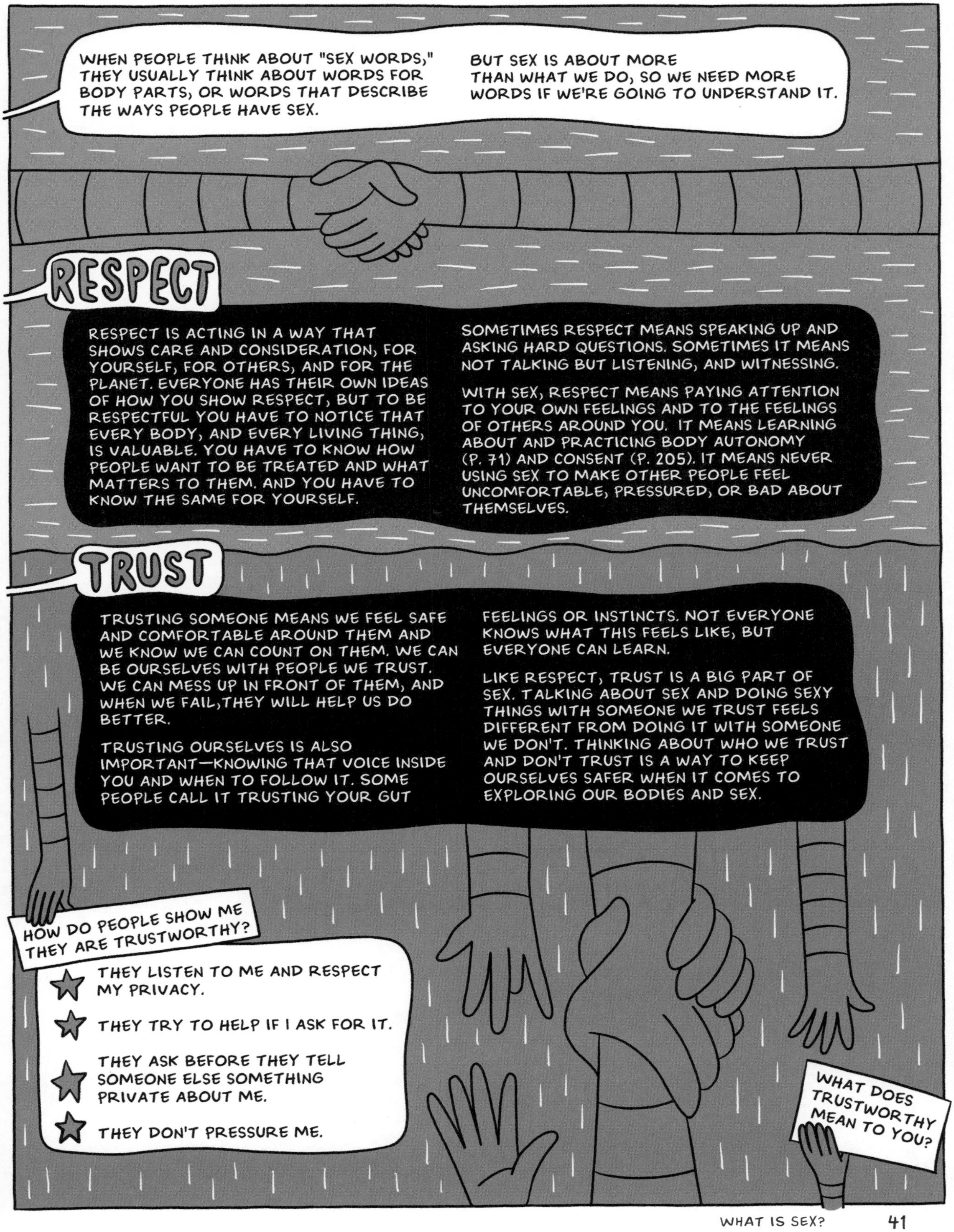
WHEN PEOPLE THINK ABOUT "SEX WORDS," THEY USUALLY THINK ABOUT WORDS FOR BODY PARTS, OR WORDS THAT DESCRIBE THE WAYS PEOPLE HAVE SEX.
BUT SEX IS ABOUT MORE THAN WHAT WE DO, SO WE NEED MORE WORDS IF WE'RE GOING TO UNDERSTAND IT.
RESPECT
RESPECT IS ACTING IN A WAY THAT SHOWS CARE AND CONSIDERATION, FOR YOURSELF, FOR OTHERS, AND FOR THE PLANET. EVERYONE HAS THEIR OWN IDEAS OF HOW YOU SHOW RESPECT, BUT TO BE RESPECTFUL YOU HAVE TO NOTICE THAT EVERY BODY, AND EVERY LIVING THING, IS VALUABLE. YOU HAVE TO KNOW HOW PEOPLE WANT TO BE TREATED AND WHAT MATTERS TO THEM. AND YOU HAVE TO KNOW THE SAME FOR YOURSELF.
SOMETIMES RESPECT MEANS SPEAKING UP AND ASKING HARD QUESTIONS. SOMETIMES IT MEANS NOT TALKING BUT LISTENING, AND WITNESSING.
WITH SEX, RESPECT MEANS PAYING ATTENTION TO YOUR OWN FEELINGS AND TO THE FEELINGS OF OTHERS AROUND YOU. IT MEANS LEARNING ABOUT AND PRACTICING BODY AUTONOMY (P. 71) AND CONSENT (P. 205). IT MEANS NEVER USING SEX TO MAKE OTHER PEOPLE FEEL UNCOMFORTABLE, PRESSURED, OR BAD ABOUT THEMSELVES.
TRUST
TRUSTING SOMEONE MEANS WE FEEL SAFE AND COMFORTABLE AROUND THEM AND WE KNOW WE CAN COUNT ON THEM. WE CAN BE OURSELVES WITH PEOPLE WE TRUST. WE CAN MESS UP IN FRONT OF THEM, AND WHEN WE FAIL,THEY WILL HELP US DO BETTER.
TRUSTING OURSELVES IS ALSO IMPORTANT—KNOWING THAT VOICE INSIDE YOU AND WHEN TO FOLLOW IT. SOME PEOPLE CALL IT TRUSTING YOUR GUT FEELINGS OR INSTINCTS. NOT EVERYONE KNOWS WHAT THIS FEELS LIKE, BUT EVERYONE CAN LEARN.
LIKE RESPECT, TRUST IS A BIG PART OF SEX. TALKING ABOUT SEX AND DOING SEXY THINGS WITH SOMEONE WE TRUST FEELS DIFFERENT FROM DOING IT WITH SOMEONE WE DON'T. THINKING ABOUT WHO WE TRUST AND DON'T TRUST IS A WAY TO KEEP OURSELVES SAFER WHEN IT COMES TO EXPLORING OUR BODIES AND SEX.
HOW DO PEOPLE SHOW ME THEY ARE TRUSTWORTHY?
THEY LISTEN TO ME AND RESPECT MY PRIVACY.
THEY TRY TO HELP IF I ASK FOR IT.
THEY ASK BEFORE THEY TELL SOMEONE ELSE SOMETHING PRIVATE ABOUT ME.
THEY DON'T PRESSURE ME.
WHAT DOES TRUSTWORTHY MEAN TO YOU?

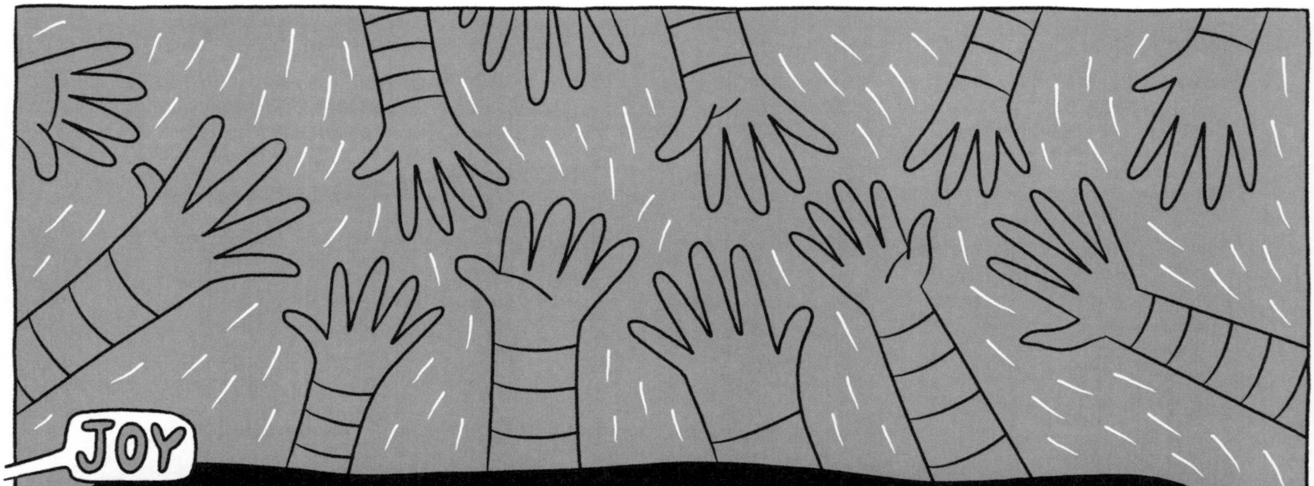

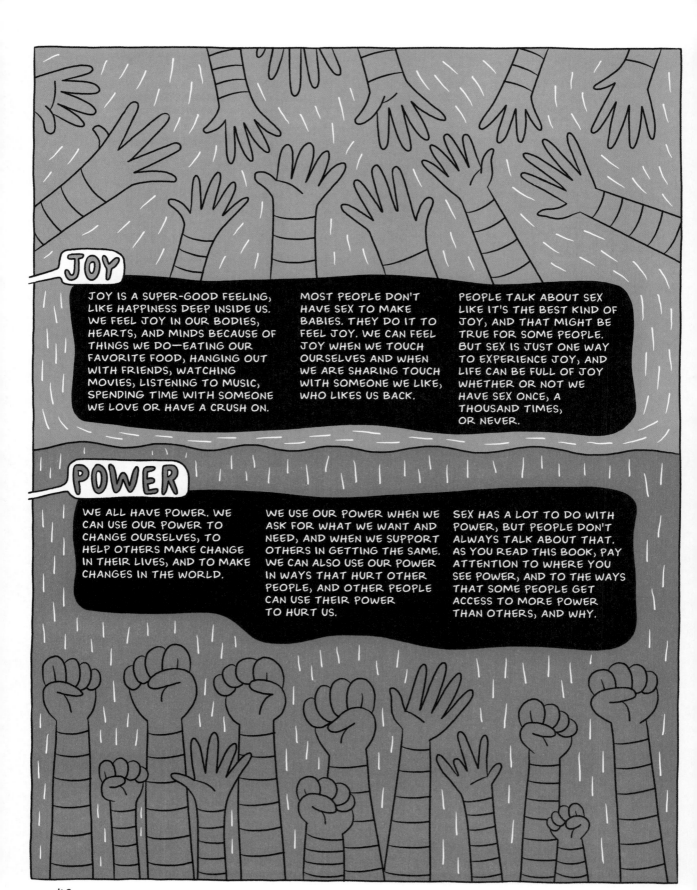

JOY

JOY IS A SUPER-GOOD FEELING, LIKE HAPPINESS DEEP INSIDE US. WE FEEL JOY IN OUR BODIES, HEARTS, AND MINDS BECAUSE OF THINGS WE DO—EATING OUR FAVORITE FOOD, HANGING OUT WITH FRIENDS, WATCHING MOVIES, LISTENING TO MUSIC, SPENDING TIME WITH SOMEONE WE LOVE OR HAVE A CRUSH ON.

MOST PEOPLE DON'T HAVE SEX TO MAKE BABIES. THEY DO IT TO FEEL JOY. WE CAN FEEL JOY WHEN WE TOUCH OURSELVES AND WHEN WE ARE SHARING TOUCH WITH SOMEONE WE LIKE, WHO LIKES US BACK.

PEOPLE TALK ABOUT SEX LIKE IT'S THE BEST KIND OF JOY, AND THAT MIGHT BE TRUE FOR SOME PEOPLE. BUT SEX IS JUST ONE WAY TO EXPERIENCE JOY, AND LIFE CAN BE FULL OF JOY WHETHER OR NOT WE HAVE SEX ONCE, A THOUSAND TIMES, OR NEVER.

POWER

WE ALL HAVE POWER. WE CAN USE OUR POWER TO CHANGE OURSELVES, TO HELP OTHERS MAKE CHANGE IN THEIR LIVES, AND TO MAKE CHANGES IN THE WORLD.

WE USE OUR POWER WHEN WE ASK FOR WHAT WE WANT AND NEED, AND WHEN WE SUPPORT OTHERS IN GETTING THE SAME. WE CAN ALSO USE OUR POWER IN WAYS THAT HURT OTHER PEOPLE, AND OTHER PEOPLE CAN USE THEIR POWER TO HURT US.

SEX HAS A LOT TO DO WITH POWER, BUT PEOPLE DON'T ALWAYS TALK ABOUT THAT. AS YOU READ THIS BOOK, PAY ATTENTION TO WHERE YOU SEE POWER, AND TO THE WAYS THAT SOME PEOPLE GET ACCESS TO MORE POWER THAN OTHERS, AND WHY.

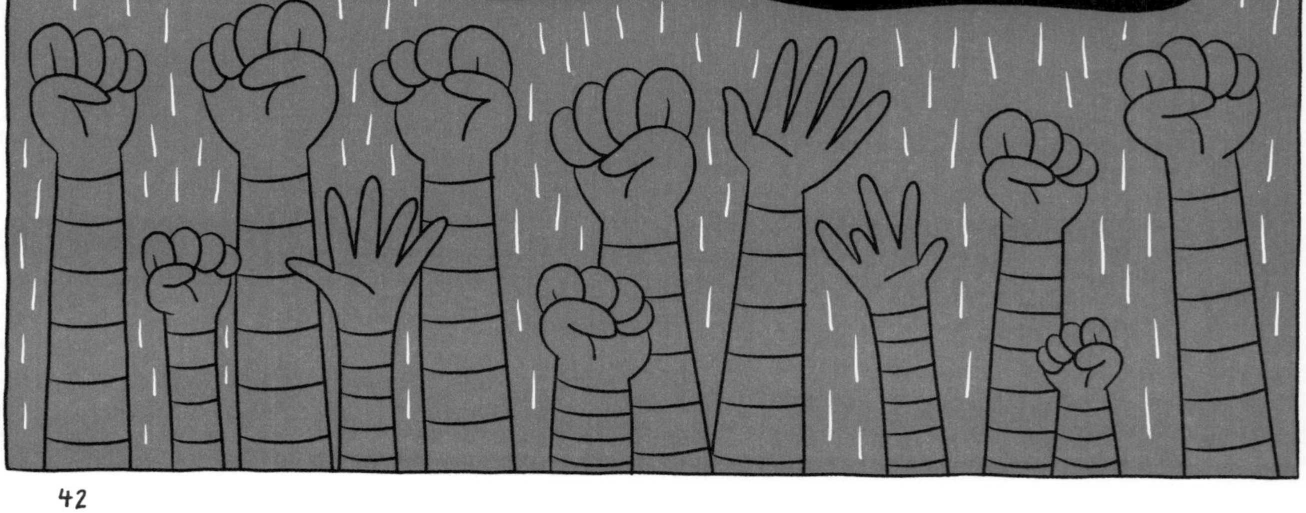

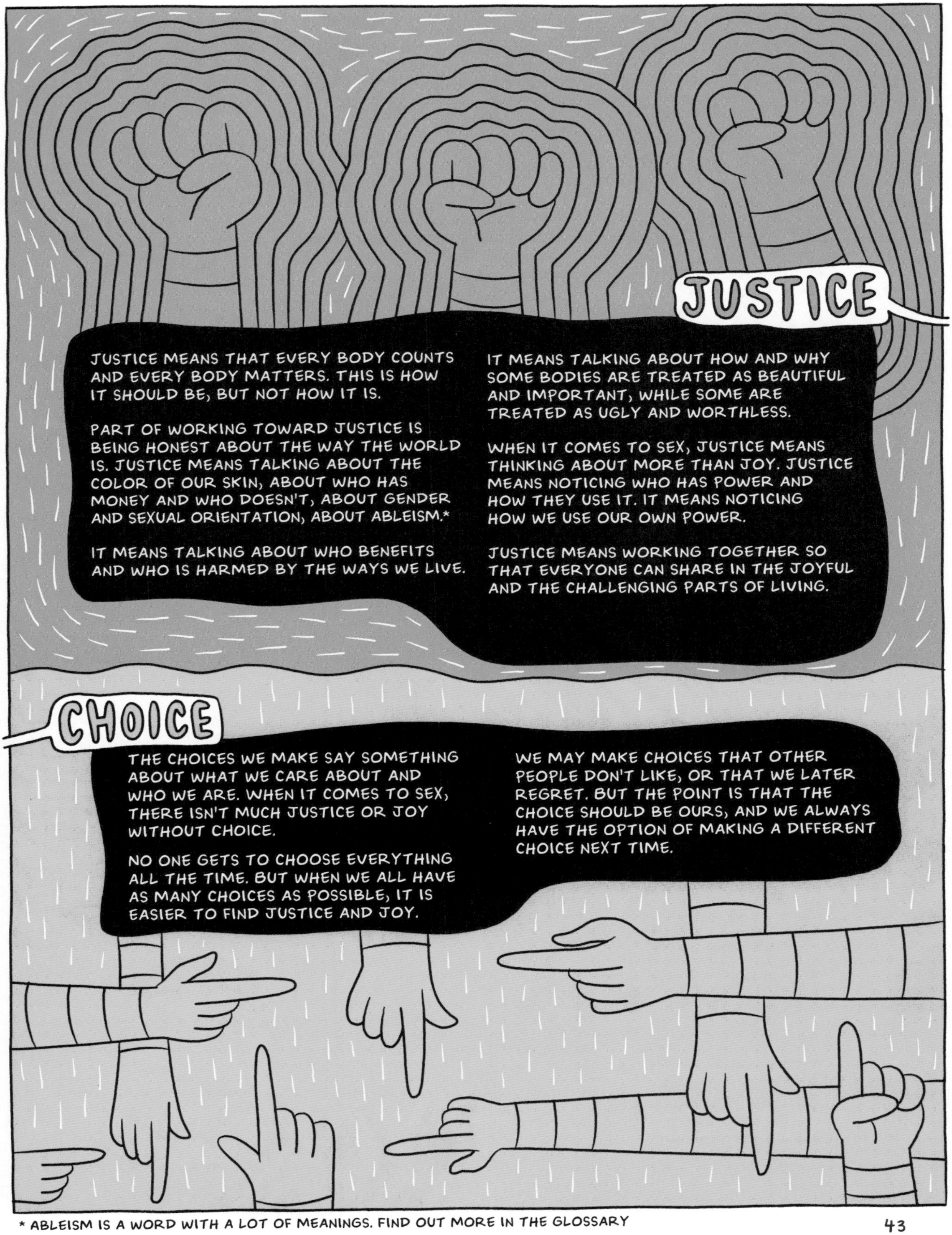
JUSTICE
JUSTICE MEANS THAT EVERY BODY COUNTS AND EVERY BODY MATTERS. THIS IS HOW IT SHOULD BE, BUT NOT HOW IT IS.
PART OF WORKING TOWARD JUSTICE IS BEING HONEST ABOUT THE WAY THE WORLD IS. JUSTICE MEANS TALKING ABOUT THE COLOR OF OUR SKIN, ABOUT WHO HAS MONEY AND WHO DOESN'T, ABOUT GENDER AND SEXUAL ORIENTATION, ABOUT ABLEISM.*
IT MEANS TALKING ABOUT WHO BENEFITS AND WHO IS HARMED BY THE WAYS WE LIVE.
IT MEANS TALKING ABOUT HOW AND WHY SOME BODIES ARE TREATED AS BEAUTIFUL AND IMPORTANT, WHILE SOME ARE TREATED AS UGLY AND WORTHLESS.
WHEN IT COMES TO SEX, JUSTICE MEANS THINKING ABOUT MORE THAN JOY. JUSTICE MEANS NOTICING WHO HAS POWER AND HOW THEY USE IT. IT MEANS NOTICING HOW WE USE OUR OWN POWER.
JUSTICE MEANS WORKING TOGETHER SO THAT EVERYONE CAN SHARE IN THE JOYFUL AND THE CHALLENGING PARTS OF LIVING.
CHOICE
THE CHOICES WE MAKE SAY SOMETHING ABOUT WHAT WE CARE ABOUT AND WHO WE ARE. WHEN IT COMES TO SEX, THERE ISN'T MUCH JUSTICE OR JOY WITHOUT CHOICE.
NO ONE GETS TO CHOOSE EVERYTHING ALL THE TIME. BUT WHEN WE ALL HAVE AS MANY CHOICES AS POSSIBLE, IT IS EASIER TO FIND JUSTICE AND JOY.
WE MAY MAKE CHOICES THAT OTHER PEOPLE DON'T LIKE, OR THAT WE LATER REGRET. BUT THE POINT IS THAT THE CHOICE SHOULD BE OURS, AND WE ALWAYS HAVE THE OPTION OF MAKING A DIFFERENT CHOICE NEXT TIME.

* ABLEISM IS A WORD WITH A LOT OF MEANINGS. FIND OUT MORE IN THE GLOSSARY

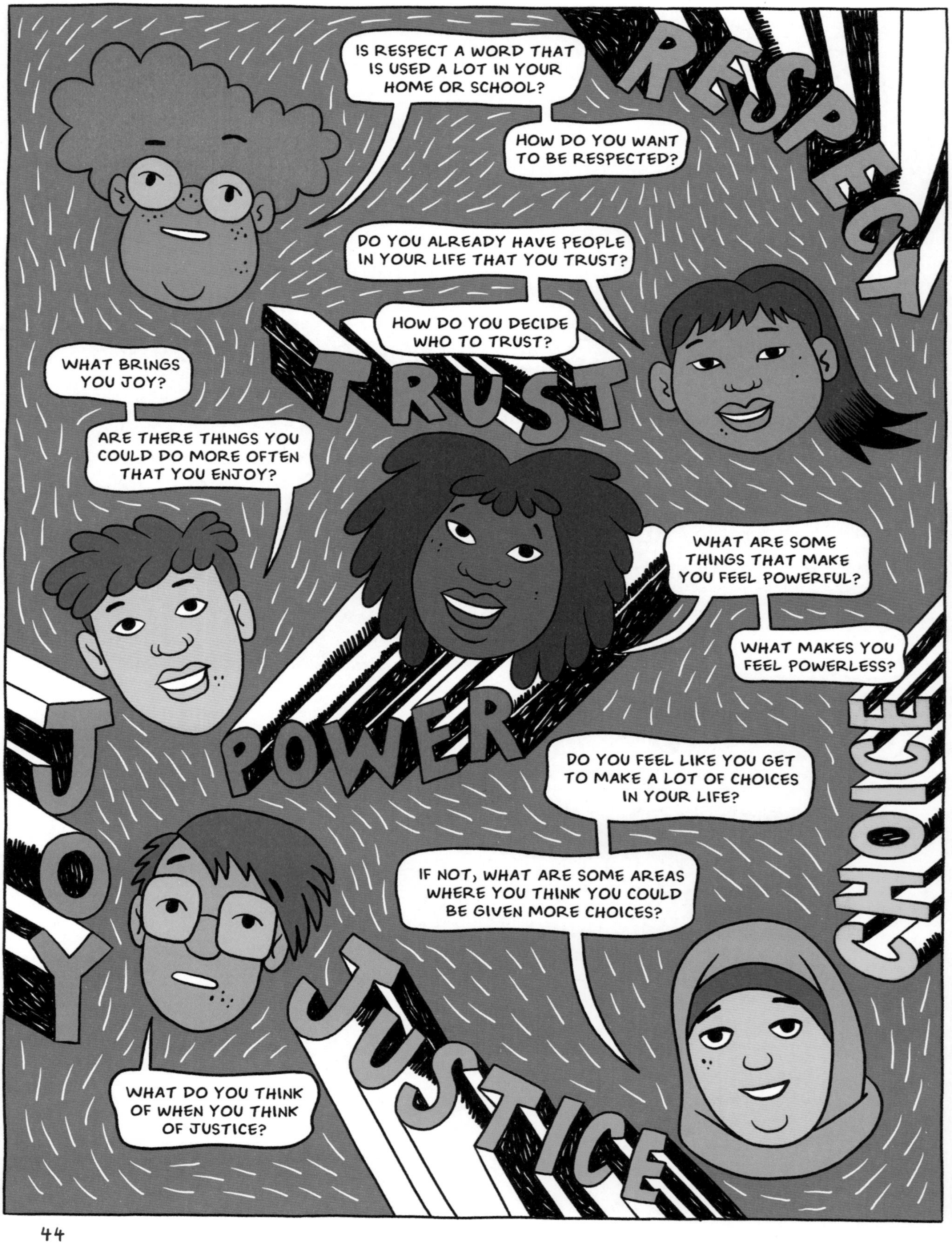
RESPECT
IS RESPECT A WORD THAT IS USED A LOT IN YOUR HOME OR SCHOOL?
HOW DO YOU WANT TO BE RESPECTED?
TRUST
DO YOU ALREADY HAVE PEOPLE IN YOUR LIFE THAT YOU TRUST?
HOW DO YOU DECIDE WHO TO TRUST?
JOY
WHAT BRINGS YOU JOY?
ARE THERE THINGS YOU COULD DO MORE OFTEN THAT YOU ENJOY?
POWER
WHAT ARE SOME THINGS THAT MAKE YOU FEEL POWERFUL?
WHAT MAKES YOU FEEL POWERLESS?
CHOICE
DO YOU FEEL LIKE YOU GET TO MAKE A LOT OF CHOICES IN YOUR LIFE?
IF NOT, WHAT ARE SOME AREAS WHERE YOU THINK YOU COULD BE GIVEN MORE CHOICES?
JUSTICE
WHAT DO YOU THINK OF WHEN YOU THINK OF JUSTICE?

2
BODIES

YAY
EEEEEEEEEEEEE

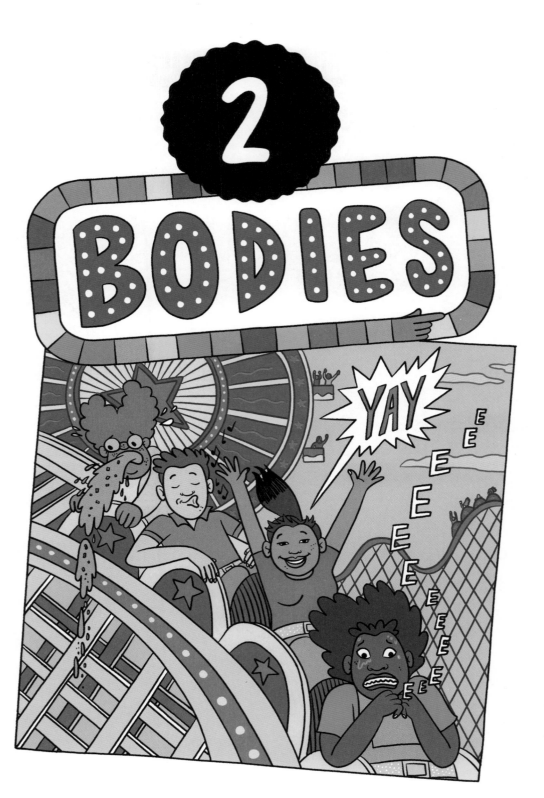

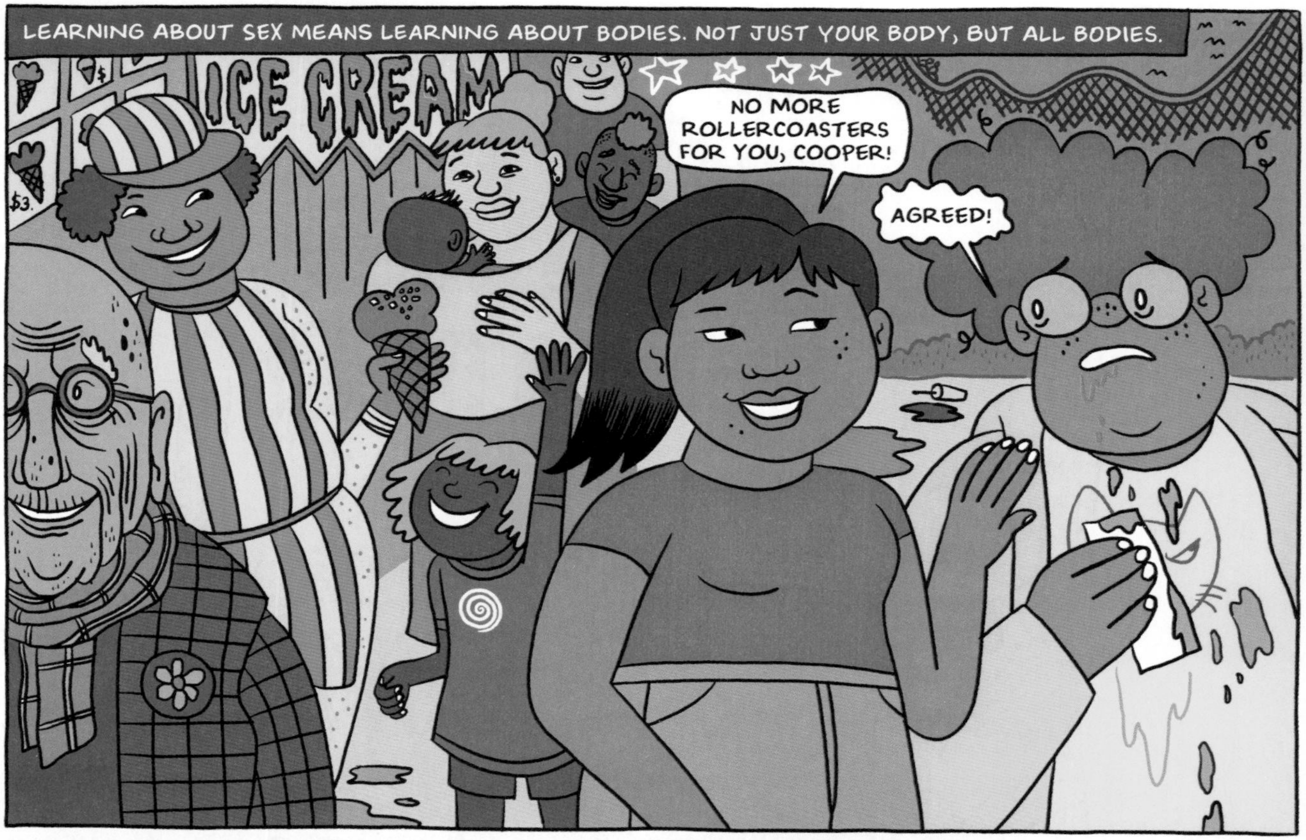
LEARNING ABOUT SEX MEANS LEARNING ABOUT BODIES. NOT JUST YOUR BODY, BUT ALL BODIES.
ICE CREAM
$3.
NO MORE ROLLERCOASTERS FOR YOU, COOPER!
AGREED!

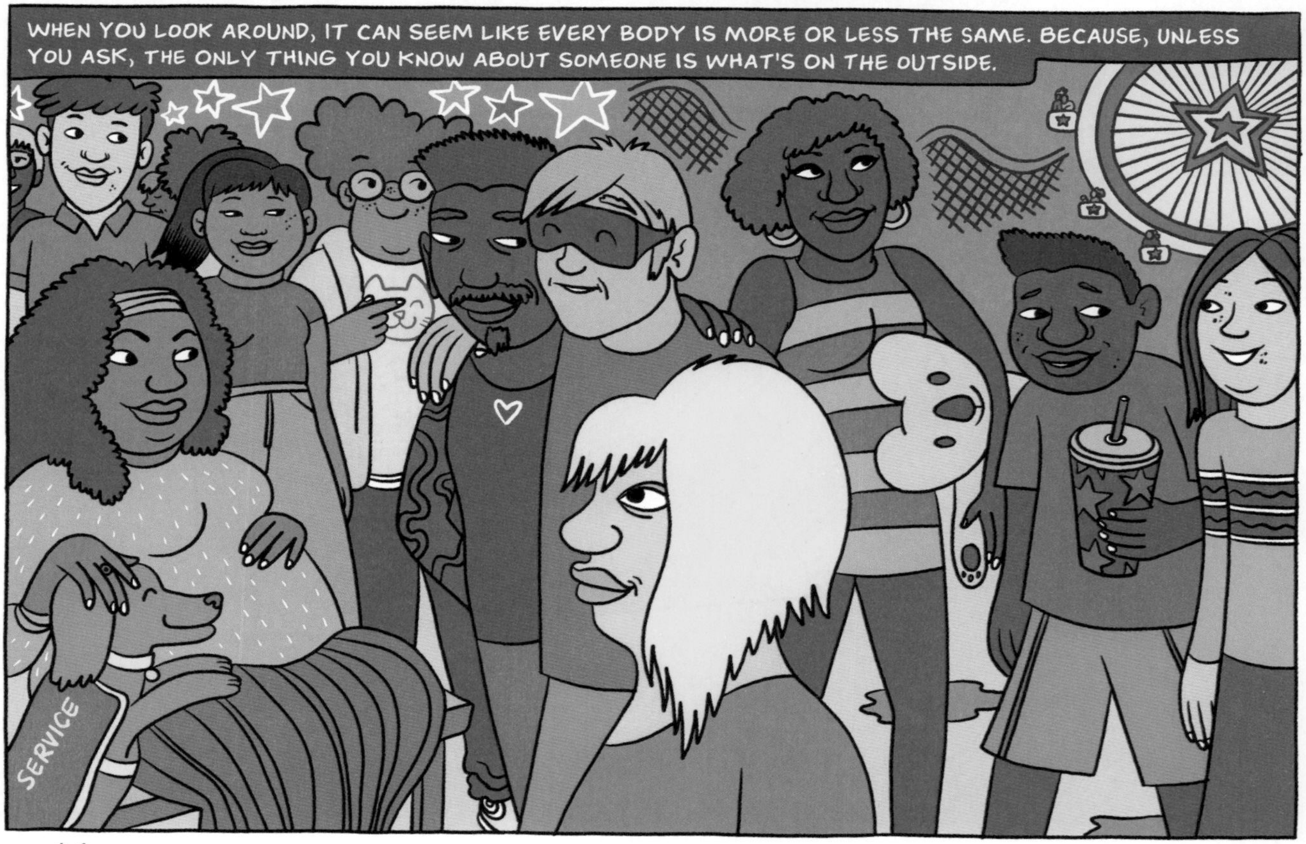
WHEN YOU LOOK AROUND, IT CAN SEEM LIKE EVERY BODY IS MORE OR LESS THE SAME. BECAUSE, UNLESS YOU ASK, THE ONLY THING YOU KNOW ABOUT SOMEONE IS WHAT'S ON THE OUTSIDE.
SERVICE

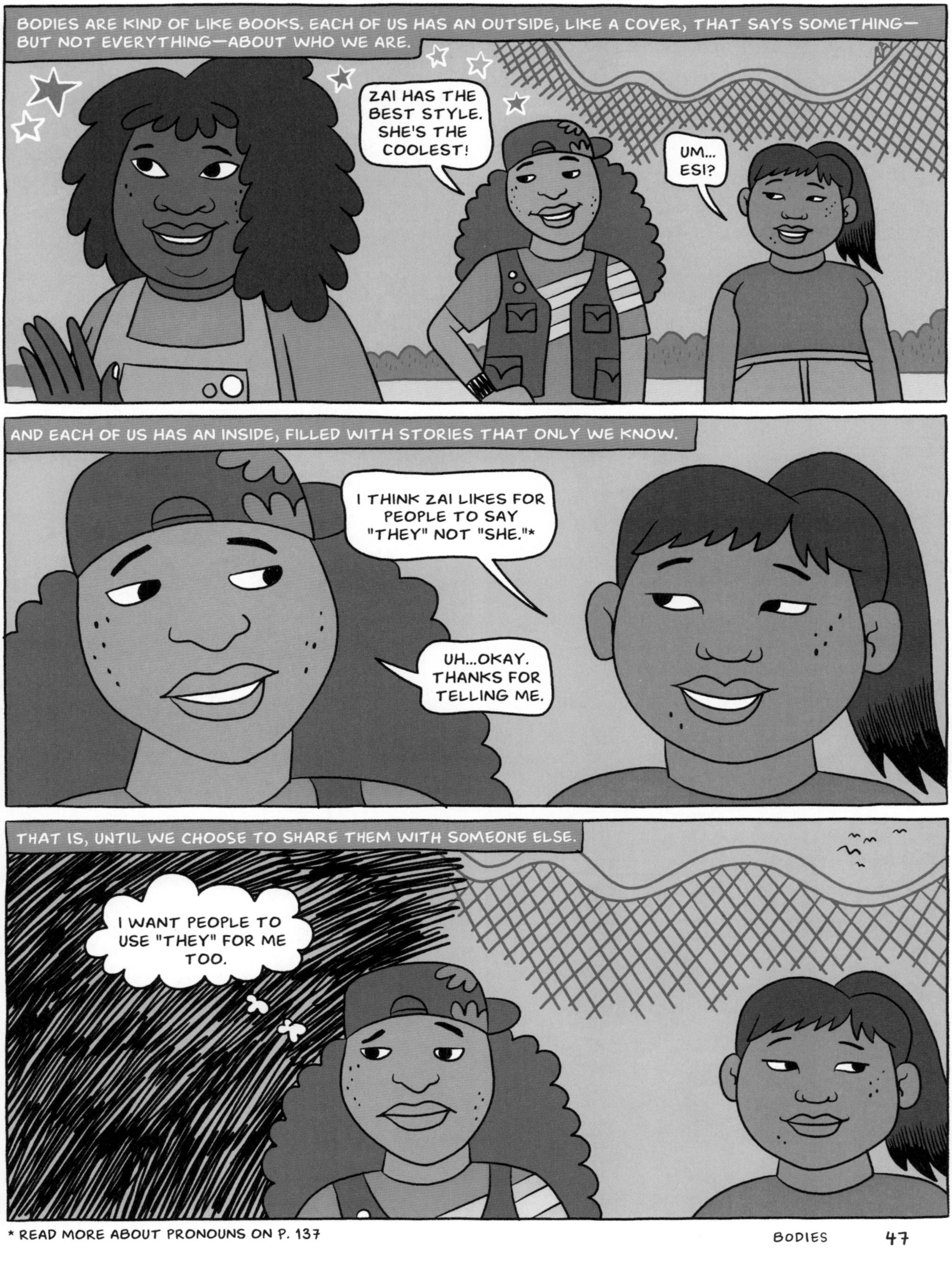
BODIES ARE KIND OF LIKE BOOKS. EACH OF US HAS AN OUTSIDE, LIKE A COVER, THAT SAYS SOMETHING—BUT NOT EVERYTHING—ABOUT WHO WE ARE.
ZAI HAS THE BEST STYLE. SHE'S THE COOLEST!
UM... ESI?
AND EACH OF US HAS AN INSIDE, FILLED WITH STORIES THAT ONLY WE KNOW.
I THINK ZAI LIKES FOR PEOPLE TO SAY "THEY" NOT "SHE."*
UH...OKAY. THANKS FOR TELLING ME.
THAT IS, UNTIL WE CHOOSE TO SHARE THEM WITH SOMEONE ELSE.
I WANT PEOPLE TO USE "THEY" FOR ME TOO.

* READ MORE ABOUT PRONOUNS ON P. 137

THOUGH EVERY BODY IS DIFFERENT, SOME THINGS ARE TRUE FOR ALL BODIES.

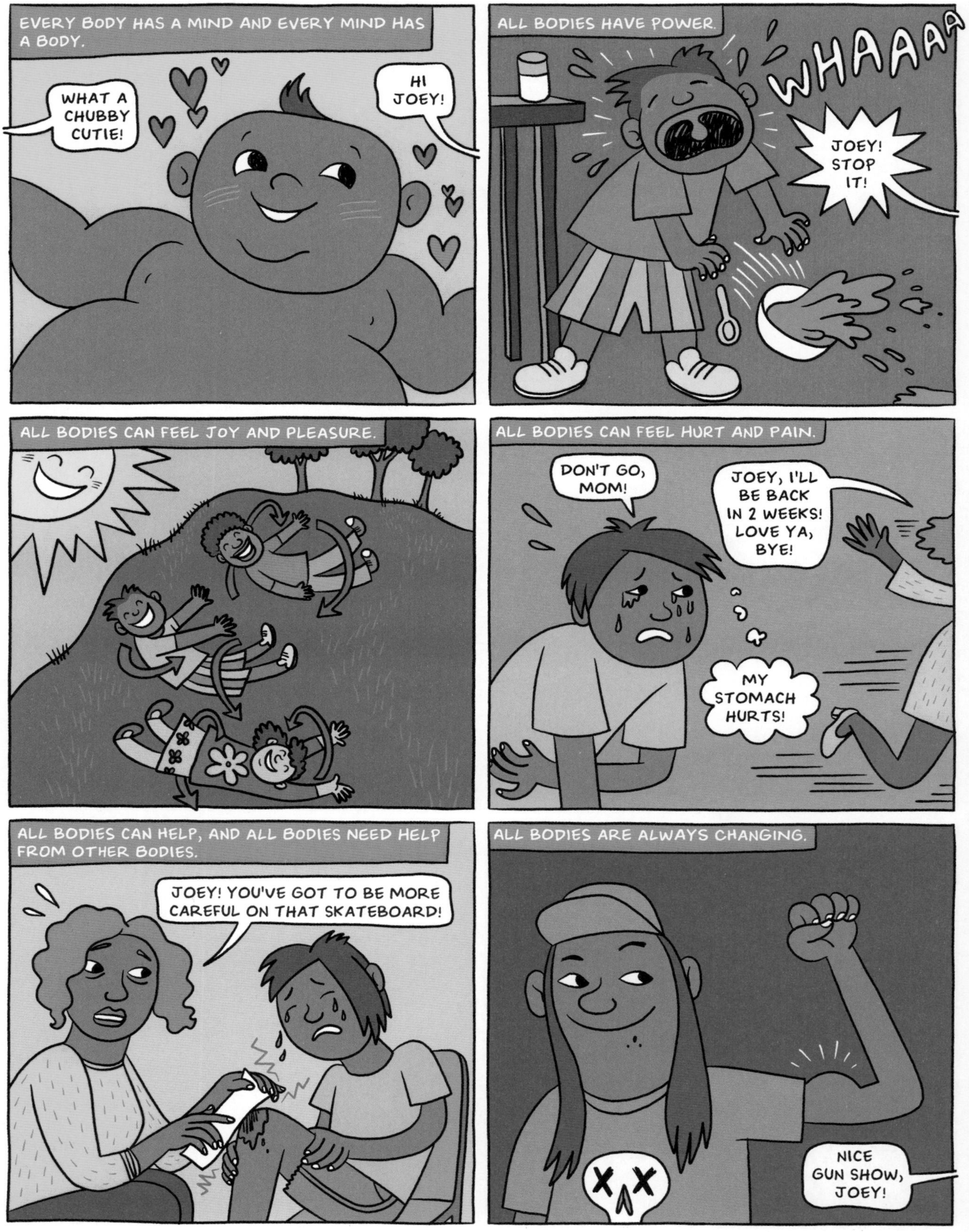
EVERY BODY HAS A MIND AND EVERY MIND HAS A BODY.
WHAT A CHUBBY CUTIE!
HI JOEY!
ALL BODIES HAVE POWER.
WHAAAA
JOEY! STOP IT!
ALL BODIES CAN FEEL JOY AND PLEASURE.
ALL BODIES CAN FEEL HURT AND PAIN.
DON'T GO, MOM!
JOEY, I'LL BE BACK IN 2 WEEKS! LOVE YA, BYE!
MY STOMACH HURTS!
ALL BODIES CAN HELP, AND ALL BODIES NEED HELP FROM OTHER BODIES.
JOEY! YOU'VE GOT TO BE MORE CAREFUL ON THAT SKATEBOARD!
ALL BODIES ARE ALWAYS CHANGING.
NICE GUN SHOW, JOEY!

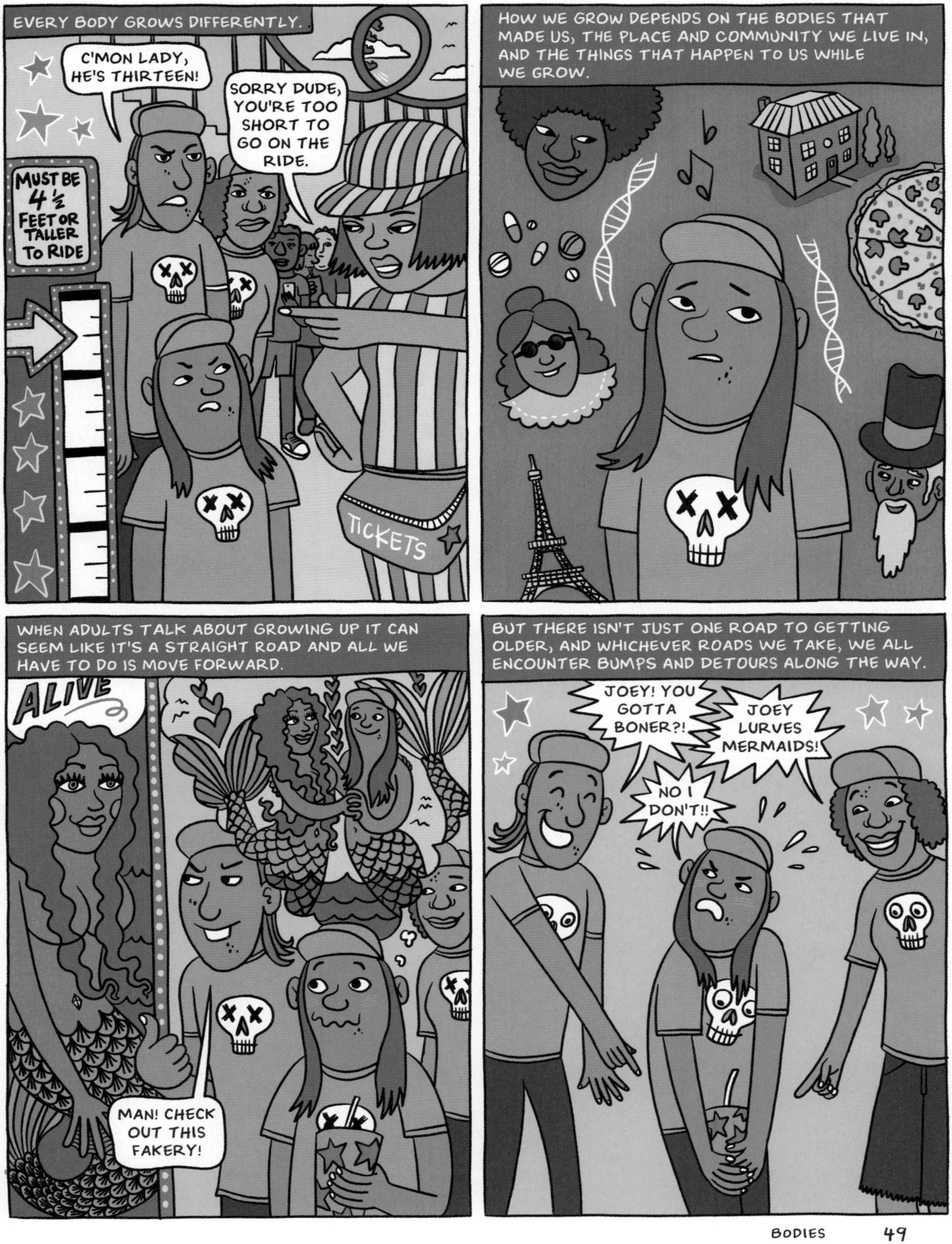
EVERY BODY GROWS DIFFERENTLY.
C'MON LADY, HE'S THIRTEEN!
SORRY DUDE, YOU'RE TOO SHORT TO GO ON THE RIDE.
MUST BE 4 1/2 FEET OR TALLER TO RIDE
TICKETS
HOW WE GROW DEPENDS ON THE BODIES THAT MADE US, THE PLACE AND COMMUNITY WE LIVE IN, AND THE THINGS THAT HAPPEN TO US WHILE WE GROW.
WHEN ADULTS TALK ABOUT GROWING UP IT CAN SEEM LIKE IT'S A STRAIGHT ROAD AND ALL WE HAVE TO DO IS MOVE FORWARD.
ALIVE
MAN! CHECK OUT THIS FAKERY!
BUT THERE ISN'T JUST ONE ROAD TO GETTING OLDER, AND WHICHEVER ROADS WE TAKE, WE ALL ENCOUNTER BUMPS AND DETOURS ALONG THE WAY.
JOEY! YOU GOTTA BONER?!
JOEY LURVES MERMAIDS!
NO I DON'T!!

BEING ALIVE CAN BE AMAZING, FUN, AND BEAUTIFUL. IT CAN ALSO BE SAD, CONFUSING AND AWKWARD.

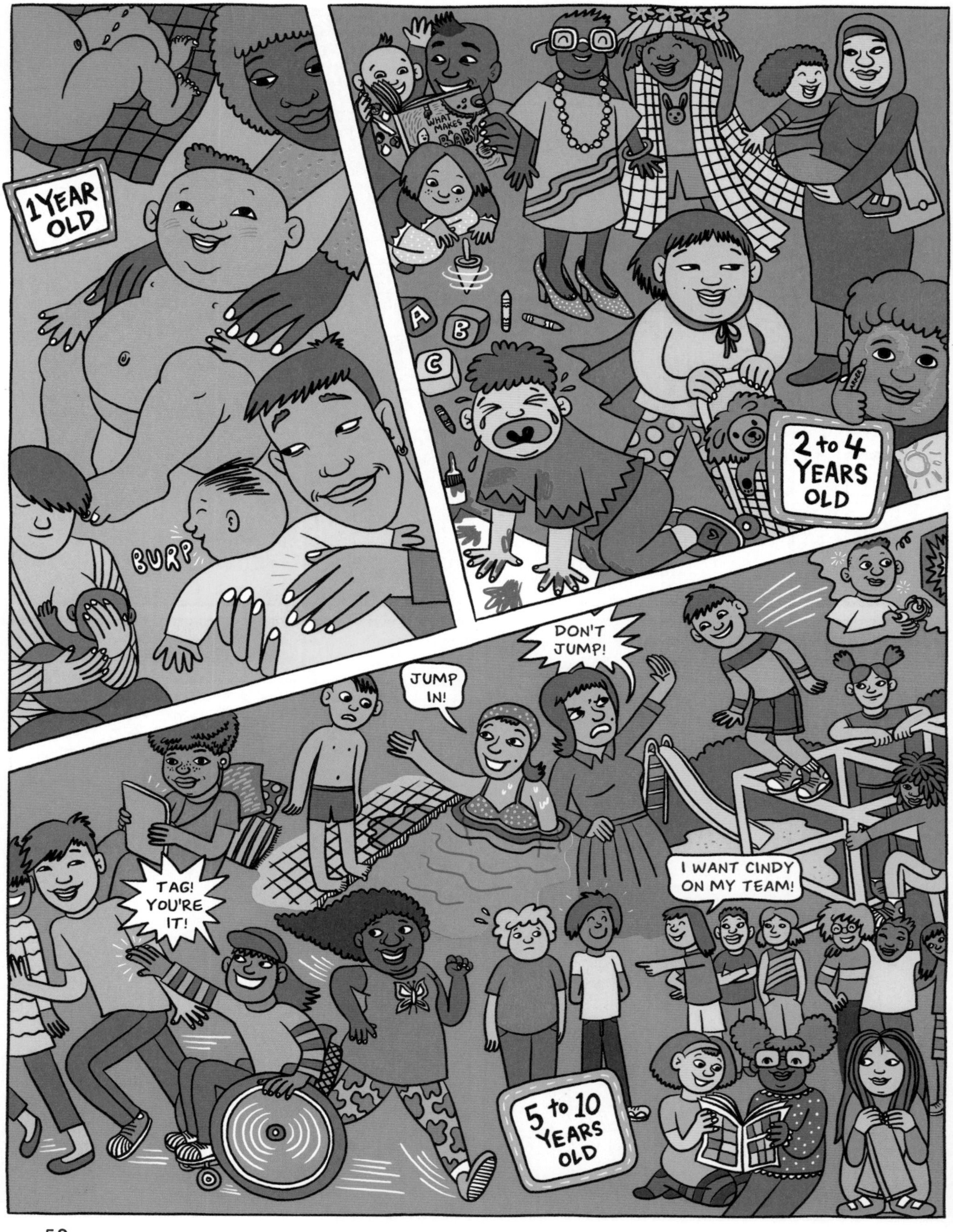
1 YEAR OLD
BURP
2 to 4 YEARS OLD
DON'T JUMP!
JUMP IN!
TAG! YOU'RE IT!
I WANT CINDY ON MY TEAM!
5 to 10 YEARS OLD

THIS ISN'T GOOD OR BAD, IT'S JUST THE WAY IT IS.

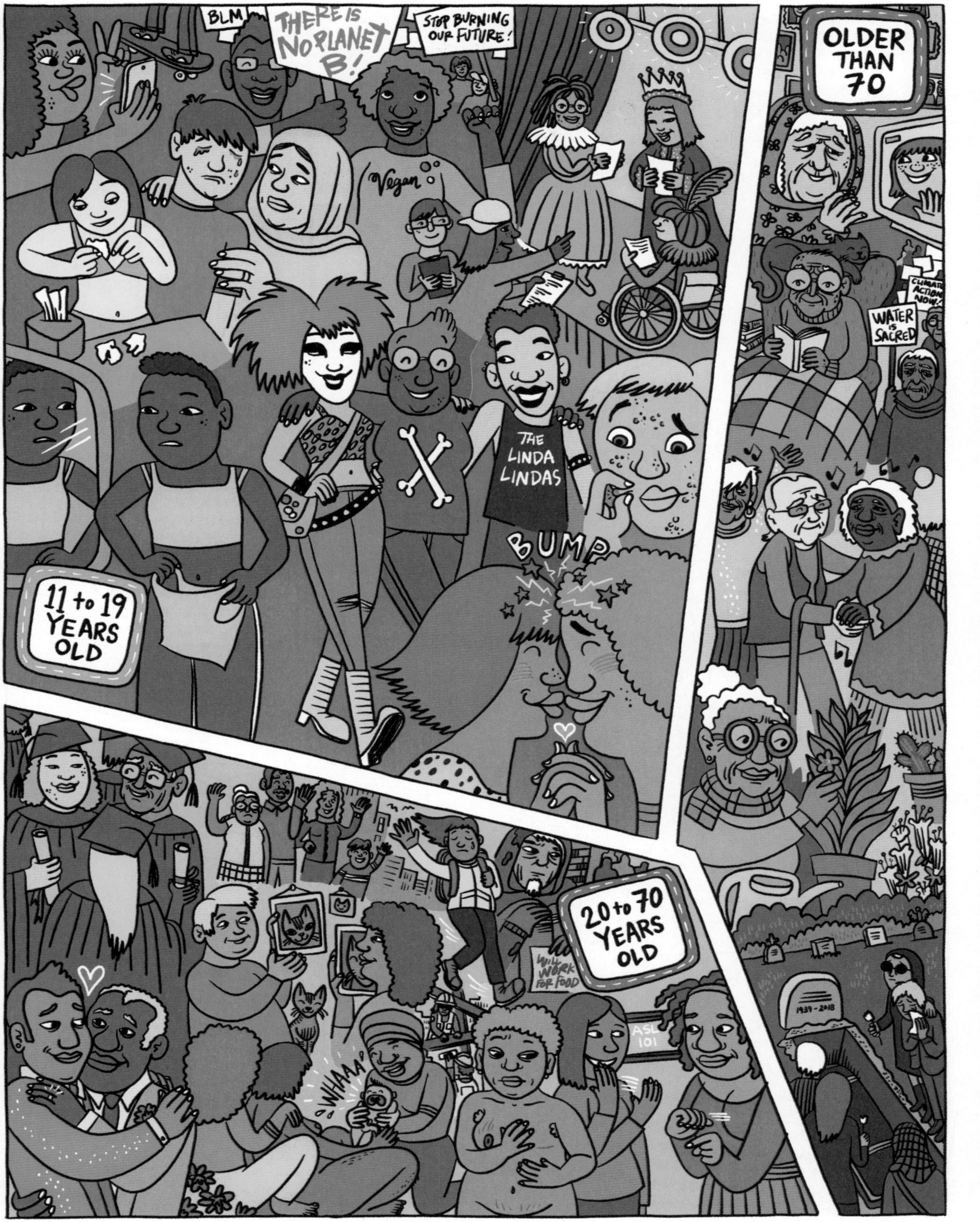
BLM
THERE IS NO PLANET B!
STOP BURNING OUR FUTURE!
Vegan
CLIMATE ACTION NOW!
WATER IS SACRED
OLDER THAN 70
THE LINDA LINDAS
BUMP
11 to 19 YEARS OLD
20 to 70 YEARS OLD
WILL WORK FOR FOOD
ASL 101
WHAAA
1939 - 2018

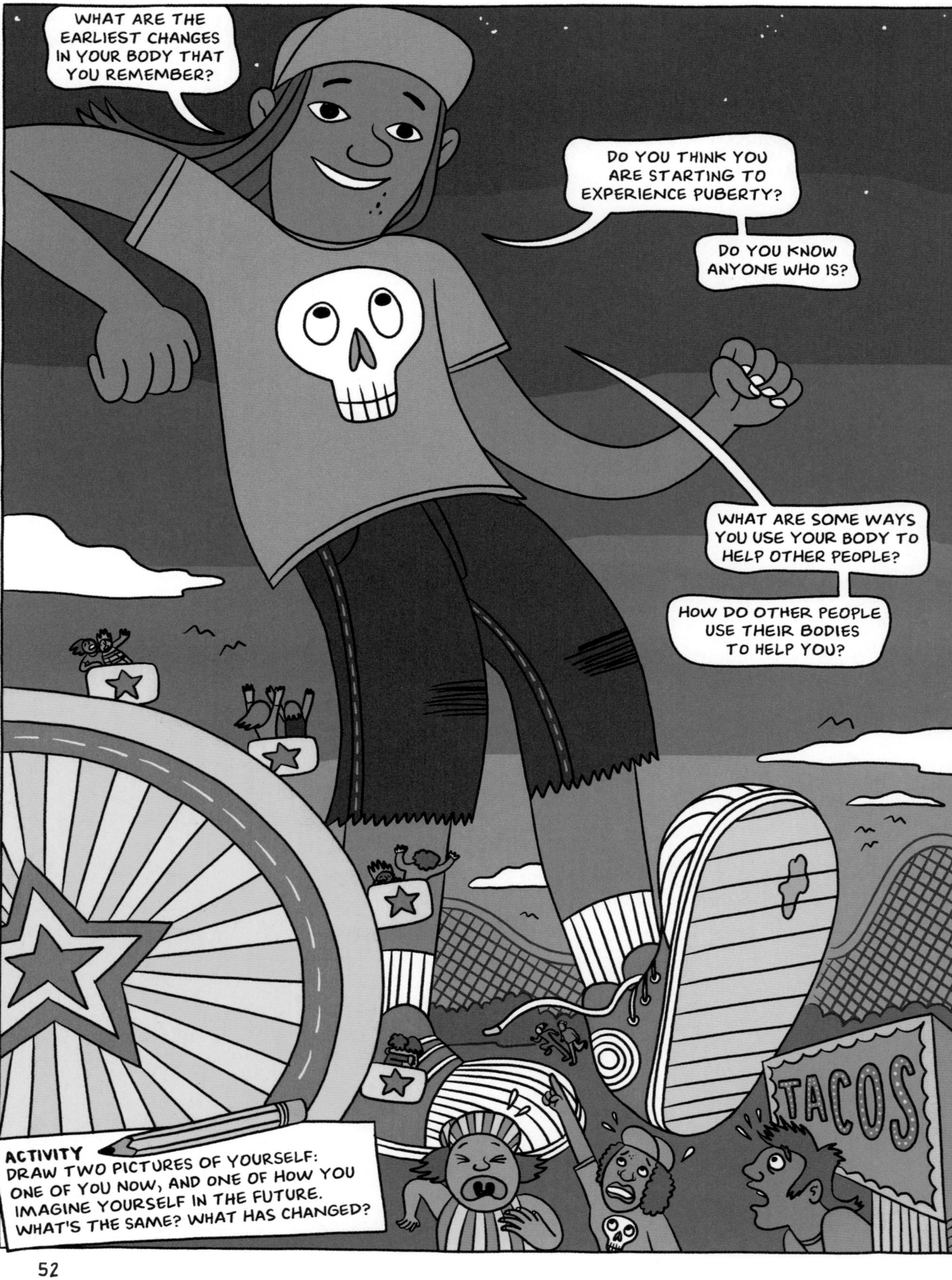
WHAT ARE THE EARLIEST CHANGES IN YOUR BODY THAT YOU REMEMBER?
DO YOU THINK YOU ARE STARTING TO EXPERIENCE PUBERTY?
DO YOU KNOW ANYONE WHO IS?
WHAT ARE SOME WAYS YOU USE YOUR BODY TO HELP OTHER PEOPLE?
HOW DO OTHER PEOPLE USE THEIR BODIES TO HELP YOU?
TACOS
ACTIVITY
DRAW TWO PICTURES OF YOURSELF: ONE OF YOU NOW, AND ONE OF HOW YOU IMAGINE YOURSELF IN THE FUTURE. WHAT'S THE SAME? WHAT HAS CHANGED?

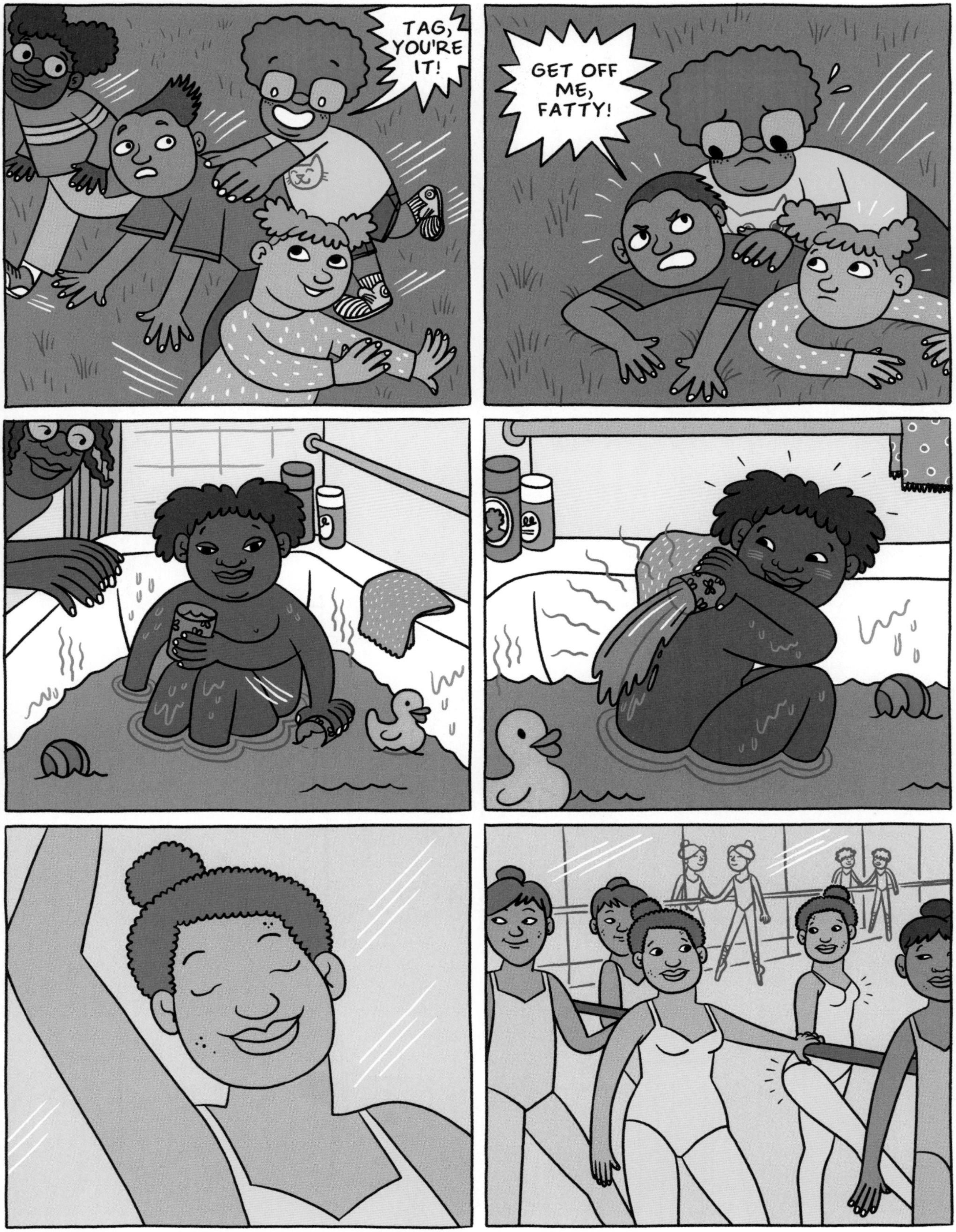
TAG, YOU'RE IT!
GET OFF ME, FATTY!

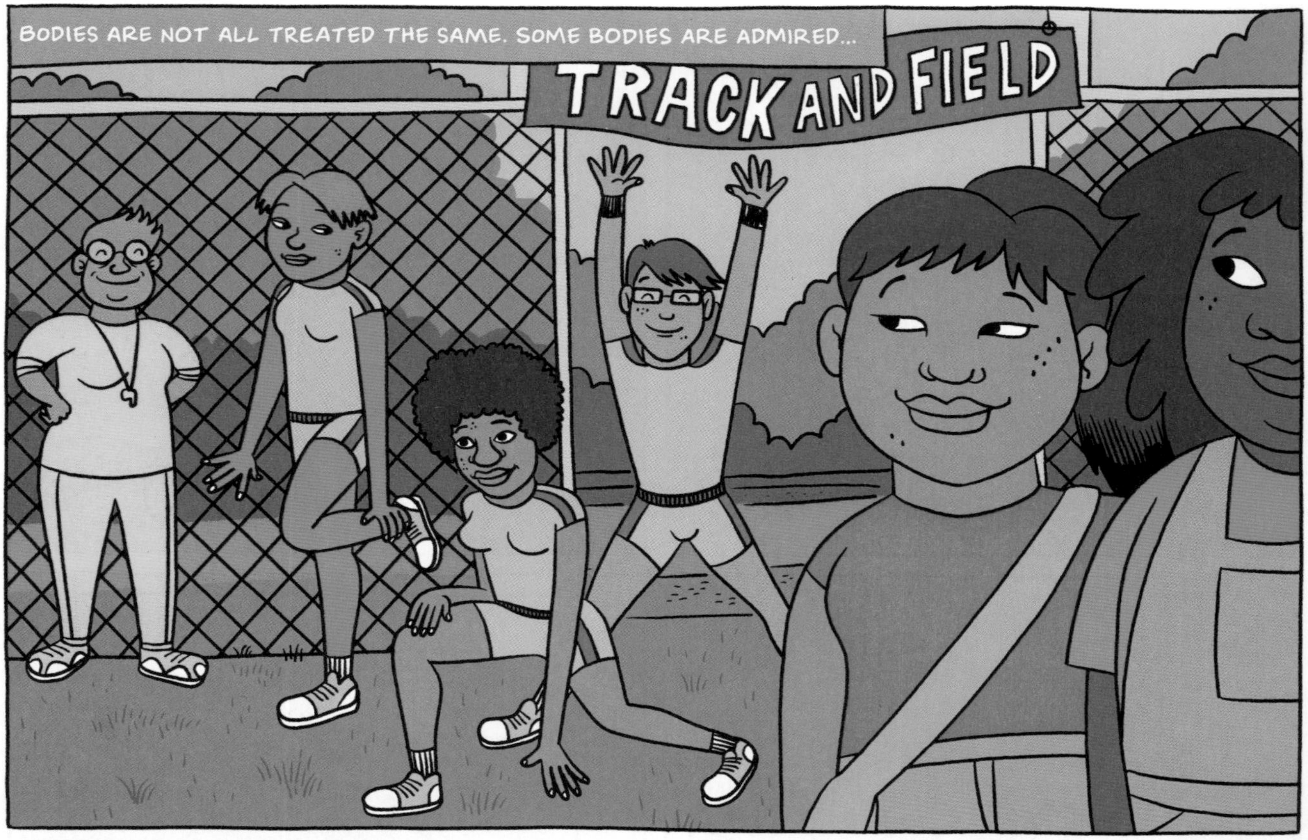
BODIES ARE NOT ALL TREATED THE SAME. SOME BODIES ARE ADMIRED...
TRACK AND FIELD

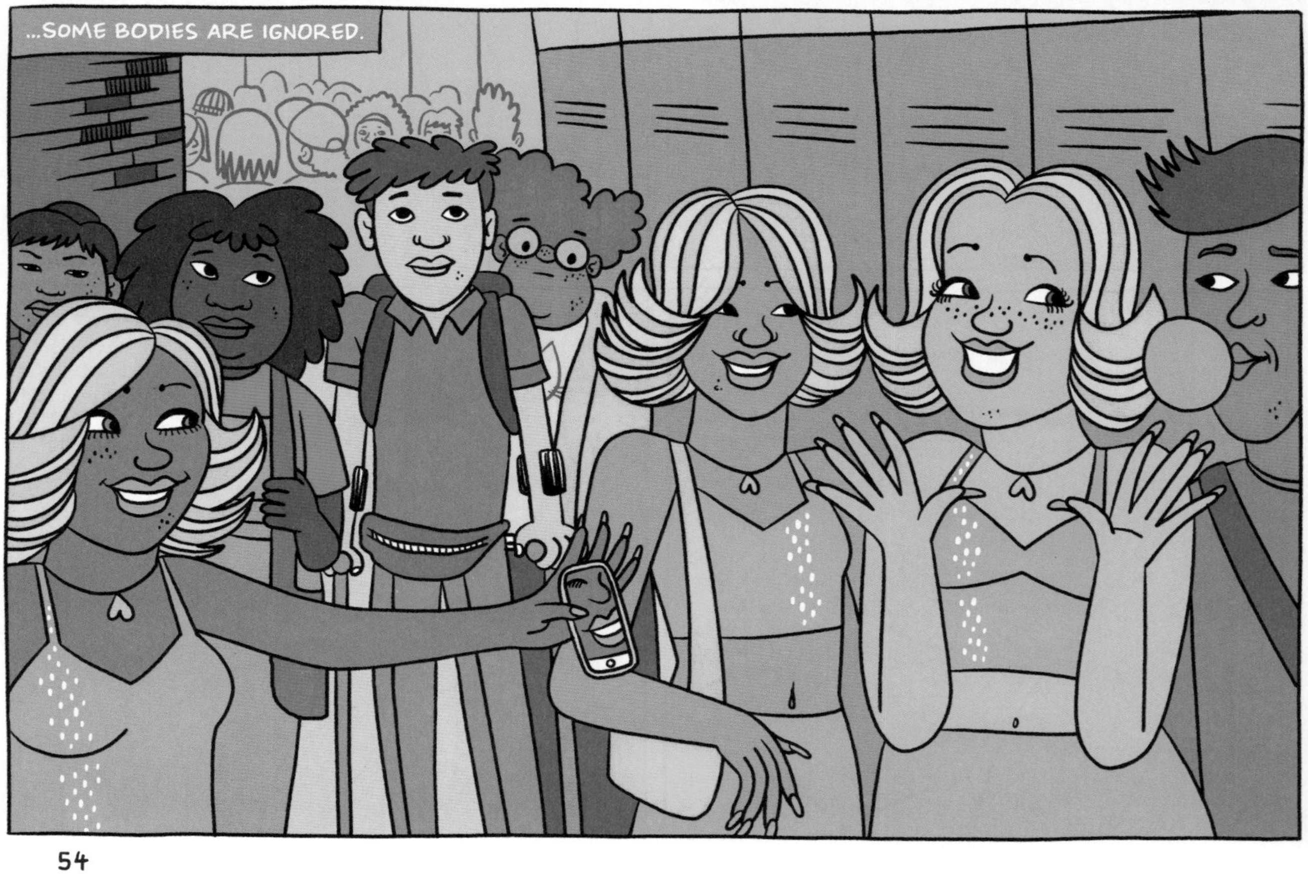
...SOME BODIES ARE IGNORED.

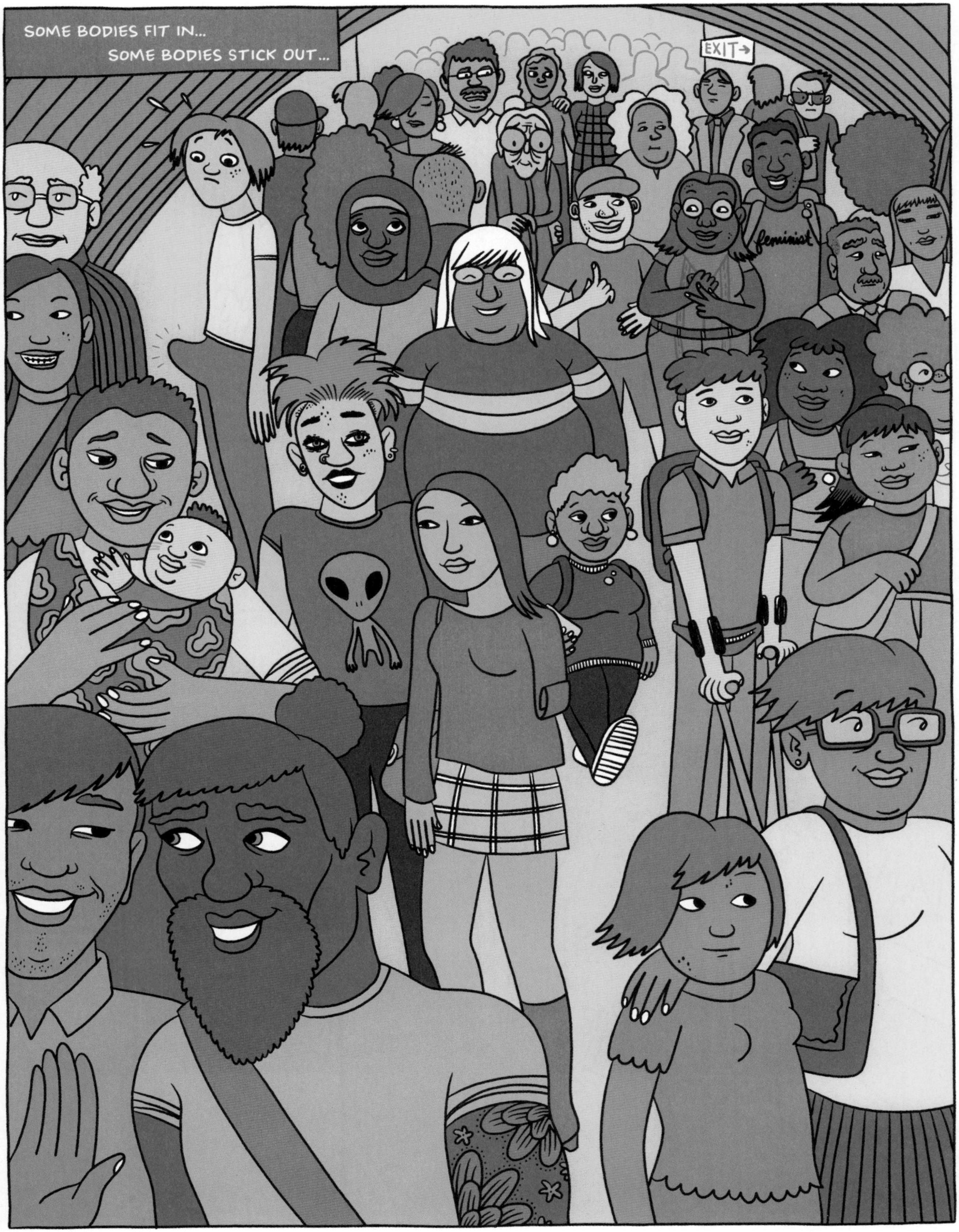
SOME BODIES FIT IN...
SOME BODIES STICK OUT...
EXIT
feminist

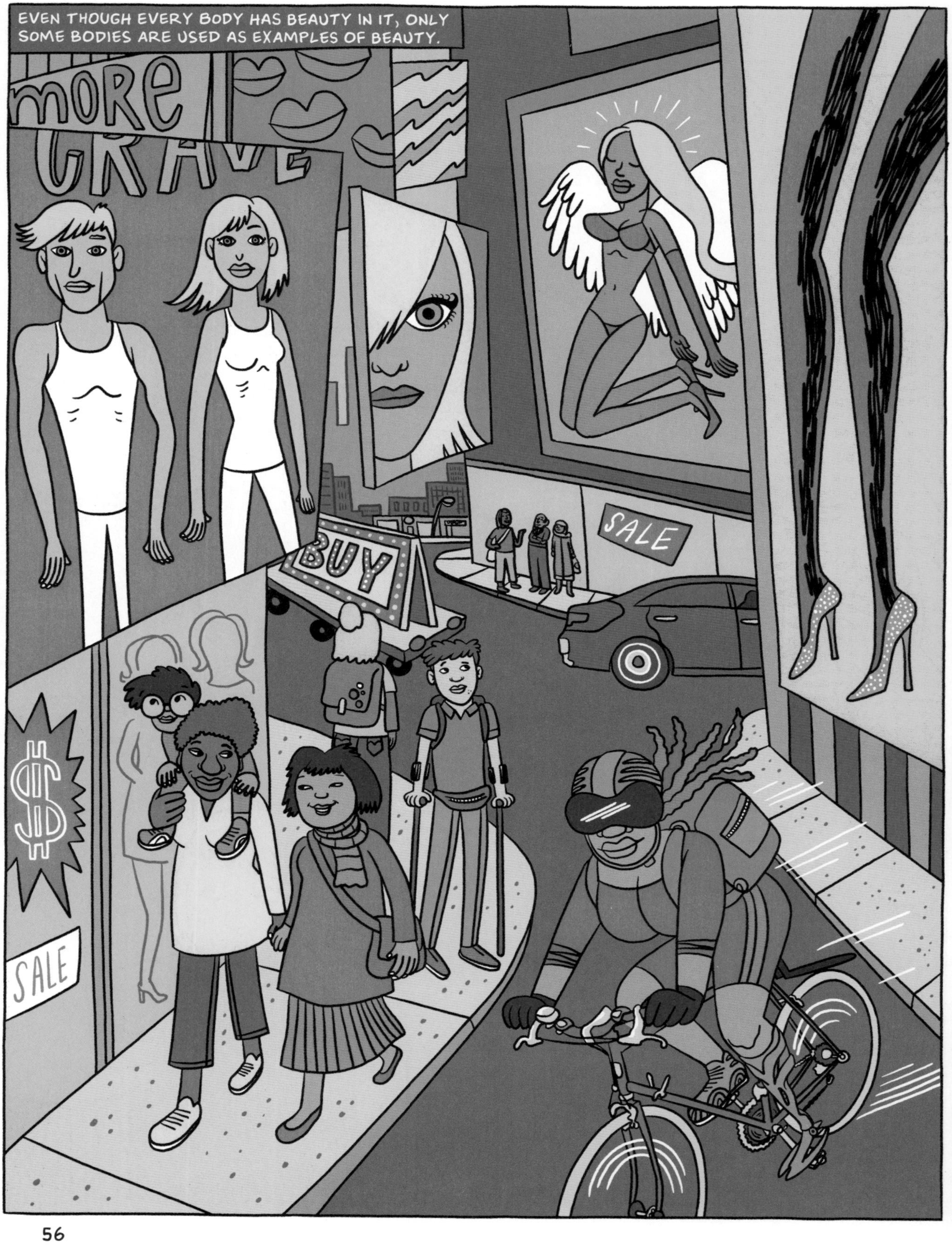
EVEN THOUGH EVERY BODY HAS BEAUTY IN IT, ONLY SOME BODIES ARE USED AS EXAMPLES OF BEAUTY.
more
CRAVE
BUY
SALE
SALE

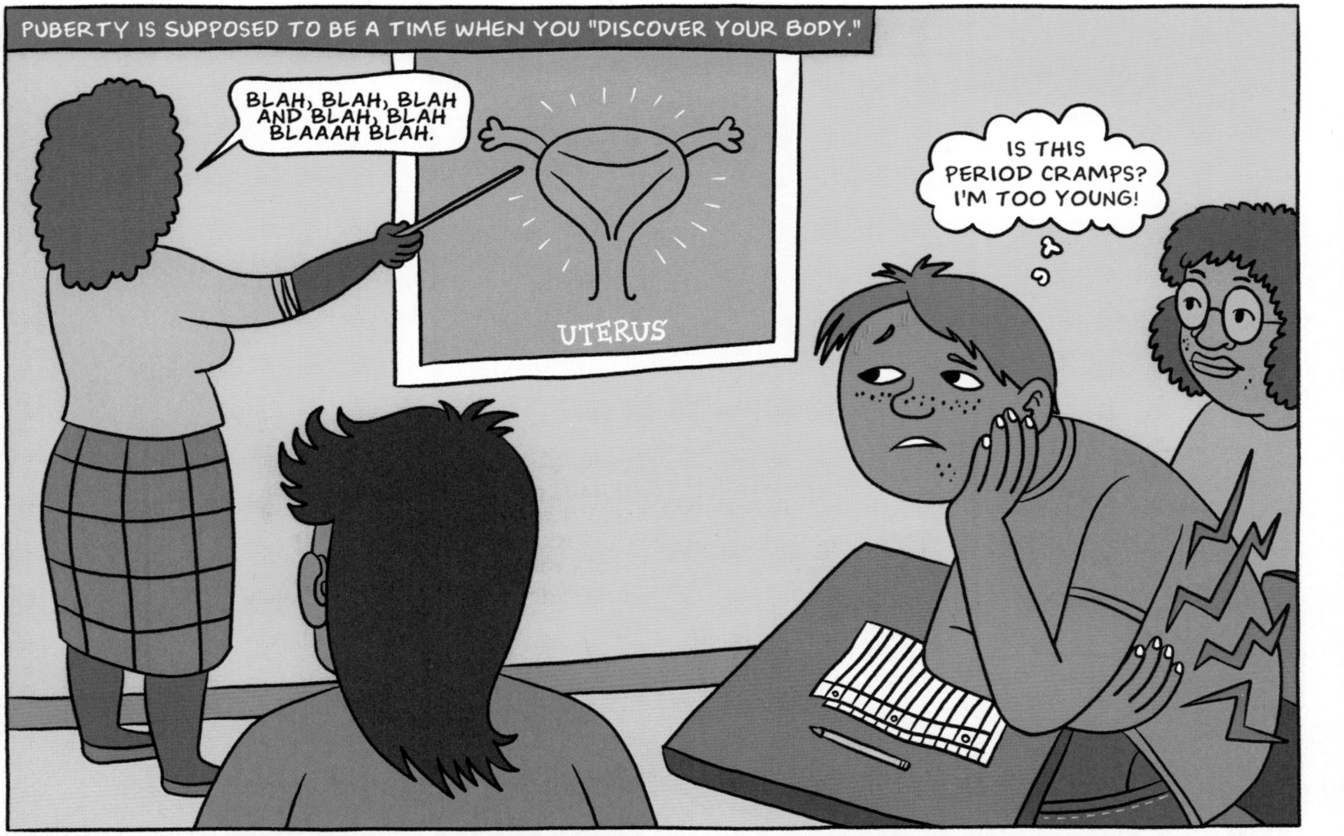
PUBERTY IS SUPPOSED TO BE A TIME WHEN YOU "DISCOVER YOUR BODY."
BLAH, BLAH, BLAH AND BLAH, BLAH BLAAAH BLAH.
UTERUS
IS THIS PERIOD CRAMPS? I'M TOO YOUNG!

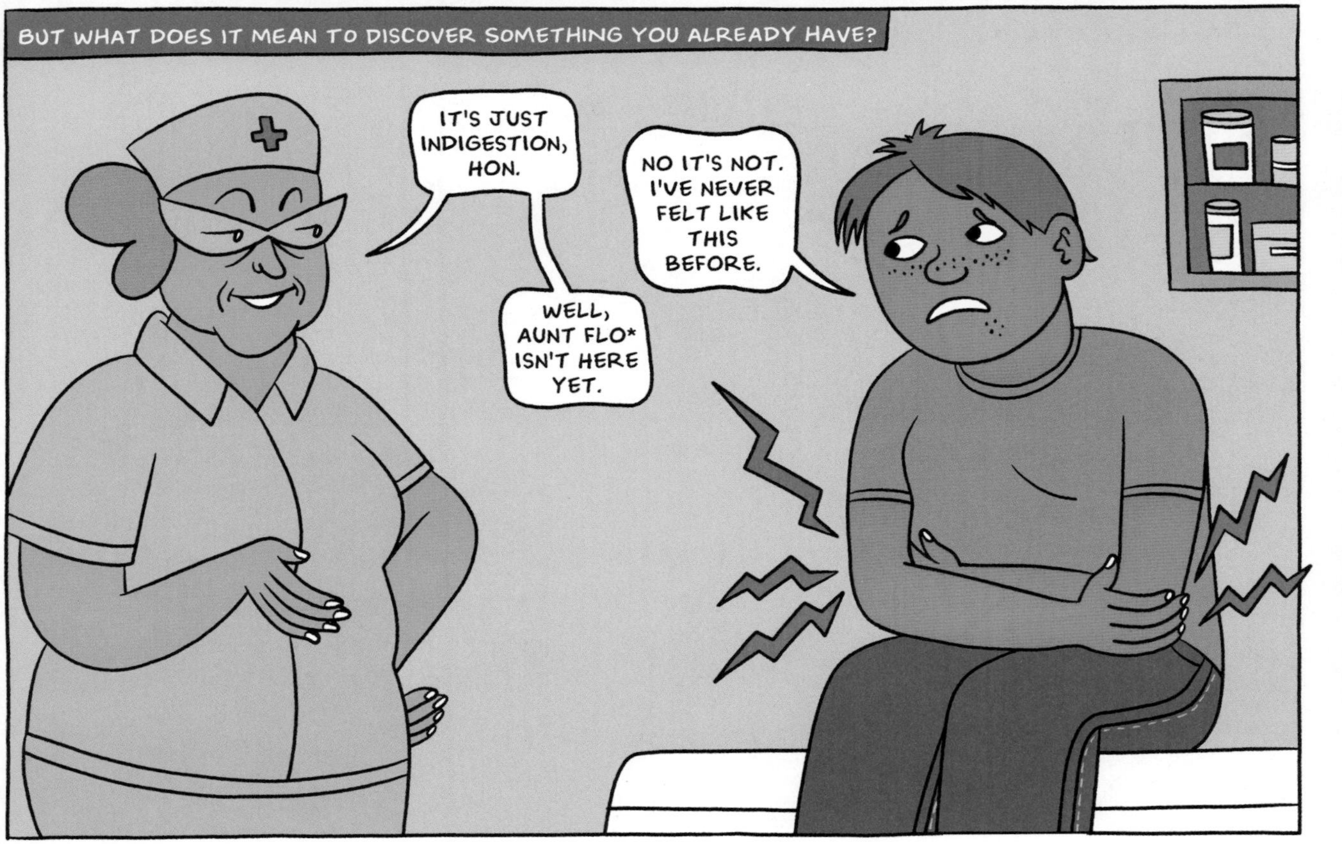
BUT WHAT DOES IT MEAN TO DISCOVER SOMETHING YOU ALREADY HAVE?
IT'S JUST INDIGESTION, HON.
NO IT'S NOT. I'VE NEVER FELT LIKE THIS BEFORE.
WELL, AUNT FLO* ISN'T HERE YET.

* MORE ABOUT CRAMPS AND AUNT FLO ON P. 172

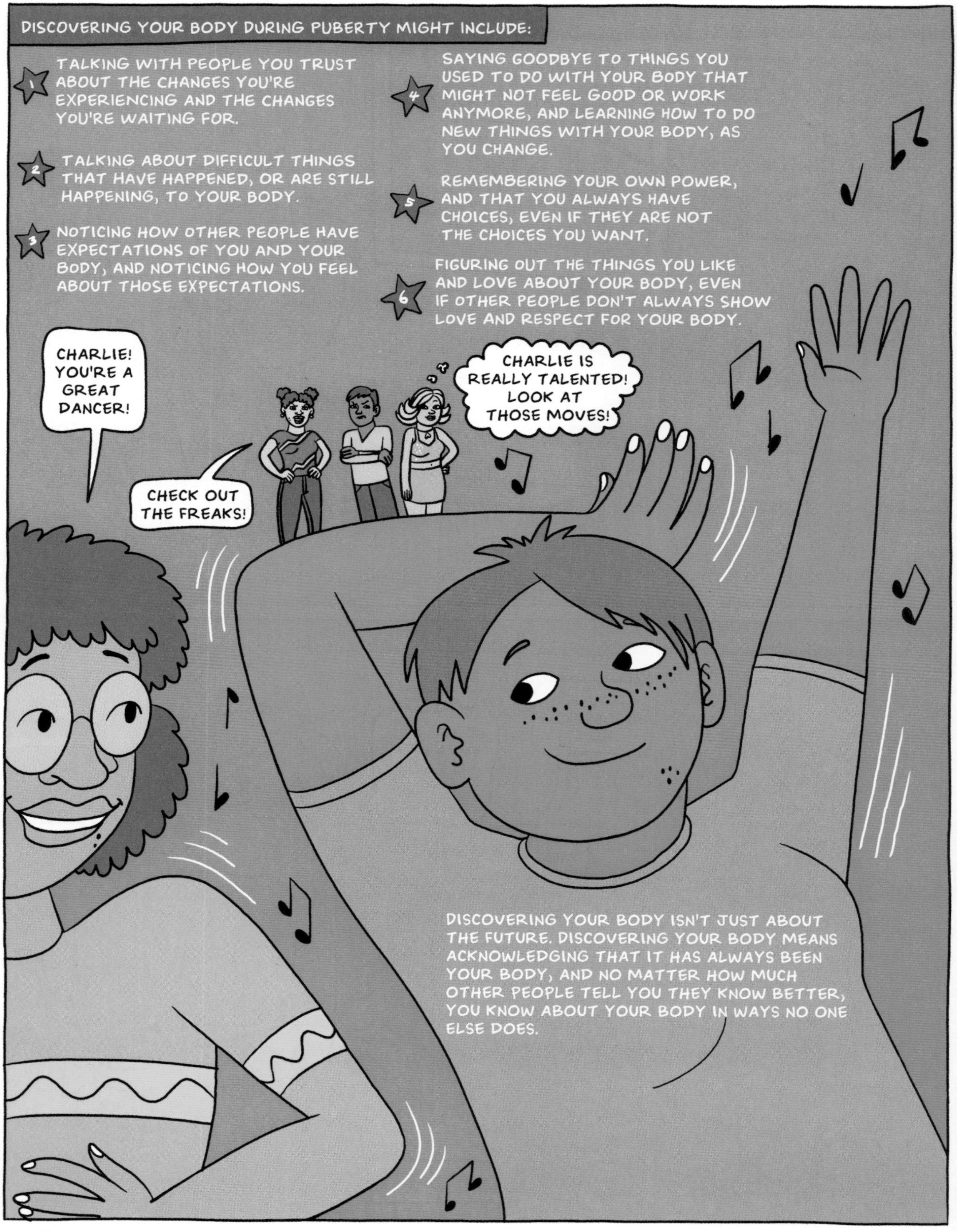
DISCOVERING YOUR BODY DURING PUBERTY MIGHT INCLUDE:
1 TALKING WITH PEOPLE YOU TRUST ABOUT THE CHANGES YOU'RE EXPERIENCING AND THE CHANGES YOU'RE WAITING FOR.
2 TALKING ABOUT DIFFICULT THINGS THAT HAVE HAPPENED, OR ARE STILL HAPPENING, TO YOUR BODY.
3 NOTICING HOW OTHER PEOPLE HAVE EXPECTATIONS OF YOU AND YOUR BODY, AND NOTICING HOW YOU FEEL ABOUT THOSE EXPECTATIONS.
4 SAYING GOODBYE TO THINGS YOU USED TO DO WITH YOUR BODY THAT MIGHT NOT FEEL GOOD OR WORK ANYMORE, AND LEARNING HOW TO DO NEW THINGS WITH YOUR BODY, AS YOU CHANGE.
5 REMEMBERING YOUR OWN POWER, AND THAT YOU ALWAYS HAVE CHOICES, EVEN IF THEY ARE NOT THE CHOICES YOU WANT.
6 FIGURING OUT THE THINGS YOU LIKE AND LOVE ABOUT YOUR BODY, EVEN IF OTHER PEOPLE DON'T ALWAYS SHOW LOVE AND RESPECT FOR YOUR BODY.
CHARLIE! YOU'RE A GREAT DANCER!
CHECK OUT THE FREAKS!
CHARLIE IS REALLY TALENTED! LOOK AT THOSE MOVES!
DISCOVERING YOUR BODY ISN'T JUST ABOUT THE FUTURE. DISCOVERING YOUR BODY MEANS ACKNOWLEDGING THAT IT HAS ALWAYS BEEN YOUR BODY, AND NO MATTER HOW MUCH OTHER PEOPLE TELL YOU THEY KNOW BETTER, YOU KNOW ABOUT YOUR BODY IN WAYS NO ONE ELSE DOES.

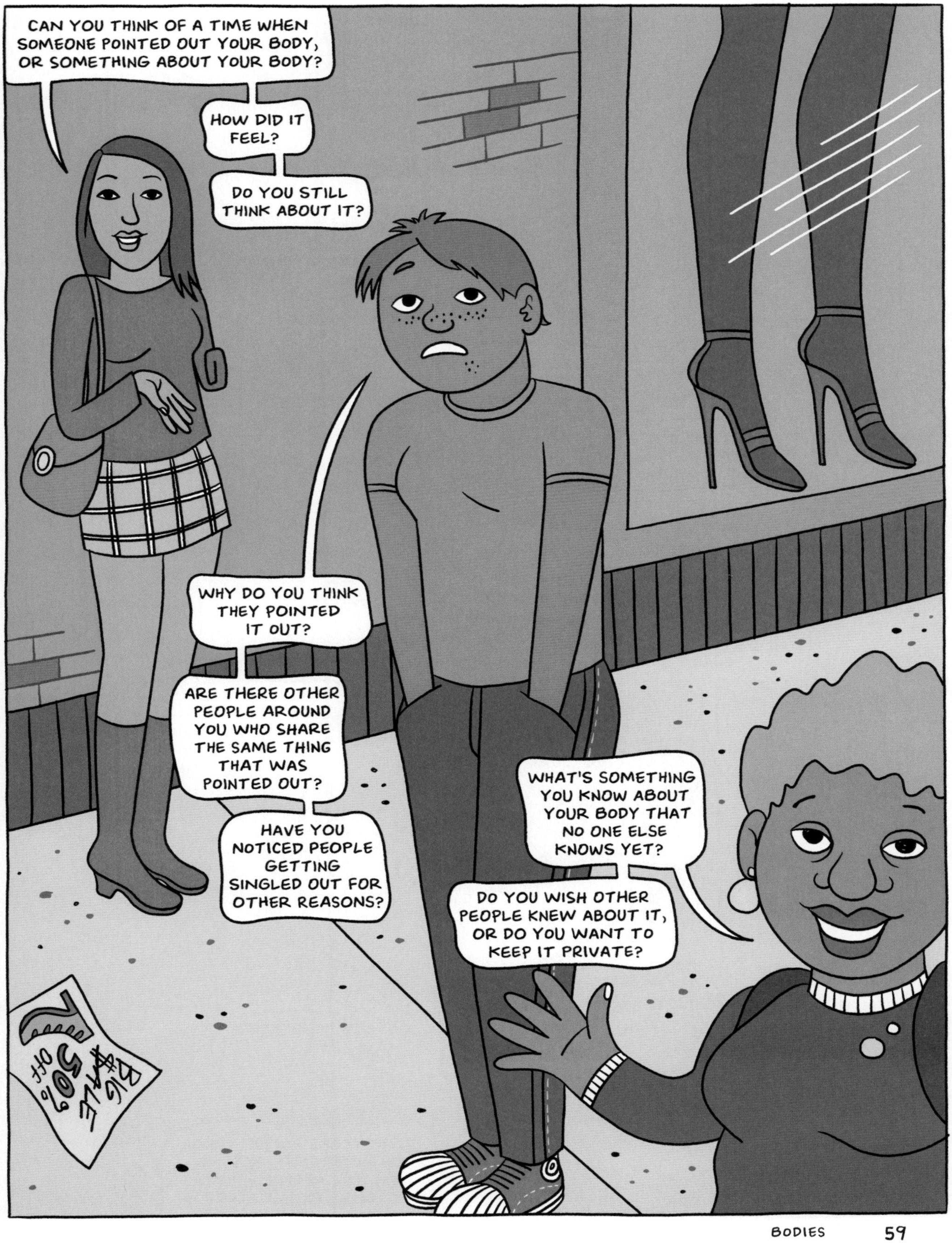
CAN YOU THINK OF A TIME WHEN SOMEONE POINTED OUT YOUR BODY, OR SOMETHING ABOUT YOUR BODY?
HOW DID IT FEEL?
DO YOU STILL THINK ABOUT IT?
WHY DO YOU THINK THEY POINTED IT OUT?
ARE THERE OTHER PEOPLE AROUND YOU WHO SHARE THE SAME THING THAT WAS POINTED OUT?
HAVE YOU NOTICED PEOPLE GETTING SINGLED OUT FOR OTHER REASONS?
WHAT'S SOMETHING YOU KNOW ABOUT YOUR BODY THAT NO ONE ELSE KNOWS YET?
DO YOU WISH OTHER PEOPLE KNEW ABOUT IT, OR DO YOU WANT TO KEEP IT PRIVATE?
BIG SALE 50% OFF

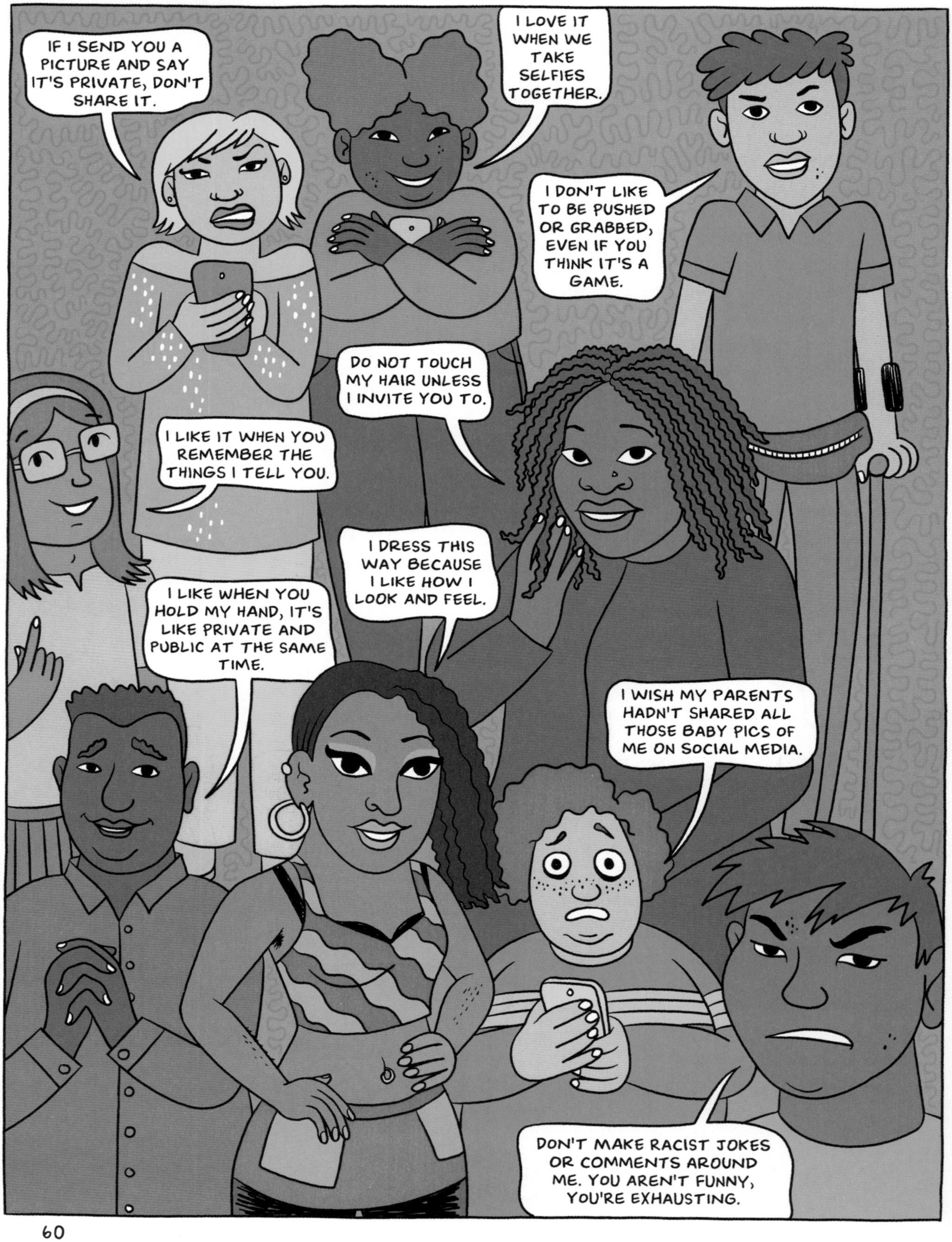
IF I SEND YOU A PICTURE AND SAY IT'S PRIVATE, DON'T SHARE IT.
I LOVE IT WHEN WE TAKE SELFIES TOGETHER.
I DON'T LIKE TO BE PUSHED OR GRABBED, EVEN IF YOU THINK IT'S A GAME.
DO NOT TOUCH MY HAIR UNLESS I INVITE YOU TO.
I LIKE IT WHEN YOU REMEMBER THE THINGS I TELL YOU.
I DRESS THIS WAY BECAUSE I LIKE HOW I LOOK AND FEEL.
I LIKE WHEN YOU HOLD MY HAND, IT'S LIKE PRIVATE AND PUBLIC AT THE SAME TIME.
I WISH MY PARENTS HADN'T SHARED ALL THOSE BABY PICS OF ME ON SOCIAL MEDIA.
DON'T MAKE RACIST JOKES OR COMMENTS AROUND ME. YOU AREN'T FUNNY, YOU'RE EXHAUSTING.

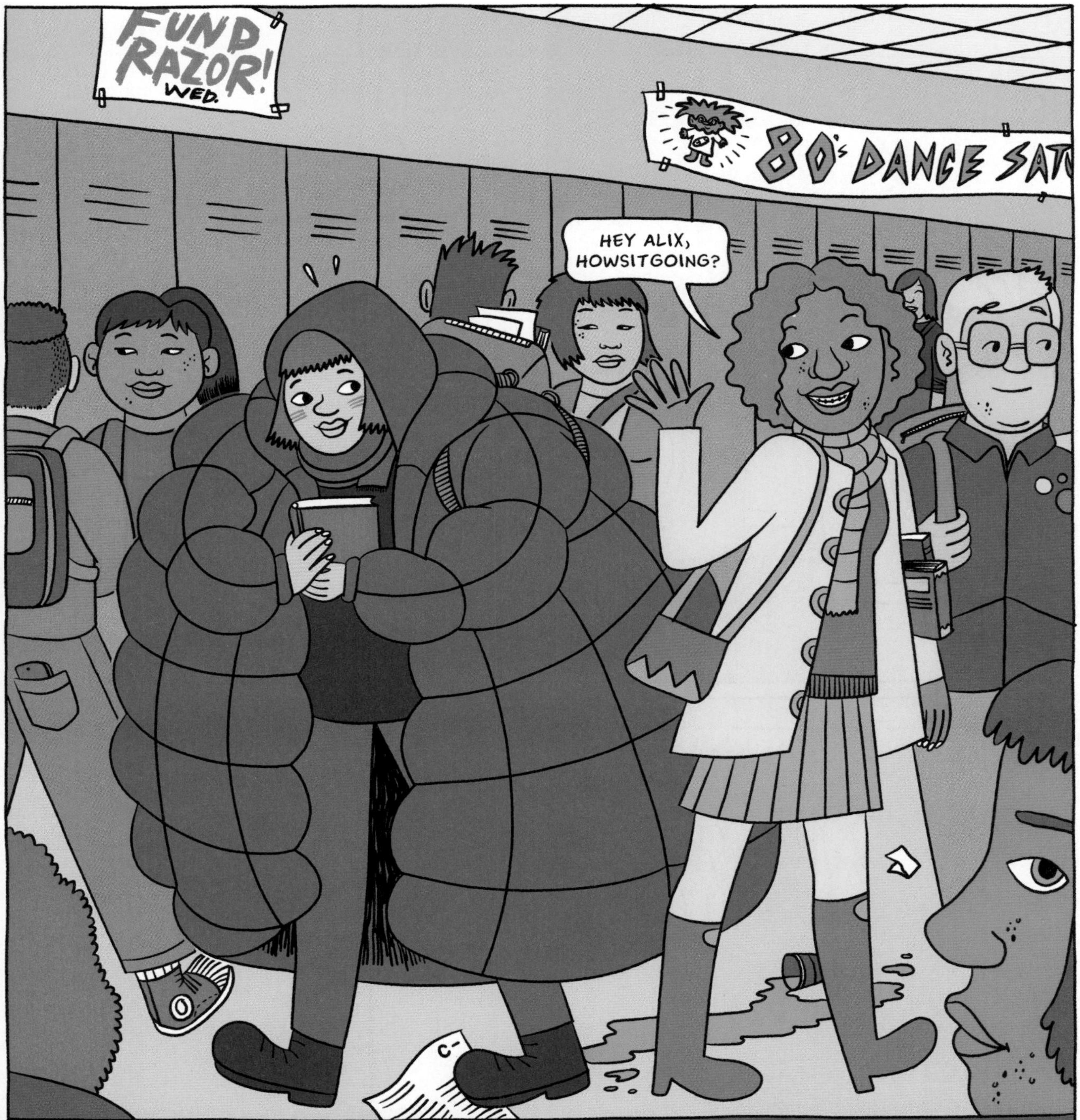
FUND RAZOR! WED.
80's DANCE SAT
HEY ALIX, HOWSITGOING?
C-

OUR BOUNDARIES ARE LIKE RULES WE MAKE FOR OUR BODIES. THEY DESCRIBE HOW WE DO AND DO NOT WANT PEOPLE TO TREAT US.

WE MAKE BOUNDARIES ABOUT THINGS LIKE WHEN, WHERE, AND WITH WHOM WE WANT TO HOLD HANDS, HUG, OR KISS. OR NOT.

WE ALSO MAKE BOUNDARIES ABOUT THE WORDS PEOPLE USE ABOUT US AND AROUND US, LIKE THE KINDS OF JOKES THAT ARE, OR ARE NOT, OKAY.

BOUNDARIES AREN'T RIGHT OR WRONG, AS LONG AS WE'RE THE ONES MAKING THEM. OTHER PEOPLE MAY RESPECT OUR BOUNDARIES OR IGNORE THEM. BUT OUR BOUNDARIES ARE REAL, AND THEY MATTER.

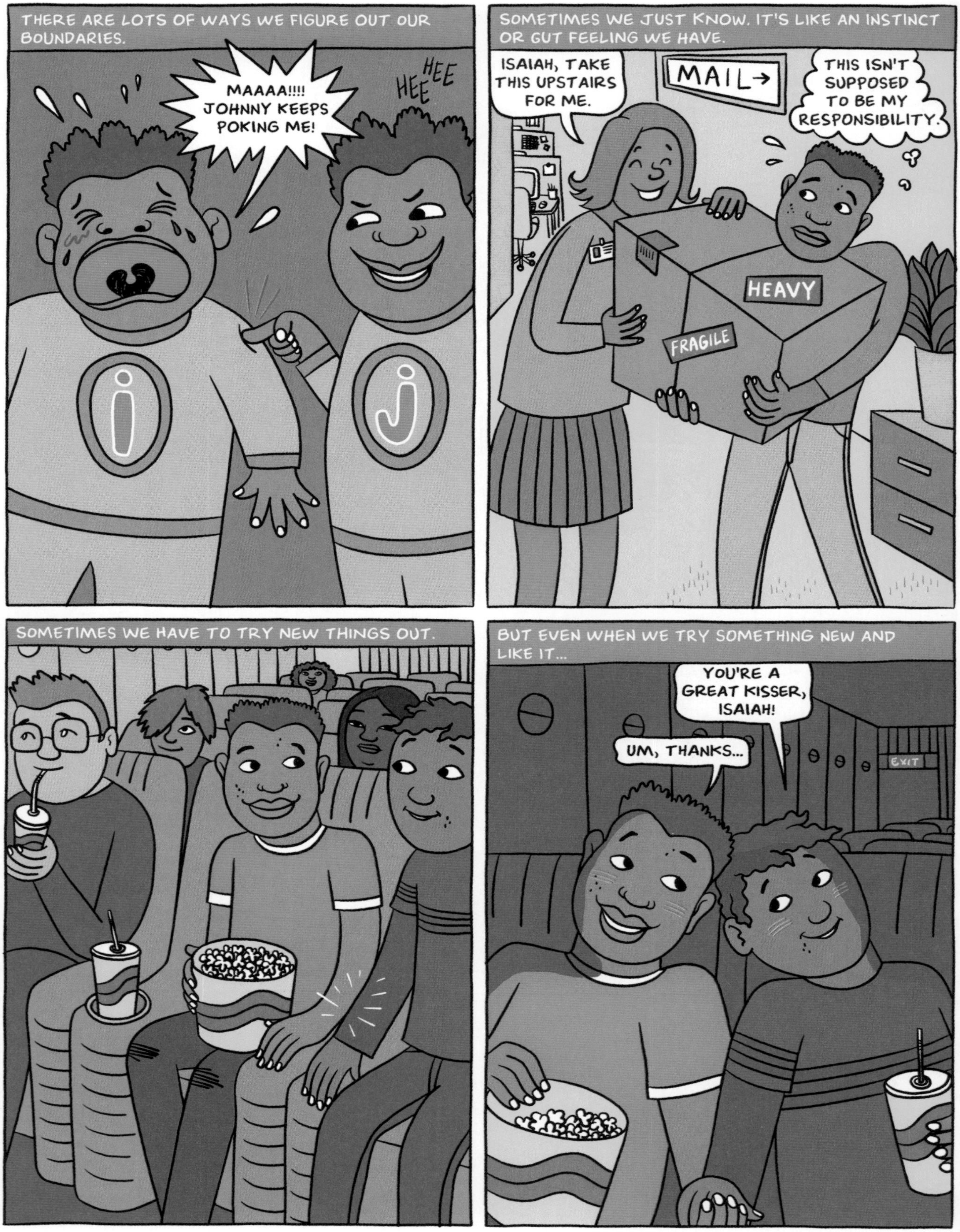
THERE ARE LOTS OF WAYS WE FIGURE OUT OUR BOUNDARIES.
MAAAA!!!! JOHNNY KEEPS POKING ME!
HEE HEE
SOMETIMES WE JUST KNOW. IT'S LIKE AN INSTINCT OR GUT FEELING WE HAVE.
ISAIAH, TAKE THIS UPSTAIRS FOR ME.
MAIL→
THIS ISN'T SUPPOSED TO BE MY RESPONSIBILITY.
HEAVY
FRAGILE
SOMETIMES WE HAVE TO TRY NEW THINGS OUT.
BUT EVEN WHEN WE TRY SOMETHING NEW AND LIKE IT...
YOU'RE A GREAT KISSER, ISAIAH!
UM, THANKS...
EXIT

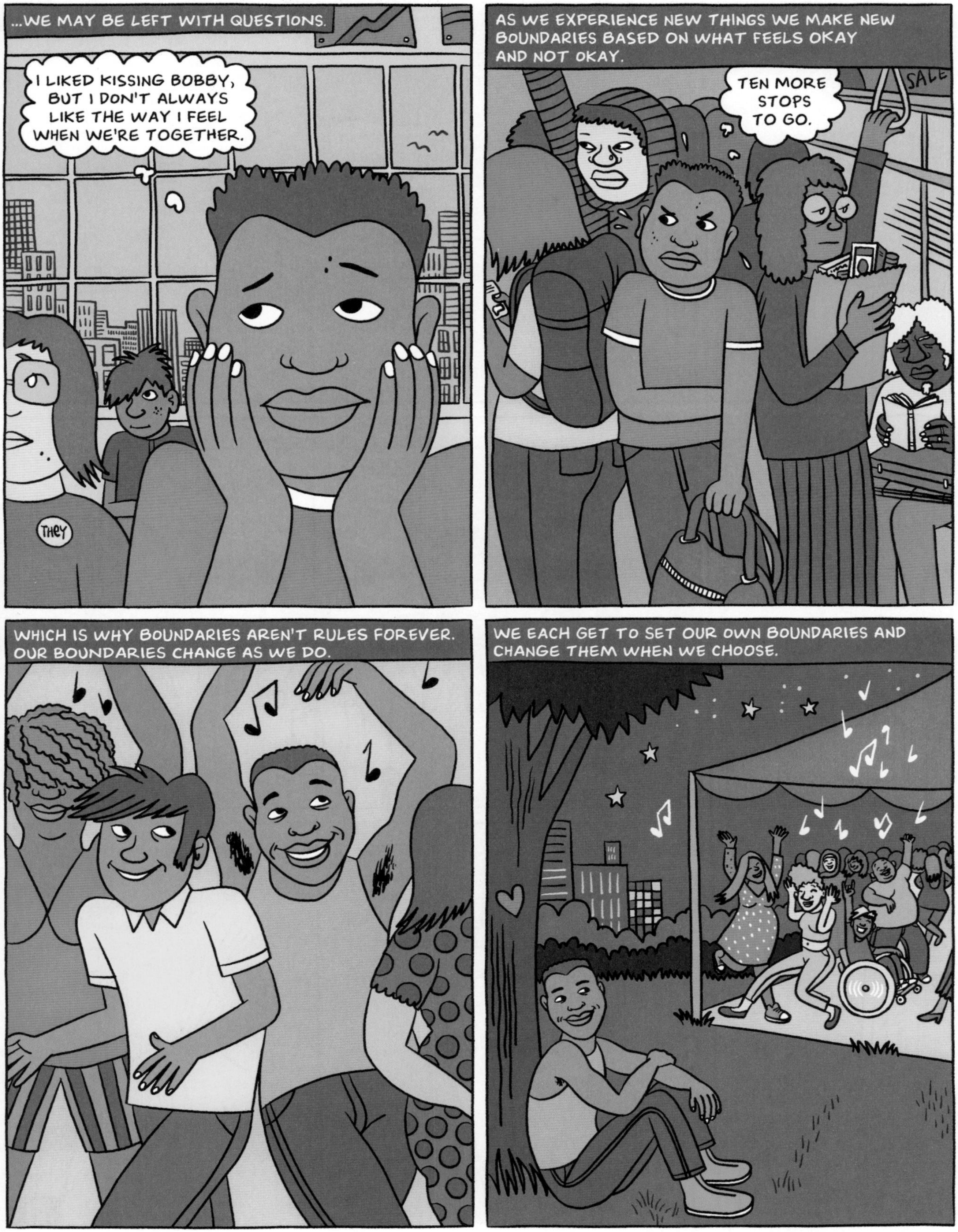
...WE MAY BE LEFT WITH QUESTIONS.
I LIKED KISSING BOBBY, BUT I DON'T ALWAYS LIKE THE WAY I FEEL WHEN WE'RE TOGETHER.
THEY
AS WE EXPERIENCE NEW THINGS WE MAKE NEW BOUNDARIES BASED ON WHAT FEELS OKAY AND NOT OKAY.
TEN MORE STOPS TO GO.
SALE
WHICH IS WHY BOUNDARIES AREN'T RULES FOREVER. OUR BOUNDARIES CHANGE AS WE DO.
WE EACH GET TO SET OUR OWN BOUNDARIES AND CHANGE THEM WHEN WE CHOOSE.

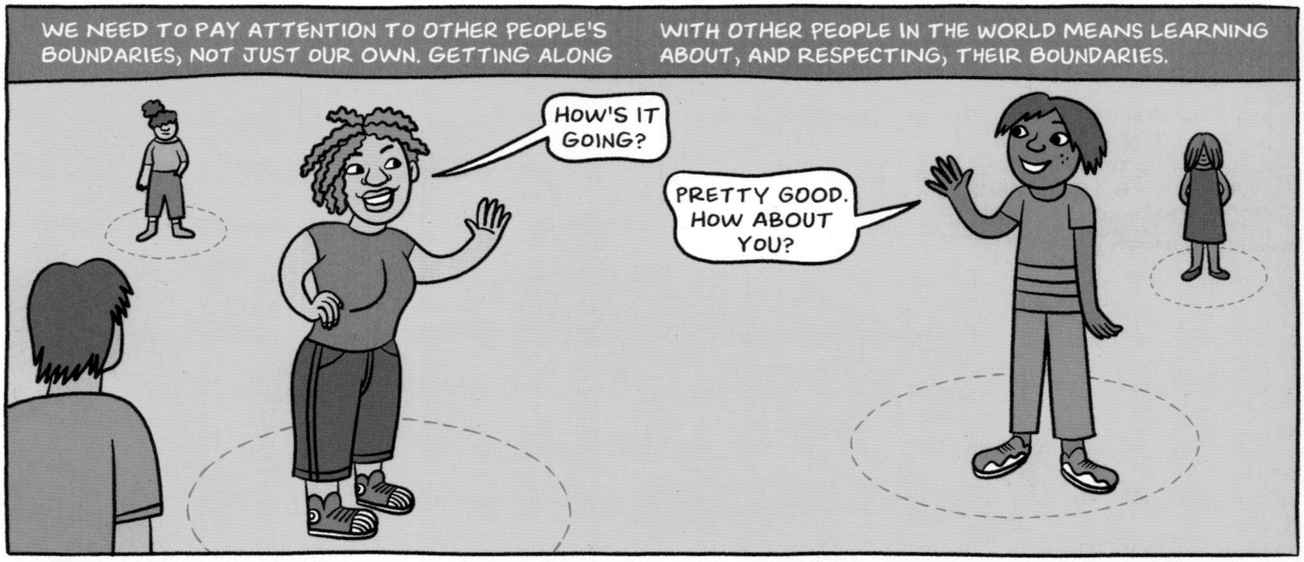

WE NEED TO PAY ATTENTION TO OTHER PEOPLE'S BOUNDARIES, NOT JUST OUR OWN. GETTING ALONG WITH OTHER PEOPLE IN THE WORLD MEANS LEARNING ABOUT, AND RESPECTING, THEIR BOUNDARIES.
HOW'S IT GOING?
PRETTY GOOD. HOW ABOUT YOU?

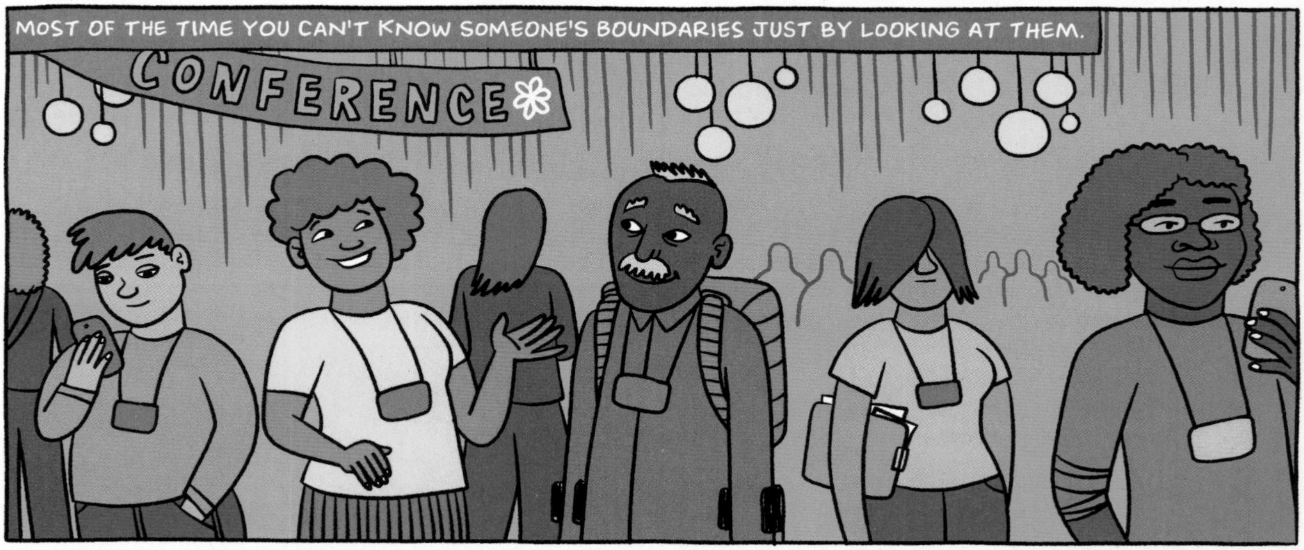

MOST OF THE TIME YOU CAN'T KNOW SOMEONE'S BOUNDARIES JUST BY LOOKING AT THEM.
CONFERENCE

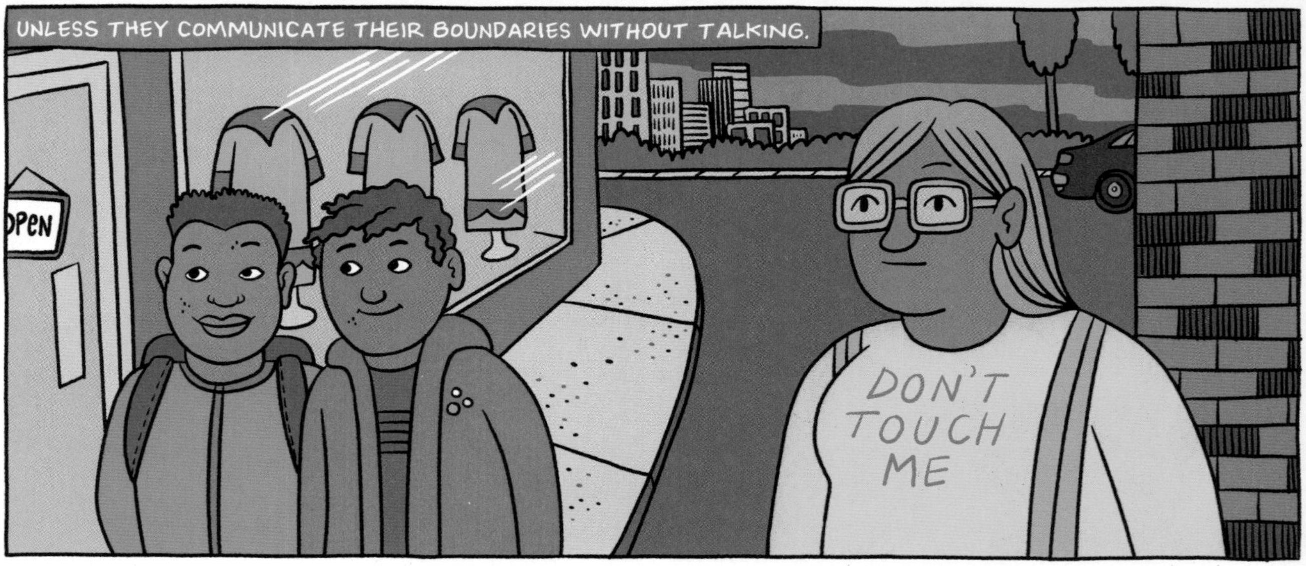

UNLESS THEY COMMUNICATE THEIR BOUNDARIES WITHOUT TALKING.
OPEN
DON'T TOUCH ME

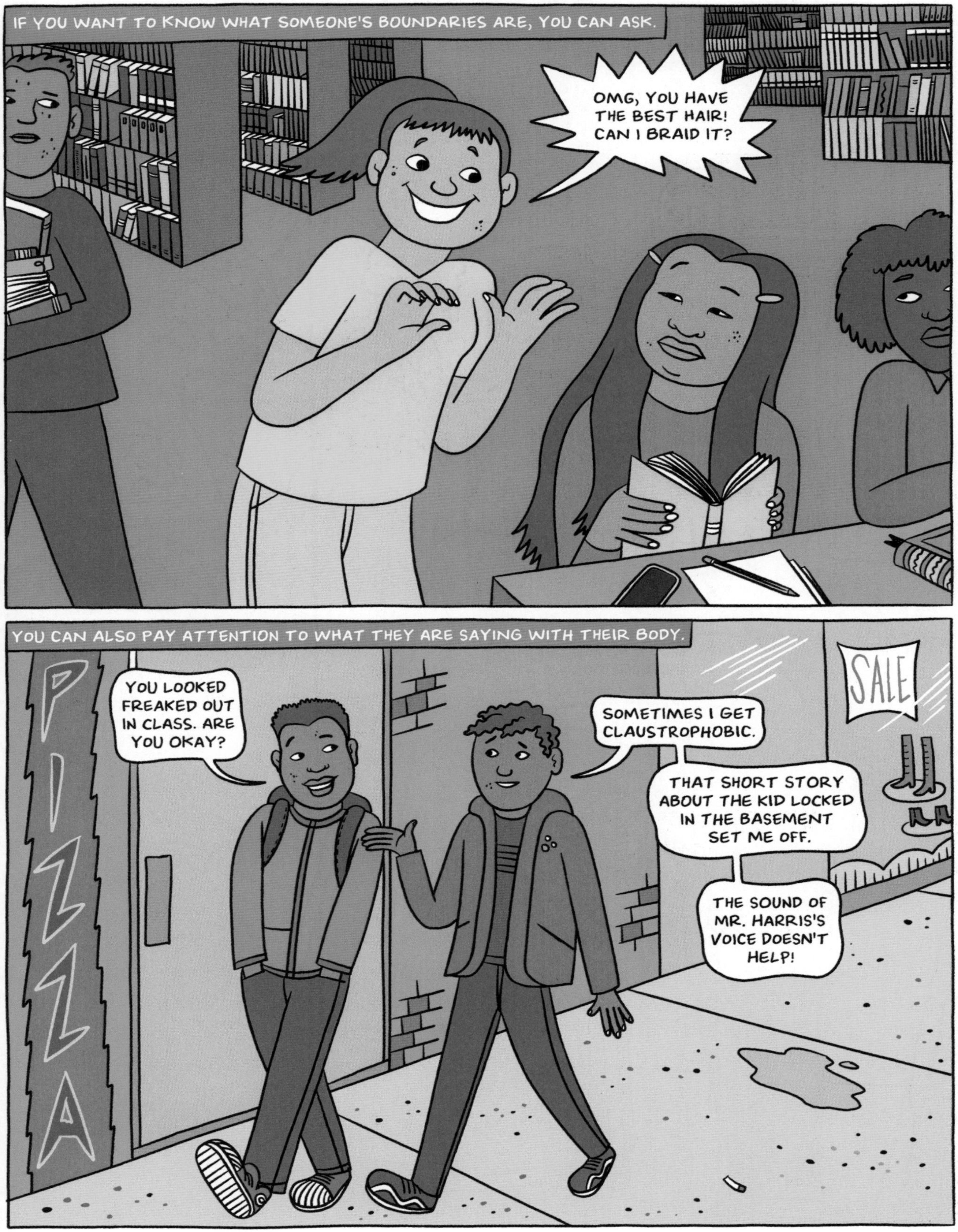
IF YOU WANT TO KNOW WHAT SOMEONE'S BOUNDARIES ARE, YOU CAN ASK.
OMG, YOU HAVE THE BEST HAIR! CAN I BRAID IT?
YOU CAN ALSO PAY ATTENTION TO WHAT THEY ARE SAYING WITH THEIR BODY.
PIZZA
SALE
YOU LOOKED FREAKED OUT IN CLASS. ARE YOU OKAY?
SOMETIMES I GET CLAUSTROPHOBIC.
THAT SHORT STORY ABOUT THE KID LOCKED IN THE BASEMENT SET ME OFF.
THE SOUND OF MR. HARRIS'S VOICE DOESN'T HELP!

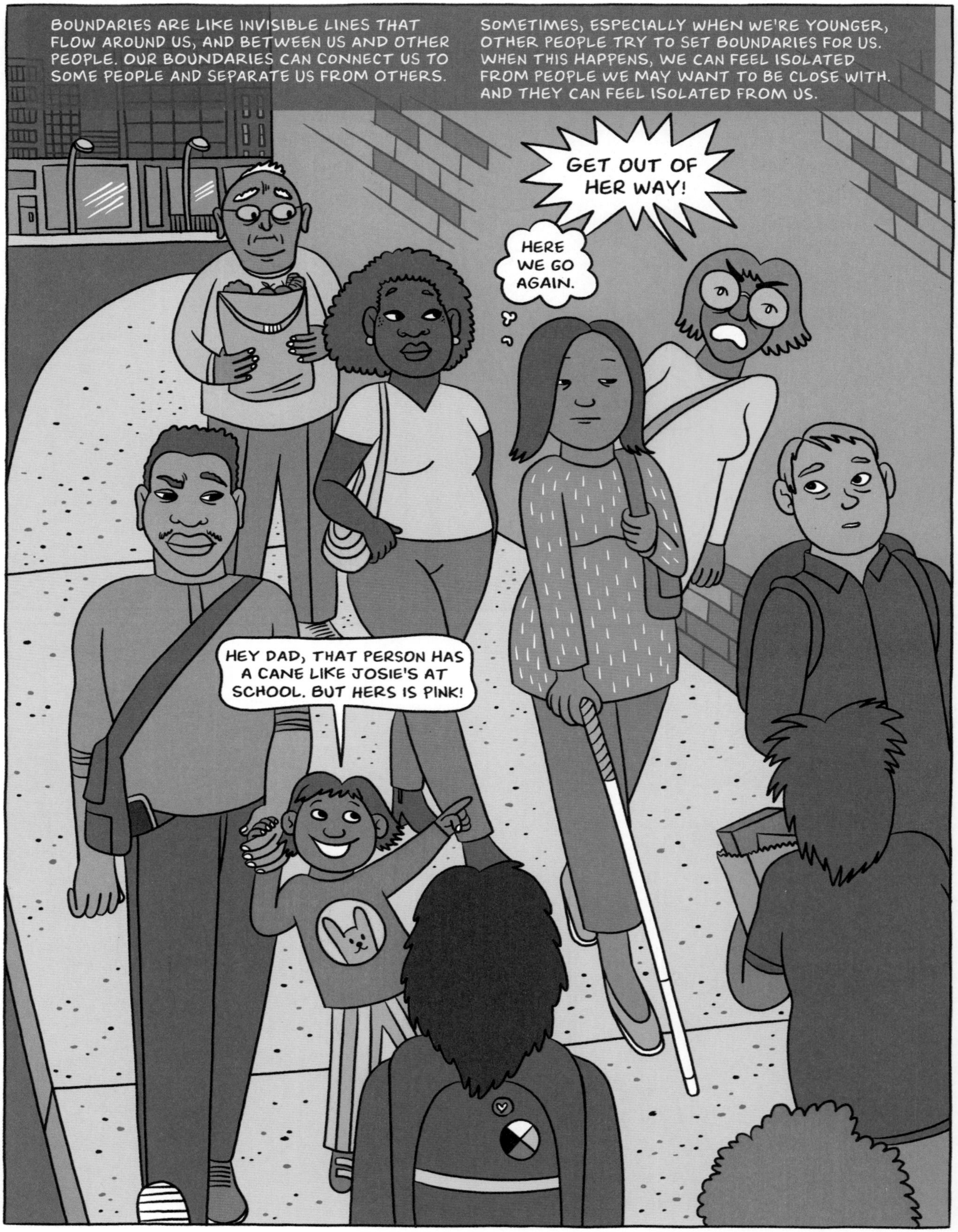
BOUNDARIES ARE LIKE INVISIBLE LINES THAT FLOW AROUND US, AND BETWEEN US AND OTHER PEOPLE. OUR BOUNDARIES CAN CONNECT US TO SOME PEOPLE AND SEPARATE US FROM OTHERS.
SOMETIMES, ESPECIALLY WHEN WE'RE YOUNGER, OTHER PEOPLE TRY TO SET BOUNDARIES FOR US. WHEN THIS HAPPENS, WE CAN FEEL ISOLATED FROM PEOPLE WE MAY WANT TO BE CLOSE WITH. AND THEY CAN FEEL ISOLATED FROM US.
GET OUT OF HER WAY!
HERE WE GO AGAIN.
HEY DAD, THAT PERSON HAS A CANE LIKE JOSIE'S AT SCHOOL. BUT HERS IS PINK!

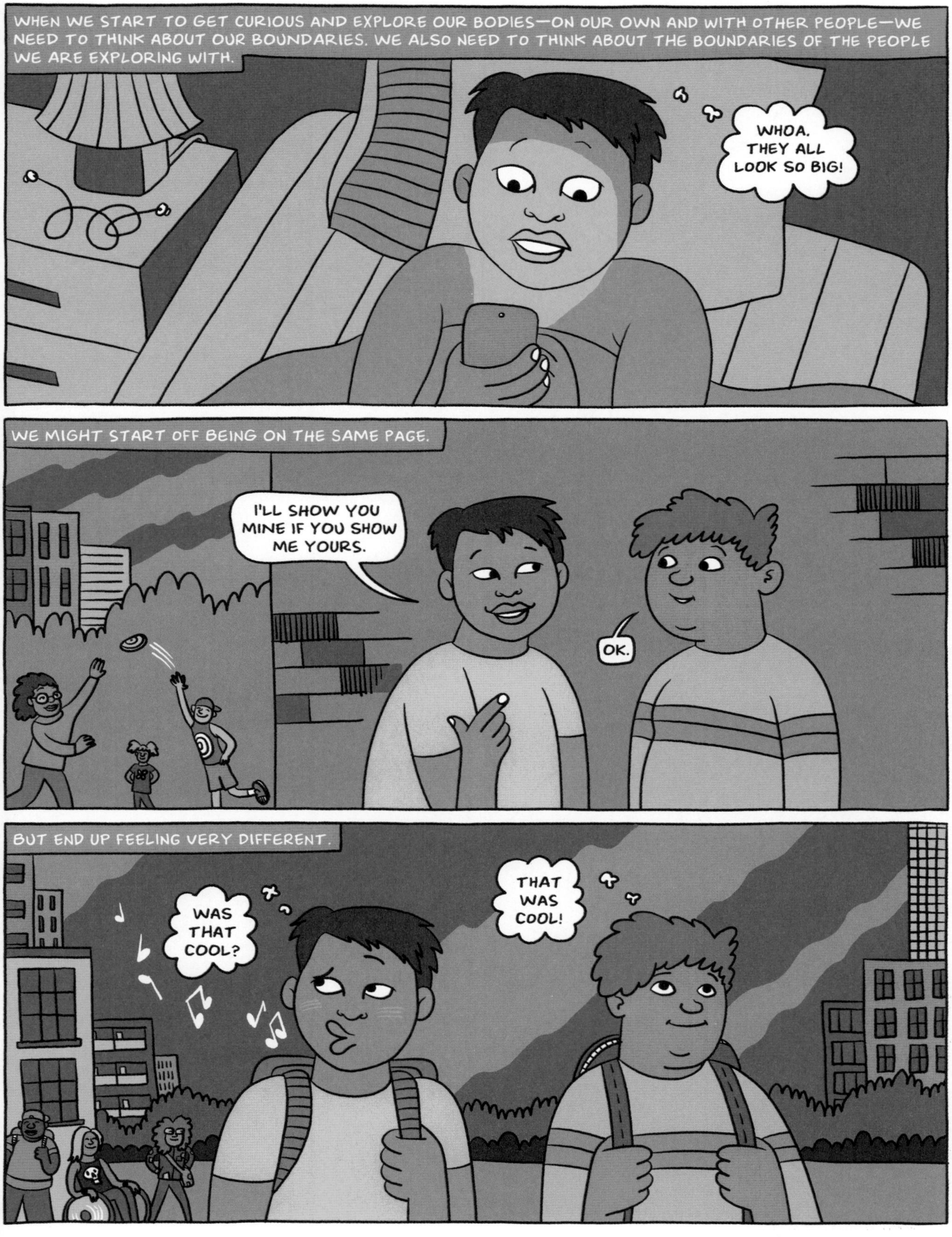
WHEN WE START TO GET CURIOUS AND EXPLORE OUR BODIES—ON OUR OWN AND WITH OTHER PEOPLE—WE NEED TO THINK ABOUT OUR BOUNDARIES. WE ALSO NEED TO THINK ABOUT THE BOUNDARIES OF THE PEOPLE WE ARE EXPLORING WITH.
WHOA. THEY ALL LOOK SO BIG!
WE MIGHT START OFF BEING ON THE SAME PAGE.
I'LL SHOW YOU MINE IF YOU SHOW ME YOURS.
OK.
BUT END UP FEELING VERY DIFFERENT.
WAS THAT COOL?
THAT WAS COOL!

SOME KINDS OF SEX INVOLVE GETTING OUR BODIES VERY CLOSE TOGETHER.

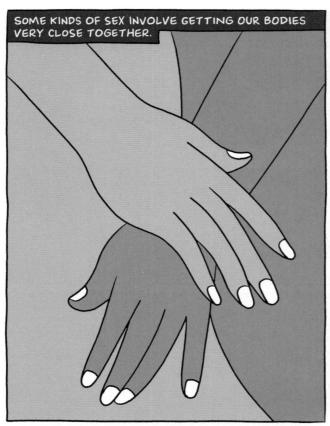

THIS CAN FEEL LIKE TAKING A RISK, BECAUSE WE ARE SHOWING OURSELVES PHYSICALLY AND EMOTIONALLY TO SOMEONE ELSE. WE MAY BE TRYING SOMETHING NEW. WE MAY NOT KNOW WHAT OUR BOUNDARIES ARE FOR THIS NEW THING.

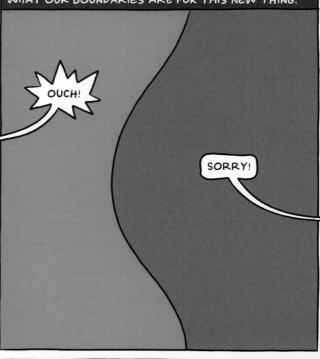

OUCH!

SORRY!

THIS IS PART OF WHAT CAN MAKE SEX FEEL EXCITING.

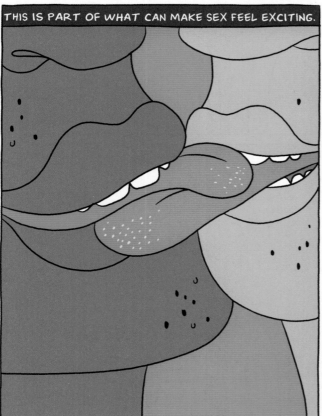

ANY TIME SOMETHING FEELS UNCOMFORTABLE OR RISKY, WE CAN TALK ABOUT OUR BOUNDARIES. WE CAN TALK ABOUT WHAT WE ARE OKAY WITH, NOT OKAY WITH, AND NOT SURE ABOUT.

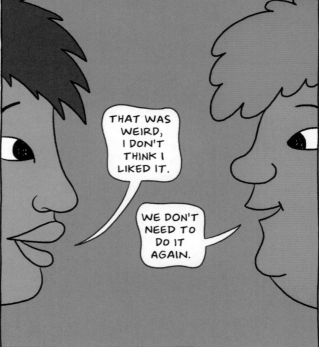

THAT WAS WEIRD, I DON'T THINK I LIKED IT.

WE DON'T NEED TO DO IT AGAIN.

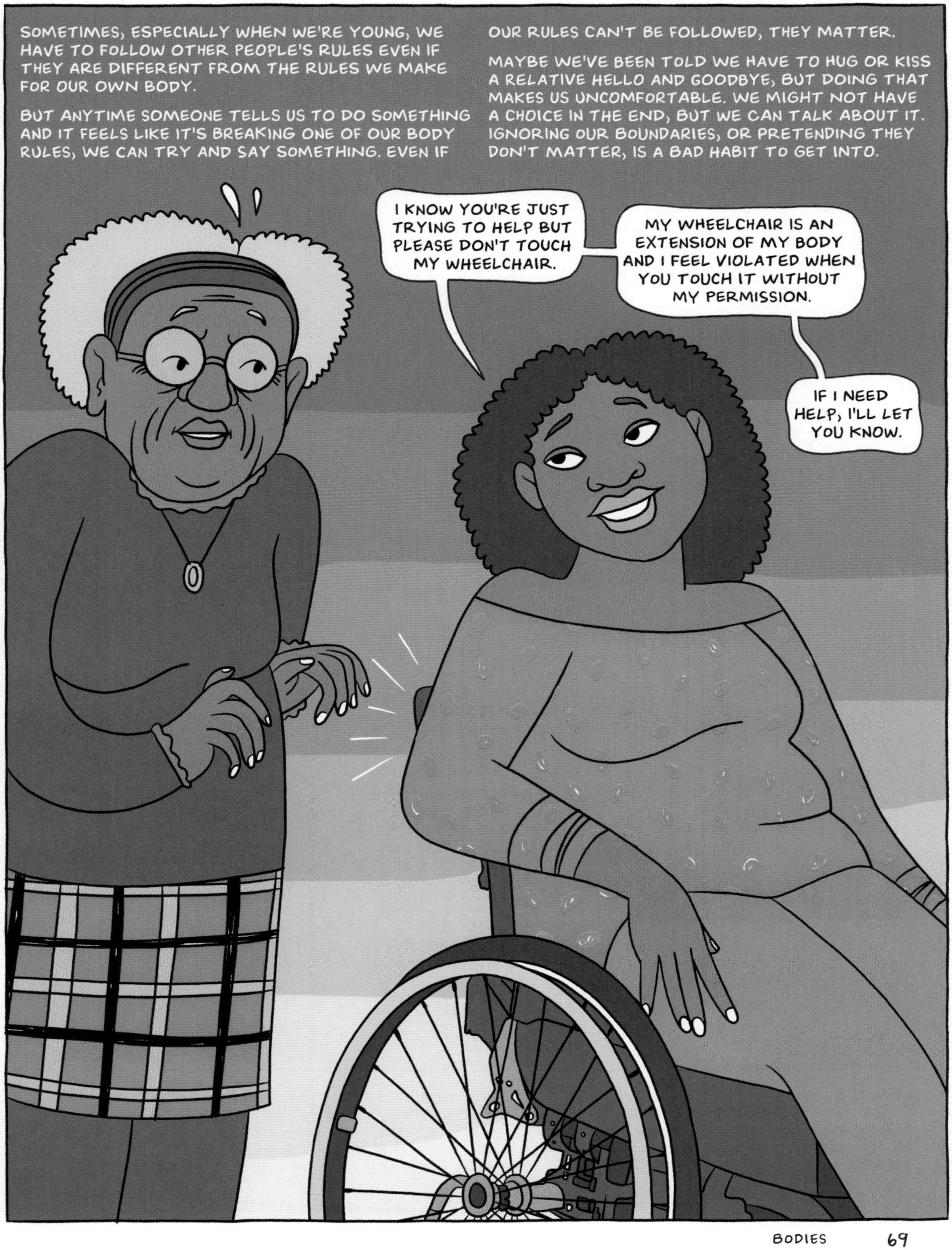
SOMETIMES, ESPECIALLY WHEN WE'RE YOUNG, WE HAVE TO FOLLOW OTHER PEOPLE'S RULES EVEN IF THEY ARE DIFFERENT FROM THE RULES WE MAKE FOR OUR OWN BODY.
BUT ANYTIME SOMEONE TELLS US TO DO SOMETHING AND IT FEELS LIKE IT'S BREAKING ONE OF OUR BODY RULES, WE CAN TRY AND SAY SOMETHING. EVEN IF OUR RULES CAN'T BE FOLLOWED, THEY MATTER.
MAYBE WE'VE BEEN TOLD WE HAVE TO HUG OR KISS A RELATIVE HELLO AND GOODBYE, BUT DOING THAT MAKES US UNCOMFORTABLE. WE MIGHT NOT HAVE A CHOICE IN THE END, BUT WE CAN TALK ABOUT IT. IGNORING OUR BOUNDARIES, OR PRETENDING THEY DON'T MATTER, IS A BAD HABIT TO GET INTO.
I KNOW YOU'RE JUST TRYING TO HELP BUT PLEASE DON'T TOUCH MY WHEELCHAIR.
MY WHEELCHAIR IS AN EXTENSION OF MY BODY AND I FEEL VIOLATED WHEN YOU TOUCH IT WITHOUT MY PERMISSION.
IF I NEED HELP, I'LL LET YOU KNOW.

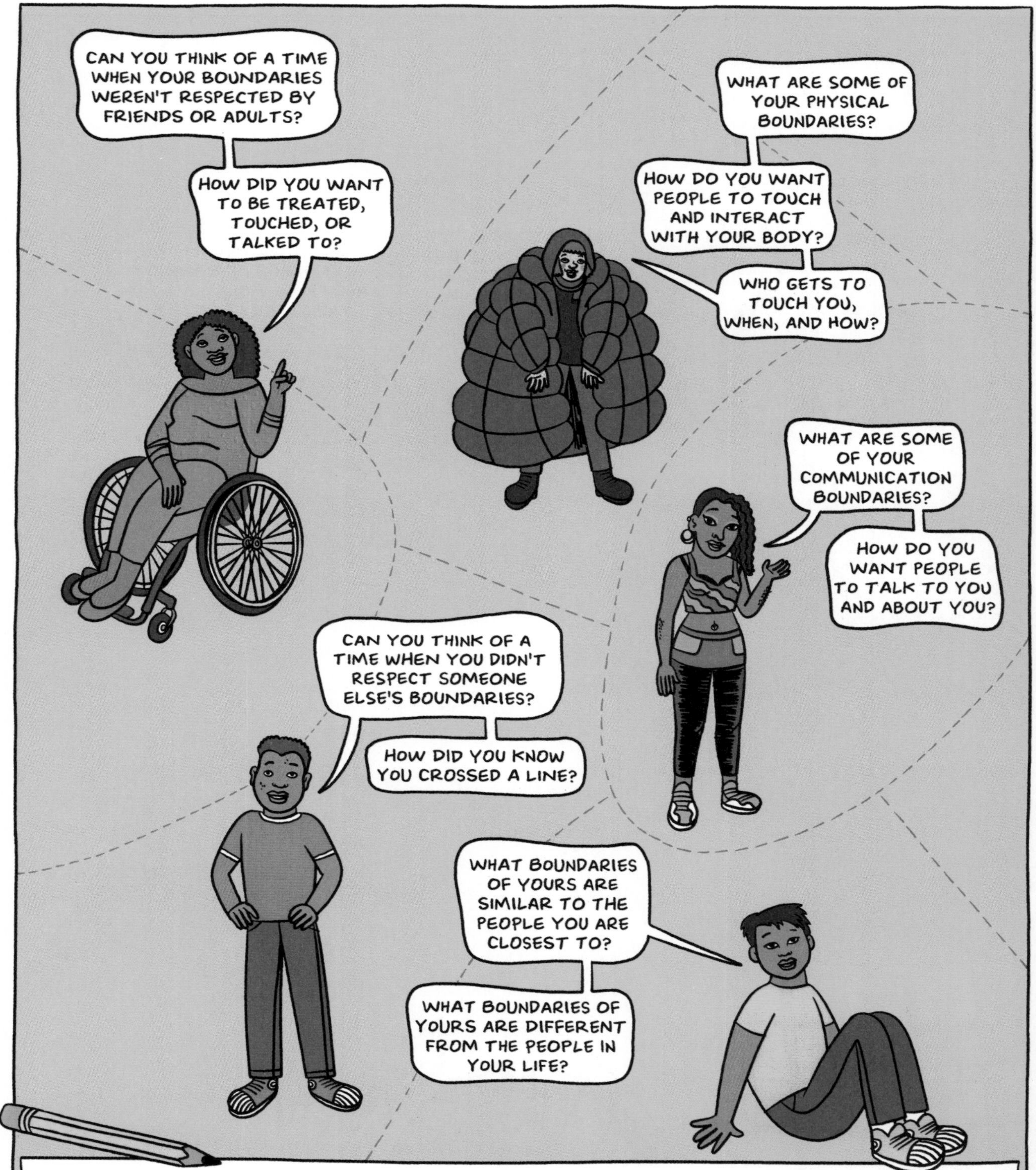
CAN YOU THINK OF A TIME WHEN YOUR BOUNDARIES WEREN'T RESPECTED BY FRIENDS OR ADULTS?
HOW DID YOU WANT TO BE TREATED, TOUCHED, OR TALKED TO?
WHAT ARE SOME OF YOUR PHYSICAL BOUNDARIES?
HOW DO YOU WANT PEOPLE TO TOUCH AND INTERACT WITH YOUR BODY?
WHO GETS TO TOUCH YOU, WHEN, AND HOW?
WHAT ARE SOME OF YOUR COMMUNICATION BOUNDARIES?
HOW DO YOU WANT PEOPLE TO TALK TO YOU AND ABOUT YOU?
CAN YOU THINK OF A TIME WHEN YOU DIDN'T RESPECT SOMEONE ELSE'S BOUNDARIES?
HOW DID YOU KNOW YOU CROSSED A LINE?
WHAT BOUNDARIES OF YOURS ARE SIMILAR TO THE PEOPLE YOU ARE CLOSEST TO?
WHAT BOUNDARIES OF YOURS ARE DIFFERENT FROM THE PEOPLE IN YOUR LIFE?

ACTIVITY

IF YOU AREN'T SURE ABOUT OTHER PEOPLE'S BOUNDARIES, AND YOU FEEL COMFORTABLE ASKING, USE THIS ACTIVITY AS AN OPPORTUNITY TO ASK. ASK SOMEONE HOW THEY LIKE AND DON'T LIKE TO BE TOUCHED, TO BE TALKED TO, AND TO BE TREATED. YOU MAY WANT TO SHARE WITH THEM SOME OF YOUR BOUNDARIES AND TALK ABOUT HOW THEY ARE SIMILAR AND DIFFERENT.

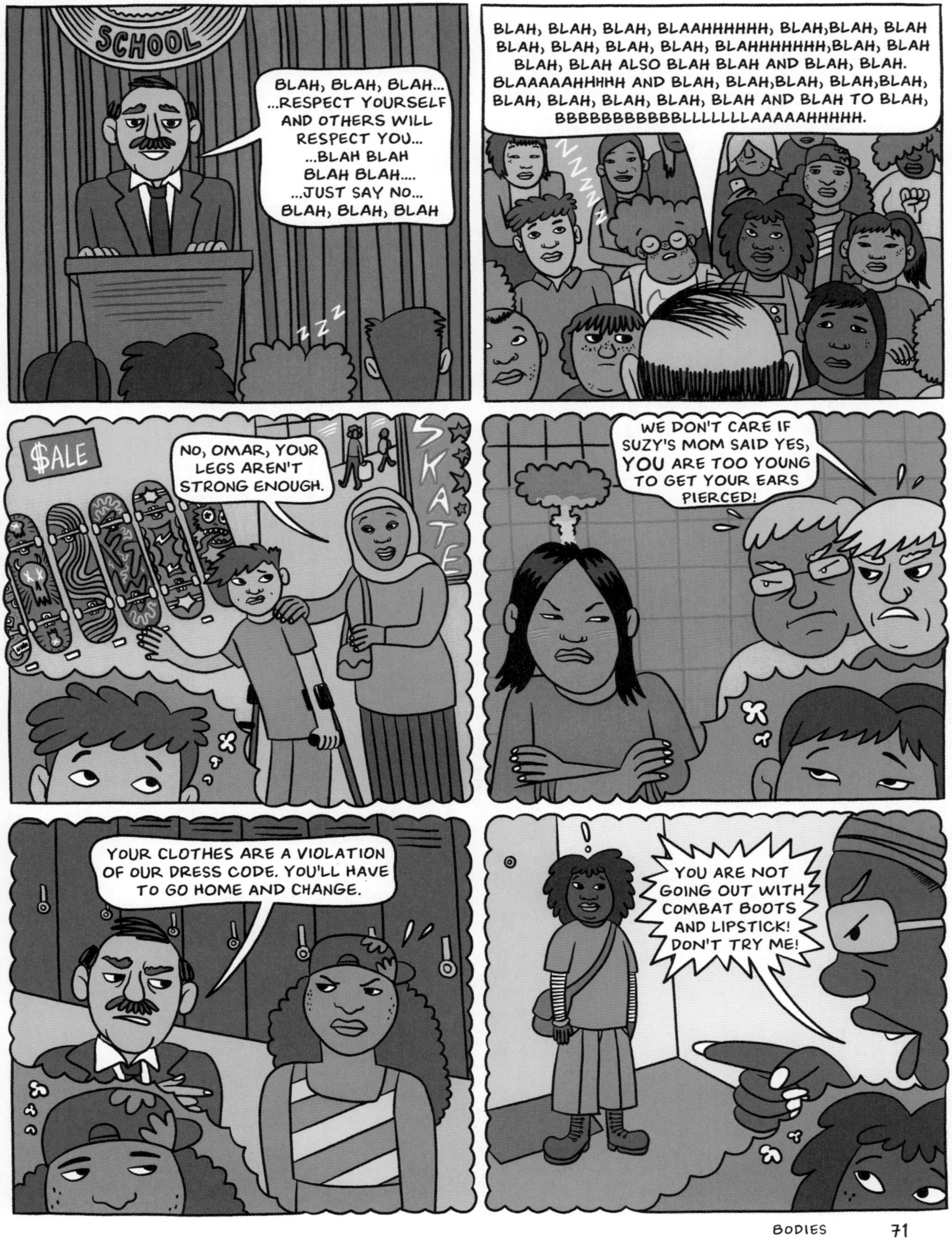
SCHOOL
BLAH, BLAH, BLAH... ...RESPECT YOURSELF AND OTHERS WILL RESPECT YOU... ...BLAH BLAH BLAH BLAH.... ...JUST SAY NO... BLAH, BLAH, BLAH
BLAH, BLAH, BLAH, BLAAHHHHHH, BLAH,BLAH, BLAH BLAH, BLAH, BLAH, BLAH, BLAHHHHHHH,BLAH, BLAH BLAH, BLAH ALSO BLAH BLAH AND BLAH, BLAH. BLAAAAAHHHHH AND BLAH, BLAH,BLAH, BLAH,BLAH, BLAH, BLAH, BLAH, BLAH, BLAH AND BLAH TO BLAH, BBBBBBBBBBBLLLLLLLAAAAAHHHHH.
$ALE
SKATE
NO, OMAR, YOUR LEGS AREN'T STRONG ENOUGH.
WE DON'T CARE IF SUZY'S MOM SAID YES, YOU ARE TOO YOUNG TO GET YOUR EARS PIERCED!
YOUR CLOTHES ARE A VIOLATION OF OUR DRESS CODE. YOU'LL HAVE TO GO HOME AND CHANGE.
YOU ARE NOT GOING OUT WITH COMBAT BOOTS AND LIPSTICK! DON'T TRY ME!

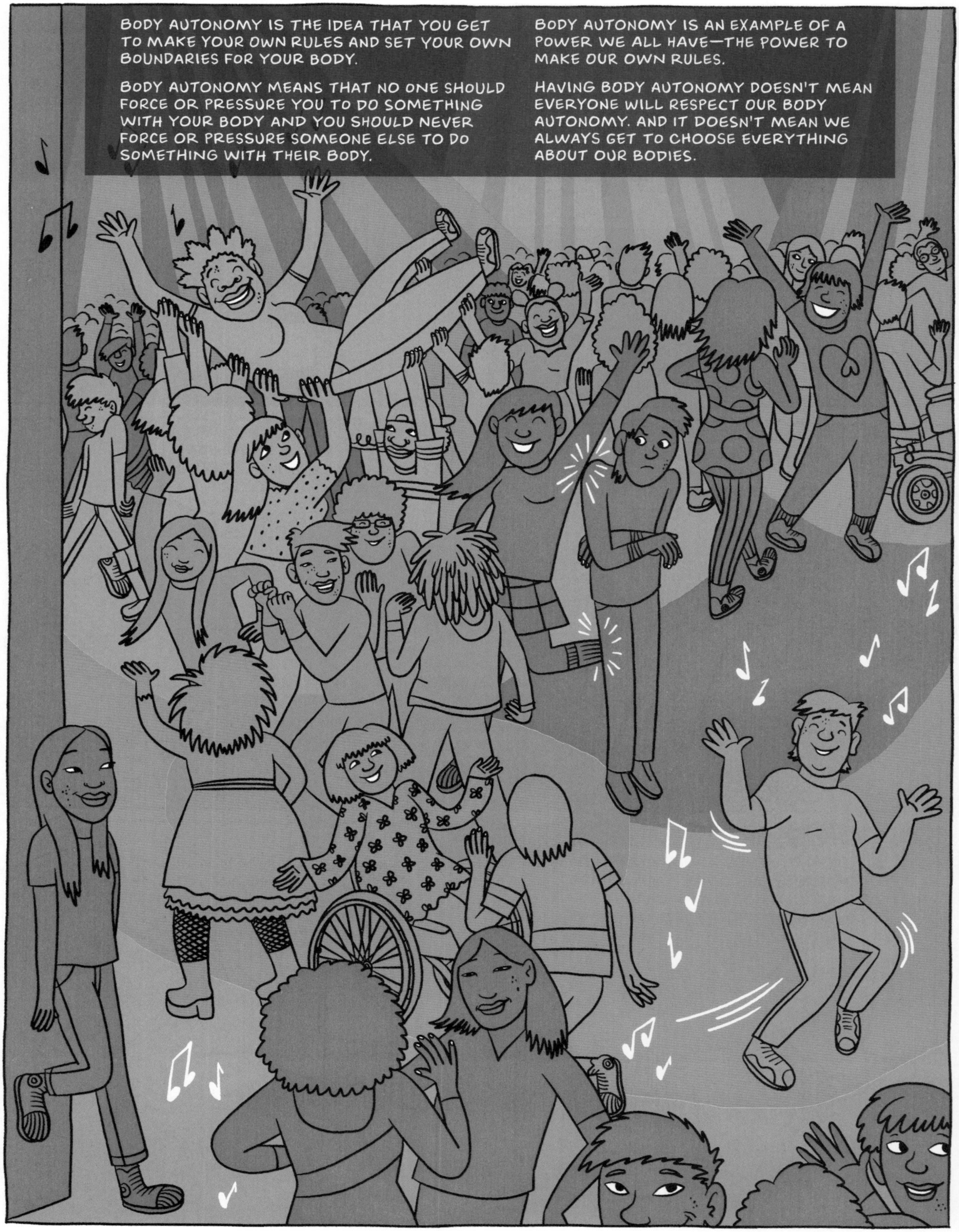
BODY AUTONOMY IS THE IDEA THAT YOU GET TO MAKE YOUR OWN RULES AND SET YOUR OWN BOUNDARIES FOR YOUR BODY.
BODY AUTONOMY MEANS THAT NO ONE SHOULD FORCE OR PRESSURE YOU TO DO SOMETHING WITH YOUR BODY AND YOU SHOULD NEVER FORCE OR PRESSURE SOMEONE ELSE TO DO SOMETHING WITH THEIR BODY.
BODY AUTONOMY IS AN EXAMPLE OF A POWER WE ALL HAVE—THE POWER TO MAKE OUR OWN RULES.
HAVING BODY AUTONOMY DOESN'T MEAN EVERYONE WILL RESPECT OUR BODY AUTONOMY. AND IT DOESN'T MEAN WE ALWAYS GET TO CHOOSE EVERYTHING ABOUT OUR BODIES.

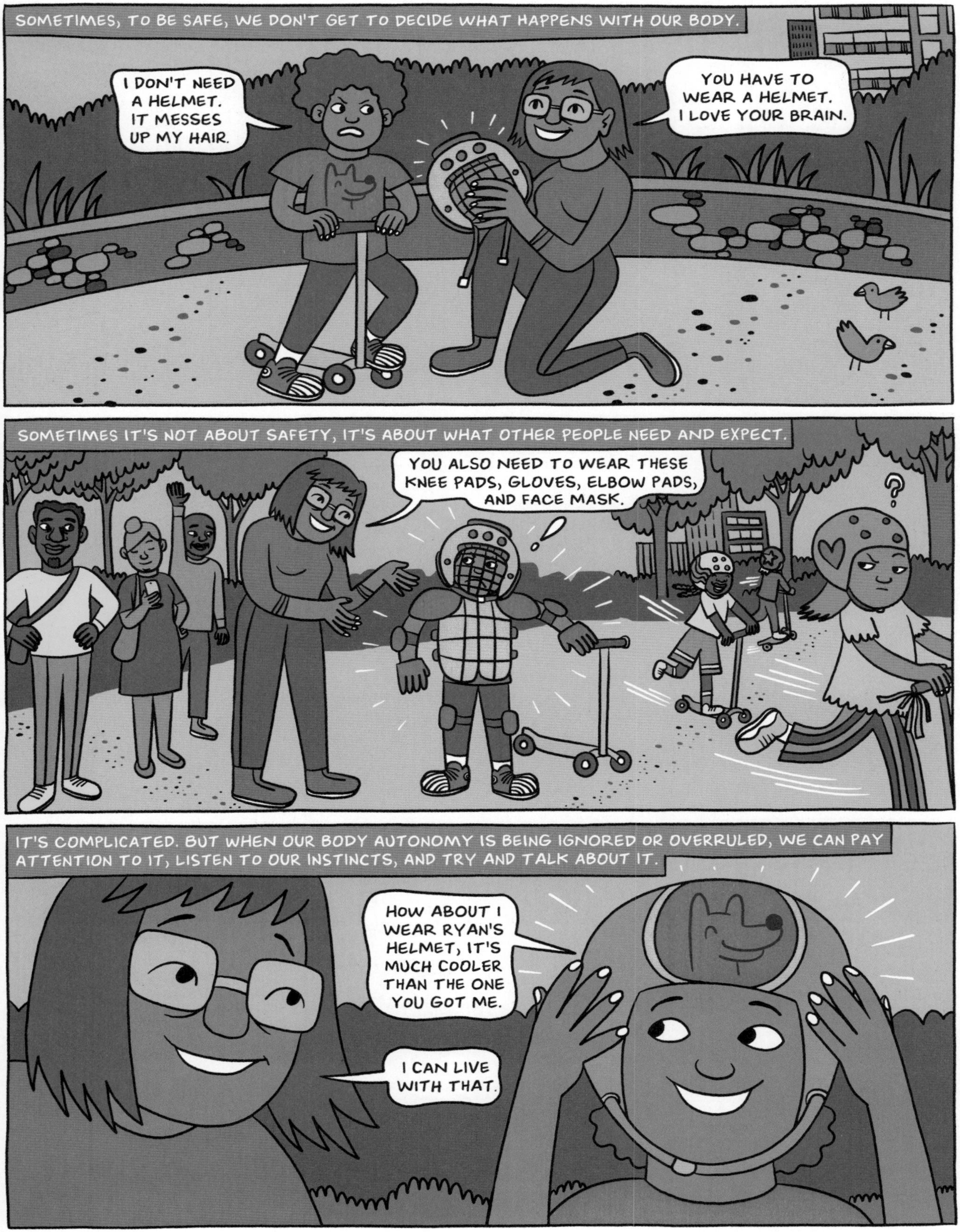
SOMETIMES, TO BE SAFE, WE DON'T GET TO DECIDE WHAT HAPPENS WITH OUR BODY.
I DON'T NEED A HELMET. IT MESSES UP MY HAIR.
YOU HAVE TO WEAR A HELMET. I LOVE YOUR BRAIN.
SOMETIMES IT'S NOT ABOUT SAFETY, IT'S ABOUT WHAT OTHER PEOPLE NEED AND EXPECT.
YOU ALSO NEED TO WEAR THESE KNEE PADS, GLOVES, ELBOW PADS, AND FACE MASK.
!
?
IT'S COMPLICATED. BUT WHEN OUR BODY AUTONOMY IS BEING IGNORED OR OVERRULED, WE CAN PAY ATTENTION TO IT, LISTEN TO OUR INSTINCTS, AND TRY AND TALK ABOUT IT.
HOW ABOUT I WEAR RYAN'S HELMET, IT'S MUCH COOLER THAN THE ONE YOU GOT ME.
I CAN LIVE WITH THAT.

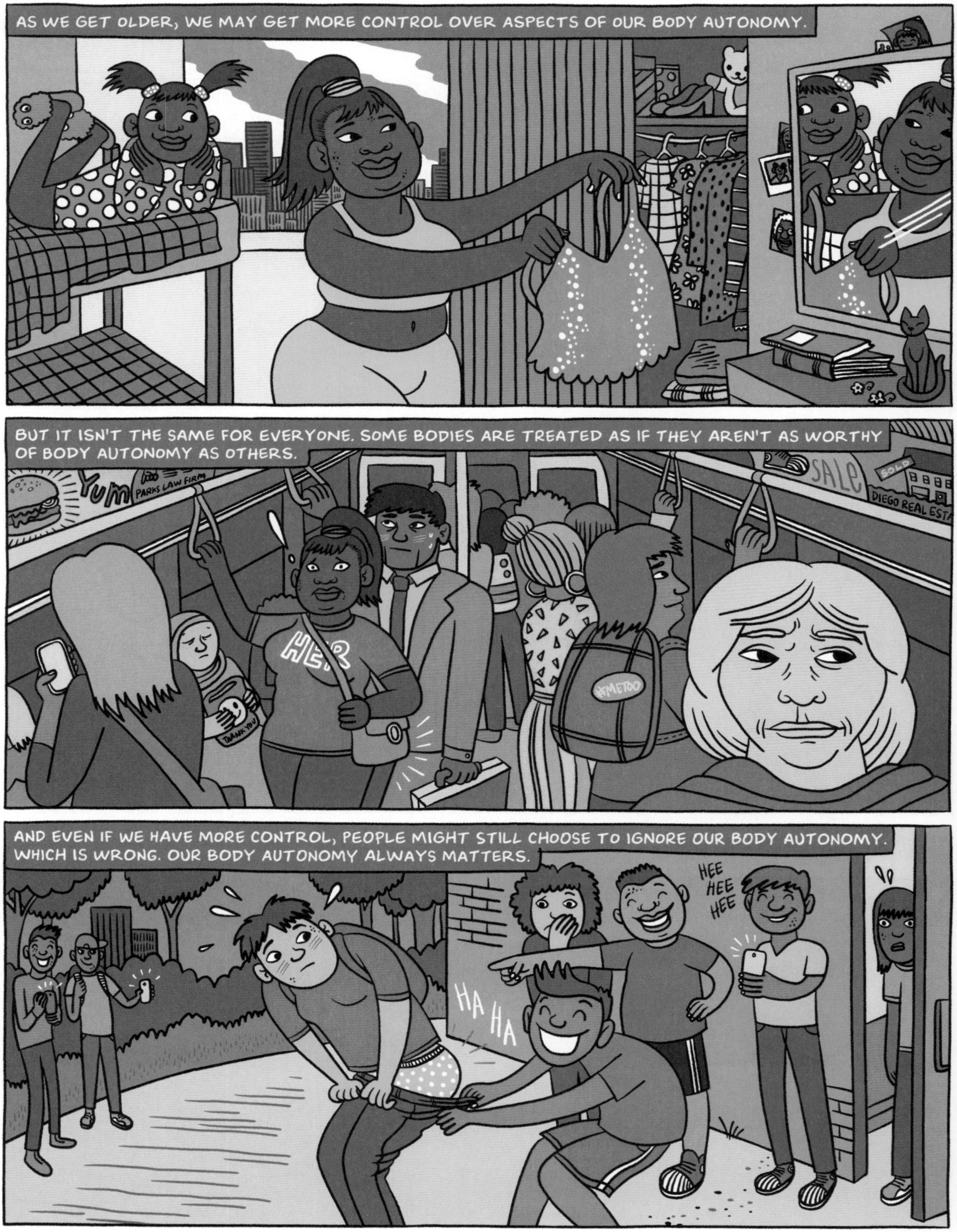
AS WE GET OLDER, WE MAY GET MORE CONTROL OVER ASPECTS OF OUR BODY AUTONOMY.
BUT IT ISN'T THE SAME FOR EVERYONE. SOME BODIES ARE TREATED AS IF THEY AREN'T AS WORTHY OF BODY AUTONOMY AS OTHERS.
Yum
PARKS LAW FIRM
SALE
SOLD
DIEGO REAL ESTA
HER
THANK YOU
#METOO
AND EVEN IF WE HAVE MORE CONTROL, PEOPLE MIGHT STILL CHOOSE TO IGNORE OUR BODY AUTONOMY. WHICH IS WRONG. OUR BODY AUTONOMY ALWAYS MATTERS.
HEE HEE HEE
HA HA

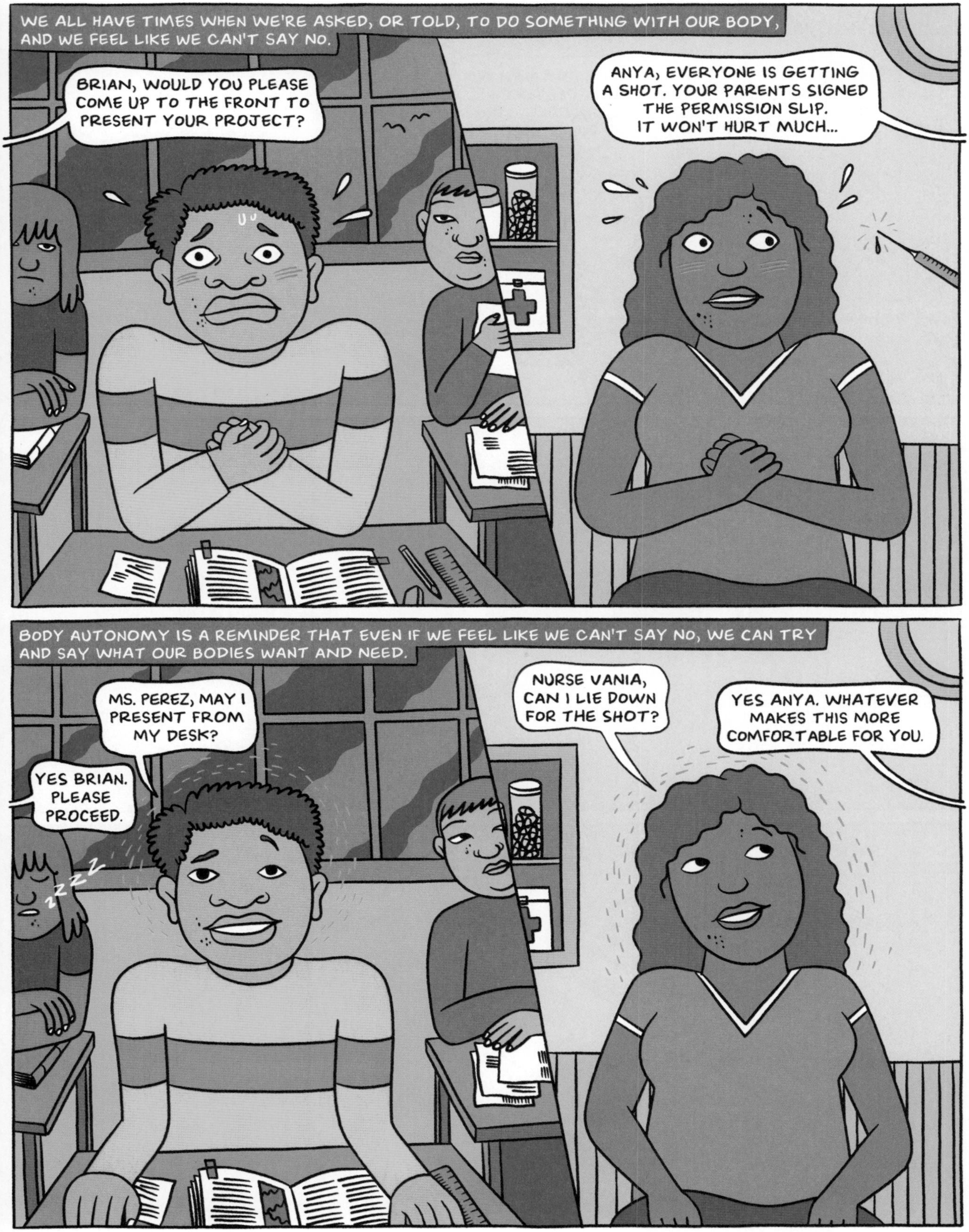
WE ALL HAVE TIMES WHEN WE'RE ASKED, OR TOLD, TO DO SOMETHING WITH OUR BODY, AND WE FEEL LIKE WE CAN'T SAY NO.
BRIAN, WOULD YOU PLEASE COME UP TO THE FRONT TO PRESENT YOUR PROJECT?
ANYA, EVERYONE IS GETTING A SHOT. YOUR PARENTS SIGNED THE PERMISSION SLIP. IT WON'T HURT MUCH...
BODY AUTONOMY IS A REMINDER THAT EVEN IF WE FEEL LIKE WE CAN'T SAY NO, WE CAN TRY AND SAY WHAT OUR BODIES WANT AND NEED.
MS. PEREZ, MAY I PRESENT FROM MY DESK?
YES BRIAN. PLEASE PROCEED.
ZZZ
NURSE VANIA, CAN I LIE DOWN FOR THE SHOT?
YES ANYA. WHATEVER MAKES THIS MORE COMFORTABLE FOR YOU.

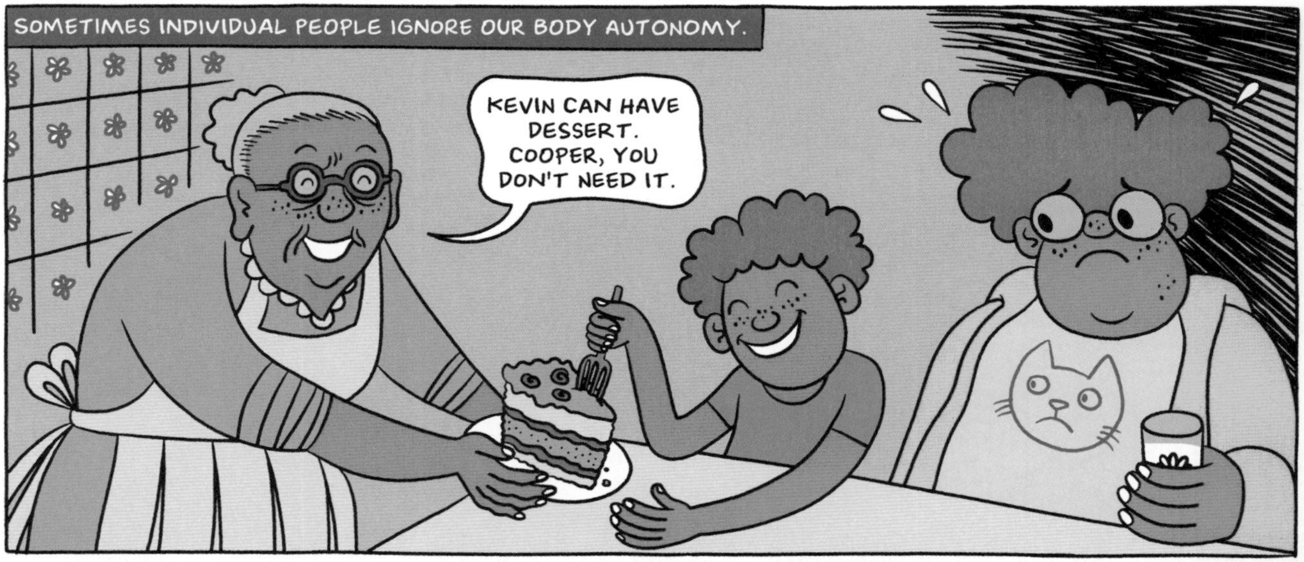
SOMETIMES INDIVIDUAL PEOPLE IGNORE OUR BODY AUTONOMY.
KEVIN CAN HAVE DESSERT. COOPER, YOU DON'T NEED IT.

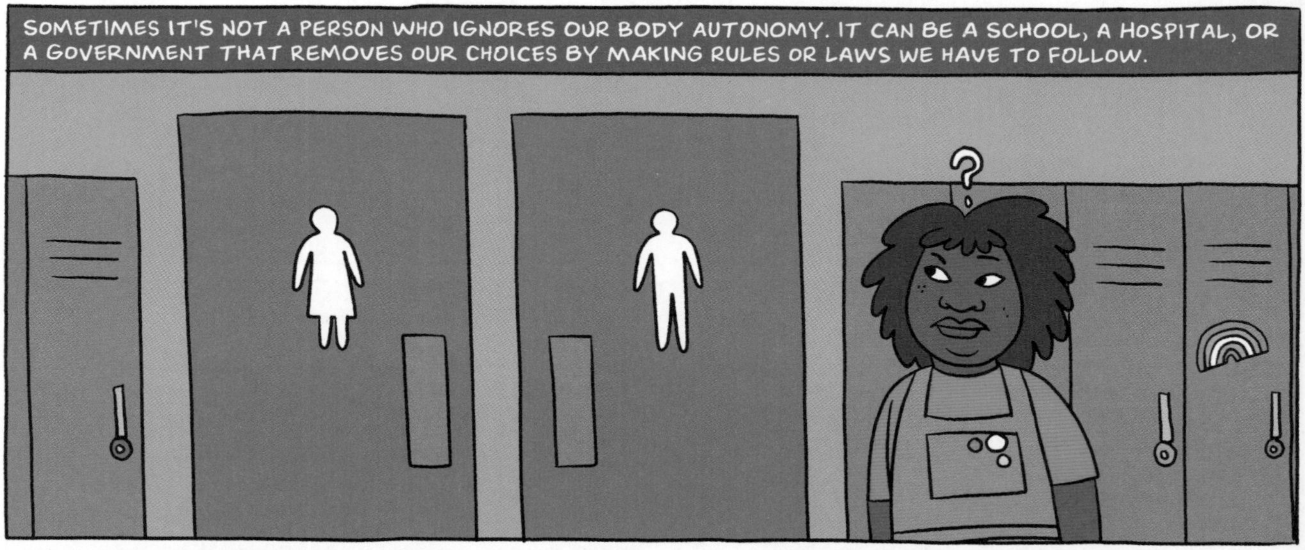
SOMETIMES IT'S NOT A PERSON WHO IGNORES OUR BODY AUTONOMY. IT CAN BE A SCHOOL, A HOSPITAL, OR A GOVERNMENT THAT REMOVES OUR CHOICES BY MAKING RULES OR LAWS WE HAVE TO FOLLOW.
?

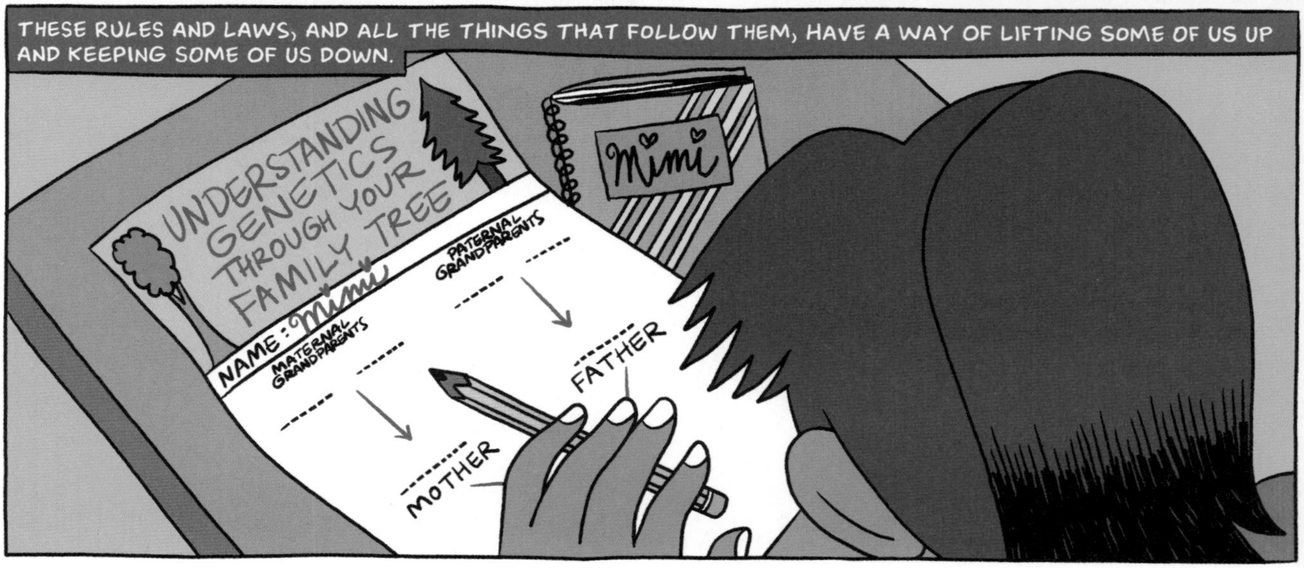
THESE RULES AND LAWS, AND ALL THE THINGS THAT FOLLOW THEM, HAVE A WAY OF LIFTING SOME OF US UP AND KEEPING SOME OF US DOWN.
UNDERSTANDING GENETICS THROUGH YOUR FAMILY TREE
Mimi
NAME: Mimi
PATERNAL GRANDPARENTS
MATERNAL GRANDPARENTS
FATHER
MOTHER

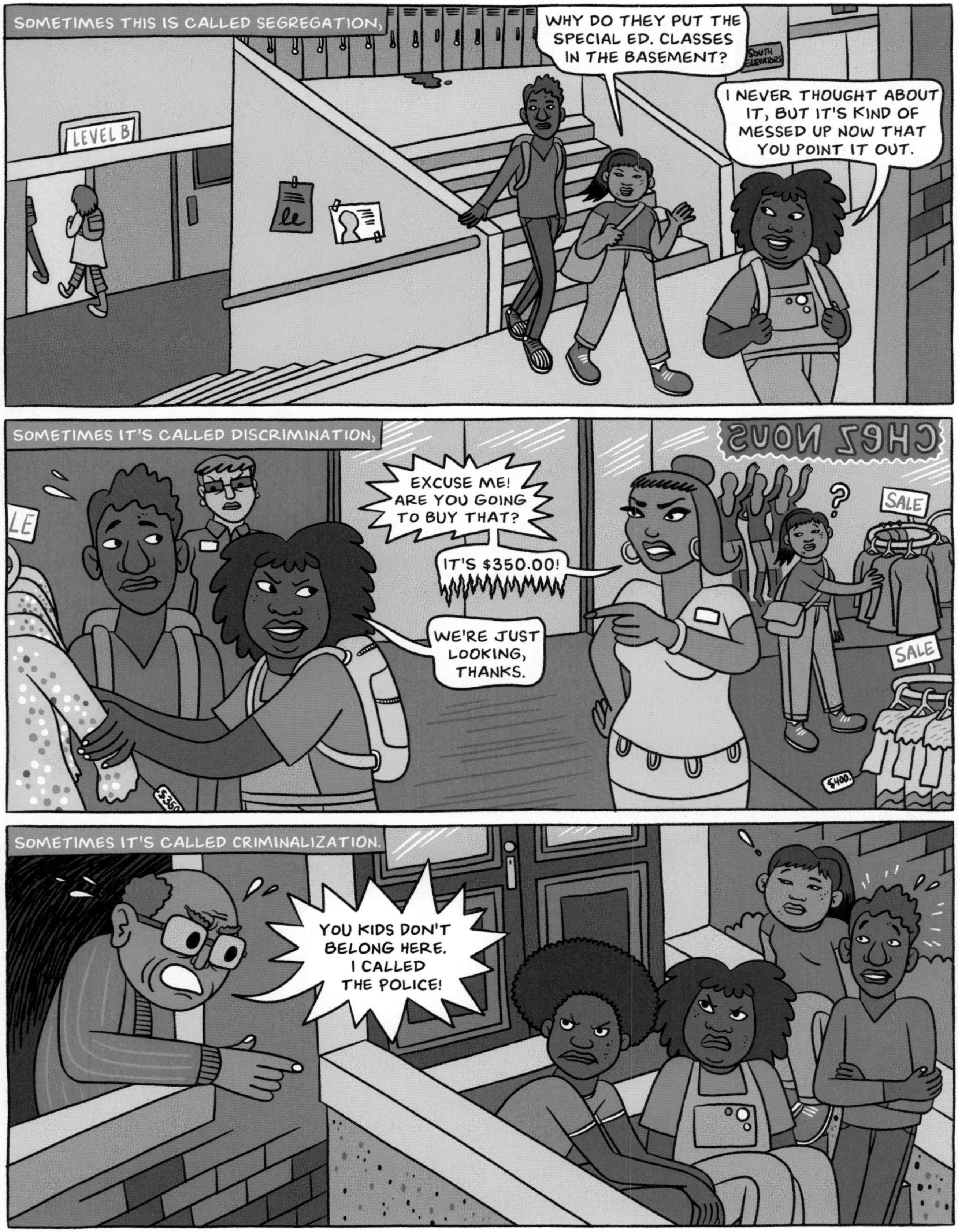
SOMETIMES THIS IS CALLED SEGREGATION,
WHY DO THEY PUT THE SPECIAL ED. CLASSES IN THE BASEMENT?
SOUTH ELEVATORS
LEVEL B
I NEVER THOUGHT ABOUT IT, BUT IT'S KIND OF MESSED UP NOW THAT YOU POINT IT OUT.
SOMETIMES IT'S CALLED DISCRIMINATION,
CHEZ NOUS
EXCUSE ME! ARE YOU GOING TO BUY THAT?
IT'S $350.00!
SALE
WE'RE JUST LOOKING, THANKS.
SALE
$400.
SOMETIMES IT'S CALLED CRIMINALIZATION.
YOU KIDS DON'T BELONG HERE. I CALLED THE POLICE!

SEGREGATION, DISCRIMINATION, AND CRIMINALIZATION ARE ALL EXAMPLES OF PEOPLE AND SYSTEMS USING POWER OVER US TO LIMIT OUR CHOICES AND BODY AUTONOMY.

EVERY BODY DESERVES BODY AUTONOMY. BUT FOR THAT TO HAPPEN, EVERYBODY HAS TO PARTICIPATE. EACH OF US NEEDS TO:

1 LISTEN TO, AND TRUST, OUR INSTINCTS WHEN WE FEEL LIKE OUR BODY AUTONOMY IS BEING DISRESPECTED.

2 TALK ABOUT WHAT OUR BODIES WANT AND NEED.

3 RESPECT OTHER PEOPLE'S BODY AUTONOMY. PAY ATTENTION AND LISTEN TO WHAT THEY ARE COMMUNICATING ABOUT THEIR BODIES.

EVEN IF THE WORLD DOESN'T ACT THIS WAY, BODY AUTONOMY IS FOR EVERY BODY.

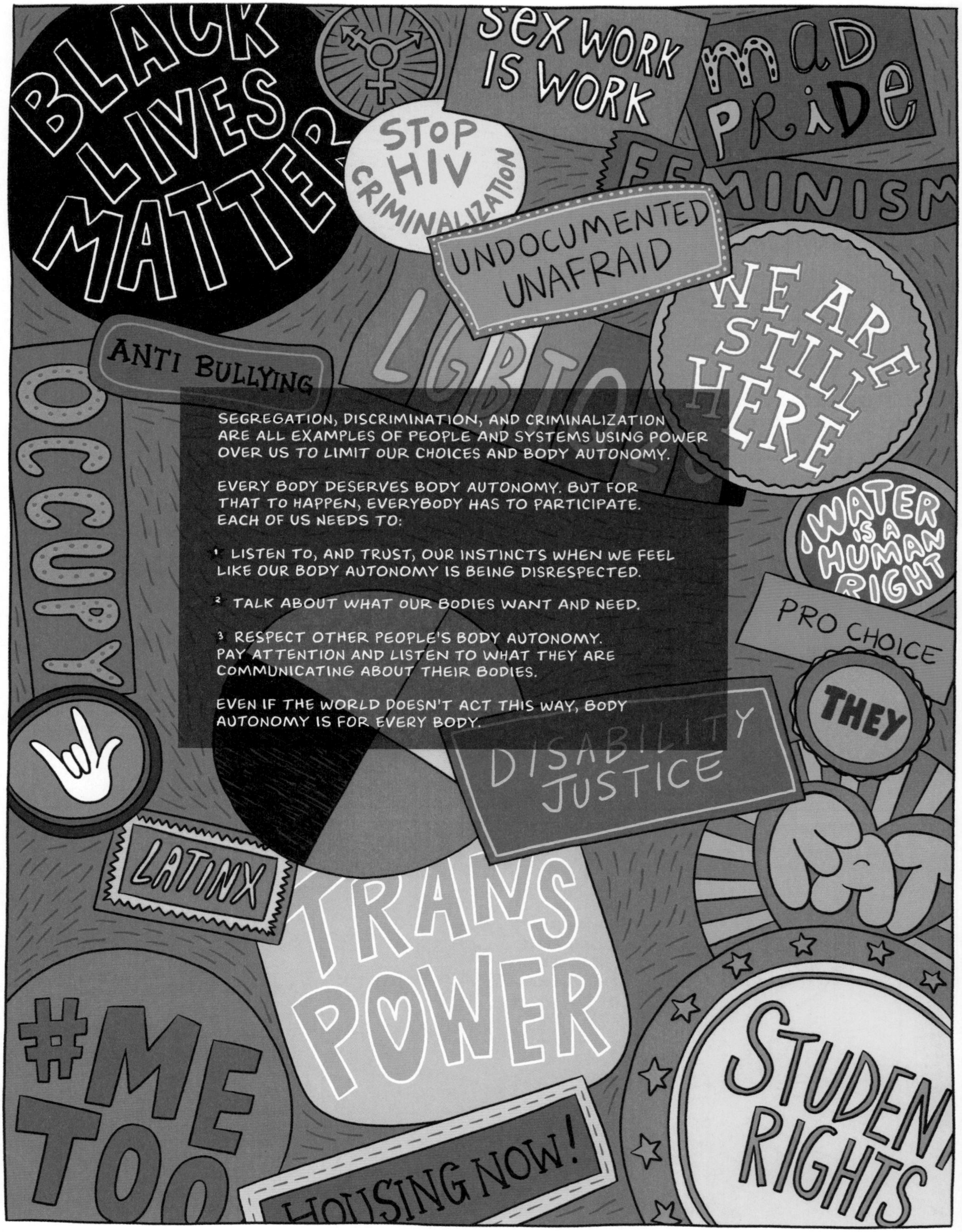
BLACK LIVES MATTER
SEX WORK IS WORK
MAD PRIDE
STOP HIV CRIMINALIZATION
FEMINISM
UNDOCUMENTED UNAFRAID
WE ARE STILL HERE
ANTI BULLYING
OCCUPY
WATER IS A HUMAN RIGHT
PRO CHOICE
THEY
DISABILITY JUSTICE
LATINX
TRANS POWER
#ME TOO
HOUSING NOW!
STUDEN
RIGHTS

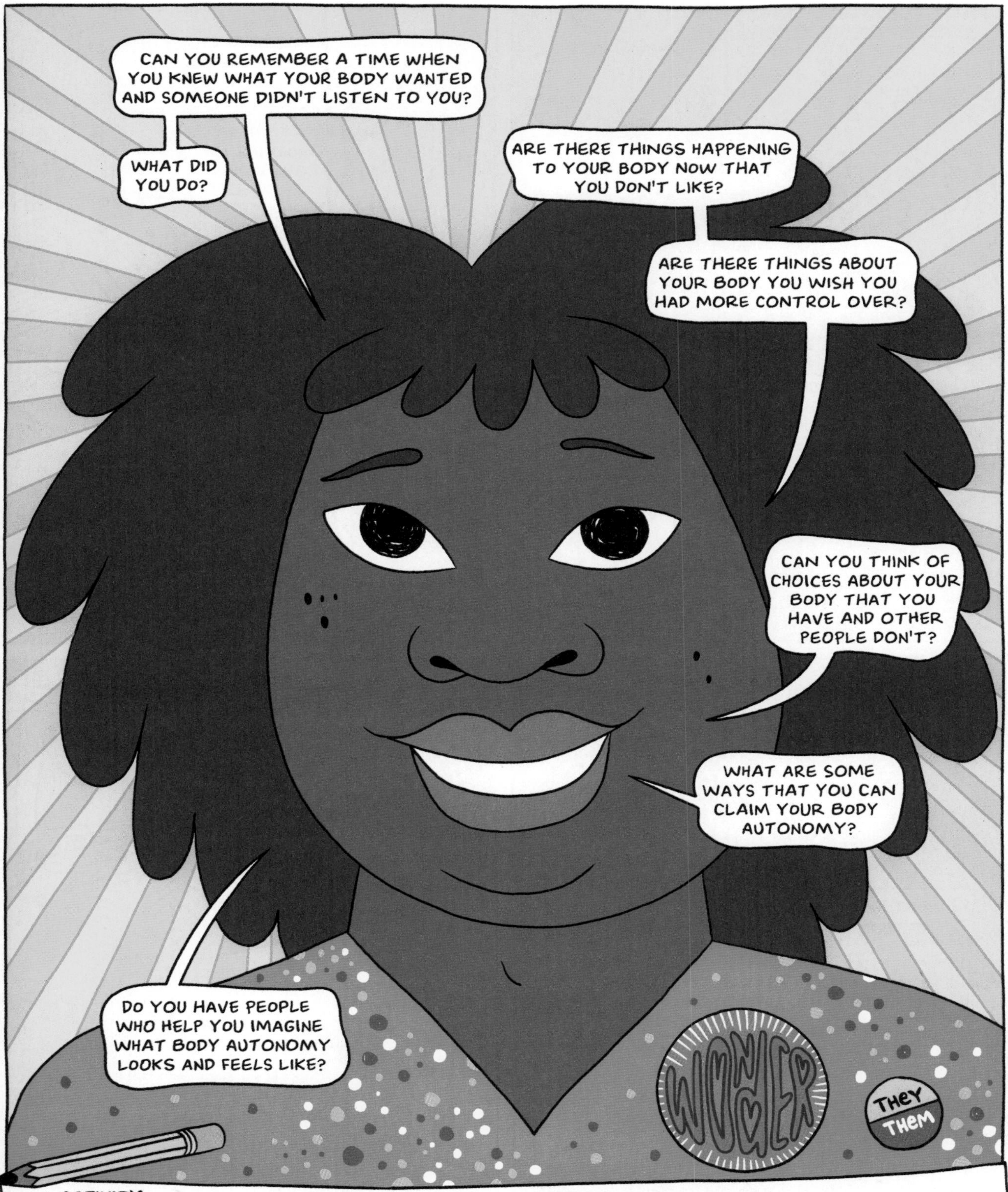
CAN YOU REMEMBER A TIME WHEN YOU KNEW WHAT YOUR BODY WANTED AND SOMEONE DIDN'T LISTEN TO YOU?
WHAT DID YOU DO?
ARE THERE THINGS HAPPENING TO YOUR BODY NOW THAT YOU DON'T LIKE?
ARE THERE THINGS ABOUT YOUR BODY YOU WISH YOU HAD MORE CONTROL OVER?
CAN YOU THINK OF CHOICES ABOUT YOUR BODY THAT YOU HAVE AND OTHER PEOPLE DON'T?
WHAT ARE SOME WAYS THAT YOU CAN CLAIM YOUR BODY AUTONOMY?
DO YOU HAVE PEOPLE WHO HELP YOU IMAGINE WHAT BODY AUTONOMY LOOKS AND FEELS LIKE?
WONDER
THEY
THEM

ACTIVITY

SPEAKING UP (LIKE BRIAN AND ANYA DO ON P. 75) ISN'T EASY, AND IT TAKES PRACTICE. THINK ABOUT A TIME WHEN SOMEONE WASN'T RESPECTING YOUR BODY AUTONOMY AND YOU WISH YOU HAD SAID SOMETHING. WHAT DO YOU WISH YOU HAD SAID?

IF YOU HAVE SOMEONE YOU TRUST, ASK THEM IF THEY CAN THINK OF A TIME IN THEIR LIFE WHEN THEY WISH THEY HAD SPOKEN UP. TRY TO COME UP WITH OTHER THINGS EACH OF YOU COULD HAVE SAID. TRY SAYING IT OUT LOUD AND SEE HOW IT FEELS!

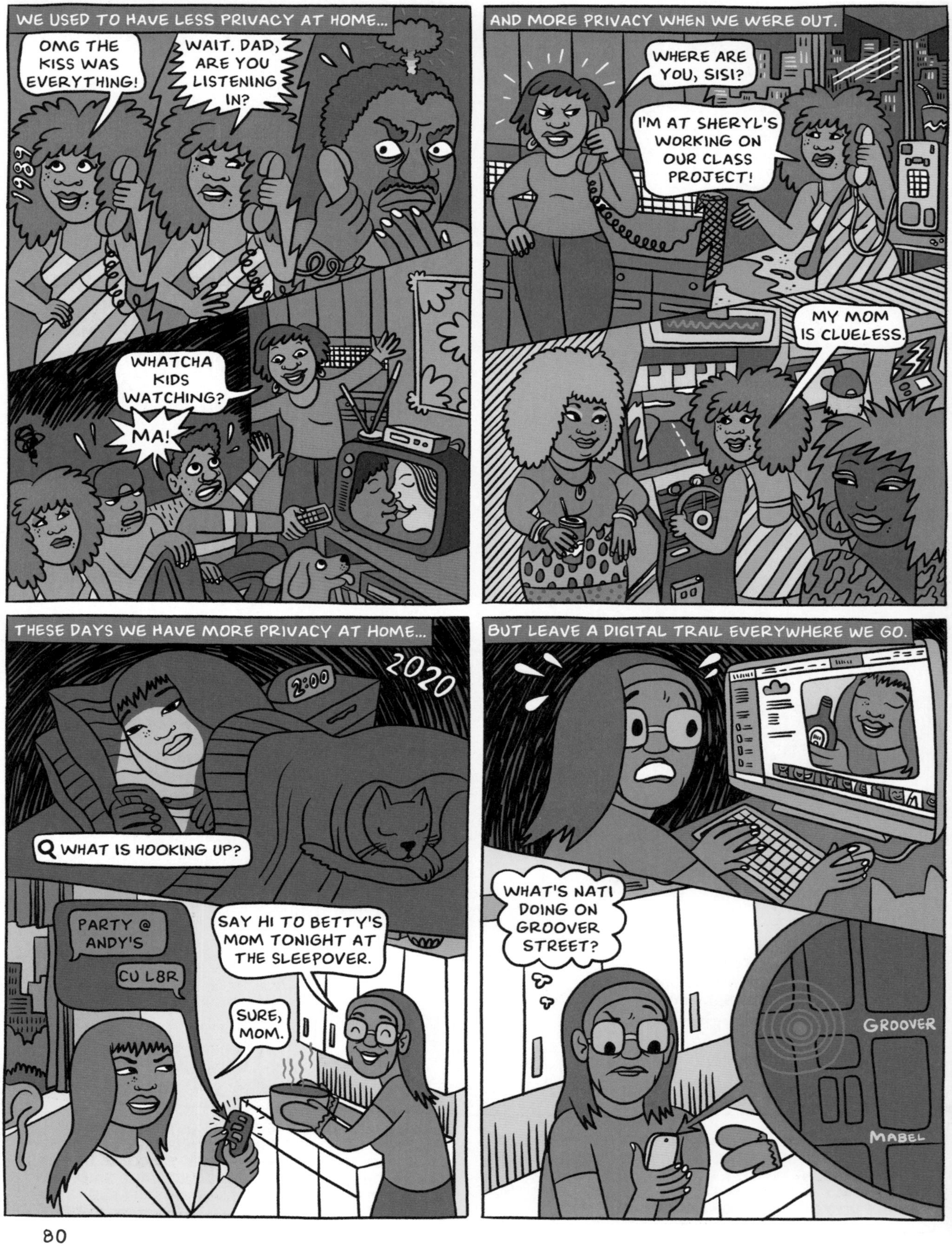
WE USED TO HAVE LESS PRIVACY AT HOME...
1989
OMG THE KISS WAS EVERYTHING!
WAIT. DAD, ARE YOU LISTENING IN?
WHATCHA KIDS WATCHING?
MA!
AND MORE PRIVACY WHEN WE WERE OUT.
WHERE ARE YOU, SISI?
I'M AT SHERYL'S WORKING ON OUR CLASS PROJECT!
MY MOM IS CLUELESS.
THESE DAYS WE HAVE MORE PRIVACY AT HOME...
2020
2:00
WHAT IS HOOKING UP?
PARTY @ ANDY'S
CU L8R
SAY HI TO BETTY'S MOM TONIGHT AT THE SLEEPOVER.
SURE, MOM.
BUT LEAVE A DIGITAL TRAIL EVERYWHERE WE GO.
WHAT'S NATI DOING ON GROOVER STREET?
GROOVER
MABEL

IT'S EASY TO CONFUSE PRIVACY AND SECRETS. BOTH WORDS HAVE SOMETHING TO DO WITH NOT TELLING PEOPLE ABOUT THINGS. BUT THEY ARE DIFFERENT.

A SECRET IS USUALLY SOMETHING WE FEEL LIKE WE HAVE TO KEEP HIDDEN.

SOME SECRETS ARE OK—LIKE WHEN WE KEEP A SURPRISE PARTY OR PRESENT A SECRET FOR A SHORT TIME. BUT WE SHOULD ALWAYS BE ABLE TO TALK TO AT LEAST ONE OTHER PERSON ABOUT A SECRET.

NO ONE SHOULD PRESSURE US TO KEEP A SECRET FROM EVERYONE, OR FOR A LONG TIME, LIKE FOREVER.*

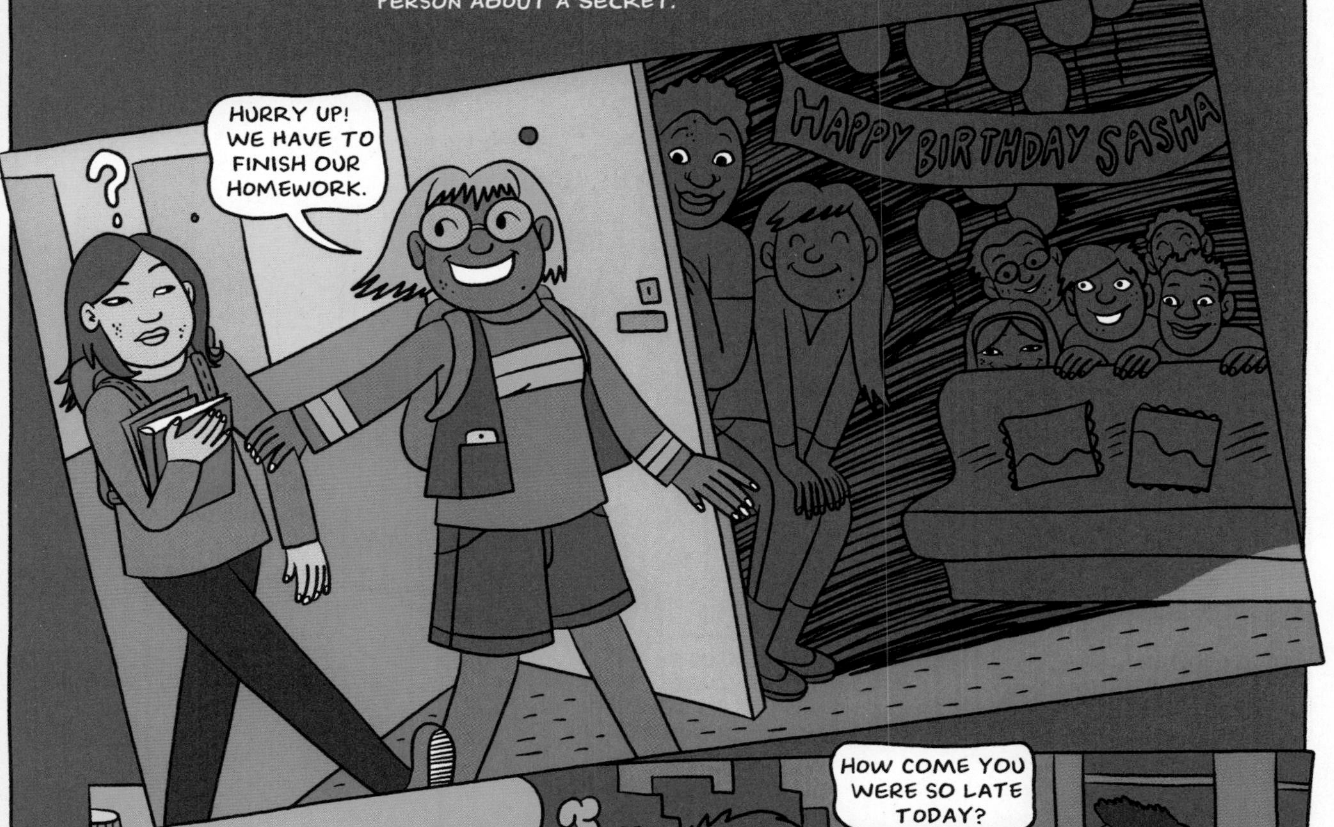

HURRY UP! WE HAVE TO FINISH OUR HOMEWORK.
HAPPY BIRTHDAY SASHA

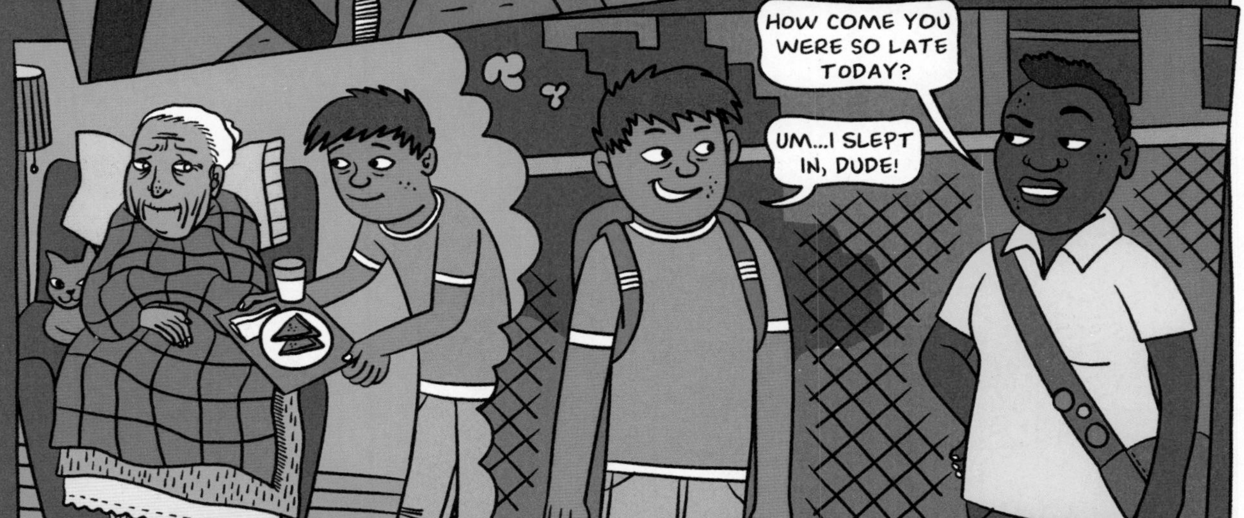

HOW COME YOU WERE SO LATE TODAY?
UM...I SLEPT IN, DUDE!

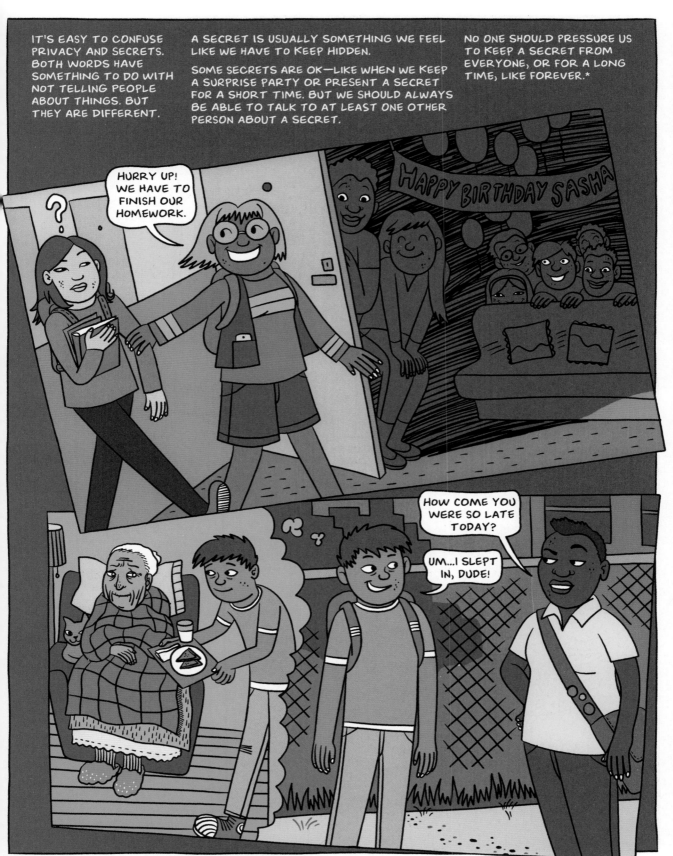

* READ MORE ABOUT HOW SECRETS CAN BE HARMFUL IN THE SAFETY CHAPTER, P. 371

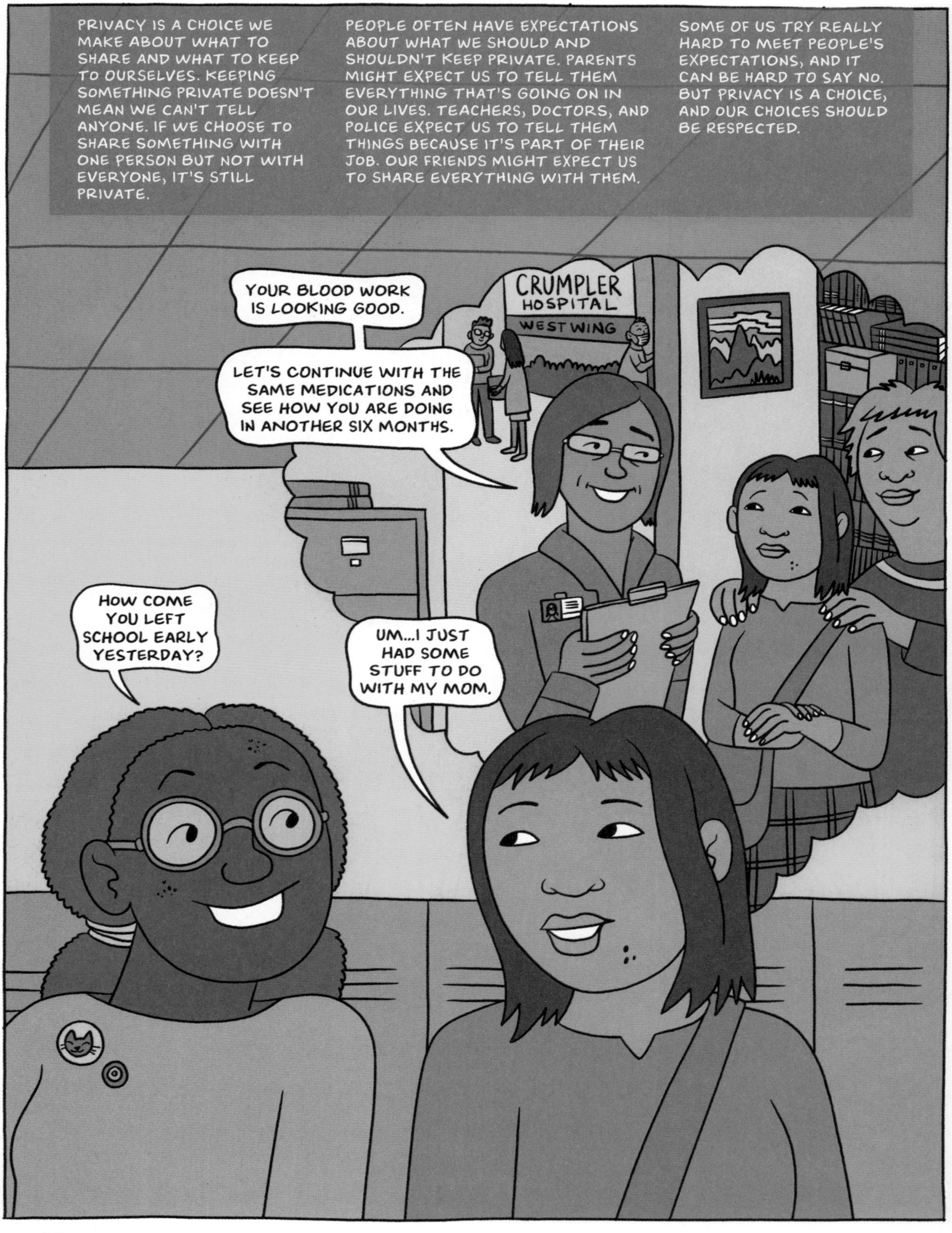
PRIVACY IS A CHOICE WE MAKE ABOUT WHAT TO SHARE AND WHAT TO KEEP TO OURSELVES. KEEPING SOMETHING PRIVATE DOESN'T MEAN WE CAN'T TELL ANYONE. IF WE CHOOSE TO SHARE SOMETHING WITH ONE PERSON BUT NOT WITH EVERYONE, IT'S STILL PRIVATE.
PEOPLE OFTEN HAVE EXPECTATIONS ABOUT WHAT WE SHOULD AND SHOULDN'T KEEP PRIVATE. PARENTS MIGHT EXPECT US TO TELL THEM EVERYTHING THAT'S GOING ON IN OUR LIVES. TEACHERS, DOCTORS, AND POLICE EXPECT US TO TELL THEM THINGS BECAUSE IT'S PART OF THEIR JOB. OUR FRIENDS MIGHT EXPECT US TO SHARE EVERYTHING WITH THEM.
SOME OF US TRY REALLY HARD TO MEET PEOPLE'S EXPECTATIONS, AND IT CAN BE HARD TO SAY NO. BUT PRIVACY IS A CHOICE, AND OUR CHOICES SHOULD BE RESPECTED.
CRUMPLER HOSPITAL
WEST WING
YOUR BLOOD WORK IS LOOKING GOOD.
LET'S CONTINUE WITH THE SAME MEDICATIONS AND SEE HOW YOU ARE DOING IN ANOTHER SIX MONTHS.
HOW COME YOU LEFT SCHOOL EARLY YESTERDAY?
UM...I JUST HAD SOME STUFF TO DO WITH MY MOM.

THERE ARE LOTS OF REASONS WE CHOOSE TO KEEP THINGS PRIVATE.

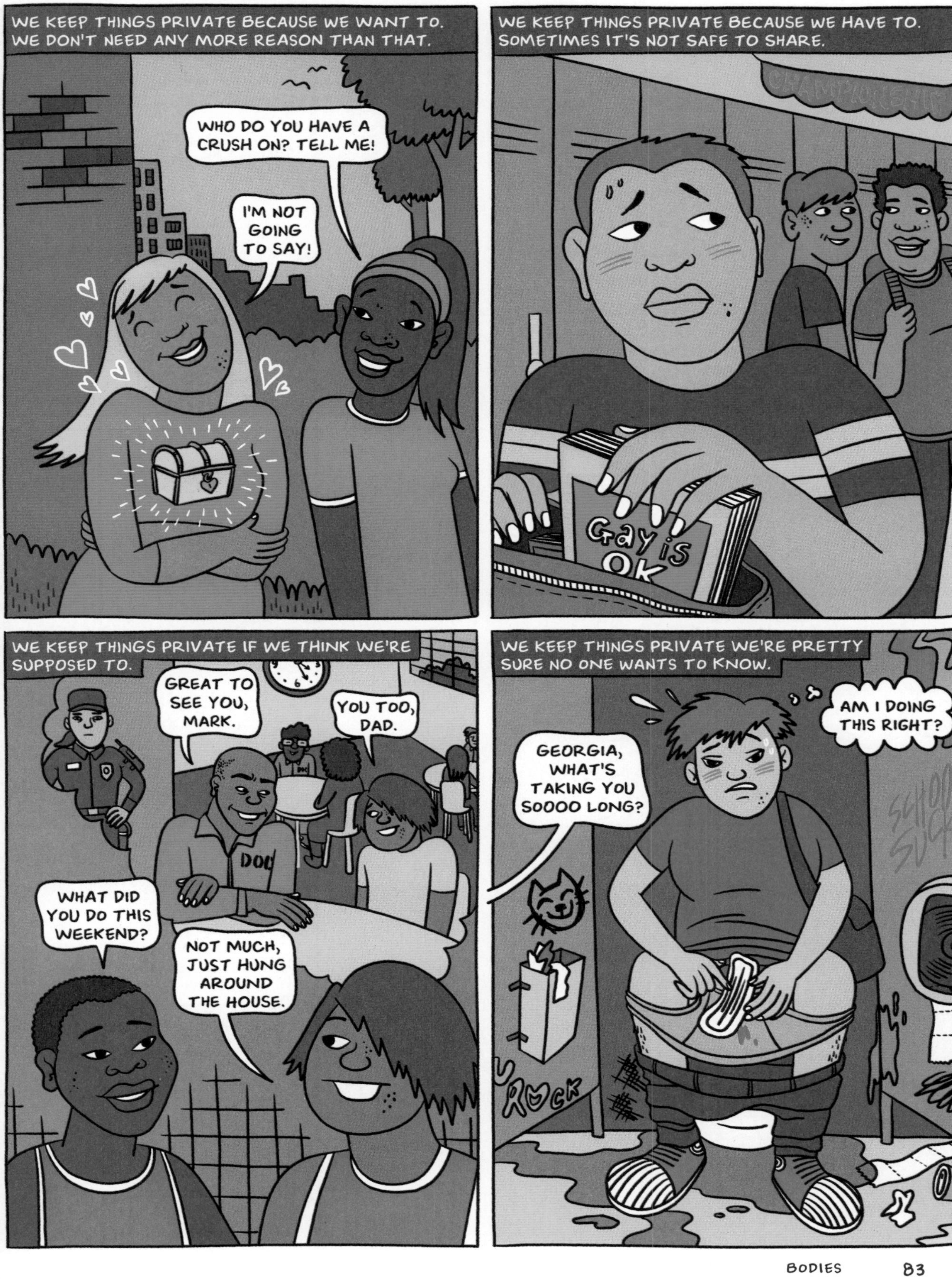
WE KEEP THINGS PRIVATE BECAUSE WE WANT TO. WE DON'T NEED ANY MORE REASON THAN THAT.
WHO DO YOU HAVE A CRUSH ON? TELL ME!
I'M NOT GOING TO SAY!
WE KEEP THINGS PRIVATE BECAUSE WE HAVE TO. SOMETIMES IT'S NOT SAFE TO SHARE.
Gay is OK
WE KEEP THINGS PRIVATE IF WE THINK WE'RE SUPPOSED TO.
GREAT TO SEE YOU, MARK.
YOU TOO, DAD.
WHAT DID YOU DO THIS WEEKEND?
NOT MUCH, JUST HUNG AROUND THE HOUSE.
WE KEEP THINGS PRIVATE WE'RE PRETTY SURE NO ONE WANTS TO KNOW.
GEORGIA, WHAT'S TAKING YOU SOOOO LONG?
AM I DOING THIS RIGHT?
U ROCK

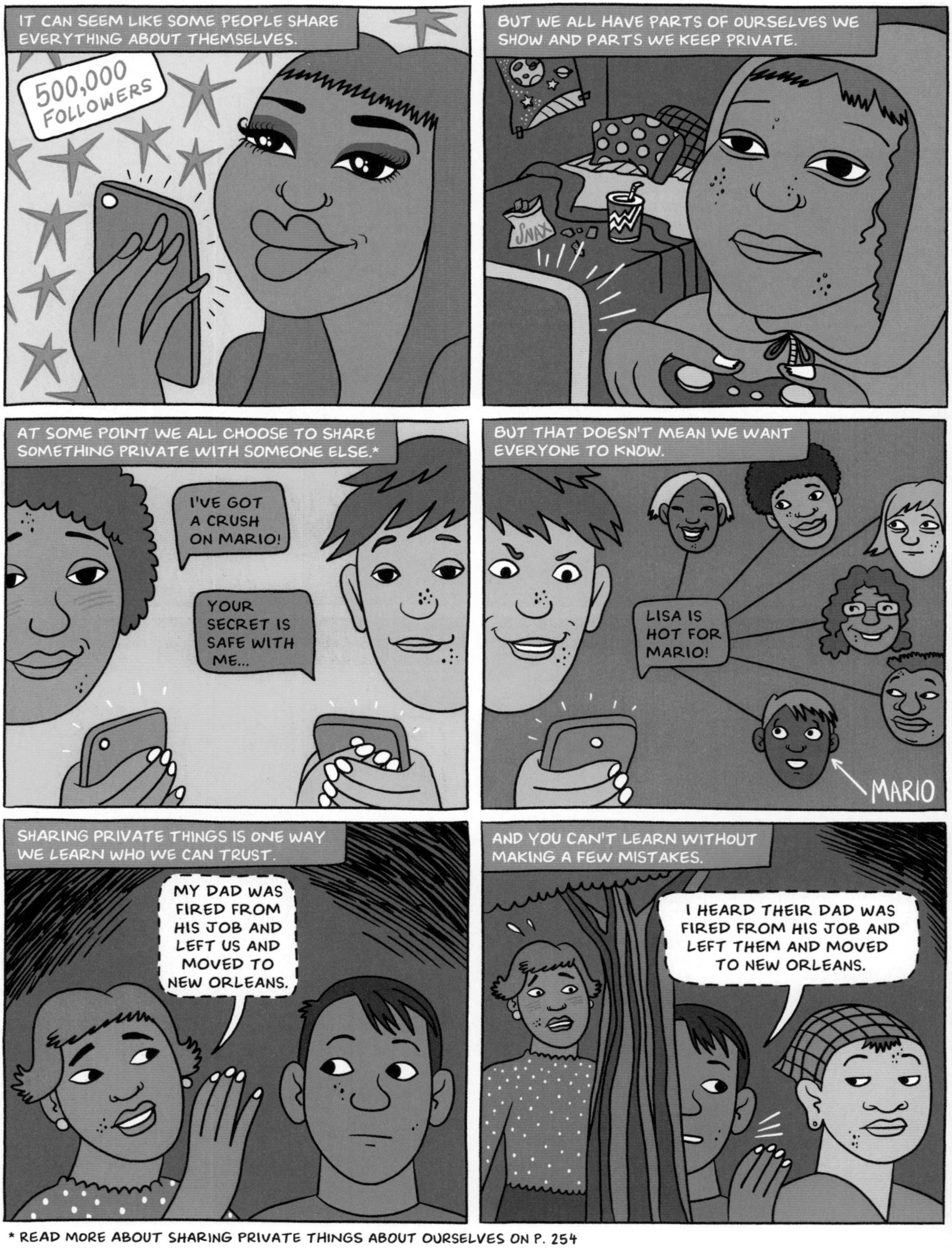
IT CAN SEEM LIKE SOME PEOPLE SHARE EVERYTHING ABOUT THEMSELVES.
500,000 FOLLOWERS
BUT WE ALL HAVE PARTS OF OURSELVES WE SHOW AND PARTS WE KEEP PRIVATE.
SNAX
AT SOME POINT WE ALL CHOOSE TO SHARE SOMETHING PRIVATE WITH SOMEONE ELSE.*
I'VE GOT A CRUSH ON MARIO!
YOUR SECRET IS SAFE WITH ME...
BUT THAT DOESN'T MEAN WE WANT EVERYONE TO KNOW.
LISA IS HOT FOR MARIO!
MARIO
SHARING PRIVATE THINGS IS ONE WAY WE LEARN WHO WE CAN TRUST.
MY DAD WAS FIRED FROM HIS JOB AND LEFT US AND MOVED TO NEW ORLEANS.
AND YOU CAN'T LEARN WITHOUT MAKING A FEW MISTAKES.
I HEARD THEIR DAD WAS FIRED FROM HIS JOB AND LEFT THEM AND MOVED TO NEW ORLEANS.

* READ MORE ABOUT SHARING PRIVATE THINGS ABOUT OURSELVES ON P. 254

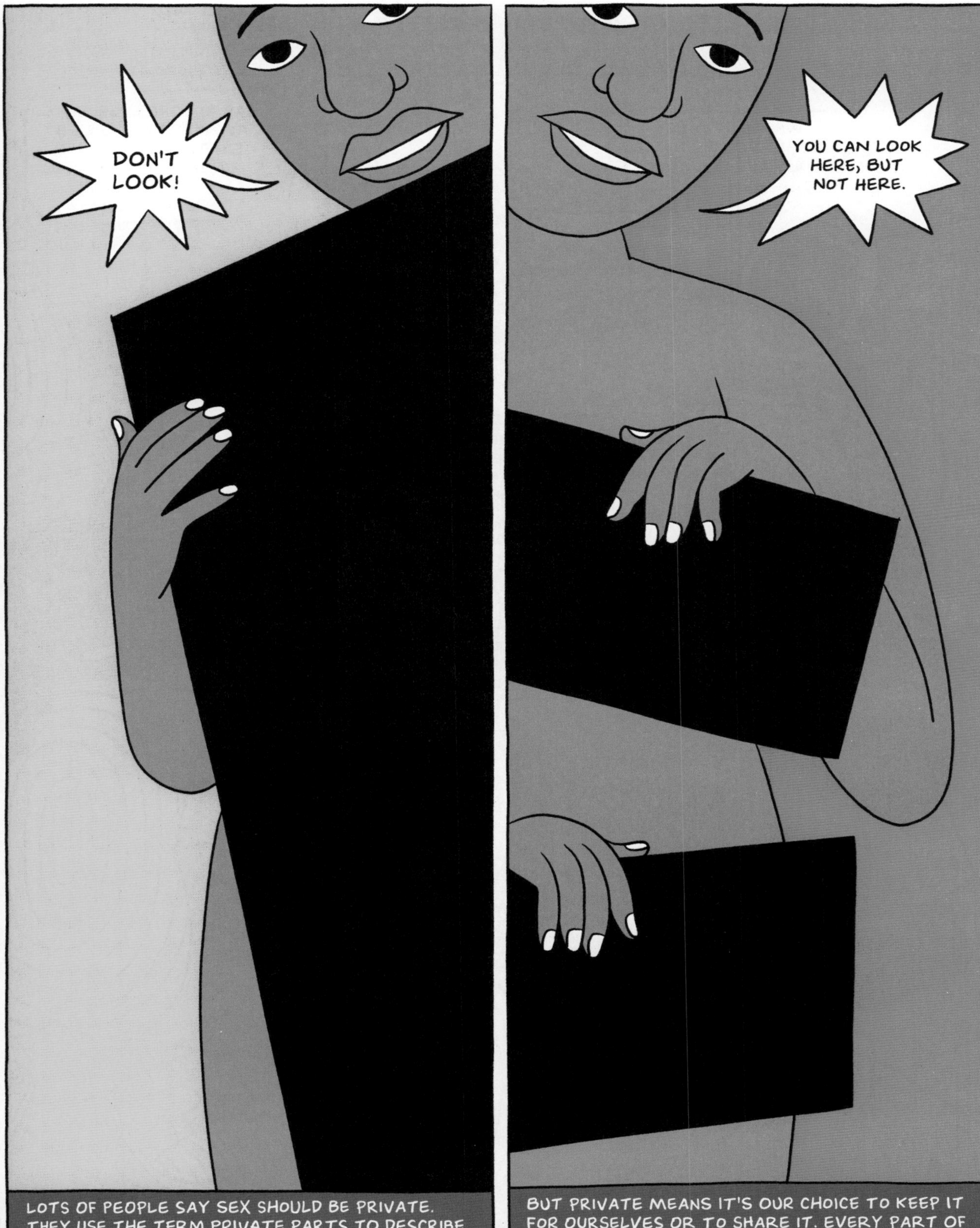
DON'T LOOK!
LOTS OF PEOPLE SAY SEX SHOULD BE PRIVATE. THEY USE THE TERM PRIVATE PARTS TO DESCRIBE PARTS OF THE BODY THAT THEY THINK ARE THE "SEX PARTS."
YOU CAN LOOK HERE, BUT NOT HERE.
BUT PRIVATE MEANS IT'S OUR CHOICE TO KEEP IT FOR OURSELVES OR TO SHARE IT. EVERY PART OF OUR BODY COULD BE PRIVATE, NOT JUST THE PARTS THAT OTHER PEOPLE THINK ARE FOR SEX.

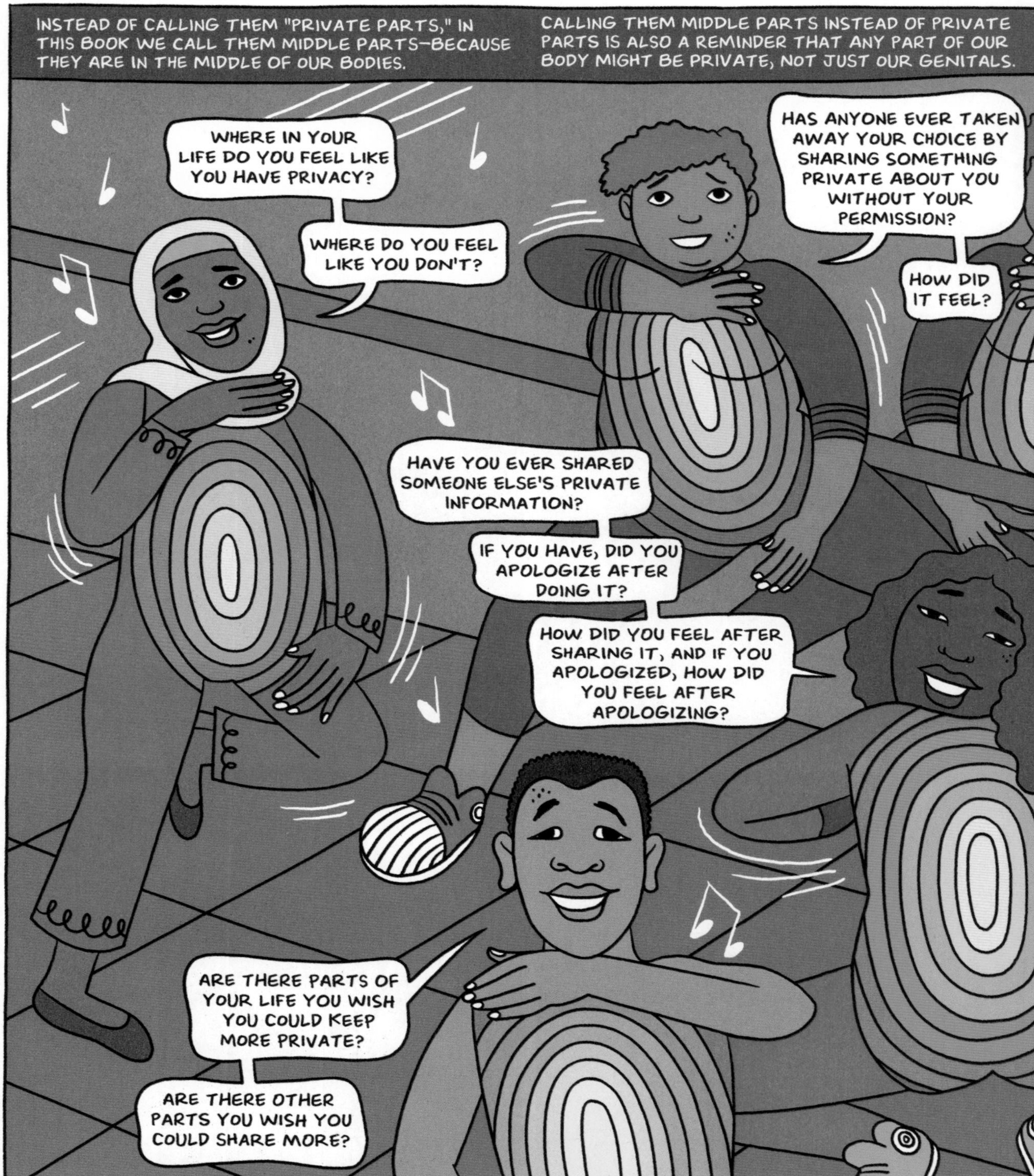

INSTEAD OF CALLING THEM "PRIVATE PARTS," IN THIS BOOK WE CALL THEM MIDDLE PARTS—BECAUSE THEY ARE IN THE MIDDLE OF OUR BODIES.
CALLING THEM MIDDLE PARTS INSTEAD OF PRIVATE PARTS IS ALSO A REMINDER THAT ANY PART OF OUR BODY MIGHT BE PRIVATE, NOT JUST OUR GENITALS.
WHERE IN YOUR LIFE DO YOU FEEL LIKE YOU HAVE PRIVACY?
WHERE DO YOU FEEL LIKE YOU DON'T?
HAS ANYONE EVER TAKEN AWAY YOUR CHOICE BY SHARING SOMETHING PRIVATE ABOUT YOU WITHOUT YOUR PERMISSION?
HOW DID IT FEEL?
HAVE YOU EVER SHARED SOMEONE ELSE'S PRIVATE INFORMATION?
IF YOU HAVE, DID YOU APOLOGIZE AFTER DOING IT?
HOW DID YOU FEEL AFTER SHARING IT, AND IF YOU APOLOGIZED, HOW DID YOU FEEL AFTER APOLOGIZING?
ARE THERE PARTS OF YOUR LIFE YOU WISH YOU COULD KEEP MORE PRIVATE?
ARE THERE OTHER PARTS YOU WISH YOU COULD SHARE MORE?

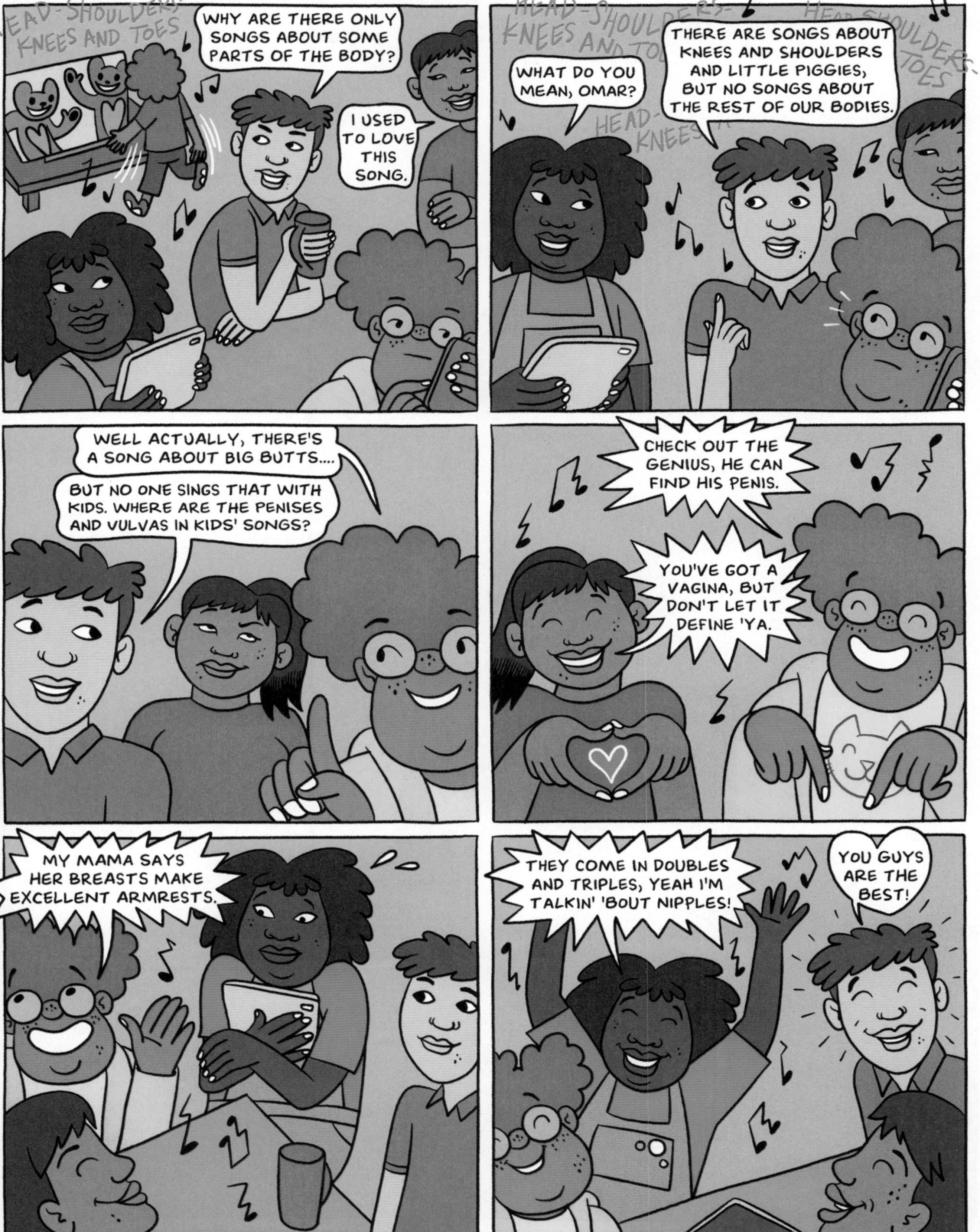
HEAD-SHOULDERS-KNEES AND TOES
WHY ARE THERE ONLY SONGS ABOUT SOME PARTS OF THE BODY?
I USED TO LOVE THIS SONG.
HEAD-SHOULDERS-KNEES AND TOES
WHAT DO YOU MEAN, OMAR?
THERE ARE SONGS ABOUT KNEES AND SHOULDERS AND LITTLE PIGGIES, BUT NO SONGS ABOUT THE REST OF OUR BODIES.
WELL ACTUALLY, THERE'S A SONG ABOUT BIG BUTTS....
BUT NO ONE SINGS THAT WITH KIDS. WHERE ARE THE PENISES AND VULVAS IN KIDS' SONGS?
CHECK OUT THE GENIUS, HE CAN FIND HIS PENIS.
YOU'VE GOT A VAGINA, BUT DON'T LET IT DEFINE 'YA.
MY MAMA SAYS HER BREASTS MAKE EXCELLENT ARMRESTS.
THEY COME IN DOUBLES AND TRIPLES, YEAH I'M TALKIN' 'BOUT NIPPLES!
YOU GUYS ARE THE BEST!

IT'S GOOD TO KNOW SOMETHING ABOUT ALL BODY PARTS: THE PARTS YOU HAVE ALREADY, THE PARTS THAT MIGHT BE STARTING TO DEVELOP, AND THE PARTS YOU DON'T HAVE NOW.

JUST LIKE PEOPLE DON'T TALK MUCH ABOUT SEX, THEY DON'T TALK MUCH ABOUT MIDDLE PARTS, EXCEPT MAYBE TO TELL YOU ABOUT MAKING BABIES. WE WANT TO CHANGE THAT. SO, IN THIS SECTION WE'RE GOING TO SHOW AND TALK ABOUT MIDDLE PARTS WITHOUT ANY BABY MAKING. IF YOU WANT TO KNOW ABOUT BABY MAKING CHECK OUT REPRODUCTION ON P. 295. IF YOU WANT TO KNOW MORE ABOUT HOW MIDDLE PARTS CHANGE DURING PUBERTY, THAT'S COMING IN THE NEXT SECTION.

IN THIS BOOK WE USE THE NAMES FOR PARTS THAT MOST TEACHERS AND HEALTH CARE PROFESSIONALS USE. BUT BODY AUTONOMY MEANS WE ALL GET TO CHOOSE WORDS AND LANGUAGE ABOUT OUR BODIES THAT FIT FOR US.

RESPECT AND JUSTICE INCLUDE LISTENING TO OTHERS WHEN THEY USE DIFFERENT WORDS, AND NOT ACTING LIKE YOUR WORDS, OR THE WORDS IN THIS BOOK, ARE THE ONLY, OR RIGHT, ONES.

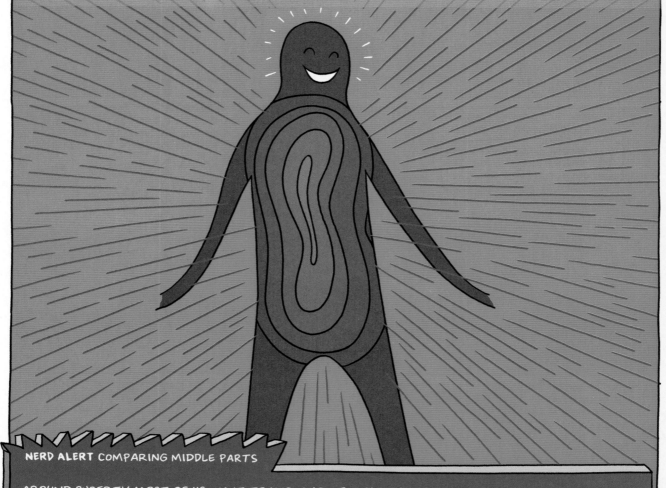

NERD ALERT COMPARING MIDDLE PARTS

AROUND PUBERTY MOST OF US WANT TO KNOW HOW BIG OUR PARTS WILL GET, ESPECIALLY BREASTS AND PENISES. IS THERE A RIGHT SIZE, OR COLOR? HOW SMALL IS TOO SMALL? HOW BIG IS TOO BIG? WHEN IT COMES TO COLOR, EVERYONE HAS DIFFERENT SKIN TONES. THE COLOR OF SKIN IN OUR MIDDLE PARTS CAN BE DIFFERENT FROM THE COLOR OF SKIN ON THE REST OF OUR BODIES.

WHEN IT COMES TO SIZE, THERE'S NO GOOD ANSWER. NO ONE CAN TELL YOU WHAT YOUR BODY IS GOING TO LOOK LIKE, AND WHATEVER IT LOOKS LIKE AT ONE POINT, IT CAN, AND PROBABLY WILL, CHANGE.

WHEN WE COMPARE OUR BODIES TO OTHER PEOPLE'S BODIES, SOMEONE ENDS UP FEELING BAD ABOUT IT. THAT'S WHY YOU WON'T FIND A LOT ABOUT THE SIZE OF YOUR MIDDLE PARTS IN THIS BOOK. SIZE COMPARISONS ARE NOT NERD ALERT—APPROVED!

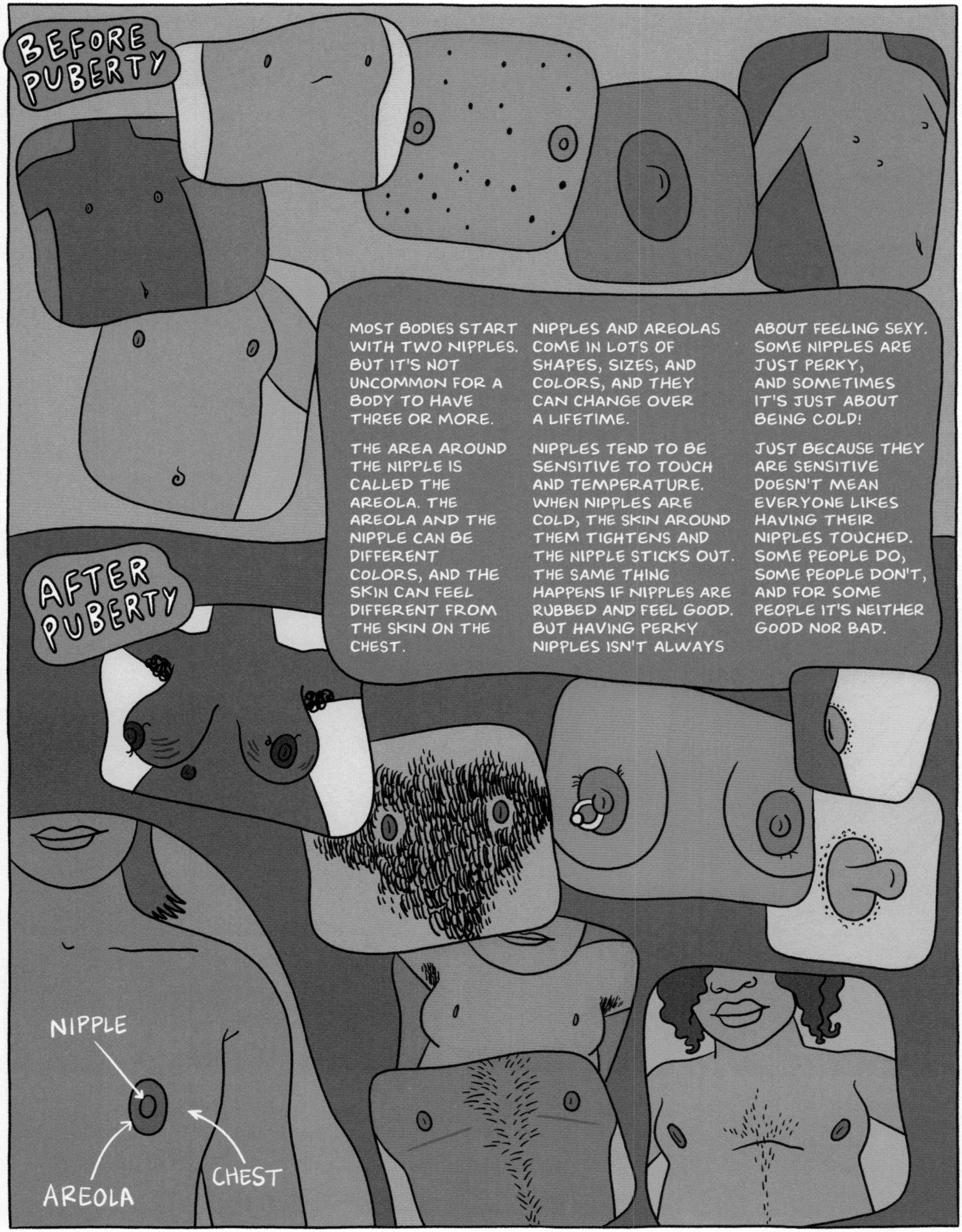
BEFORE PUBERTY
MOST BODIES START WITH TWO NIPPLES. BUT IT'S NOT UNCOMMON FOR A BODY TO HAVE THREE OR MORE.
THE AREA AROUND THE NIPPLE IS CALLED THE AREOLA. THE AREOLA AND THE NIPPLE CAN BE DIFFERENT COLORS, AND THE SKIN CAN FEEL DIFFERENT FROM THE SKIN ON THE CHEST.
NIPPLES AND AREOLAS COME IN LOTS OF SHAPES, SIZES, AND COLORS, AND THEY CAN CHANGE OVER A LIFETIME.
NIPPLES TEND TO BE SENSITIVE TO TOUCH AND TEMPERATURE. WHEN NIPPLES ARE COLD, THE SKIN AROUND THEM TIGHTENS AND THE NIPPLE STICKS OUT. THE SAME THING HAPPENS IF NIPPLES ARE RUBBED AND FEEL GOOD. BUT HAVING PERKY NIPPLES ISN'T ALWAYS ABOUT FEELING SEXY. SOME NIPPLES ARE JUST PERKY, AND SOMETIMES IT'S JUST ABOUT BEING COLD!
JUST BECAUSE THEY ARE SENSITIVE DOESN'T MEAN EVERYONE LIKES HAVING THEIR NIPPLES TOUCHED. SOME PEOPLE DO, SOME PEOPLE DON'T, AND FOR SOME PEOPLE IT'S NEITHER GOOD NOR BAD.
AFTER PUBERTY
NIPPLE
AREOLA
CHEST

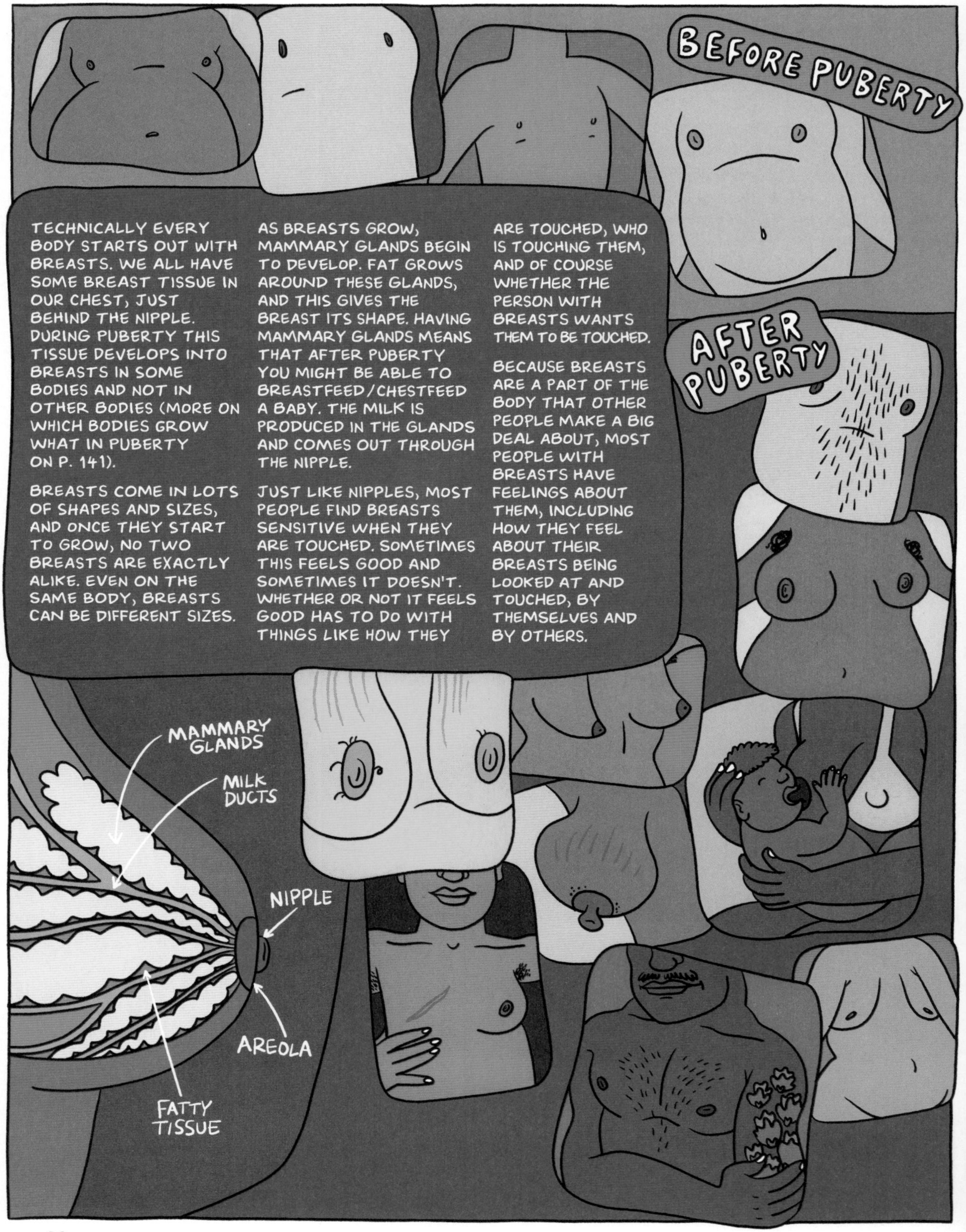
BEFORE PUBERTY
AFTER PUBERTY
MAMMARY GLANDS
MILK DUCTS
NIPPLE
AREOLA
FATTY TISSUE

TECHNICALLY EVERY BODY STARTS OUT WITH BREASTS. WE ALL HAVE SOME BREAST TISSUE IN OUR CHEST, JUST BEHIND THE NIPPLE. DURING PUBERTY THIS TISSUE DEVELOPS INTO BREASTS IN SOME BODIES AND NOT IN OTHER BODIES (MORE ON WHICH BODIES GROW WHAT IN PUBERTY ON P. 141).

BREASTS COME IN LOTS OF SHAPES AND SIZES, AND ONCE THEY START TO GROW, NO TWO BREASTS ARE EXACTLY ALIKE. EVEN ON THE SAME BODY, BREASTS CAN BE DIFFERENT SIZES.

AS BREASTS GROW, MAMMARY GLANDS BEGIN TO DEVELOP. FAT GROWS AROUND THESE GLANDS, AND THIS GIVES THE BREAST ITS SHAPE. HAVING MAMMARY GLANDS MEANS THAT AFTER PUBERTY YOU MIGHT BE ABLE TO BREASTFEED/CHESTFEED A BABY. THE MILK IS PRODUCED IN THE GLANDS AND COMES OUT THROUGH THE NIPPLE.

JUST LIKE NIPPLES, MOST PEOPLE FIND BREASTS SENSITIVE WHEN THEY ARE TOUCHED. SOMETIMES THIS FEELS GOOD AND SOMETIMES IT DOESN'T. WHETHER OR NOT IT FEELS GOOD HAS TO DO WITH THINGS LIKE HOW THEY ARE TOUCHED, WHO IS TOUCHING THEM, AND OF COURSE WHETHER THE PERSON WITH BREASTS WANTS THEM TO BE TOUCHED.

BECAUSE BREASTS ARE A PART OF THE BODY THAT OTHER PEOPLE MAKE A BIG DEAL ABOUT, MOST PEOPLE WITH BREASTS HAVE FEELINGS ABOUT THEM, INCLUDING HOW THEY FEEL ABOUT THEIR BREASTS BEING LOOKED AT AND TOUCHED, BY THEMSELVES AND BY OTHERS.

BUTTOCKS

EVERY BODY HAS BUTTOCKS. THEY GO BY MANY NAMES INCLUDING BUTT—THE SHORT FORM OF BUTTOCKS—BOTTOM, REAR END, BEHIND, BUM, AND MORE.

EVERY BUTT IS A LITTLE BIT DIFFERENT IN SIZE AND SHAPE, AND EVERY BUTT CHANGES DURING PUBERTY AND BEYOND. BUMS CAN GET BIGGER AND ROUNDER, THEY CAN GET SMALLER AND FLATTER, THEY CAN DEVELOP WRINKLES AND STRETCH MARKS AND MORE.

BETWEEN THE TWO CHEEKS IS THE ANUS. THIS IS THE HOLE WHERE, FOR MOST OF US, FECES (A.K.A. POOP) COMES OUT.

INSIDE THE ANUS THERE ARE TWO SPHINCTER MUSCLES, WHICH CONTROL WHEN THE ANUS TIGHTENS AND WHEN IT RELAXES.

BECAUSE THE ANUS IS ONE OF THE PLACES WHERE THE OUTSIDE OF THE BODY MEETS THE INSIDE, AND IT IS WHERE FECES COMES OUT, IT'S IMPORTANT TO WASH HANDS BEFORE AND AFTER TOUCHING IT. GETTING FECES IN ANY OTHER OPENING (MOUTH, EYES, VAGINA) CAN LEAD TO AN INFECTION, WHICH CAN BE ANNOYING OR BECOME A SERIOUS HEALTH PROBLEM.

LIKE OTHER HOLES IN THE BODY, THE ANUS IS USUALLY VERY SENSITIVE, WHICH MEANS IT CAN FEEL GOOD TO TOUCH BUT CAN ALSO HURT IF IT IS TOUCHED ROUGHLY. SPHINCTER MUSCLES ALSO CAN FEEL GOOD OR HURT DEPENDING ON HOW THEY ARE TOUCHED.

THE AREA BETWEEN THE ANUS AND THE GENITALS IS CALLED THE PERINEUM. LIKE OTHER MIDDLE PARTS, THE PERINEUM IS OFTEN SENSITIVE TO PRESSURE AND TOUCH, AND CAN FEEL GOOD WHEN TOUCHED.

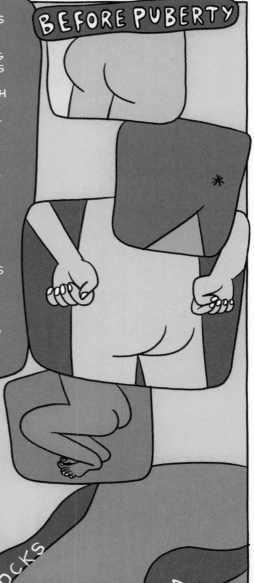

BEFORE PUBERTY

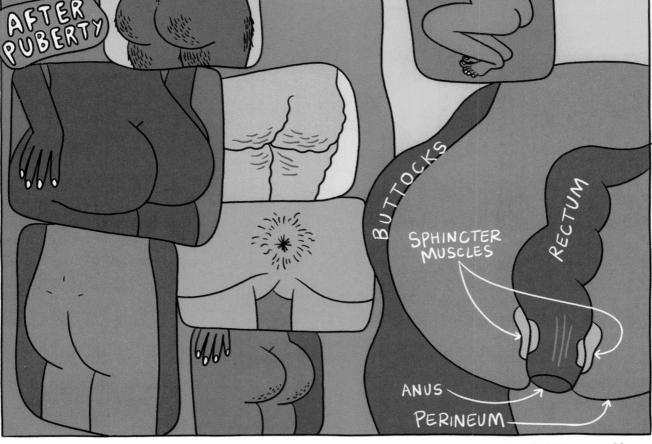

AFTER PUBERTY

BUTTOCKS

SPHINCTER MUSCLES

RECTUM

ANUS

PERINEUM

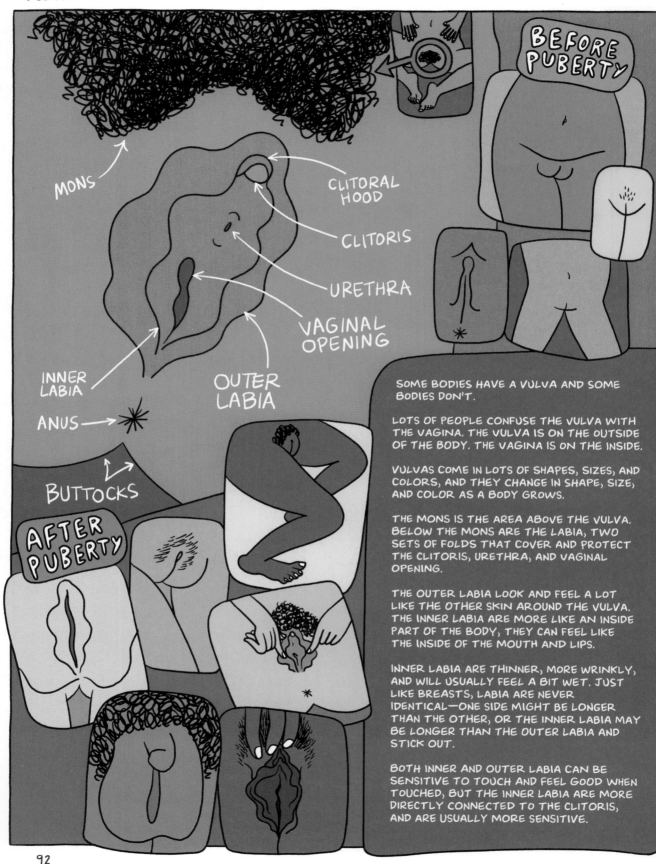

BEFORE PUBERTY

MONS

CLITORAL HOOD

CLITORIS

URETHRA

VAGINAL OPENING

INNER LABIA

OUTER LABIA

ANUS

BUTTOCKS

AFTER PUBERTY

SOME BODIES HAVE A VULVA AND SOME BODIES DON'T.

LOTS OF PEOPLE CONFUSE THE VULVA WITH THE VAGINA. THE VULVA IS ON THE OUTSIDE OF THE BODY. THE VAGINA IS ON THE INSIDE.

VULVAS COME IN LOTS OF SHAPES, SIZES, AND COLORS, AND THEY CHANGE IN SHAPE, SIZE, AND COLOR AS A BODY GROWS.

THE MONS IS THE AREA ABOVE THE VULVA. BELOW THE MONS ARE THE LABIA, TWO SETS OF FOLDS THAT COVER AND PROTECT THE CLITORIS, URETHRA, AND VAGINAL OPENING.

THE OUTER LABIA LOOK AND FEEL A LOT LIKE THE OTHER SKIN AROUND THE VULVA. THE INNER LABIA ARE MORE LIKE AN INSIDE PART OF THE BODY, THEY CAN FEEL LIKE THE INSIDE OF THE MOUTH AND LIPS.

INNER LABIA ARE THINNER, MORE WRINKLY, AND WILL USUALLY FEEL A BIT WET. JUST LIKE BREASTS, LABIA ARE NEVER IDENTICAL—ONE SIDE MIGHT BE LONGER THAN THE OTHER, OR THE INNER LABIA MAY BE LONGER THAN THE OUTER LABIA AND STICK OUT.

BOTH INNER AND OUTER LABIA CAN BE SENSITIVE TO TOUCH AND FEEL GOOD WHEN TOUCHED, BUT THE INNER LABIA ARE MORE DIRECTLY CONNECTED TO THE CLITORIS, AND ARE USUALLY MORE SENSITIVE.

CLITORIS

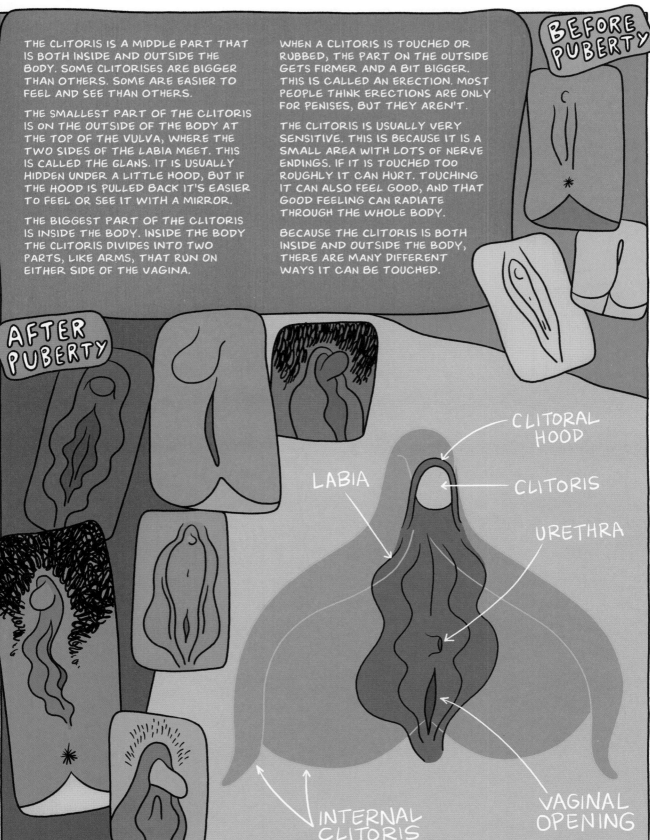

THE CLITORIS IS A MIDDLE PART THAT IS BOTH INSIDE AND OUTSIDE THE BODY. SOME CLITORISES ARE BIGGER THAN OTHERS. SOME ARE EASIER TO FEEL AND SEE THAN OTHERS.

THE SMALLEST PART OF THE CLITORIS IS ON THE OUTSIDE OF THE BODY AT THE TOP OF THE VULVA, WHERE THE TWO SIDES OF THE LABIA MEET. THIS IS CALLED THE GLANS. IT IS USUALLY HIDDEN UNDER A LITTLE HOOD, BUT IF THE HOOD IS PULLED BACK IT'S EASIER TO FEEL OR SEE IT WITH A MIRROR.

THE BIGGEST PART OF THE CLITORIS IS INSIDE THE BODY. INSIDE THE BODY THE CLITORIS DIVIDES INTO TWO PARTS, LIKE ARMS, THAT RUN ON EITHER SIDE OF THE VAGINA.

WHEN A CLITORIS IS TOUCHED OR RUBBED, THE PART ON THE OUTSIDE GETS FIRMER AND A BIT BIGGER. THIS IS CALLED AN ERECTION. MOST PEOPLE THINK ERECTIONS ARE ONLY FOR PENISES, BUT THEY AREN'T.

THE CLITORIS IS USUALLY VERY SENSITIVE. THIS IS BECAUSE IT IS A SMALL AREA WITH LOTS OF NERVE ENDINGS. IF IT IS TOUCHED TOO ROUGHLY IT CAN HURT. TOUCHING IT CAN ALSO FEEL GOOD, AND THAT GOOD FEELING CAN RADIATE THROUGH THE WHOLE BODY.

BECAUSE THE CLITORIS IS BOTH INSIDE AND OUTSIDE THE BODY, THERE ARE MANY DIFFERENT WAYS IT CAN BE TOUCHED.

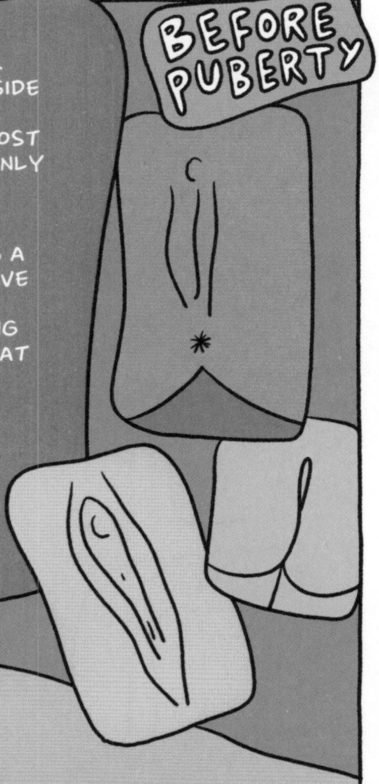
BEFORE PUBERTY

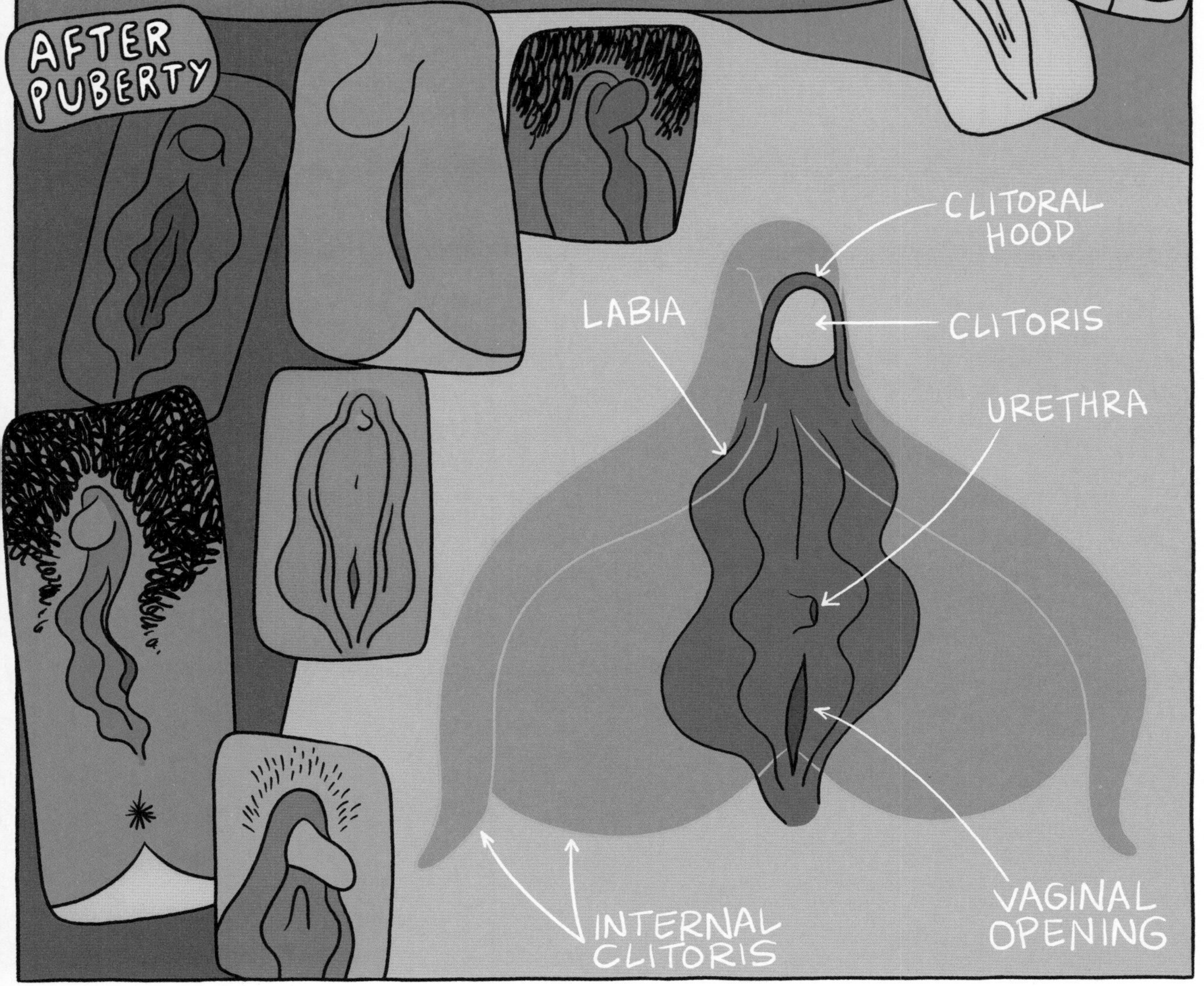
AFTER PUBERTY
CLITORAL HOOD
LABIA
CLITORIS
URETHRA
VAGINAL OPENING
INTERNAL CLITORIS

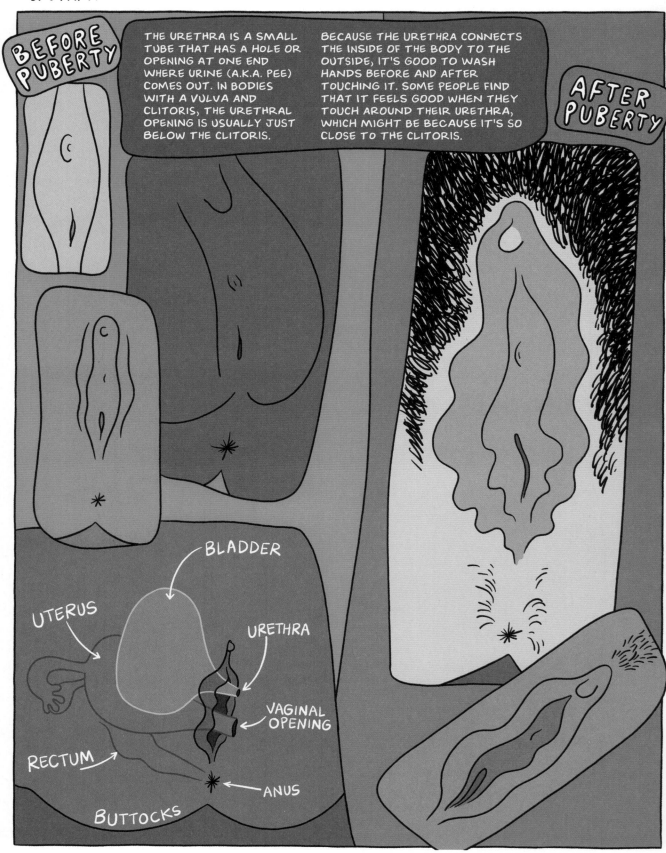

BEFORE PUBERTY

AFTER PUBERTY

THE URETHRA IS A SMALL TUBE THAT HAS A HOLE OR OPENING AT ONE END WHERE URINE (A.K.A. PEE) COMES OUT. IN BODIES WITH A VULVA AND CLITORIS, THE URETHRAL OPENING IS USUALLY JUST BELOW THE CLITORIS.

BECAUSE THE URETHRA CONNECTS THE INSIDE OF THE BODY TO THE OUTSIDE, IT'S GOOD TO WASH HANDS BEFORE AND AFTER TOUCHING IT. SOME PEOPLE FIND THAT IT FEELS GOOD WHEN THEY TOUCH AROUND THEIR URETHRA, WHICH MIGHT BE BECAUSE IT'S SO CLOSE TO THE CLITORIS.

BLADDER

UTERUS

URETHRA

VAGINAL OPENING

RECTUM

ANUS

BUTTOCKS

BELOW THE URETHRA IS THE OPENING TO THE VAGINA. THE VAGINA IS A STRONG AND STRETCHY TUBE THAT GOES FROM THE OUTSIDE OF THE BODY (THE VAGINAL OPENING) UP TO THE CERVIX, WHICH IS THE AREA THAT CONNECTS THE VAGINA TO THE UTERUS (MORE ABOUT THE UTERUS IN THE REPRODUCTION SECTION, P. 295).

THE WALLS OF THE VAGINA ARE MUSCULAR. THEY CAN STRETCH A LOT AND THEN RETURN TO THEIR ORIGINAL RESTING SHAPE AND PLACE.

BEHIND THE VAGINAL WALLS ARE GLANDS, WHICH PRODUCE FLUID OR LUBRICATION. THESE GLANDS KEEP THE INSIDE OF THE VAGINA A LITTLE WET, WHICH IS ONE WAY THE BODY TAKES CARE OF ITSELF. THE CERVIX ALSO PRODUCES FLUID, CALLED CERVICAL MUCUS.

IN YOUNGER BODIES, JUST INSIDE THE VAGINAL OPENING THERE IS A THIN MEMBRANE THAT PARTLY COVERS THE OPENING OF THE VAGINAL CANAL. THIS MEMBRANE IS CALLED THE HYMEN. SOME PEOPLE THINK OF THE HYMEN AS A BARRIER OR SHIELD, BUT IT ISN'T.

BECAUSE THE VAGINA, CLITORIS, PERINEUM, AND ANUS ARE ALL SO CLOSE TOGETHER, TOUCHING INSIDE THE VAGINA CAN FEEL GOOD.

UTERUS
CERVIX
BUTTOCK
BLADDER
LABIA
CLITORIS
VAGINAL CANAL
RECTUM
URETHRA
ANUS
VAGINAL OPENING
GLANDS
HYMEN
HYMEN

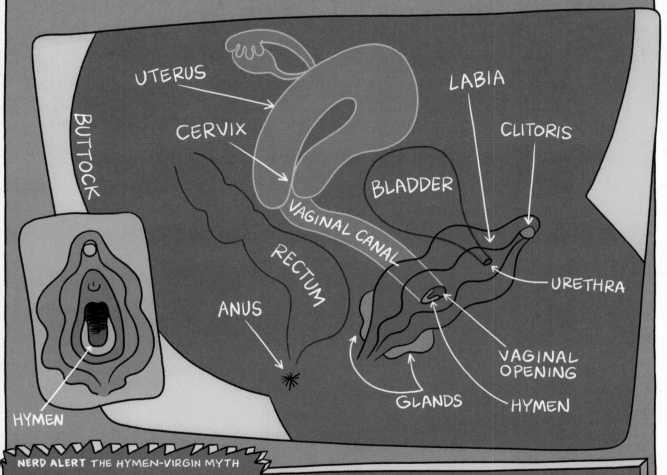

NERD ALERT THE HYMEN-VIRGIN MYTH

THERE'S A VERY OLD IDEA THAT THE HYMEN IS LIKE SOME KIND OF SEAL IN THE VAGINA, AND THE WAY SOMEONE STOPS BEING A VIRGIN IS BY HAVING THAT SEAL BROKEN DURING INTERCOURSE. SOME PEOPLE STILL CALL THIS "POPPING YOUR CHERRY." BUT THAT'S NOT HOW THE HYMEN WORKS.

THE HYMEN IS A RING OF STRETCHY TISSUE AROUND THE ENTRANCE OF THE VAGINA. HYMENS CAN COME IN DIFFERENT SHAPES, BUT THE MOST COMMON IS A HALF-MOON THAT ALLOWS MENSTRUAL BLOOD TO FLOW OUT. THE HYMEN DOESN'T BREAK OR DISAPPEAR AT PUBERTY OR AFTER SOMEONE STARTS HAVING SEX. IT THINS OUT AND WEARS DOWN, BUT PARTS OF THE HYMEN REMAIN IN THE VAGINAL WALLS.

YOU CAN'T TELL IF SOMEONE IS A VIRGIN OR NOT BASED ON THEIR HYMEN. YOU CAN READ MORE ABOUT VIRGINITY ON P. 370.

SOME BODIES HAVE A PENIS AND SOME BODIES DON'T. EVERY PENIS LOOKS A BIT DIFFERENT IN SHAPE, SIZE, AND COLOR. AND EVERY PENIS LOOKS DIFFERENT WHEN IT'S SOFT AND WHEN IT'S HARD.

THE SHAFT IS THE LONGEST PART OF THE PENIS. IT ENDS AT THE HEAD, ALSO CALLED THE GLANS. THIS IS USUALLY THE MOST SENSITIVE PART OF THE PENIS. MOST PENISES AREN'T COMPLETELY STRAIGHT; THEY BEND ONE WAY OR ANOTHER.

JUST LIKE THE CLITORIS, WHEN A PENIS IS TOUCHED OR RUBBED IT CAN GET FIRMER AND BIGGER, WHICH IS CALLED AN ERECTION.

AS THE BODY GROWS, THE PENIS GROWS TOO.

LIKE THE CLITORIS, THE PENIS CAN BE VERY SENSITIVE, ESPECIALLY AROUND THE GLANS OR TIP. TOUCHING IT CAN FEEL WARM AND TINGLY NOT JUST IN AND AROUND THE PENIS BUT THROUGH THE WHOLE BODY.

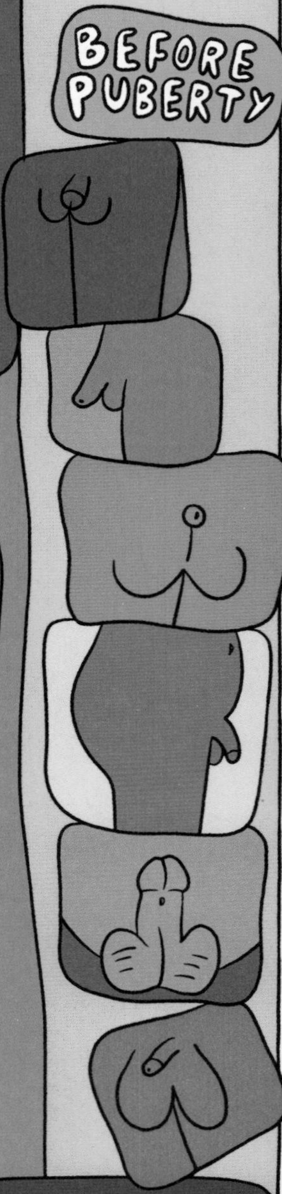
BEFORE PUBERTY

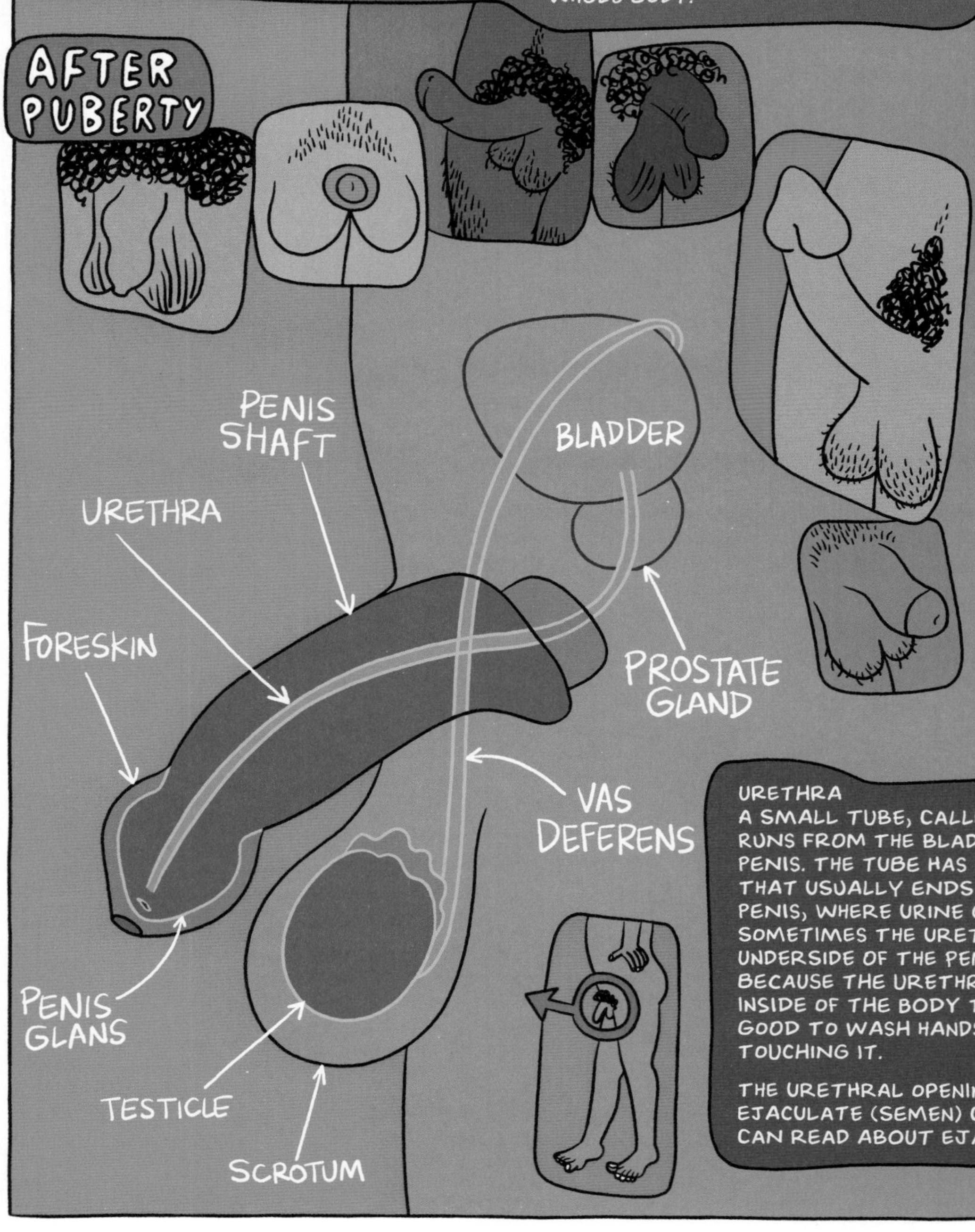
AFTER PUBERTY
PENIS SHAFT
BLADDER
URETHRA
FORESKIN
PROSTATE GLAND
VAS DEFERENS
PENIS GLANS
TESTICLE
SCROTUM

URETHRA
A SMALL TUBE, CALLED THE URETHRA, RUNS FROM THE BLADDER THROUGH THE PENIS. THE TUBE HAS A HOLE OR OPENING THAT USUALLY ENDS AT THE TIP OF THE PENIS, WHERE URINE COMES OUT. SOMETIMES THE URETHRA ENDS ON THE UNDERSIDE OF THE PENIS AND NOT THE TIP. BECAUSE THE URETHRA CONNECTS THE INSIDE OF THE BODY TO THE OUTSIDE, IT'S GOOD TO WASH HANDS BEFORE AND AFTER TOUCHING IT.

THE URETHRAL OPENING IS ALSO WHERE EJACULATE (SEMEN) CAN COME OUT. YOU CAN READ ABOUT EJACULATION ON P. 170.

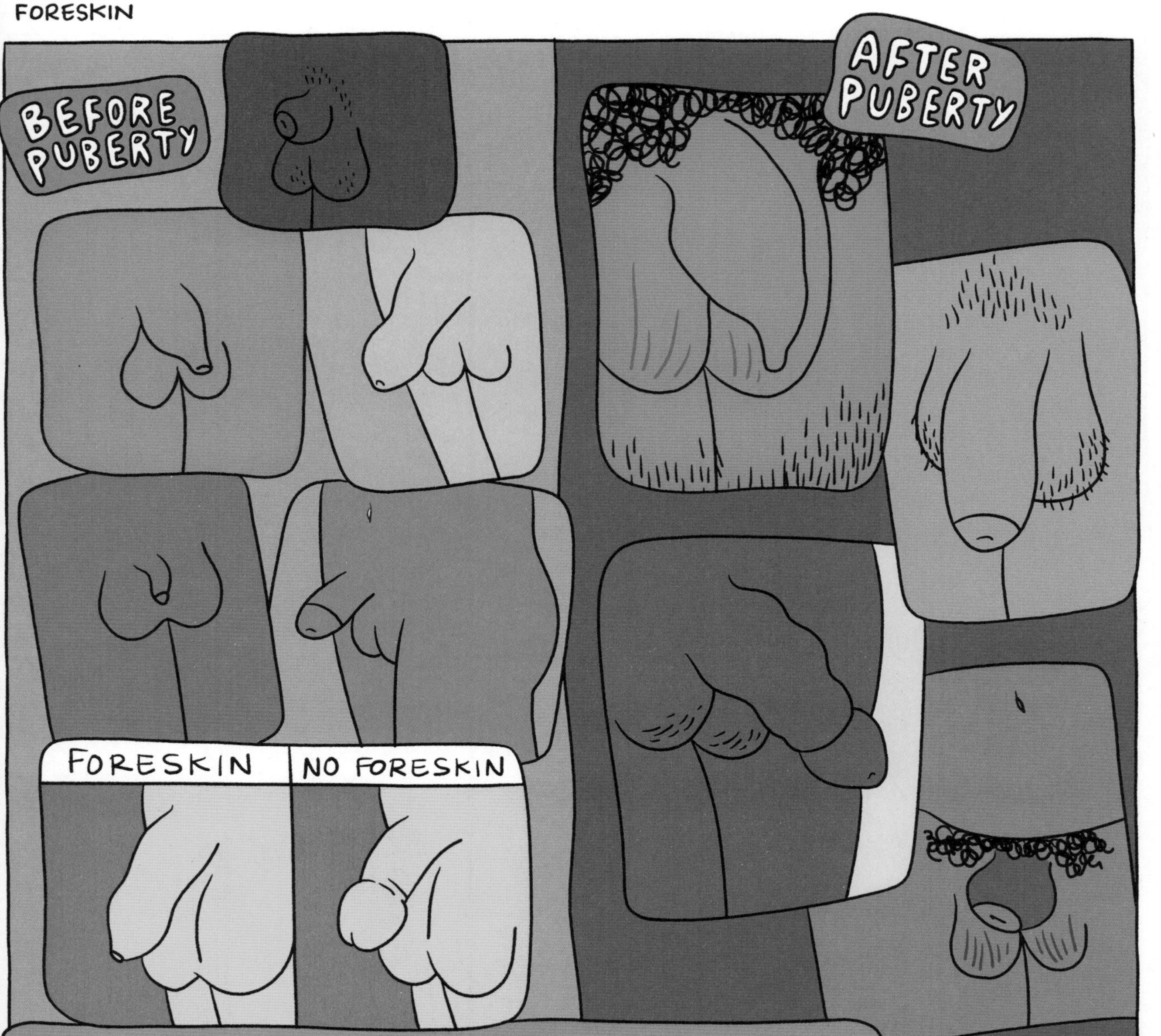
BEFORE PUBERTY
AFTER PUBERTY
FORESKIN
NO FORESKIN

IF A BABY IS BORN WITH A PENIS, THERE WILL USUALLY BE A LAYER OF SKIN THAT COVERS THE END OF THE PENIS LIKE A HOOD. THIS IS CALLED THE FORESKIN. THE FORESKIN PROTECTS THE HEAD OF THE PENIS WHEN A PENIS IS SOFT.

WHEN A BODY IS YOUNG, THE FORESKIN IS OFTEN TIGHT AND MAY NOT MOVE A LOT. IT'S IMPORTANT NOT TO PULL IT TOO HARD BEFORE IT LOOSENS ON ITS OWN.

SOMETIMES A FORESKIN THAT'S TOO TIGHT CAN CAUSE PAIN. WHEN THIS HAPPENS THERE ARE THINGS A DOCTOR CAN DO TO REDUCE THE PAIN.

SOME FAMILIES CHOOSE TO HAVE THE FORESKIN REMOVED, USUALLY FOR RELIGIOUS REASONS, OR BECAUSE OTHER PEOPLE IN THEIR FAMILY AND COMMUNITY HAD IT REMOVED. THE PROCEDURE OF REMOVING THE FORESKIN IS CALLED CIRCUMCISION, AND IT'S USUALLY DONE SHORTLY AFTER A BABY IS BORN.

WHEN A PENIS IS SOFT, YOU CAN TELL IF IT'S CIRCUMCISED BECAUSE THE HEAD IS ALWAYS VISIBLE ON A CIRCUMCISED PENIS. WHEN ERECT, CIRCUMCISED AND INTACT PENISES LOOK MORE SIMILAR TO EACH OTHER.

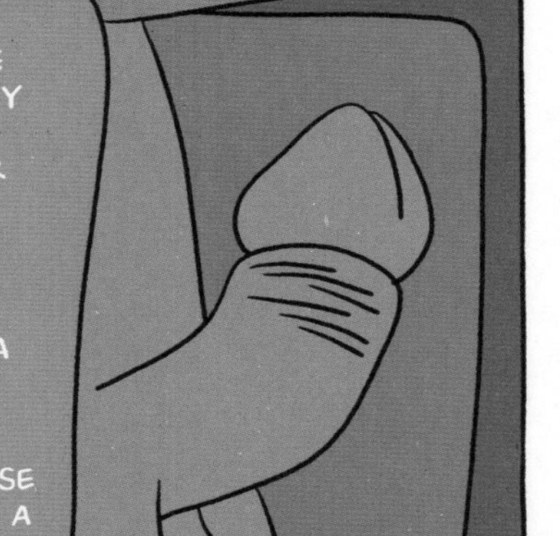

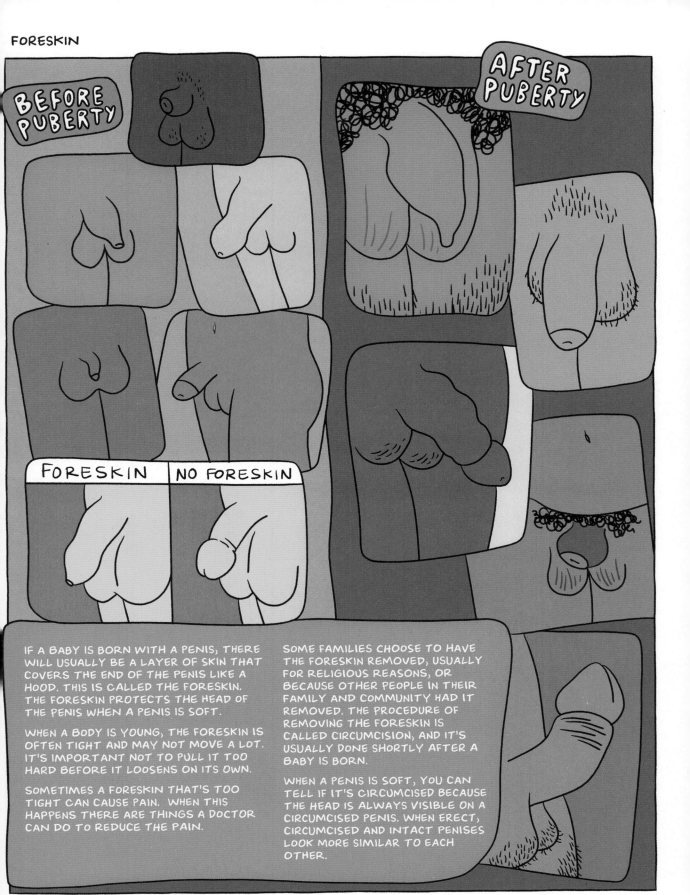

SCROTUM AND TESTICLES

THE SCROTUM LOOKS KIND OF LIKE A LITTLE BAG OR SAC MADE OF WRINKLY SKIN THAT SITS BELOW AND BEHIND THE PENIS. THE SCROTUM HOLDS AND PROTECTS THE TESTICLES, ALSO CALLED BALLS.

MOST BODIES WITH TESTICLES HAVE TWO OF THEM, SOME HAVE ONE. LIKE BREASTS AND LABIA, TESTICLES AREN'T EXACTLY THE SAME. EVEN ON THE SAME BODY ONE CAN BE A BIT BIGGER THAN THE OTHER, AND ONE MIGHT HANG LOWER THAN THE OTHER.

TESTICLES ARE VERY SENSITIVE TO PRESSURE AND TEMPERATURE, WHICH IS WHY THEY ARE PROTECTED INSIDE THE SCROTUM. THE SCROTUM PROTECTS THE TESTICLES FROM BEING HIT OR HURT, AND IT ALSO ACTS AS A KIND OF HEATING/COOLING SYSTEM TO MAKE SURE THE TESTICLES STAY AT THE RIGHT TEMPERATURE ALL THE TIME.

WHEN IT'S COLD, THE SCROTUM TIGHTENS AND PULLS CLOSER TO THE BODY, MAKING BOTH THE SCROTUM AND PENIS LOOK SMALLER. WHEN IT'S HOT, THE SKIN GETS LOOSER AND THE SCROTUM GETS LARGER, GIVING THE TESTICLES MORE ROOM TO COOL DOWN.

EVEN WITH THE SCROTUM PROTECTING THEM, TESTICLES CAN BE HURT IF THEY ARE TOUCHED ROUGHLY, WHICH IS WHY SOME PEOPLE WITH TESTICLES WEAR PROTECTIVE GEAR WHEN PLAYING SPORTS.

JUST LIKE THE PENIS, THE SCROTUM IS SENSITIVE TO TOUCH AND CAN FEEL VERY GOOD WHEN TOUCHED.

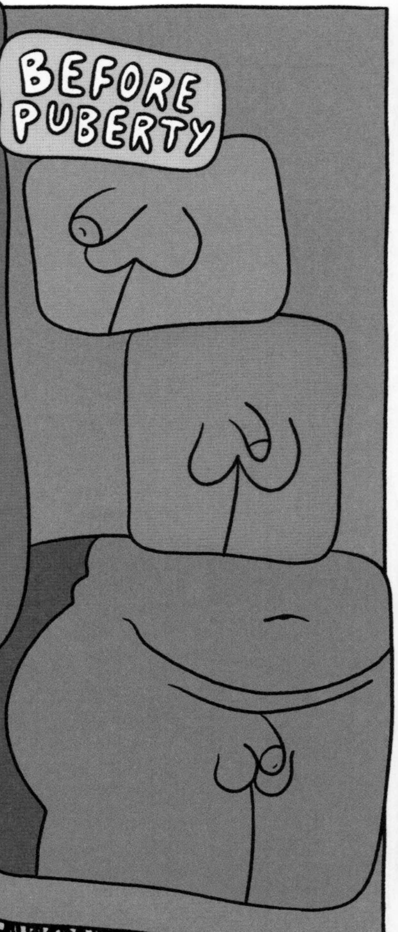
BEFORE PUBERTY

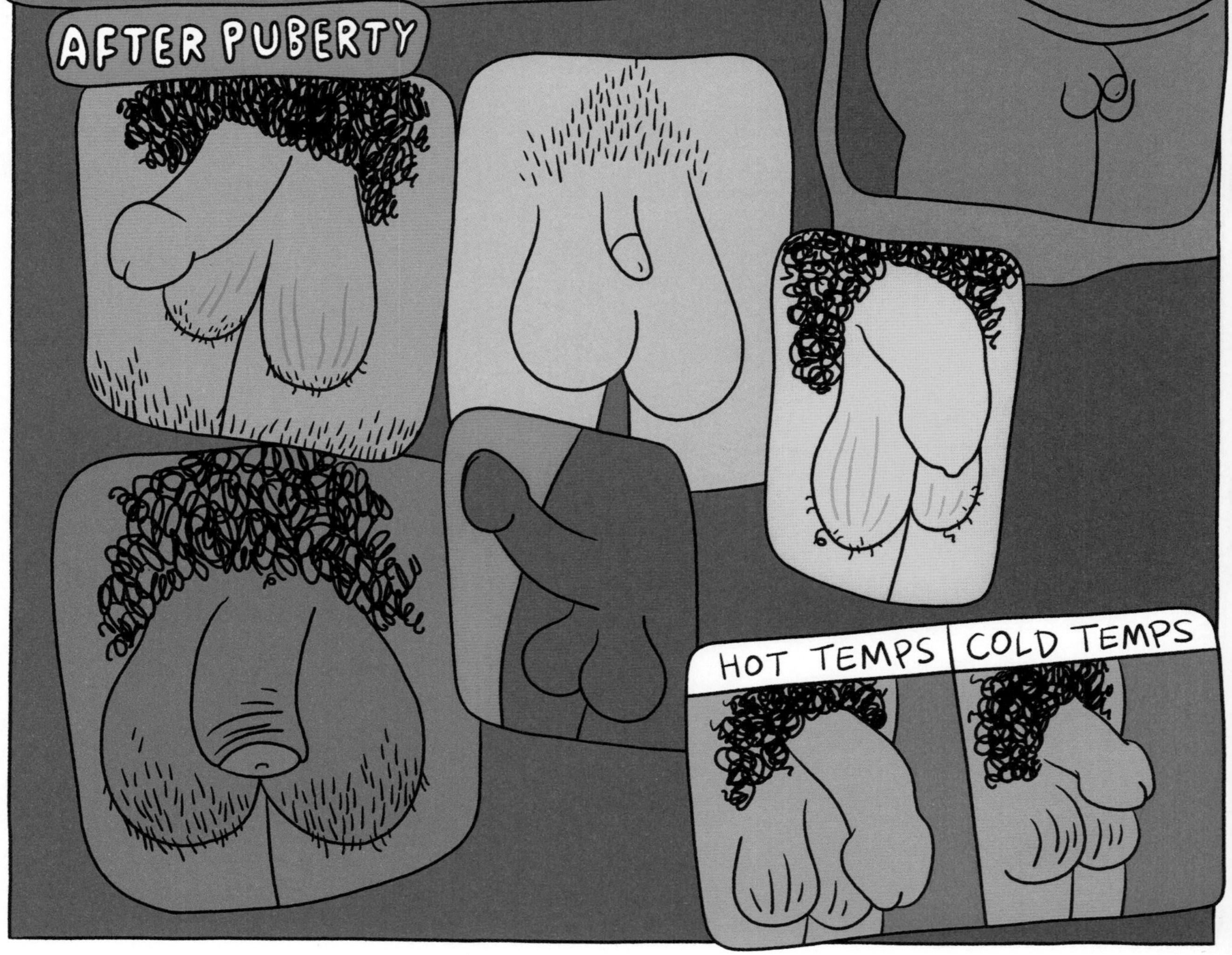
AFTER PUBERTY
HOT TEMPS
COLD TEMPS

ERECTIONS

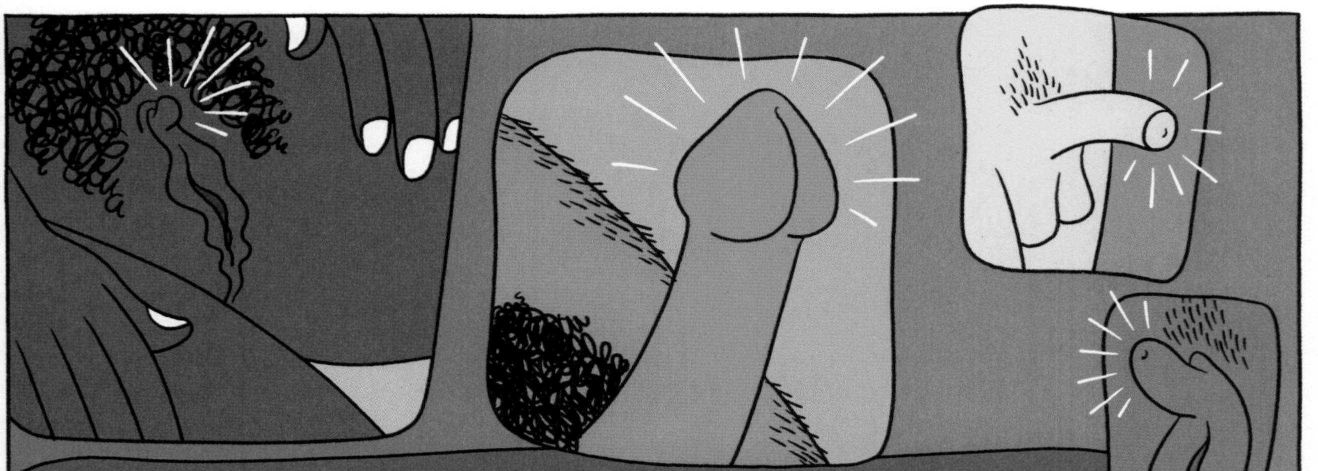

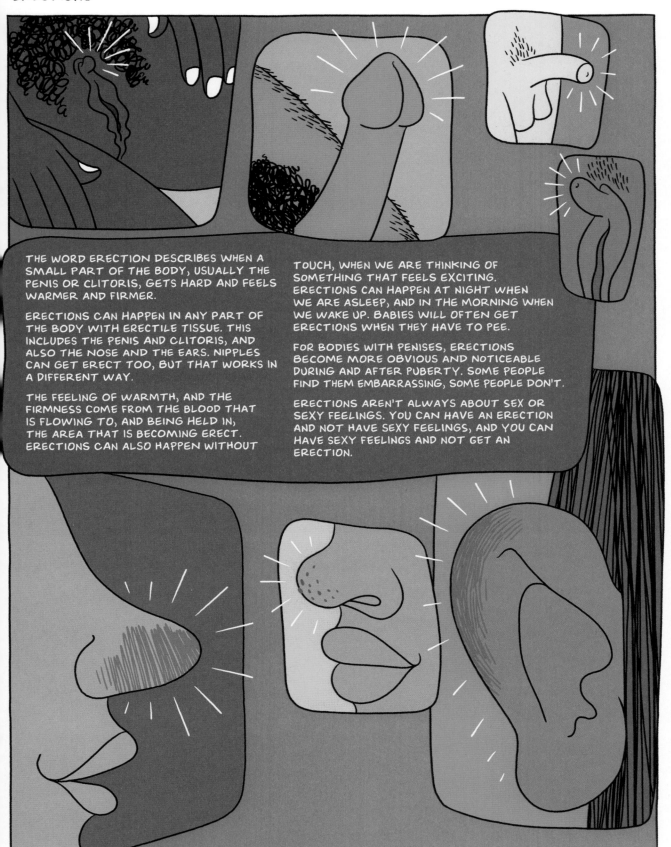

THE WORD ERECTION DESCRIBES WHEN A SMALL PART OF THE BODY, USUALLY THE PENIS OR CLITORIS, GETS HARD AND FEELS WARMER AND FIRMER.

ERECTIONS CAN HAPPEN IN ANY PART OF THE BODY WITH ERECTILE TISSUE. THIS INCLUDES THE PENIS AND CLITORIS, AND ALSO THE NOSE AND THE EARS. NIPPLES CAN GET ERECT TOO, BUT THAT WORKS IN A DIFFERENT WAY.

THE FEELING OF WARMTH, AND THE FIRMNESS COME FROM THE BLOOD THAT IS FLOWING TO, AND BEING HELD IN, THE AREA THAT IS BECOMING ERECT. ERECTIONS CAN ALSO HAPPEN WITHOUT TOUCH, WHEN WE ARE THINKING OF SOMETHING THAT FEELS EXCITING. ERECTIONS CAN HAPPEN AT NIGHT WHEN WE ARE ASLEEP, AND IN THE MORNING WHEN WE WAKE UP. BABIES WILL OFTEN GET ERECTIONS WHEN THEY HAVE TO PEE.

FOR BODIES WITH PENISES, ERECTIONS BECOME MORE OBVIOUS AND NOTICEABLE DURING AND AFTER PUBERTY. SOME PEOPLE FIND THEM EMBARRASSING, SOME PEOPLE DON'T.

ERECTIONS AREN'T ALWAYS ABOUT SEX OR SEXY FEELINGS. YOU CAN HAVE AN ERECTION AND NOT HAVE SEXY FEELINGS, AND YOU CAN HAVE SEXY FEELINGS AND NOT GET AN ERECTION.

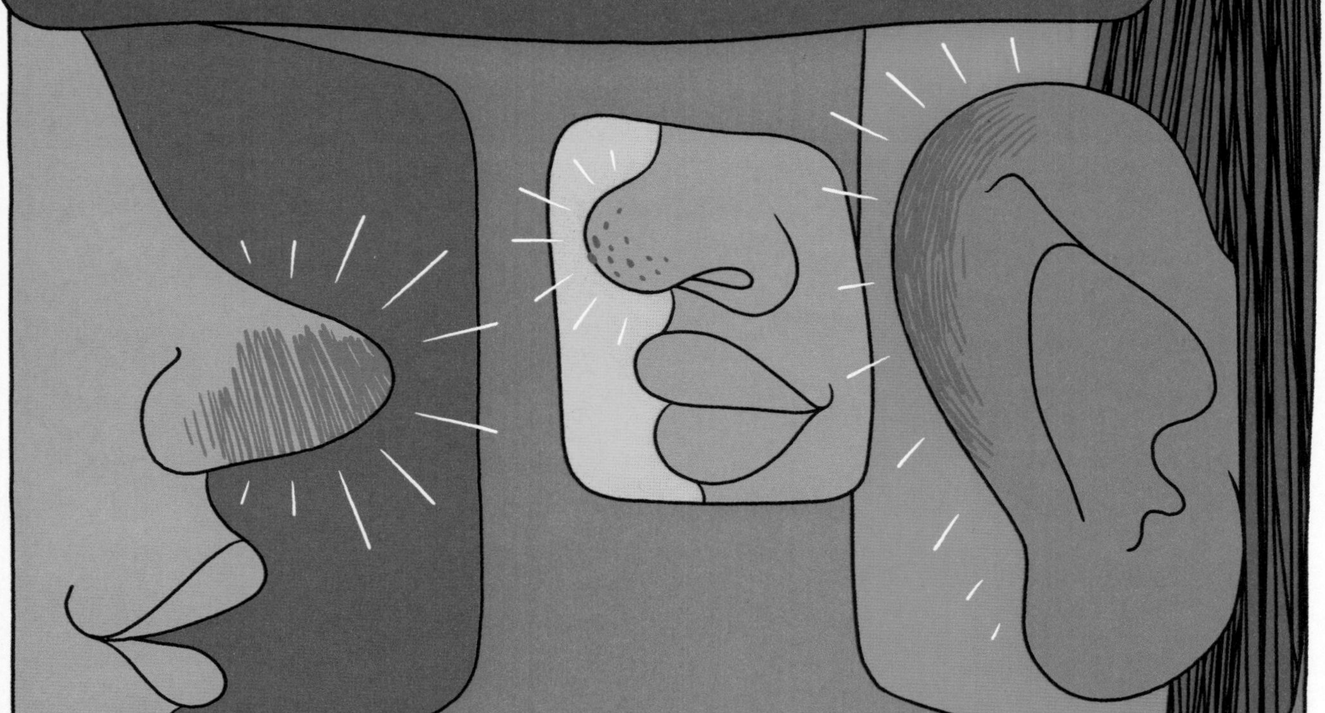

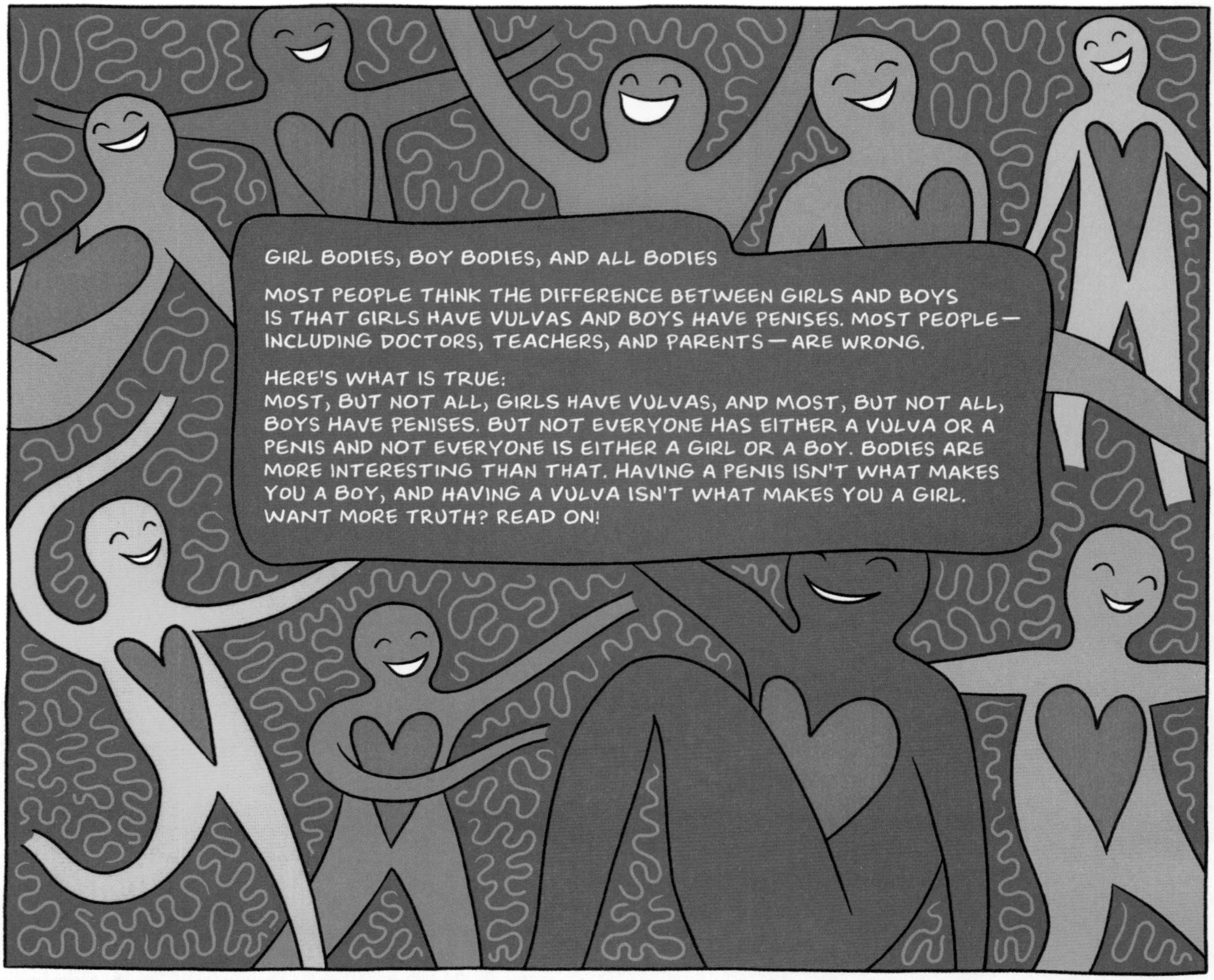
GIRL BODIES, BOY BODIES, AND ALL BODIES
MOST PEOPLE THINK THE DIFFERENCE BETWEEN GIRLS AND BOYS IS THAT GIRLS HAVE VULVAS AND BOYS HAVE PENISES. MOST PEOPLE—INCLUDING DOCTORS, TEACHERS, AND PARENTS—ARE WRONG.
HERE'S WHAT IS TRUE:
MOST, BUT NOT ALL, GIRLS HAVE VULVAS, AND MOST, BUT NOT ALL, BOYS HAVE PENISES. BUT NOT EVERYONE HAS EITHER A VULVA OR A PENIS AND NOT EVERYONE IS EITHER A GIRL OR A BOY. BODIES ARE MORE INTERESTING THAN THAT. HAVING A PENIS ISN'T WHAT MAKES YOU A BOY, AND HAVING A VULVA ISN'T WHAT MAKES YOU A GIRL. WANT MORE TRUTH? READ ON!

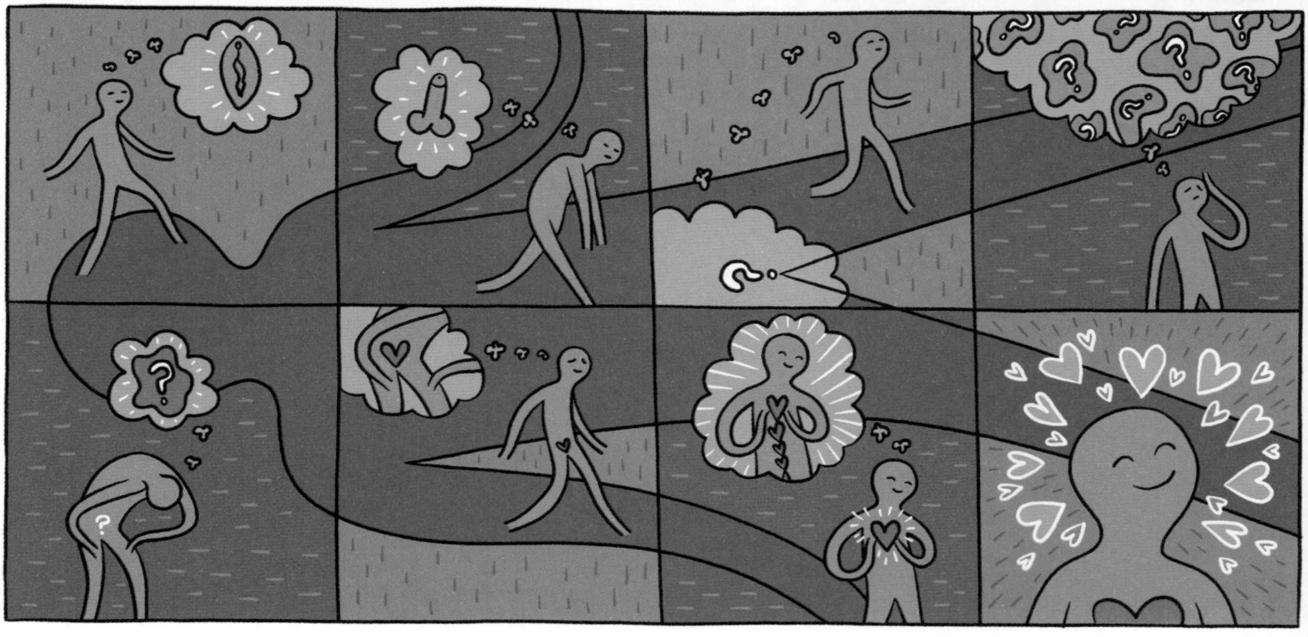

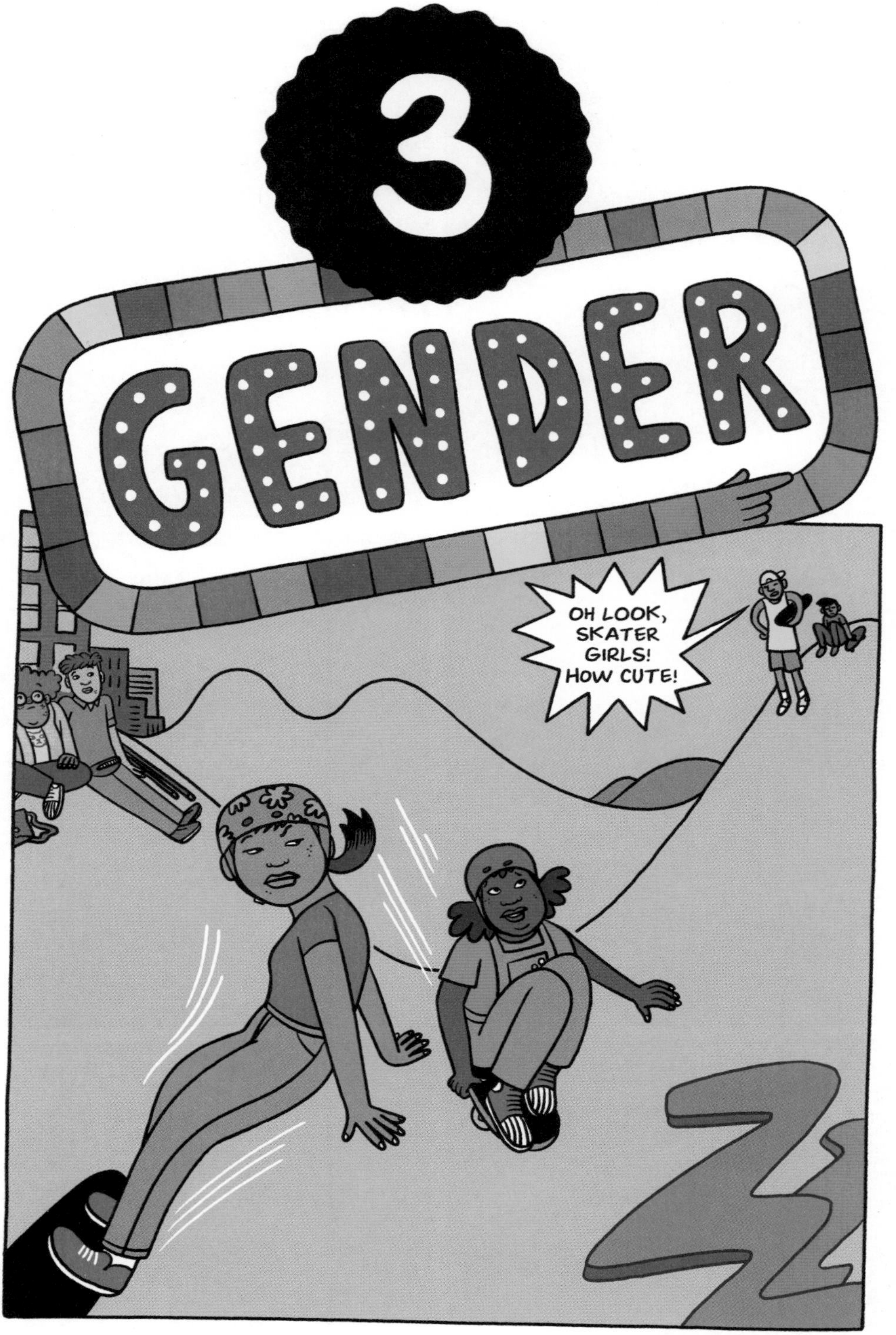
3
GENDER
OH LOOK, SKATER GIRLS! HOW CUTE!

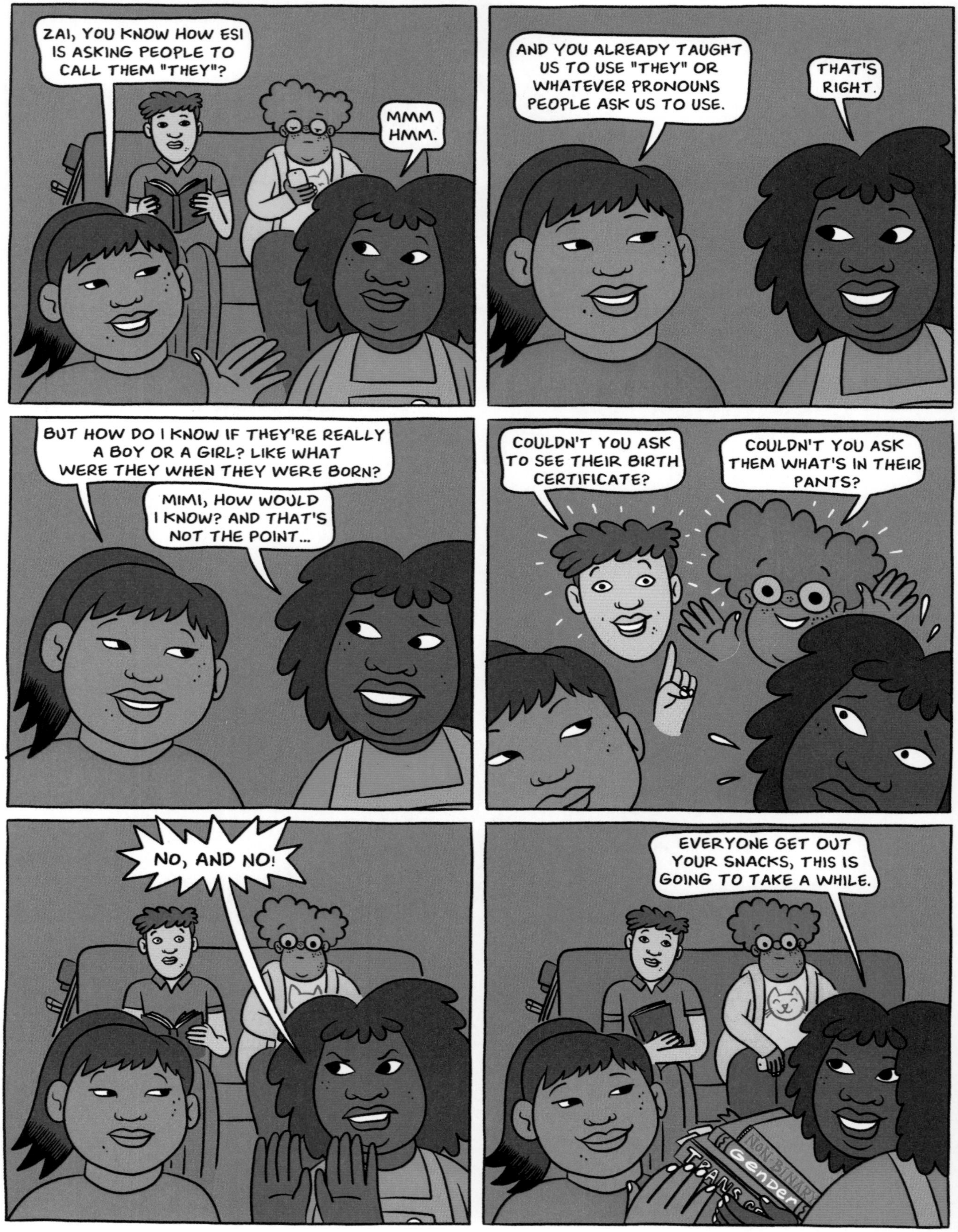
ZAI, YOU KNOW HOW ESI IS ASKING PEOPLE TO CALL THEM "THEY"?
MMM HMM.
AND YOU ALREADY TAUGHT US TO USE "THEY" OR WHATEVER PRONOUNS PEOPLE ASK US TO USE.
THAT'S RIGHT.
BUT HOW DO I KNOW IF THEY'RE REALLY A BOY OR A GIRL? LIKE WHAT WERE THEY WHEN THEY WERE BORN?
MIMI, HOW WOULD I KNOW? AND THAT'S NOT THE POINT...
COULDN'T YOU ASK TO SEE THEIR BIRTH CERTIFICATE?
COULDN'T YOU ASK THEM WHAT'S IN THEIR PANTS?
NO, AND NO!
EVERYONE GET OUT YOUR SNACKS, THIS IS GOING TO TAKE A WHILE.
NON-BINARY
Gender

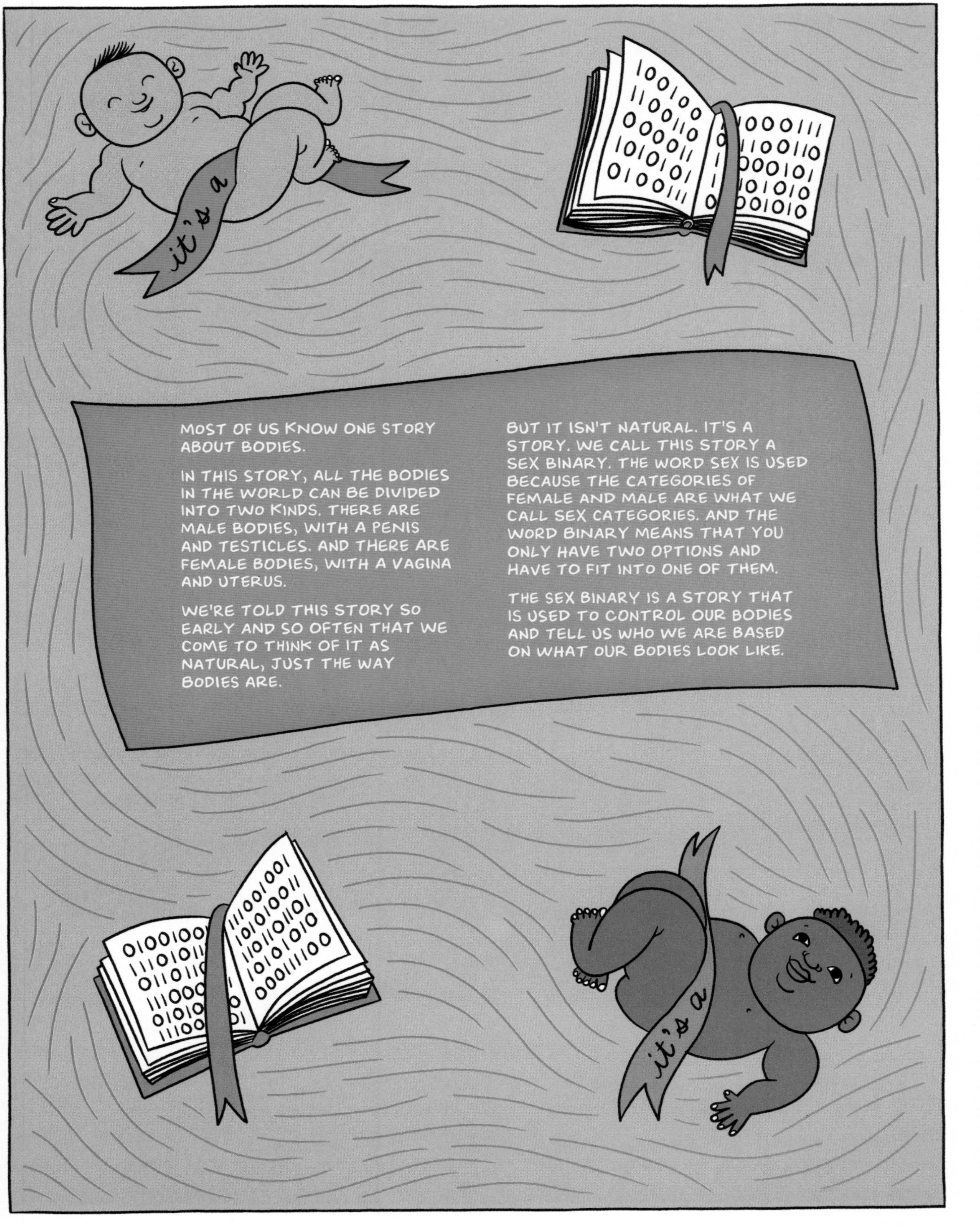
it's a
MOST OF US KNOW ONE STORY ABOUT BODIES.
IN THIS STORY, ALL THE BODIES IN THE WORLD CAN BE DIVIDED INTO TWO KINDS. THERE ARE MALE BODIES, WITH A PENIS AND TESTICLES. AND THERE ARE FEMALE BODIES, WITH A VAGINA AND UTERUS.
WE'RE TOLD THIS STORY SO EARLY AND SO OFTEN THAT WE COME TO THINK OF IT AS NATURAL, JUST THE WAY BODIES ARE.
BUT IT ISN'T NATURAL. IT'S A STORY. WE CALL THIS STORY A SEX BINARY. THE WORD SEX IS USED BECAUSE THE CATEGORIES OF FEMALE AND MALE ARE WHAT WE CALL SEX CATEGORIES. AND THE WORD BINARY MEANS THAT YOU ONLY HAVE TWO OPTIONS AND HAVE TO FIT INTO ONE OF THEM.
THE SEX BINARY IS A STORY THAT IS USED TO CONTROL OUR BODIES AND TELL US WHO WE ARE BASED ON WHAT OUR BODIES LOOK LIKE.
it's a

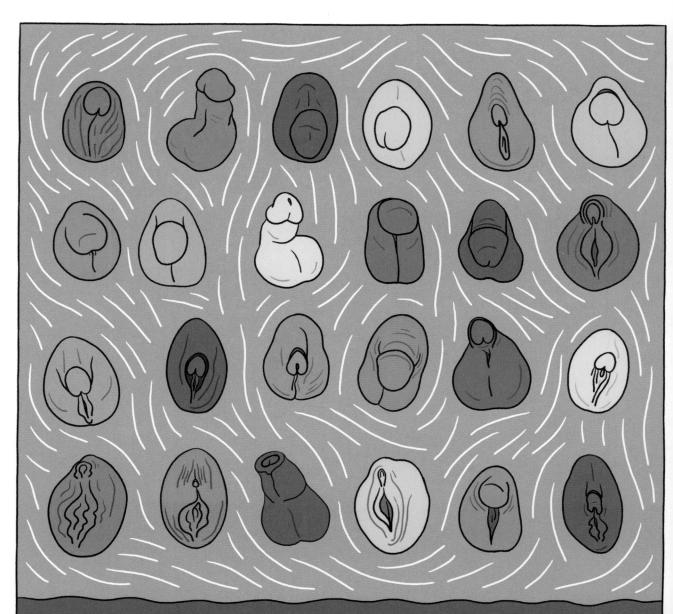

HERE'S HOW THE SEX BINARY WORKS TODAY. WHEN A BABY IS BORN, THE PERSON WHO HELPED IT BE BORN — USUALLY A DOCTOR OR MIDWIFE—LOOKS AT ITS NAKED BODY. IF THEY SEE A VULVA THEY SAY, "CONGRATULATIONS, IT'S A GIRL!" IF THEY SEE A PENIS THEY SAY, "CONGRATULATIONS, IT'S A BOY!"

THIS IS A LABEL YOU'RE GIVEN BASED ON WHAT THE DOCTOR OR MIDWIFE SEES ON THE OUTSIDE. IT'S CALLED YOUR SEX ASSIGNMENT AT BIRTH.

THERE ARE MANY PROBLEMS WITH SEX ASSIGNMENT. ONE OF THEM IS THAT A LOT OF BABIES ARE BORN WITH GENITALS THAT ARE NOT OBVIOUSLY ONE THING OR THE OTHER.

VULVAS AND SCROTUMS, CLITORISES AND PENISES ALL DEVELOP FROM THE SAME STUFF. LOTS OF PEOPLE MAKING THESE SEX ASSIGNMENTS FORGET ABOUT THAT.

SOME BABIES HAVE A LARGER CLITORIS THAT LOOKS LIKE A PENIS, OR A SMALLER PENIS THAT LOOKS LIKE A CLITORIS. SOMETIMES THE PERSON LOOKING ISN'T SURE IF THEY ARE LOOKING AT A SCROTUM OR A VULVA.

THE PROBLEM IS NOT OUR BODIES. THE PROBLEM IS THE IDEA THAT ALL THE STUFF THAT MAKES UP OUR BODIES CAN BE DIVIDED INTO TWO OPPOSITE CATEGORIES—A BINARY. THAT'S NOT HOW BODIES REALLY WORK.

* THESE ILLUSTRATIONS ARE INSPIRED BY THE WORK OF ARTIST AND SEXUALITY EDUCATOR VIELMA (STEFANIE GRÜBL)

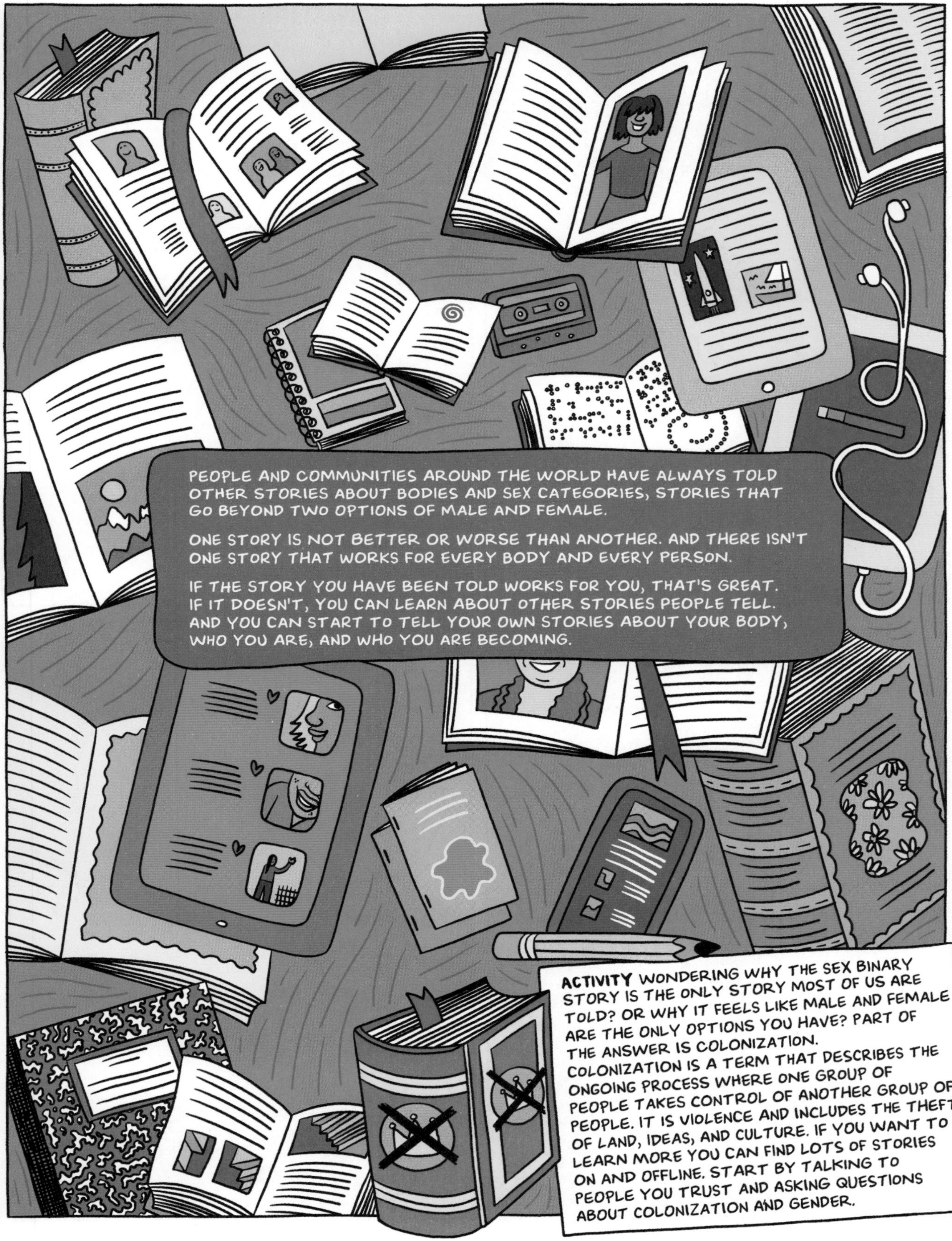
PEOPLE AND COMMUNITIES AROUND THE WORLD HAVE ALWAYS TOLD OTHER STORIES ABOUT BODIES AND SEX CATEGORIES, STORIES THAT GO BEYOND TWO OPTIONS OF MALE AND FEMALE.
ONE STORY IS NOT BETTER OR WORSE THAN ANOTHER. AND THERE ISN'T ONE STORY THAT WORKS FOR EVERY BODY AND EVERY PERSON.
IF THE STORY YOU HAVE BEEN TOLD WORKS FOR YOU, THAT'S GREAT. IF IT DOESN'T, YOU CAN LEARN ABOUT OTHER STORIES PEOPLE TELL. AND YOU CAN START TO TELL YOUR OWN STORIES ABOUT YOUR BODY, WHO YOU ARE, AND WHO YOU ARE BECOMING.
ACTIVITY WONDERING WHY THE SEX BINARY STORY IS THE ONLY STORY MOST OF US ARE TOLD? OR WHY IT FEELS LIKE MALE AND FEMALE ARE THE ONLY OPTIONS YOU HAVE? PART OF THE ANSWER IS COLONIZATION.
THE COLONIZATION IS A TERM THAT DESCRIBES THE ONGOING PROCESS WHERE ONE GROUP OF PEOPLE TAKES CONTROL OF ANOTHER GROUP OF PEOPLE. IT IS VIOLENCE AND INCLUDES THE THEFT OF LAND, IDEAS, AND CULTURE. IF YOU WANT TO LEARN MORE YOU CAN FIND LOTS OF STORIES ON AND OFFLINE. START BY TALKING TO PEOPLE YOU TRUST AND ASKING QUESTIONS ABOUT COLONIZATION AND GENDER.

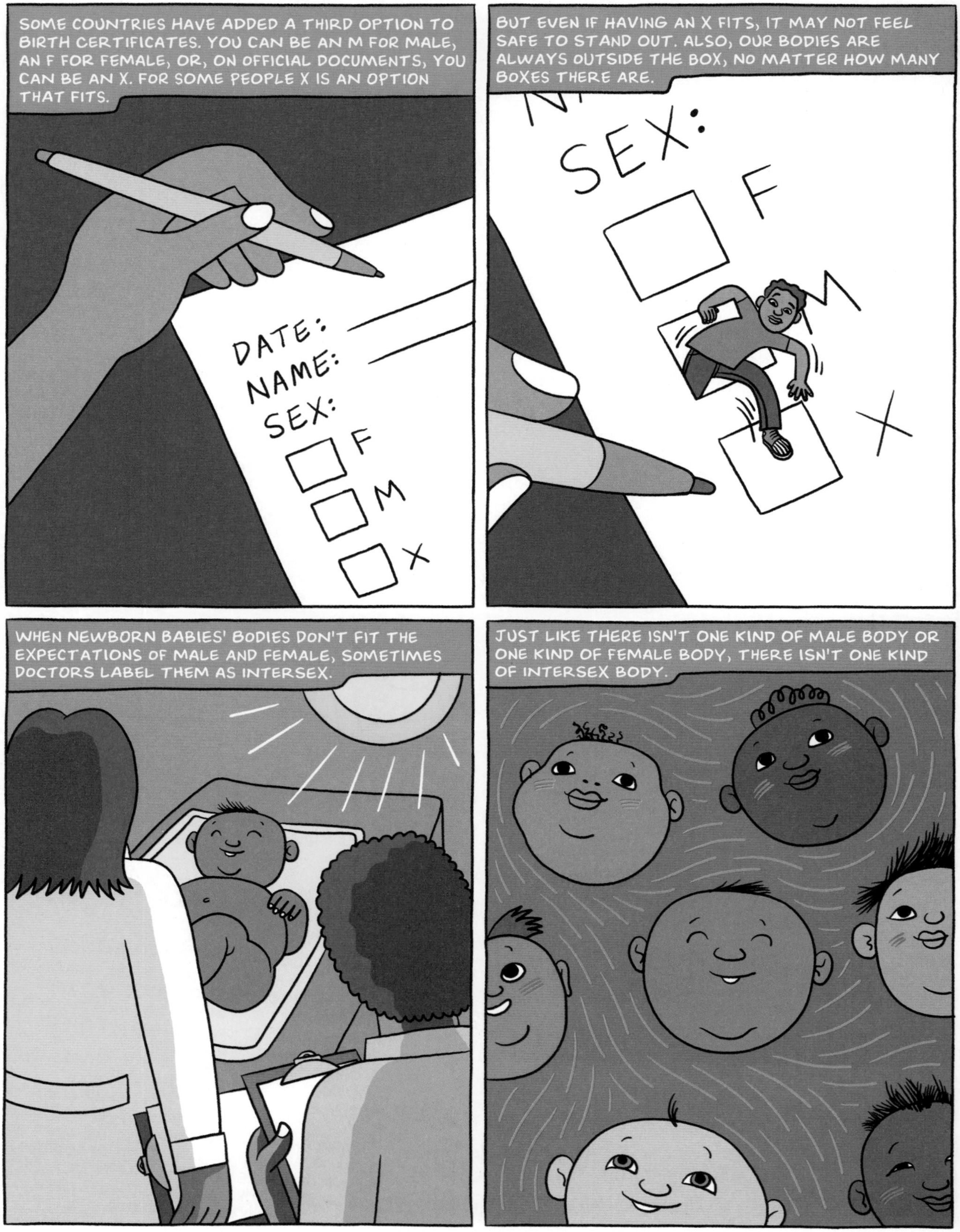
SOME COUNTRIES HAVE ADDED A THIRD OPTION TO BIRTH CERTIFICATES. YOU CAN BE AN M FOR MALE, AN F FOR FEMALE, OR, ON OFFICIAL DOCUMENTS, YOU CAN BE AN X. FOR SOME PEOPLE X IS AN OPTION THAT FITS.
DATE:
NAME:
SEX:
F
M
X
BUT EVEN IF HAVING AN X FITS, IT MAY NOT FEEL SAFE TO STAND OUT. ALSO, OUR BODIES ARE ALWAYS OUTSIDE THE BOX, NO MATTER HOW MANY BOXES THERE ARE.
SEX:
F
M
X
WHEN NEWBORN BABIES' BODIES DON'T FIT THE EXPECTATIONS OF MALE AND FEMALE, SOMETIMES DOCTORS LABEL THEM AS INTERSEX.
JUST LIKE THERE ISN'T ONE KIND OF MALE BODY OR ONE KIND OF FEMALE BODY, THERE ISN'T ONE KIND OF INTERSEX BODY.

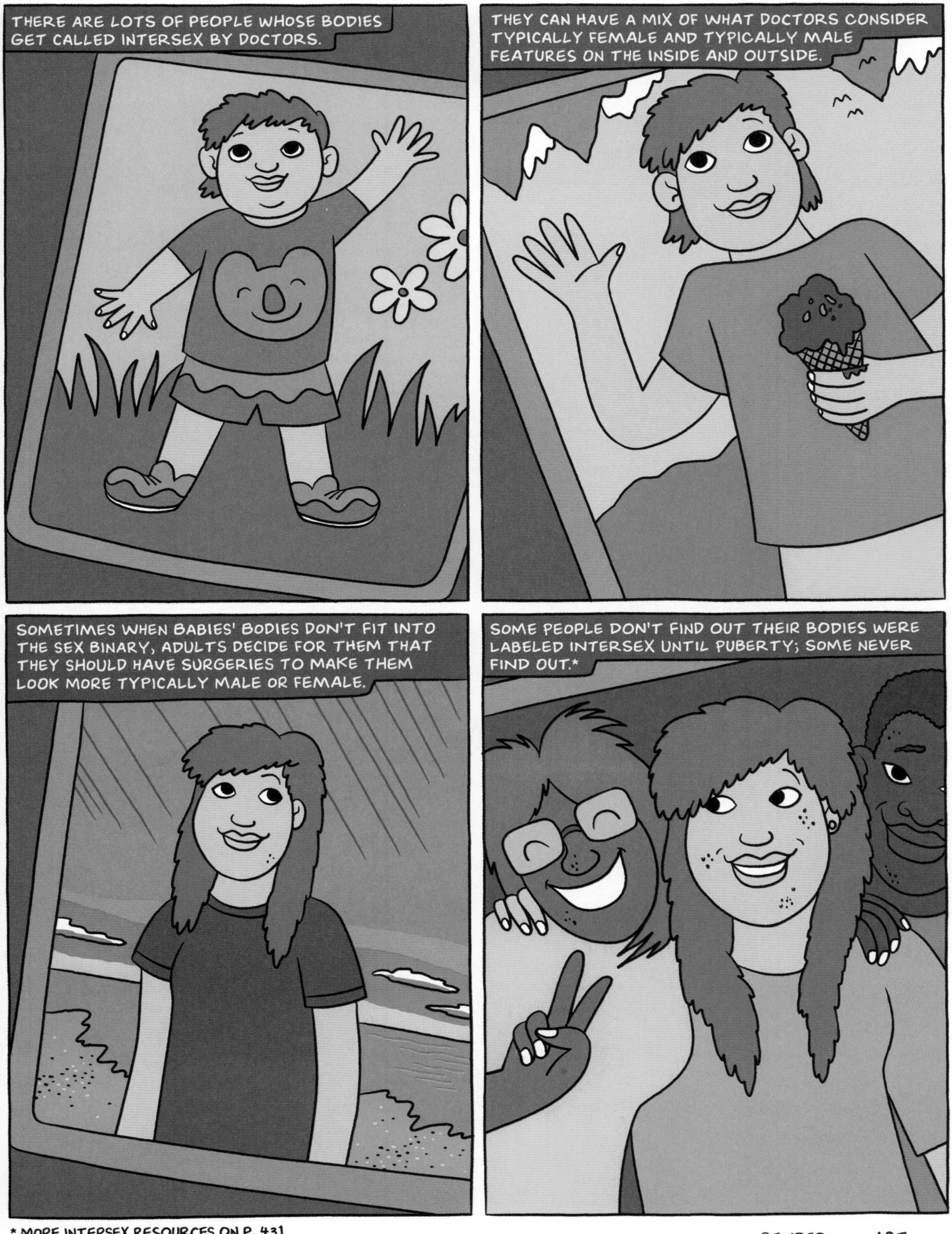
THERE ARE LOTS OF PEOPLE WHOSE BODIES GET CALLED INTERSEX BY DOCTORS.
THEY CAN HAVE A MIX OF WHAT DOCTORS CONSIDER TYPICALLY FEMALE AND TYPICALLY MALE FEATURES ON THE INSIDE AND OUTSIDE.
SOMETIMES WHEN BABIES' BODIES DON'T FIT INTO THE SEX BINARY, ADULTS DECIDE FOR THEM THAT THEY SHOULD HAVE SURGERIES TO MAKE THEM LOOK MORE TYPICALLY MALE OR FEMALE.
SOME PEOPLE DON'T FIND OUT THEIR BODIES WERE LABELED INTERSEX UNTIL PUBERTY; SOME NEVER FIND OUT.*

* MORE INTERSEX RESOURCES ON P. 431

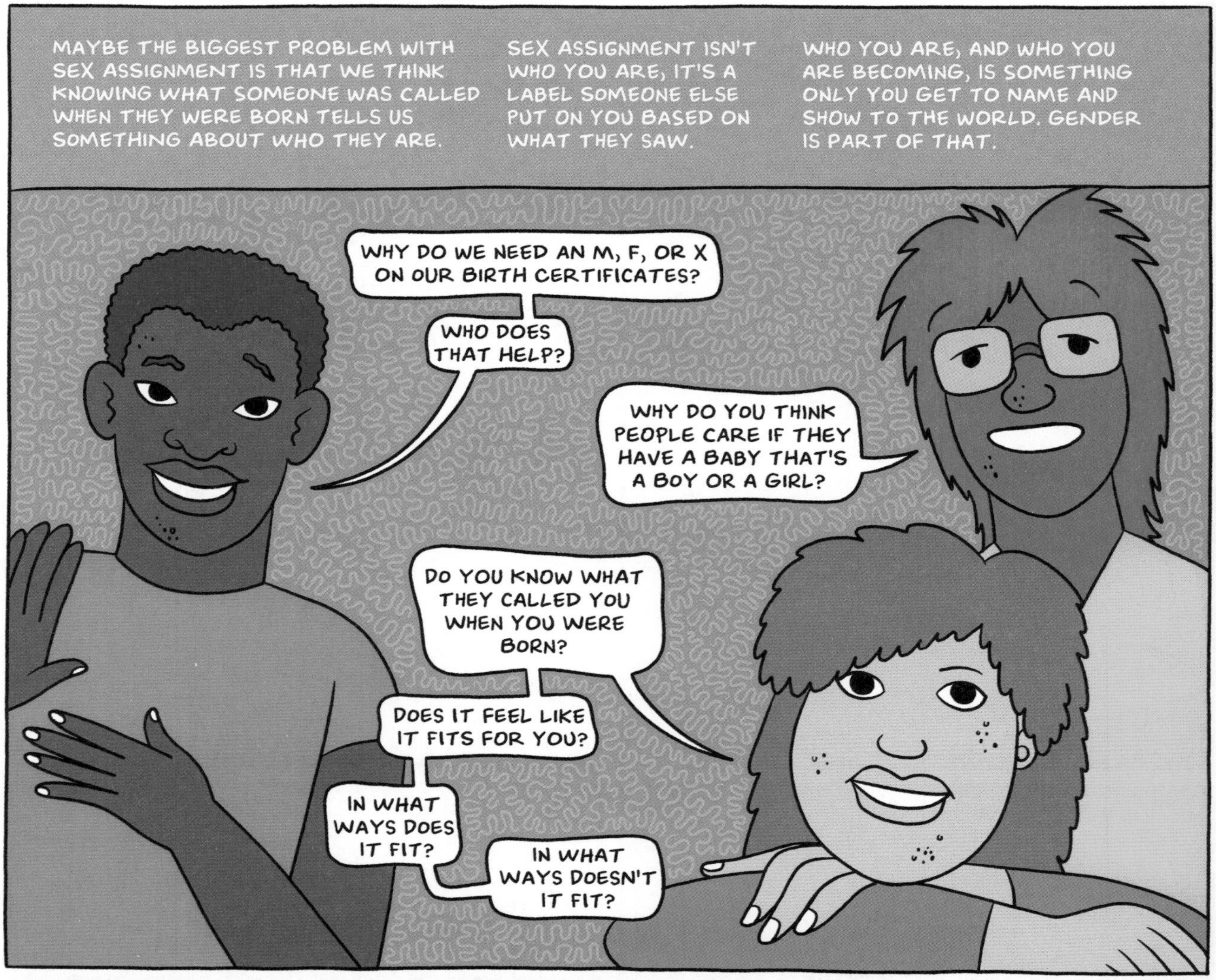
MAYBE THE BIGGEST PROBLEM WITH SEX ASSIGNMENT IS THAT WE THINK KNOWING WHAT SOMEONE WAS CALLED WHEN THEY WERE BORN TELLS US SOMETHING ABOUT WHO THEY ARE.
SEX ASSIGNMENT ISN'T WHO YOU ARE, IT'S A LABEL SOMEONE ELSE PUT ON YOU BASED ON WHAT THEY SAW.
WHO YOU ARE, AND WHO YOU ARE BECOMING, IS SOMETHING ONLY YOU GET TO NAME AND SHOW TO THE WORLD. GENDER IS PART OF THAT.
WHY DO WE NEED AN M, F, OR X ON OUR BIRTH CERTIFICATES?
WHO DOES THAT HELP?
WHY DO YOU THINK PEOPLE CARE IF THEY HAVE A BABY THAT'S A BOY OR A GIRL?
DO YOU KNOW WHAT THEY CALLED YOU WHEN YOU WERE BORN?
DOES IT FEEL LIKE IT FITS FOR YOU?
IN WHAT WAYS DOES IT FIT?
IN WHAT WAYS DOESN'T IT FIT?

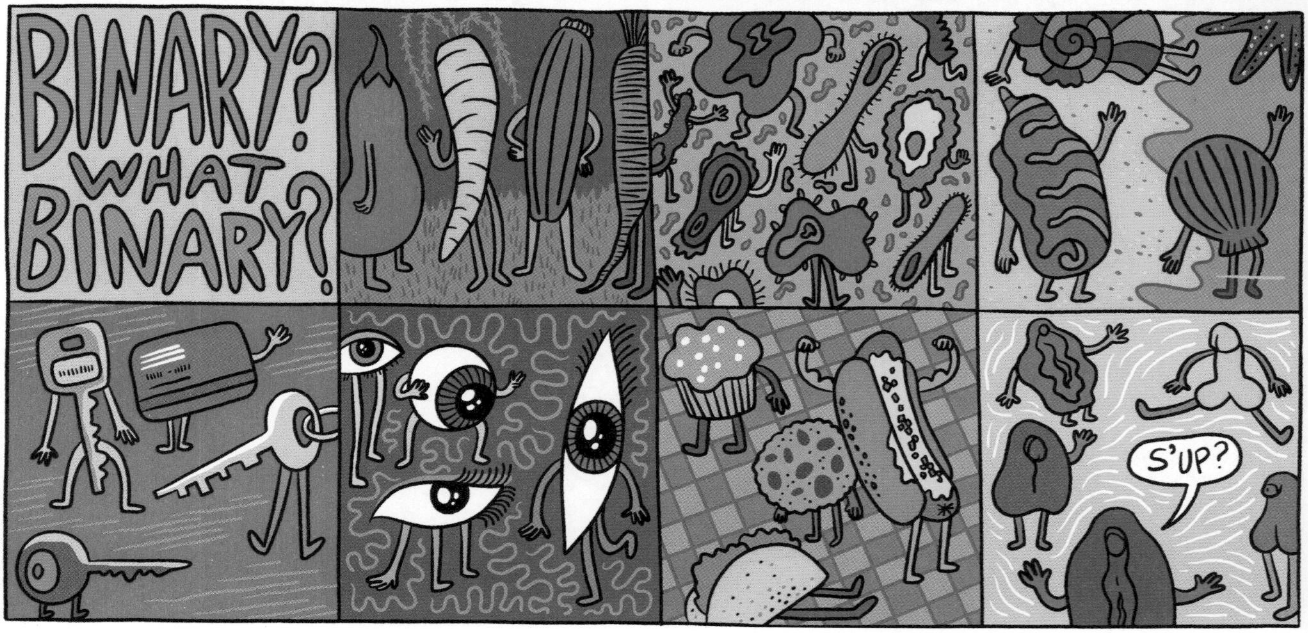
BINARY? WHAT BINARY?
S'UP?

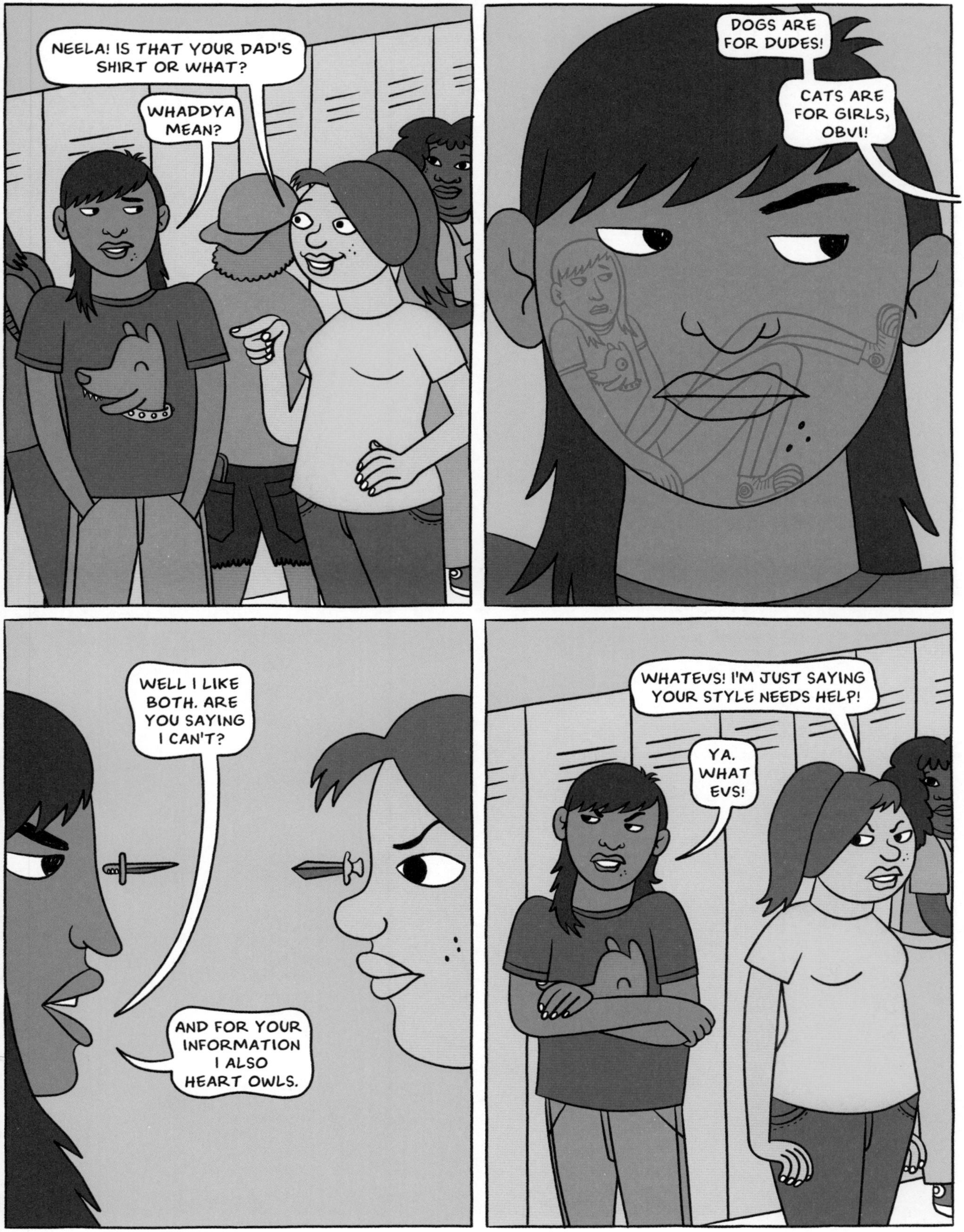
NEELA! IS THAT YOUR DAD'S SHIRT OR WHAT?
WHADDYA MEAN?
DOGS ARE FOR DUDES!
CATS ARE FOR GIRLS, OBVI!
WELL I LIKE BOTH. ARE YOU SAYING I CAN'T?
AND FOR YOUR INFORMATION I ALSO HEART OWLS.
WHATEVS! I'M JUST SAYING YOUR STYLE NEEDS HELP!
YA. WHAT EVS!

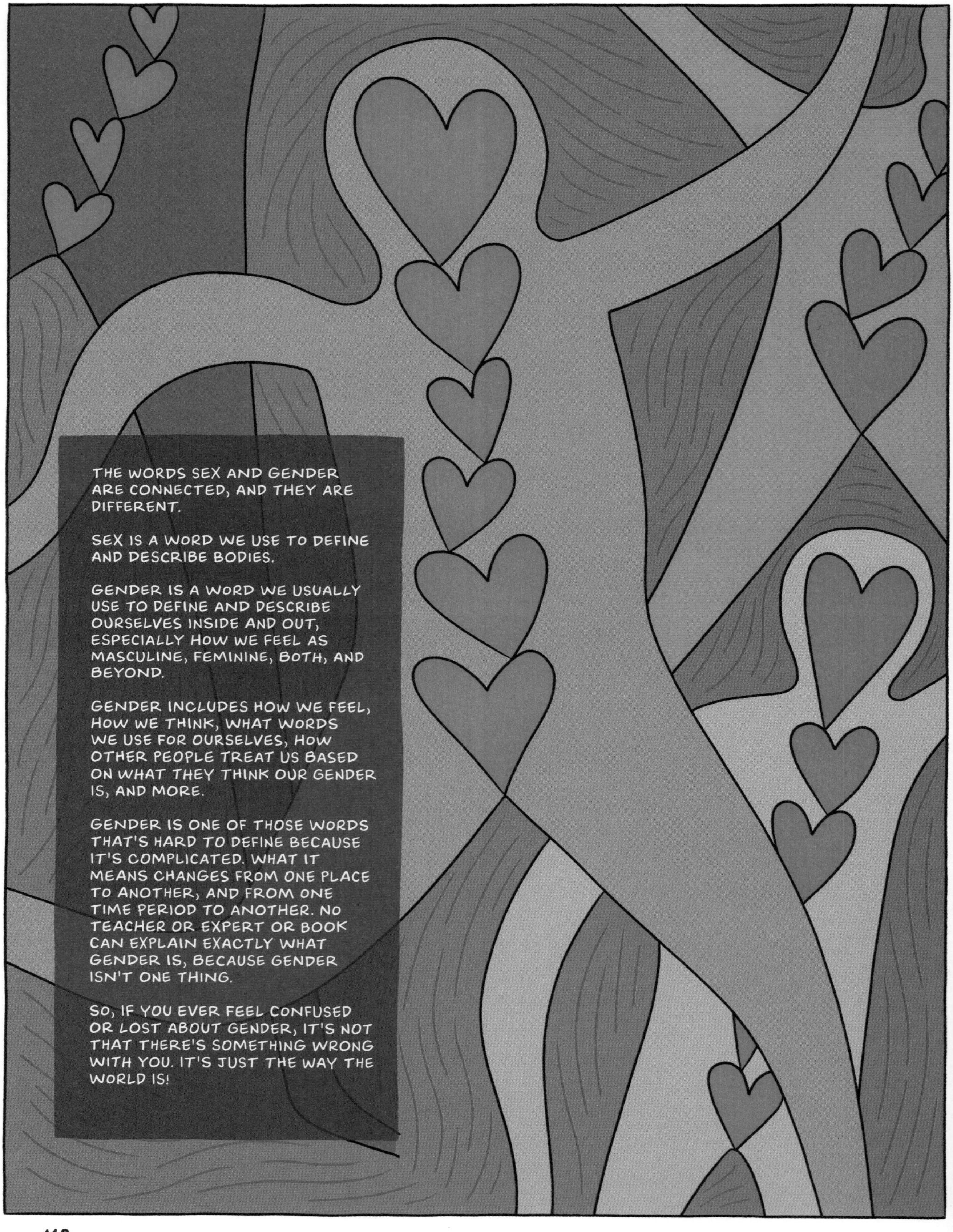
THE WORDS SEX AND GENDER ARE CONNECTED, AND THEY ARE DIFFERENT.
SEX IS A WORD WE USE TO DEFINE AND DESCRIBE BODIES.
GENDER IS A WORD WE USUALLY USE TO DEFINE AND DESCRIBE OURSELVES INSIDE AND OUT, ESPECIALLY HOW WE FEEL AS MASCULINE, FEMININE, BOTH, AND BEYOND.
GENDER INCLUDES HOW WE FEEL, HOW WE THINK, WHAT WORDS WE USE FOR OURSELVES, HOW OTHER PEOPLE TREAT US BASED ON WHAT THEY THINK OUR GENDER IS, AND MORE.
GENDER IS ONE OF THOSE WORDS THAT'S HARD TO DEFINE BECAUSE IT'S COMPLICATED. WHAT IT MEANS CHANGES FROM ONE PLACE TO ANOTHER, AND FROM ONE TIME PERIOD TO ANOTHER. NO TEACHER OR EXPERT OR BOOK CAN EXPLAIN EXACTLY WHAT GENDER IS, BECAUSE GENDER ISN'T ONE THING.
SO, IF YOU EVER FEEL CONFUSED OR LOST ABOUT GENDER, IT'S NOT THAT THERE'S SOMETHING WRONG WITH YOU. IT'S JUST THE WAY THE WORLD IS!

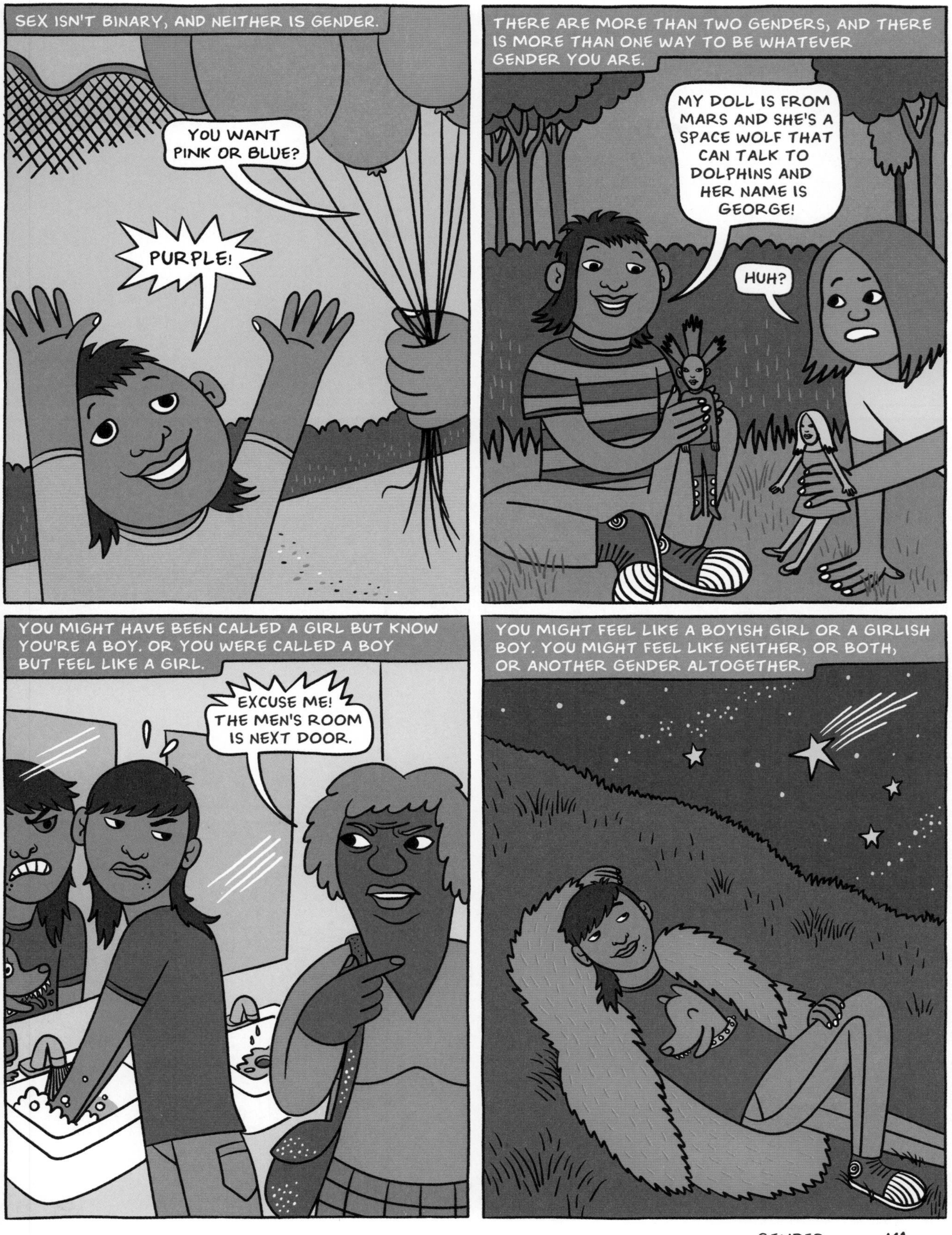
SEX ISN'T BINARY, AND NEITHER IS GENDER.
YOU WANT PINK OR BLUE?
PURPLE!
THERE ARE MORE THAN TWO GENDERS, AND THERE IS MORE THAN ONE WAY TO BE WHATEVER GENDER YOU ARE.
MY DOLL IS FROM MARS AND SHE'S A SPACE WOLF THAT CAN TALK TO DOLPHINS AND HER NAME IS GEORGE!
HUH?
YOU MIGHT HAVE BEEN CALLED A GIRL BUT KNOW YOU'RE A BOY. OR YOU WERE CALLED A BOY BUT FEEL LIKE A GIRL.
EXCUSE ME! THE MEN'S ROOM IS NEXT DOOR.
YOU MIGHT FEEL LIKE A BOYISH GIRL OR A GIRLISH BOY. YOU MIGHT FEEL LIKE NEITHER, OR BOTH, OR ANOTHER GENDER ALTOGETHER.

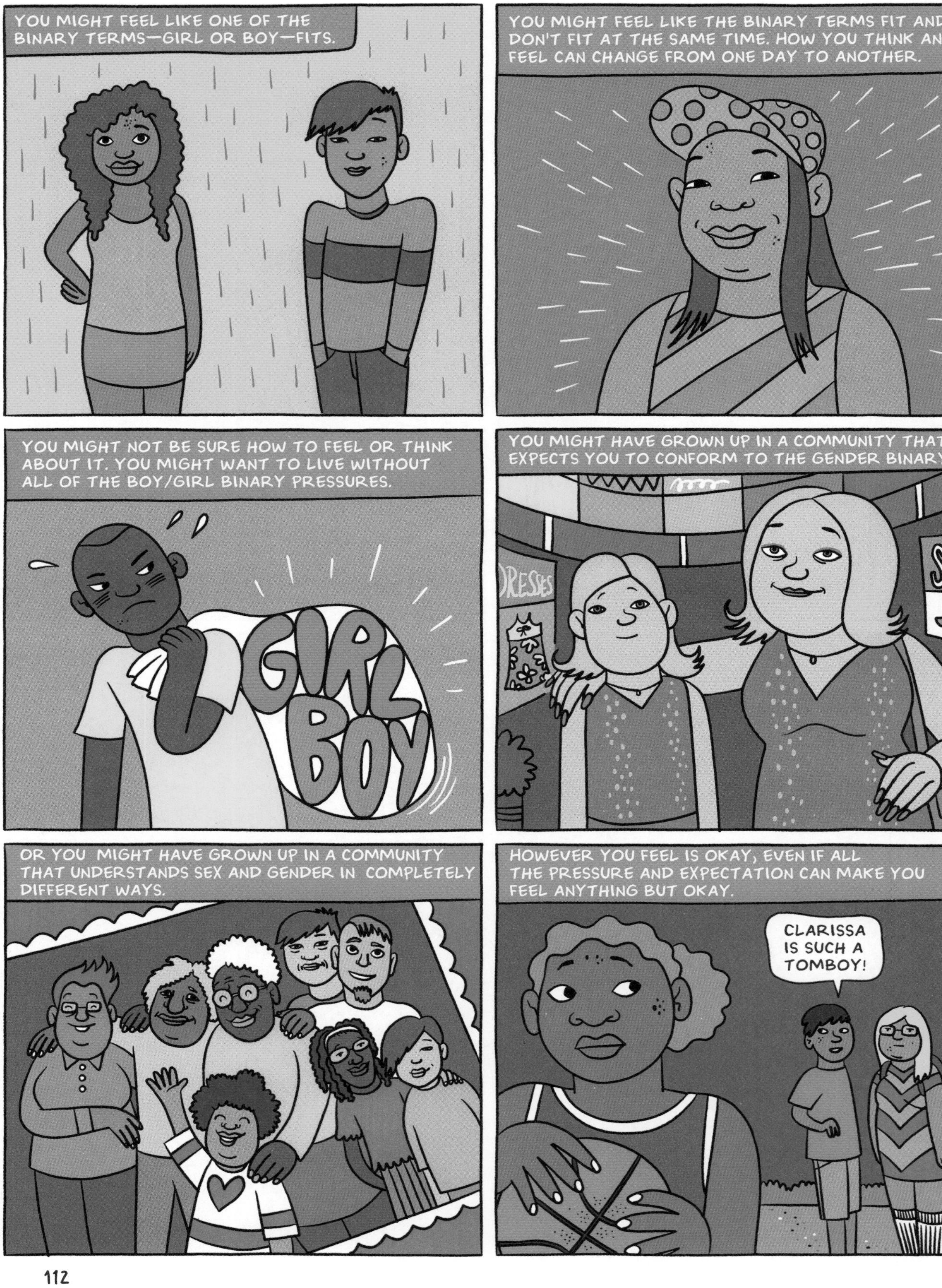
YOU MIGHT FEEL LIKE ONE OF THE BINARY TERMS—GIRL OR BOY—FITS.
YOU MIGHT FEEL LIKE THE BINARY TERMS FIT AND DON'T FIT AT THE SAME TIME. HOW YOU THINK AND FEEL CAN CHANGE FROM ONE DAY TO ANOTHER.
YOU MIGHT NOT BE SURE HOW TO FEEL OR THINK ABOUT IT. YOU MIGHT WANT TO LIVE WITHOUT ALL OF THE BOY/GIRL BINARY PRESSURES.
GIRL
BOY
YOU MIGHT HAVE GROWN UP IN A COMMUNITY THAT EXPECTS YOU TO CONFORM TO THE GENDER BINARY.
DRESSES
SH
OR YOU MIGHT HAVE GROWN UP IN A COMMUNITY THAT UNDERSTANDS SEX AND GENDER IN COMPLETELY DIFFERENT WAYS.
HOWEVER YOU FEEL IS OKAY, EVEN IF ALL THE PRESSURE AND EXPECTATION CAN MAKE YOU FEEL ANYTHING BUT OKAY.
CLARISSA IS SUCH A TOMBOY!

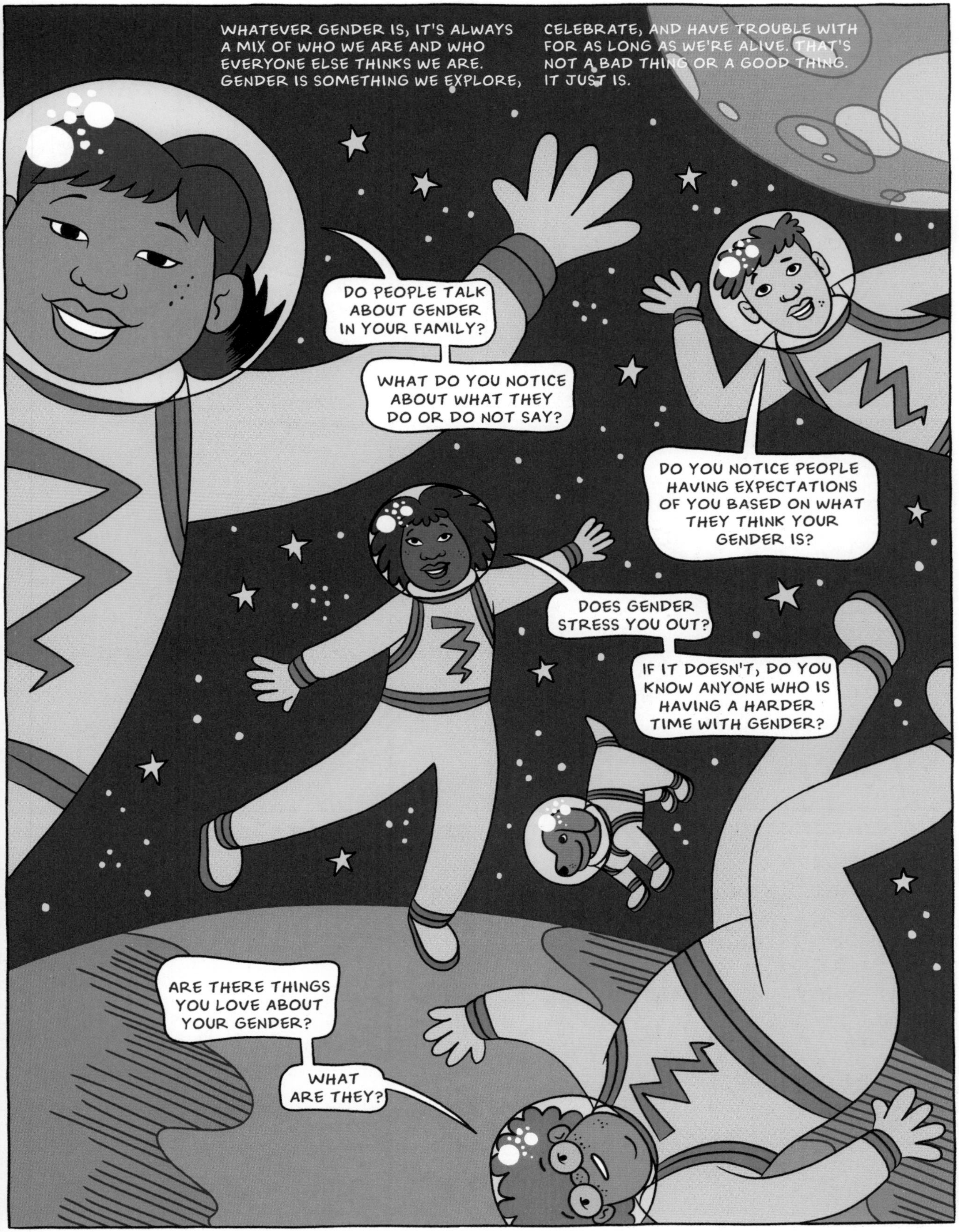
WHATEVER GENDER IS, IT'S ALWAYS A MIX OF WHO WE ARE AND WHO EVERYONE ELSE THINKS WE ARE. GENDER IS SOMETHING WE EXPLORE, CELEBRATE, AND HAVE TROUBLE WITH FOR AS LONG AS WE'RE ALIVE. THAT'S NOT A BAD THING OR A GOOD THING. IT JUST IS.
DO PEOPLE TALK ABOUT GENDER IN YOUR FAMILY?
WHAT DO YOU NOTICE ABOUT WHAT THEY DO OR DO NOT SAY?
DO YOU NOTICE PEOPLE HAVING EXPECTATIONS OF YOU BASED ON WHAT THEY THINK YOUR GENDER IS?
DOES GENDER STRESS YOU OUT?
IF IT DOESN'T, DO YOU KNOW ANYONE WHO IS HAVING A HARDER TIME WITH GENDER?
ARE THERE THINGS YOU LOVE ABOUT YOUR GENDER?
WHAT ARE THEY?

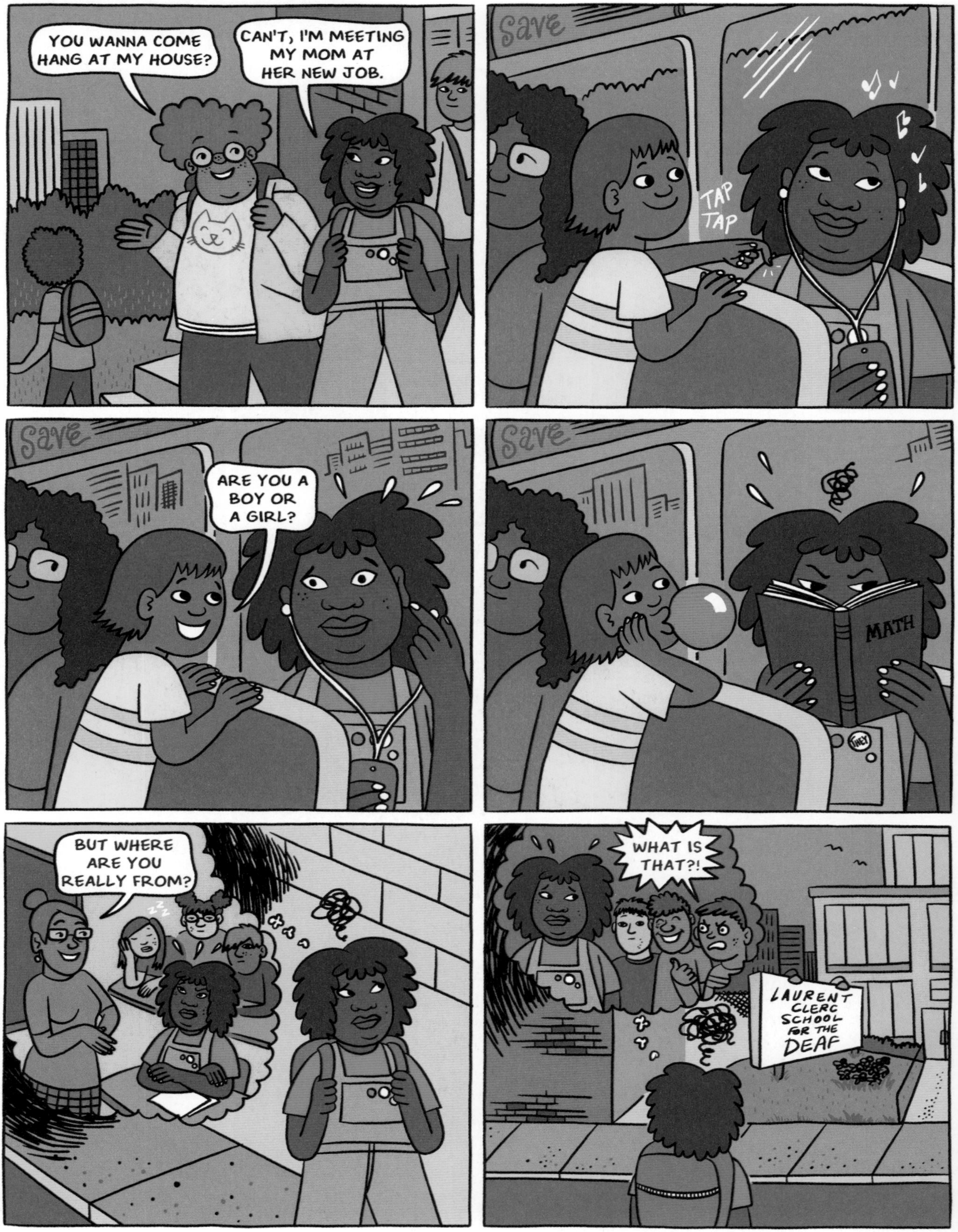
YOU WANNA COME HANG AT MY HOUSE?
CAN'T, I'M MEETING MY MOM AT HER NEW JOB.
save
TAP TAP
save
ARE YOU A BOY OR A GIRL?
save
MATH
BUT WHERE ARE YOU REALLY FROM?
WHAT IS THAT?!
LAURENT CLERC SCHOOL FOR THE DEAF

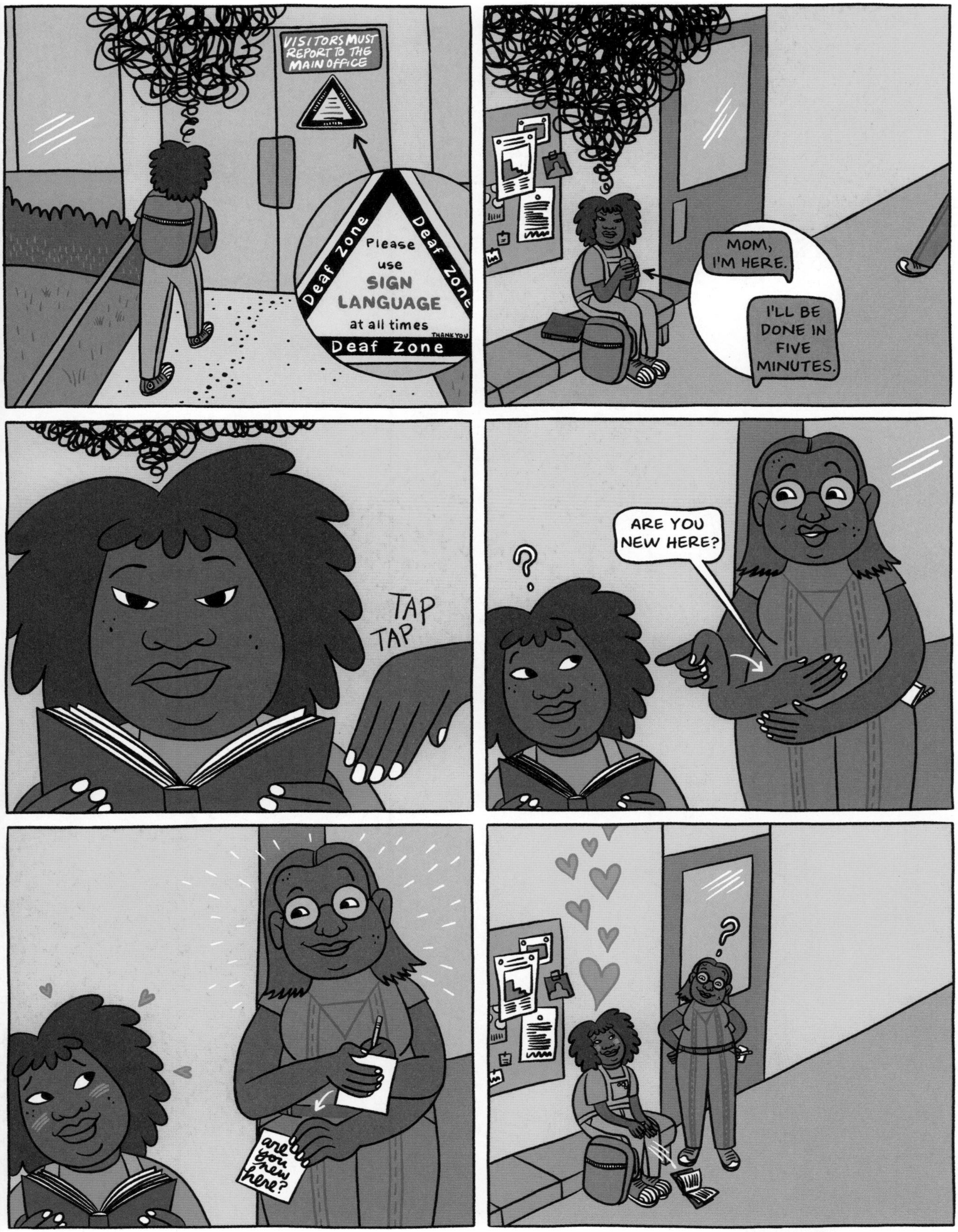
VISITORS MUST REPORT TO THE MAIN OFFICE
Deaf Zone
Deaf Zone
Please use SIGN LANGUAGE at all times
THANK YOU
Deaf Zone
MOM, I'M HERE.
I'LL BE DONE IN FIVE MINUTES.
TAP TAP
ARE YOU NEW HERE?
are you new here?

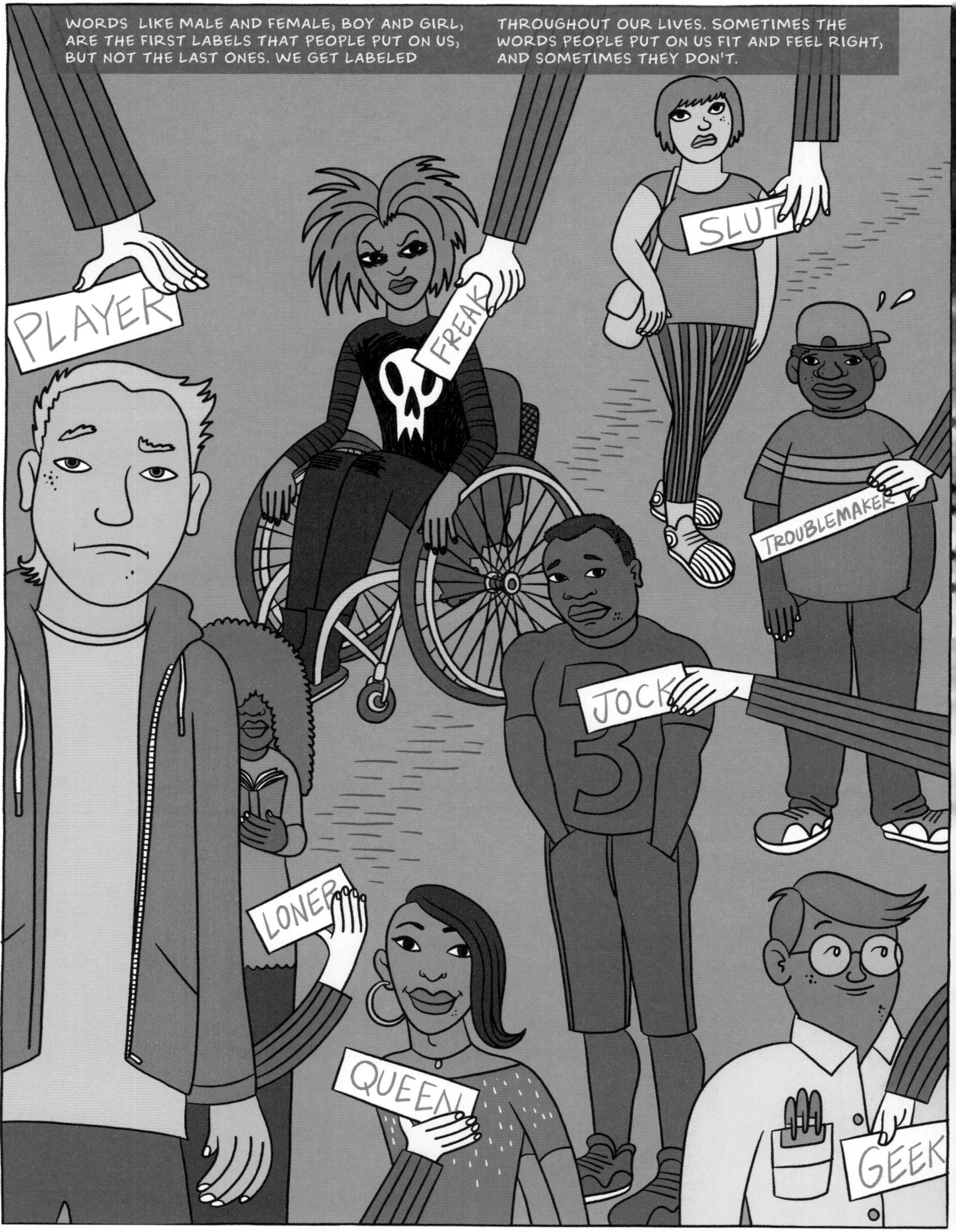
WORDS LIKE MALE AND FEMALE, BOY AND GIRL, ARE THE FIRST LABELS THAT PEOPLE PUT ON US, BUT NOT THE LAST ONES. WE GET LABELED THROUGHOUT OUR LIVES. SOMETIMES THE WORDS PEOPLE PUT ON US FIT AND FEEL RIGHT, AND SOMETIMES THEY DON'T.
PLAYER
FREAK
SLUT
TROUBLEMAKER
JOCK
LONER
QUEEN
GEEK

WHEN WE CHOOSE WORDS TO DESCRIBE A PART OF OURSELVES, WE DON'T CALL THEM LABELS, WE CALL THEM IDENTITIES. OUR IDENTITIES RELATE TO EVERY PART OF WHO WE ARE.

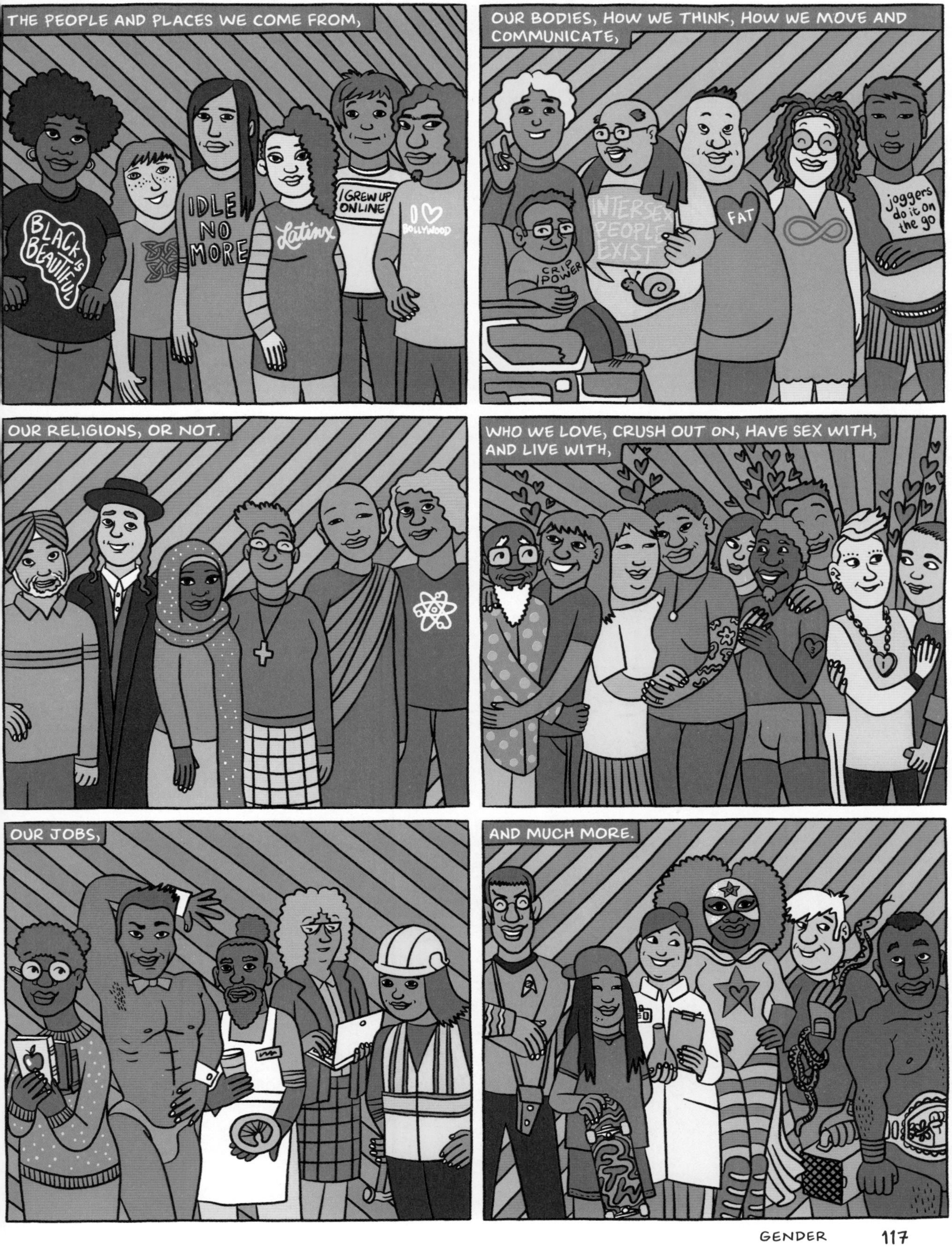
THE PEOPLE AND PLACES WE COME FROM,
BLACK IS BEAUTIFUL
IDLE NO MORE
Latinx
I GREW UP ONLINE
I ♡ BOLLYWOOD
OUR BODIES, HOW WE THINK, HOW WE MOVE AND COMMUNICATE,
INTERSEX PEOPLE EXIST
CRIP POWER
FAT
joggers do it on the go
OUR RELIGIONS, OR NOT.
WHO WE LOVE, CRUSH OUT ON, HAVE SEX WITH, AND LIVE WITH,
OUR JOBS,
AND MUCH MORE.

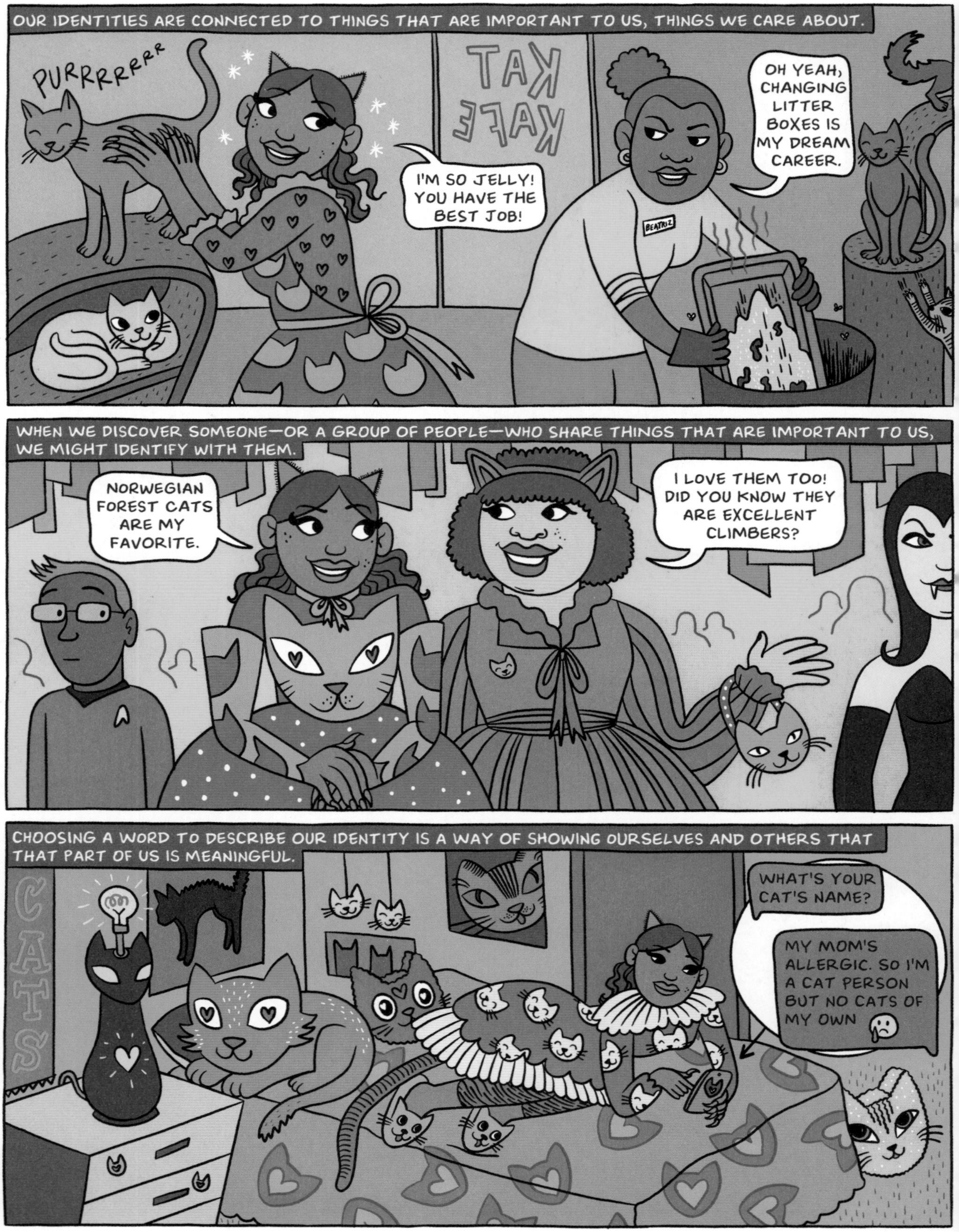
OUR IDENTITIES ARE CONNECTED TO THINGS THAT ARE IMPORTANT TO US, THINGS WE CARE ABOUT.
PURRRRRRR
KAT KAFE
I'M SO JELLY! YOU HAVE THE BEST JOB!
OH YEAH, CHANGING LITTER BOXES IS MY DREAM CAREER.
BEATRIZ
WHEN WE DISCOVER SOMEONE—OR A GROUP OF PEOPLE—WHO SHARE THINGS THAT ARE IMPORTANT TO US, WE MIGHT IDENTIFY WITH THEM.
NORWEGIAN FOREST CATS ARE MY FAVORITE.
I LOVE THEM TOO! DID YOU KNOW THEY ARE EXCELLENT CLIMBERS?
CHOOSING A WORD TO DESCRIBE OUR IDENTITY IS A WAY OF SHOWING OURSELVES AND OTHERS THAT THAT PART OF US IS MEANINGFUL.
CATS
WHAT'S YOUR CAT'S NAME?
MY MOM'S ALLERGIC. SO I'M A CAT PERSON BUT NO CATS OF MY OWN

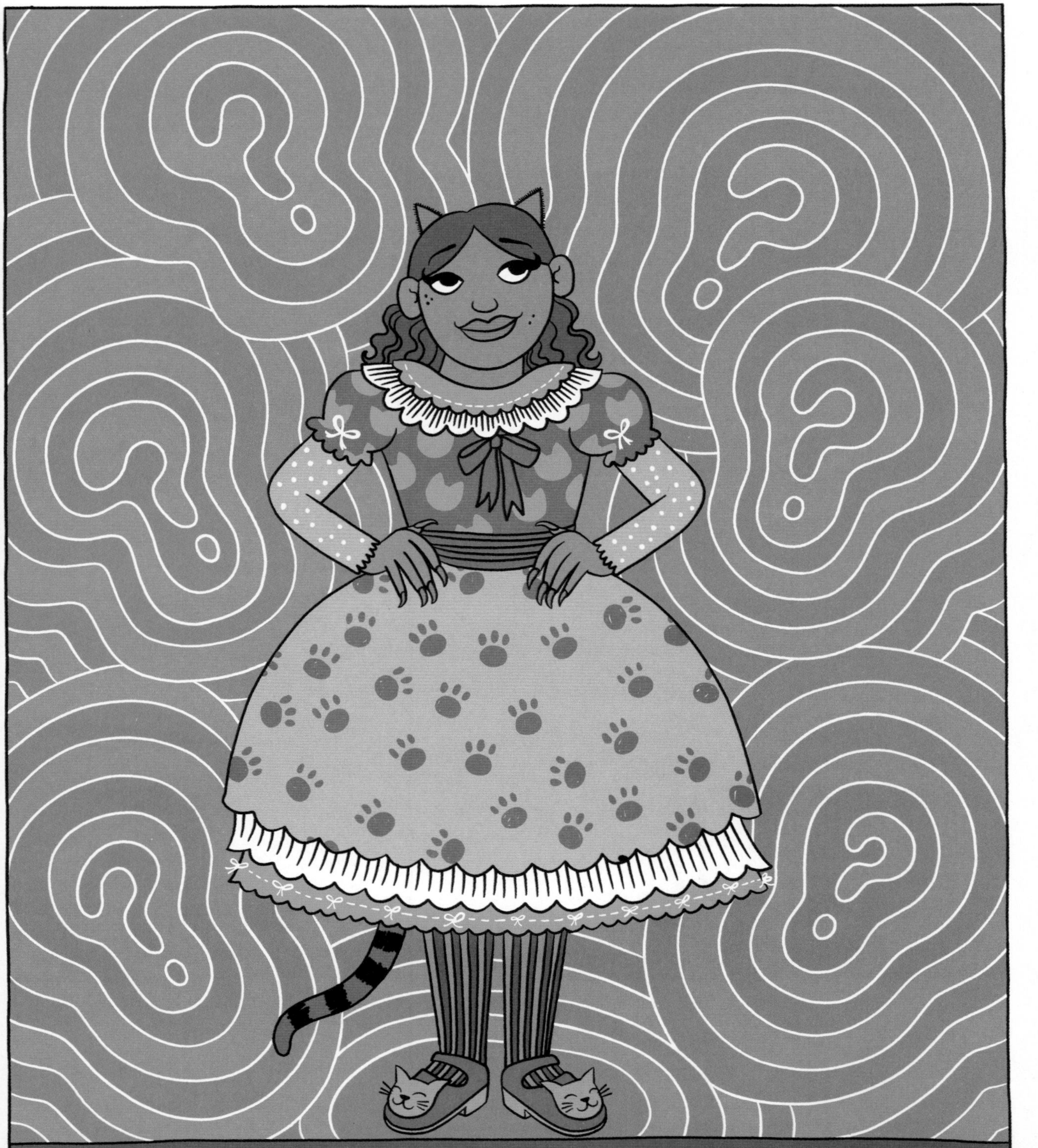

YOUR GENDER IDENTITY DESCRIBES HOW YOU THINK AND FEEL ABOUT YOURSELF, AND HOW YOU WANT OTHERS TO THINK AND FEEL ABOUT YOU, WHEN IT COMES TO MASCULINITY AND FEMININITY.

THERE ISN'T ONE COMPLETE LIST OF GENDER IDENTITIES. EVERY COMMUNITY HAS ITS OWN WORDS FOR GENDER AND FOR PEOPLE WHO ARE INSIDE, OUTSIDE, AND BETWEEN THE BINARY. ON THE NEXT TWO PAGES YOU'LL FIND DEFINITIONS OF SOME GENDER IDENTITIES.

YOU MAY USE ONE, OR MORE THAN ONE, OF THESE TERMS. YOU MAY USE A TERM THAT ISN'T HERE. THERE MAY NOT BE A TERM, YET, FOR THE WAY YOU FEEL.

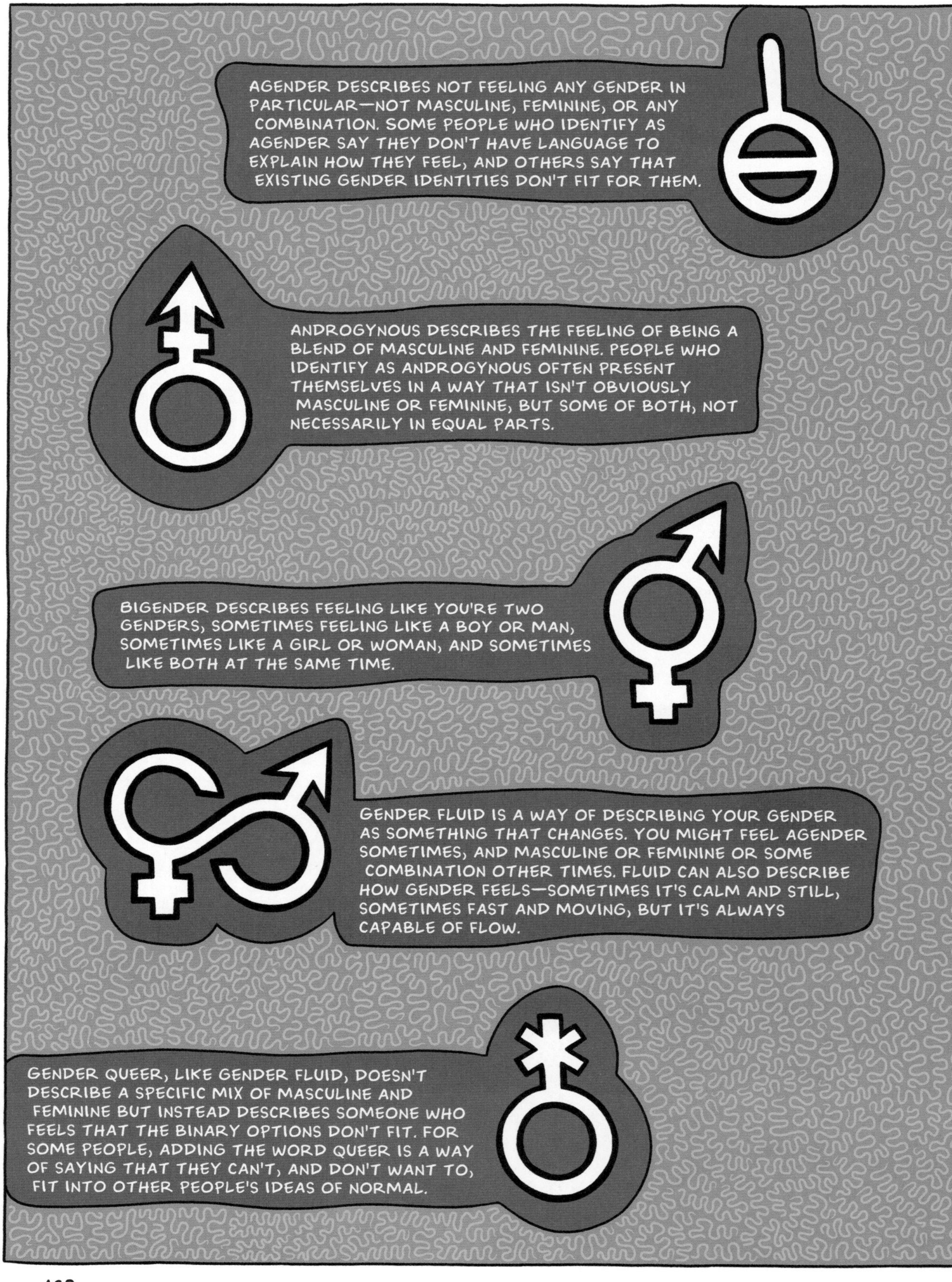
AGENDER DESCRIBES NOT FEELING ANY GENDER IN PARTICULAR—NOT MASCULINE, FEMININE, OR ANY COMBINATION. SOME PEOPLE WHO IDENTIFY AS AGENDER SAY THEY DON'T HAVE LANGUAGE TO EXPLAIN HOW THEY FEEL, AND OTHERS SAY THAT EXISTING GENDER IDENTITIES DON'T FIT FOR THEM.
ANDROGYNOUS DESCRIBES THE FEELING OF BEING A BLEND OF MASCULINE AND FEMININE. PEOPLE WHO IDENTIFY AS ANDROGYNOUS OFTEN PRESENT THEMSELVES IN A WAY THAT ISN'T OBVIOUSLY MASCULINE OR FEMININE, BUT SOME OF BOTH, NOT NECESSARILY IN EQUAL PARTS.
BIGENDER DESCRIBES FEELING LIKE YOU'RE TWO GENDERS, SOMETIMES FEELING LIKE A BOY OR MAN, SOMETIMES LIKE A GIRL OR WOMAN, AND SOMETIMES LIKE BOTH AT THE SAME TIME.
GENDER FLUID IS A WAY OF DESCRIBING YOUR GENDER AS SOMETHING THAT CHANGES. YOU MIGHT FEEL AGENDER SOMETIMES, AND MASCULINE OR FEMININE OR SOME COMBINATION OTHER TIMES. FLUID CAN ALSO DESCRIBE HOW GENDER FEELS—SOMETIMES IT'S CALM AND STILL, SOMETIMES FAST AND MOVING, BUT IT'S ALWAYS CAPABLE OF FLOW.
GENDER QUEER, LIKE GENDER FLUID, DOESN'T DESCRIBE A SPECIFIC MIX OF MASCULINE AND FEMININE BUT INSTEAD DESCRIBES SOMEONE WHO FEELS THAT THE BINARY OPTIONS DON'T FIT. FOR SOME PEOPLE, ADDING THE WORD QUEER IS A WAY OF SAYING THAT THEY CAN'T, AND DON'T WANT TO, FIT INTO OTHER PEOPLE'S IDEAS OF NORMAL.

MAN, OR BOY, IS A WORD THAT IS USUALLY CONNECTED TO THE GENDER BINARY. EVERY COMMUNITY HAS ITS OWN IDEAS OF WHAT IT MEANS TO BE MASCULINE. AND PEOPLE WHO CALL THEMSELVES BOY OR MAN MAY FIT THOSE IDEAS. BUT THERE ARE AS MANY WAYS OF BEING A BOY OR A MAN AS THERE ARE OF BEING ANY GENDER.

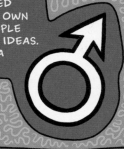

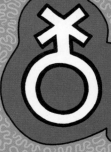

NONBINARY (SOMETIMES "NB" OR "ENBY") DESCRIBES SOMEONE WHO MAY PRESENT AS FEMININE, MASCULINE, ANDROGYNOUS, AND MAY CHANGE AMONG THOSE. IDENTIFYING AS NONBINARY CAN MEAN A LOT OF THINGS, BUT THE IDEA THAT CONNECTS THEM IS THAT HAVING ONLY TWO CHOICES, AND HAVING TO MAKE A DECISION AND STICK WITH IT, DOESN'T WORK.

TRANS (SOMETIMES SHORT FOR TRANSGENDER OR TRANSSEXUAL) IS A WORD THAT PEOPLE USUALLY USE IF THEY WERE ASSIGNED ONE SEX AT BIRTH, BUT THAT ASSIGNED SEX AND THE GENDER EXPECTED TO GO WITH IT DON'T FIT WHO THEY ARE. SOME TRANS PEOPLE IDENTIFY AS A MAN OR A WOMAN. OTHER PEOPLE USE TRANS AS ITS OWN GENDER IDENTITY, RELATED TO BUT SEPARATE FROM MAN OR WOMAN. LIKE ALL GENDERS, THERE ISN'T ONE WAY TO BE TRANS. BEING TRANS DOESN'T MEAN YOU WANT TO, OR ALREADY HAVE, USED HORMONES OR SURGERY TO CHANGE YOUR BODY. HORMONES AND SURGERY ARE PART OF SOME TRANS PEOPLE'S EXPERIENCE.

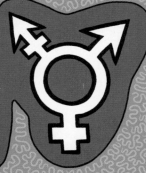

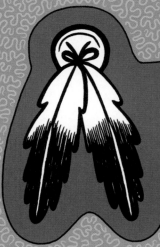

TWO-SPIRIT IS A TERM THAT INCLUDES MANY DIFFERENT SEXUAL AND GENDER IDENTITIES OF INDIGENOUS PEOPLE, INSIDE, OUTSIDE, AND BETWEEN BINARY GENDERS AND SEXUAL IDENTITIES. TWO-SPIRIT HAS DIFFERENT MEANINGS IN DIFFERENT COMMUNITIES. TWO-SPIRIT IS MORE THAN A GENDER OR SEXUAL IDENTITY, IT'S A TERM THAT IS CONNECTED TO BEING INDIGENOUS IN A LAND THAT IS COLONIZED. THIS IS WHY, IF YOU ARE NOT INDIGENOUS, YOU SHOULD NOT USE TWO-SPIRIT FOR YOURSELF.

WOMAN, OR GIRL, IS A GENDER IDENTITY THAT IS USUALLY CONNECTED TO THE GENDER BINARY. EVERY COMMUNITY HAS ITS OWN IDEAS OF WHAT IT MEANS TO BE FEMININE. AND PEOPLE WHO CALL THEMSELVES GIRL OR WOMAN MAY FIT THOSE IDEAS. BUT THERE ARE AS MANY WAYS OF BEING A GIRL OR A WOMAN AS THERE ARE OF BEING ANY GENDER.

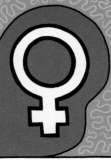

UNITY CENTE
MAKE YOUR OWN STICKERS
PROTECT TRANS KIDS
CHESS CLUB
GENDER WORKSHOP

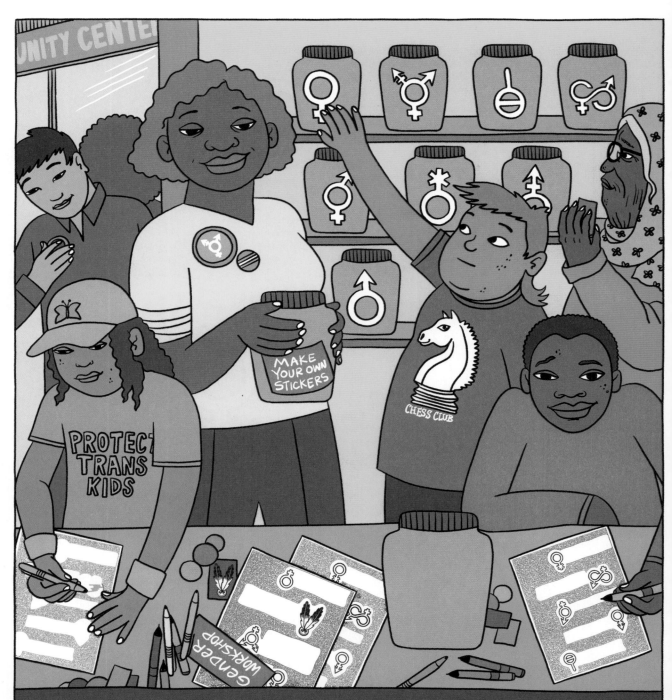

THE GENDER IDENTITY WORDS IN THIS BOOK AREN'T THE BEST ONES OR THE RIGHT ONES, THEY ARE JUST A PLACE TO START. LANGUAGE IS SUPPOSED TO CHANGE. IF YOU DON'T FIND YOURSELF IN THESE TERMS, OR IF YOU THINK THERE'S SOMETHING WRONG WITH ONE OF THEM, YOU GET TO CHANGE IT.

SOME PEOPLE USE THE SAME GENDER IDENTITY THEY WERE CALLED AT BIRTH FOR THEIR WHOLE LIVES. SOME PEOPLE FIND OTHER IDENTITY WORDS THAT ARE A BETTER FIT. AND SOME PEOPLE HAVEN'T FOUND THE WORD THAT FITS FOR THEM, AND INSTEAD FIND THEMSELVES IN THE SPACES BETWEEN OTHER PEOPLE'S DEFINITIONS.

FOR A LOT OF US, GENDER IDENTITY ISN'T SOMETHING WE FIGURE OUT ONCE, AND THEN WE'RE DONE. HOW WE FEEL ABOUT GENDER CAN CHANGE AS WE CHANGE. HOW WE FEEL CAN CHANGE FROM DAY TO DAY AND YEAR TO YEAR.

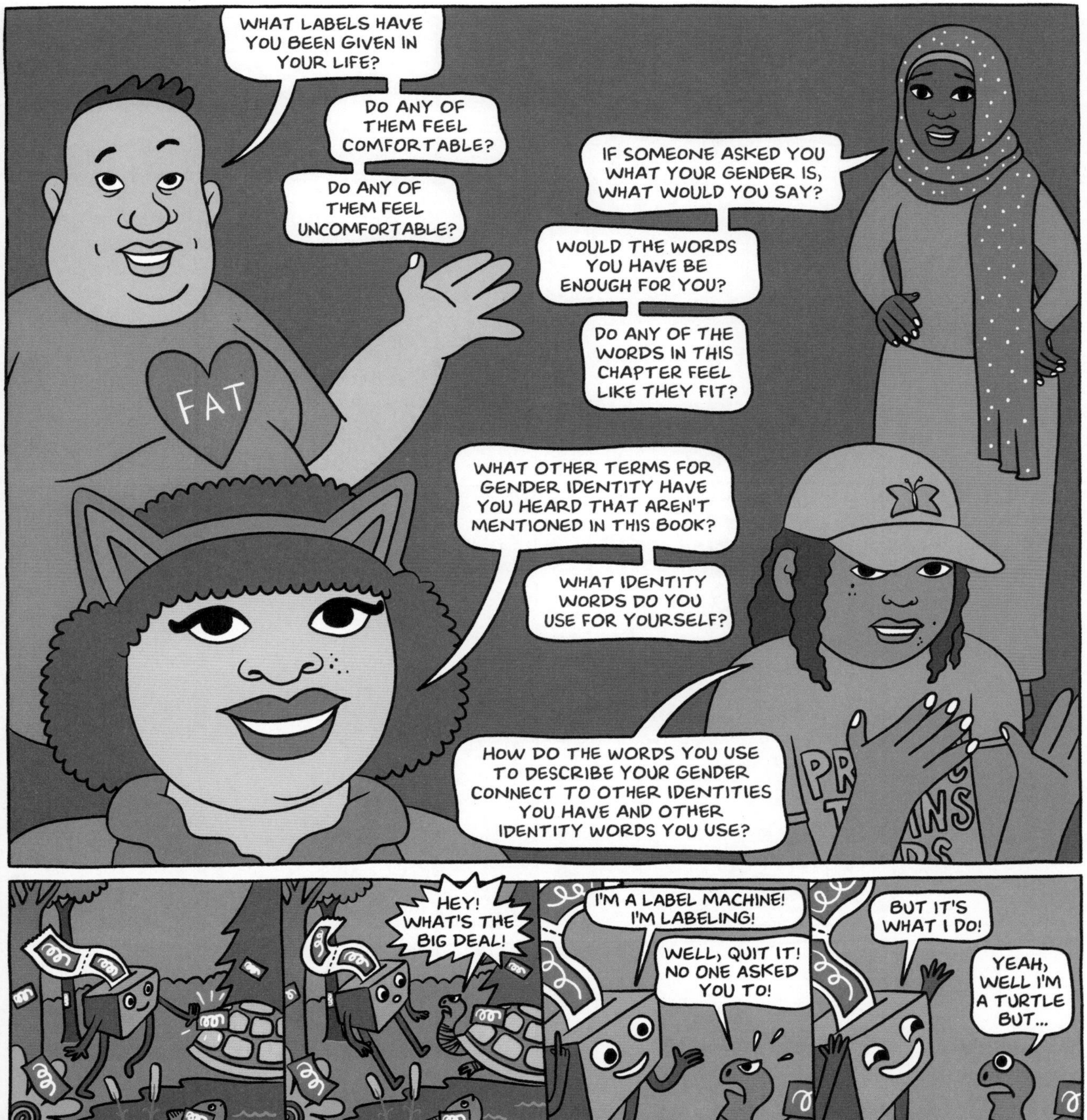
WHAT LABELS HAVE YOU BEEN GIVEN IN YOUR LIFE?
DO ANY OF THEM FEEL COMFORTABLE?
DO ANY OF THEM FEEL UNCOMFORTABLE?
FAT
IF SOMEONE ASKED YOU WHAT YOUR GENDER IS, WHAT WOULD YOU SAY?
WOULD THE WORDS YOU HAVE BE ENOUGH FOR YOU?
DO ANY OF THE WORDS IN THIS CHAPTER FEEL LIKE THEY FIT?
WHAT OTHER TERMS FOR GENDER IDENTITY HAVE YOU HEARD THAT AREN'T MENTIONED IN THIS BOOK?
WHAT IDENTITY WORDS DO YOU USE FOR YOURSELF?
HOW DO THE WORDS YOU USE TO DESCRIBE YOUR GENDER CONNECT TO OTHER IDENTITIES YOU HAVE AND OTHER IDENTITY WORDS YOU USE?
HEY! WHAT'S THE BIG DEAL!
I'M A LABEL MACHINE! I'M LABELING!
WELL, QUIT IT! NO ONE ASKED YOU TO!
BUT IT'S WHAT I DO!
YEAH, WELL I'M A TURTLE BUT...
YOU DON'T SEE ME EATING PIZZA!
YOU ARE MAKING A FICTIONAL TURTLE REFERENCE...
BUT YOU'RE A TURTLE LIVING BESIDE A POND.
AND YOU'RE A TALKING MACHINE!
POINT TAKEN!

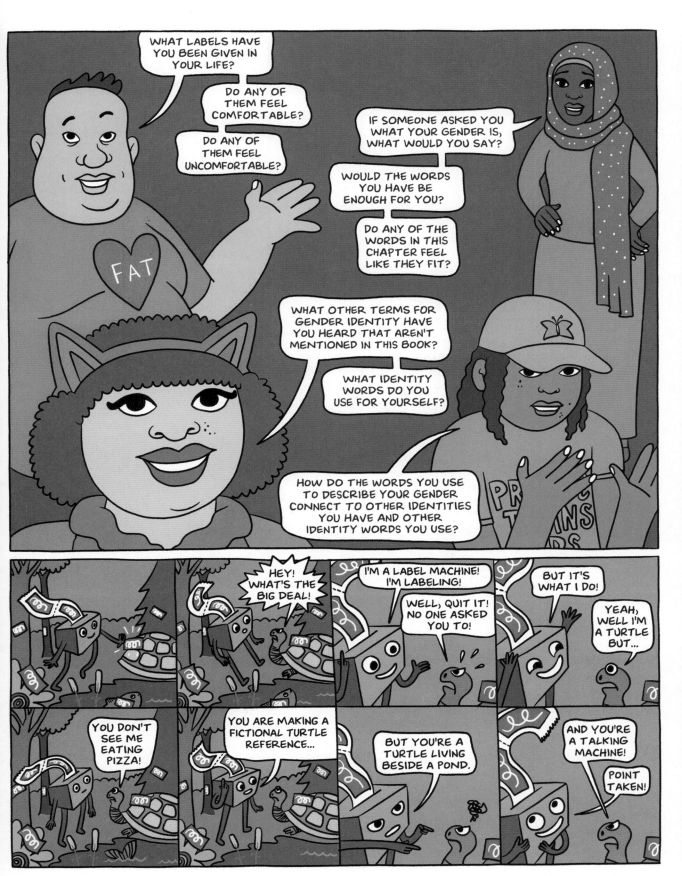

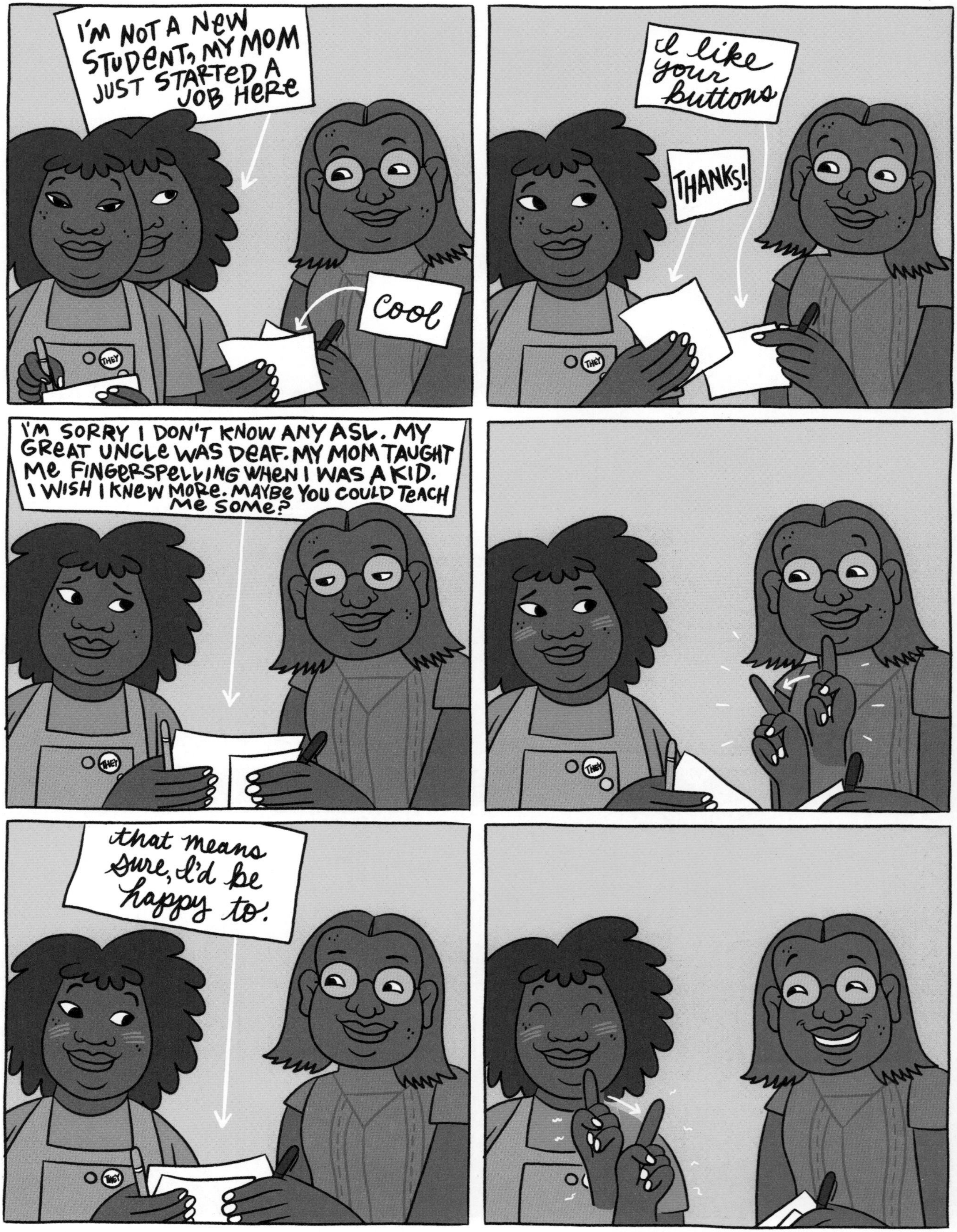
I'M NOT A NEW STUDENT, MY MOM JUST STARTED A JOB HERE
Cool
I like your buttons
THANKS!
I'M SORRY I DON'T KNOW ANY ASL. MY GREAT UNCLE WAS DEAF. MY MOM TAUGHT ME FINGERSPELLING WHEN I WAS A KID. I WISH I KNEW MORE. MAYBE YOU COULD TEACH ME SOME?
THEY
that means sure, I'd be happy to.

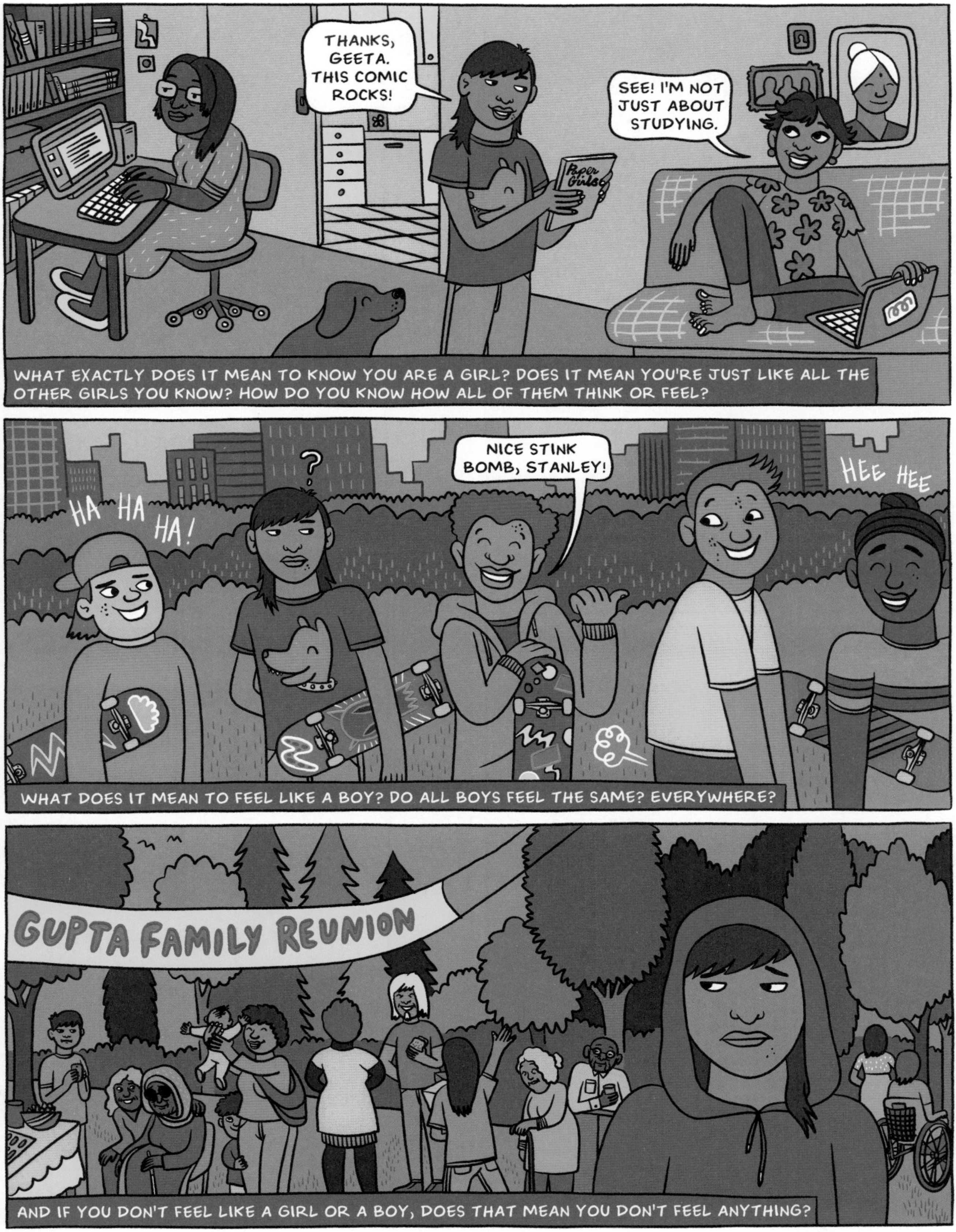
THANKS, GEETA. THIS COMIC ROCKS!
Paper Girls
SEE! I'M NOT JUST ABOUT STUDYING.
WHAT EXACTLY DOES IT MEAN TO KNOW YOU ARE A GIRL? DOES IT MEAN YOU'RE JUST LIKE ALL THE OTHER GIRLS YOU KNOW? HOW DO YOU KNOW HOW ALL OF THEM THINK OR FEEL?
HA HA HA!
?
NICE STINK BOMB, STANLEY!
HEE HEE
WHAT DOES IT MEAN TO FEEL LIKE A BOY? DO ALL BOYS FEEL THE SAME? EVERYWHERE?
GUPTA FAMILY REUNION
AND IF YOU DON'T FEEL LIKE A GIRL OR A BOY, DOES THAT MEAN YOU DON'T FEEL ANYTHING?

WE ALL HAVE FEELINGS ABOUT WHO WE ARE, AND ABOUT WHO OTHER PEOPLE THINK WE ARE. THESE FEELINGS ARE PART OF GENDER.

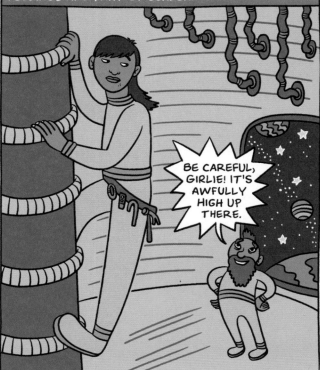

BE CAREFUL, GIRLIE! IT'S AWFULLY HIGH UP THERE.

GENDER CAN FEEL LIKE A BIG DEAL DURING PUBERTY BECAUSE LOTS OF PEOPLE TREAT PUBERTY LIKE IT'S ONLY ABOUT BECOMING A MAN OR A WOMAN.

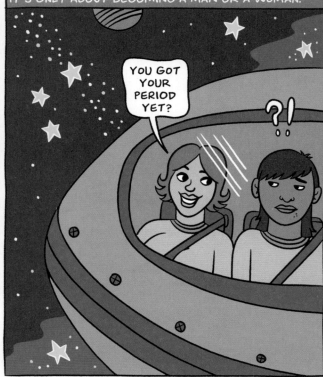

YOU GOT YOUR PERIOD YET?

?!

THERE'S SO MUCH PRESSURE TO FIT IN THAT IT CAN FEEL LIKE WE'RE NEVER COOL ENOUGH, INTERESTING ENOUGH, OR GOOD ENOUGH.

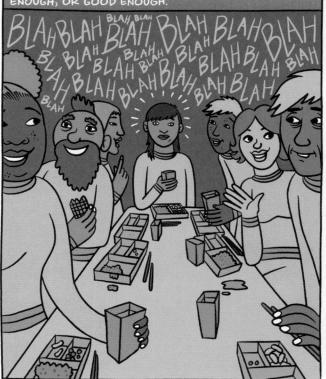

BLAH BLAH BLAH BLAH BLAH BLAH BLAH BLAH BLAH BLAH BLAH BLAH BLAH BLAH BLAH BLAH BLAH BLAH BLAH BLAH BLAH BLAH

FEELING LIKE WE AREN'T RIGHT OR AREN'T ENOUGH IS EXHAUSTING. IT CAN LEAVE US FEELING LIKE AN ALIEN OR LIKE A "THING," NOT A PERSON AT ALL.

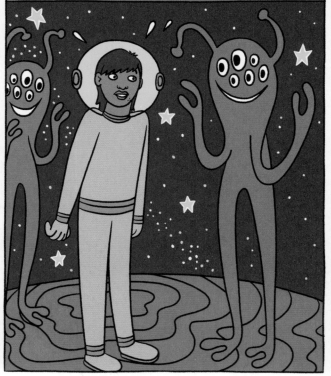

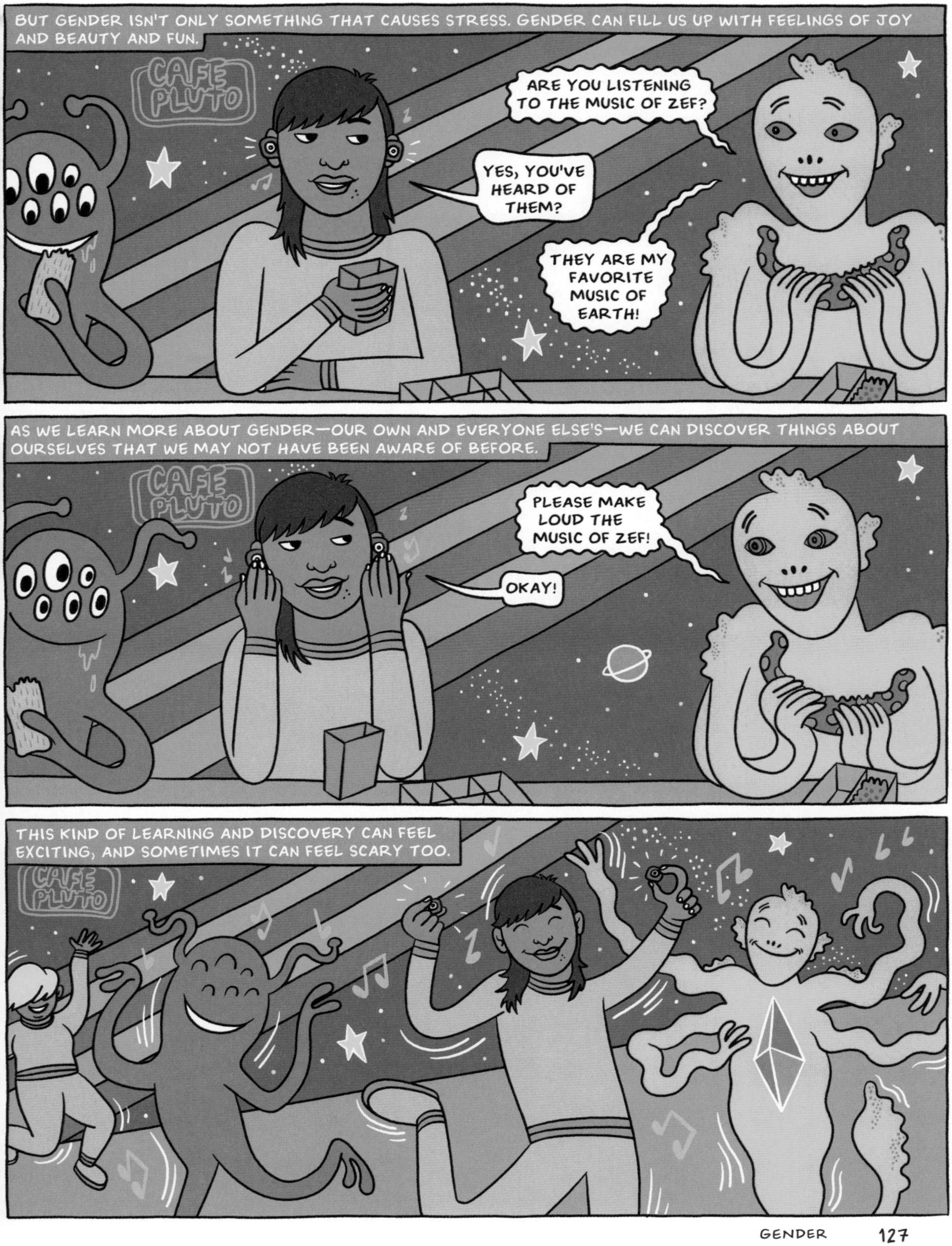
BUT GENDER ISN'T ONLY SOMETHING THAT CAUSES STRESS. GENDER CAN FILL US UP WITH FEELINGS OF JOY AND BEAUTY AND FUN.
CAFE PLUTO
ARE YOU LISTENING TO THE MUSIC OF ZEF?
YES, YOU'VE HEARD OF THEM?
THEY ARE MY FAVORITE MUSIC OF EARTH!
AS WE LEARN MORE ABOUT GENDER—OUR OWN AND EVERYONE ELSE'S—WE CAN DISCOVER THINGS ABOUT OURSELVES THAT WE MAY NOT HAVE BEEN AWARE OF BEFORE.
CAFE PLUTO
PLEASE MAKE LOUD THE MUSIC OF ZEF!
OKAY!
THIS KIND OF LEARNING AND DISCOVERY CAN FEEL EXCITING, AND SOMETIMES IT CAN FEEL SCARY TOO.
CAFE PLUTO

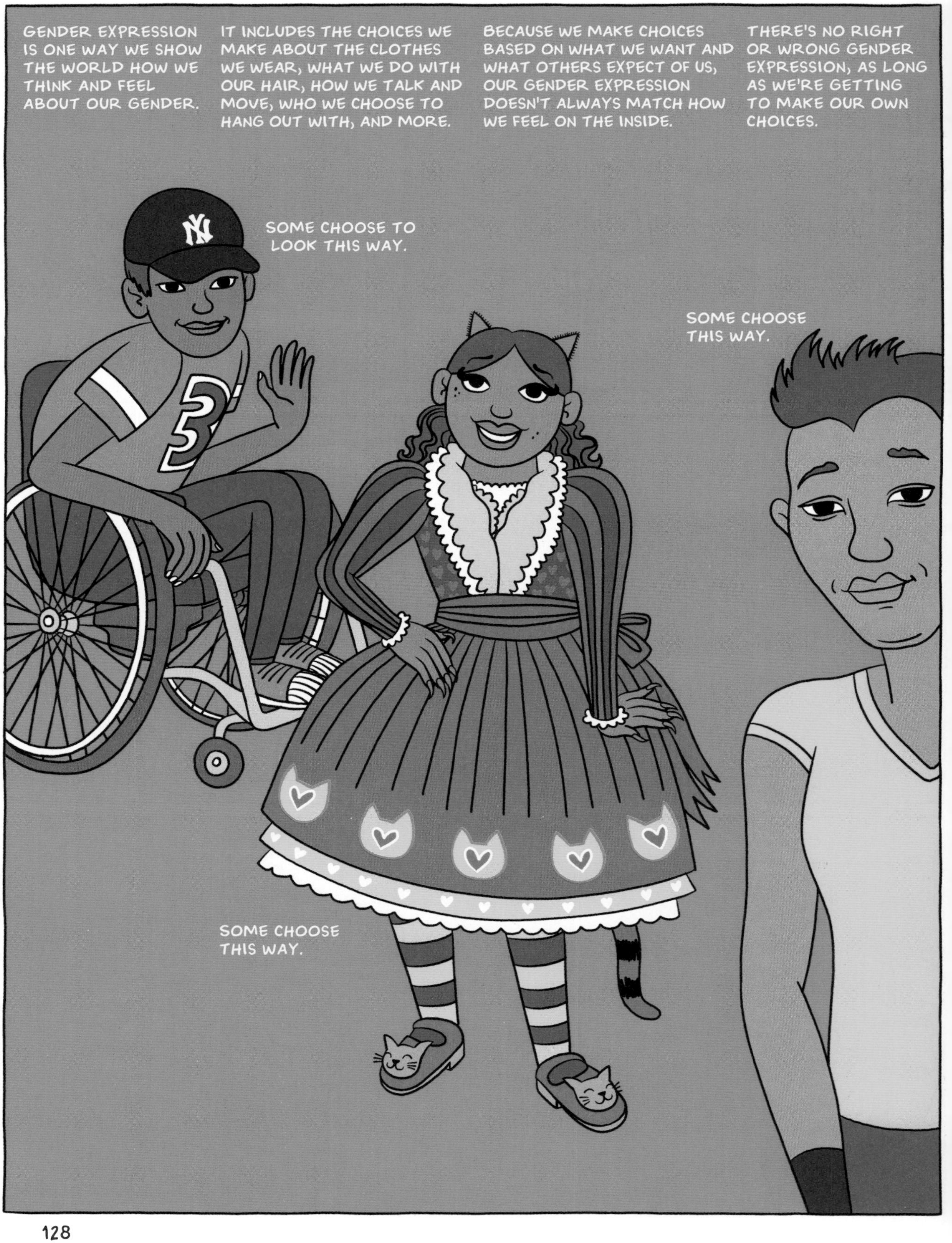
GENDER EXPRESSION IS ONE WAY WE SHOW THE WORLD HOW WE THINK AND FEEL ABOUT OUR GENDER.
IT INCLUDES THE CHOICES WE MAKE ABOUT THE CLOTHES WE WEAR, WHAT WE DO WITH OUR HAIR, HOW WE TALK AND MOVE, WHO WE CHOOSE TO HANG OUT WITH, AND MORE.
BECAUSE WE MAKE CHOICES BASED ON WHAT WE WANT AND WHAT OTHERS EXPECT OF US, OUR GENDER EXPRESSION DOESN'T ALWAYS MATCH HOW WE FEEL ON THE INSIDE.
THERE'S NO RIGHT OR WRONG GENDER EXPRESSION, AS LONG AS WE'RE GETTING TO MAKE OUR OWN CHOICES.
SOME CHOOSE TO LOOK THIS WAY.
SOME CHOOSE THIS WAY.
SOME CHOOSE THIS WAY.

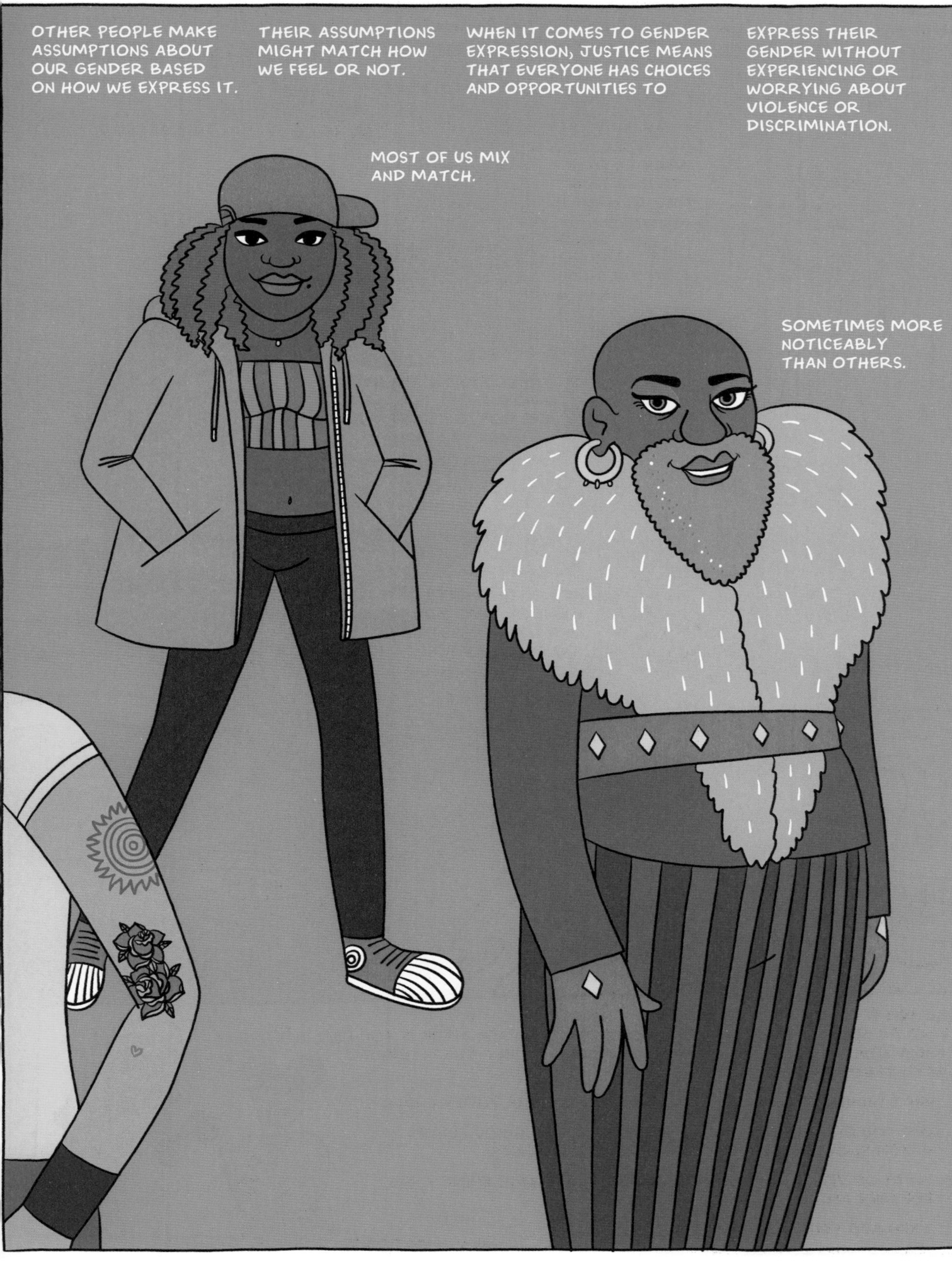
OTHER PEOPLE MAKE ASSUMPTIONS ABOUT OUR GENDER BASED ON HOW WE EXPRESS IT.
THEIR ASSUMPTIONS MIGHT MATCH HOW WE FEEL OR NOT.
WHEN IT COMES TO GENDER EXPRESSION, JUSTICE MEANS THAT EVERYONE HAS CHOICES AND OPPORTUNITIES TO
EXPRESS THEIR GENDER WITHOUT EXPERIENCING OR WORRYING ABOUT VIOLENCE OR DISCRIMINATION.
MOST OF US MIX AND MATCH.
SOMETIMES MORE NOTICEABLY THAN OTHERS.

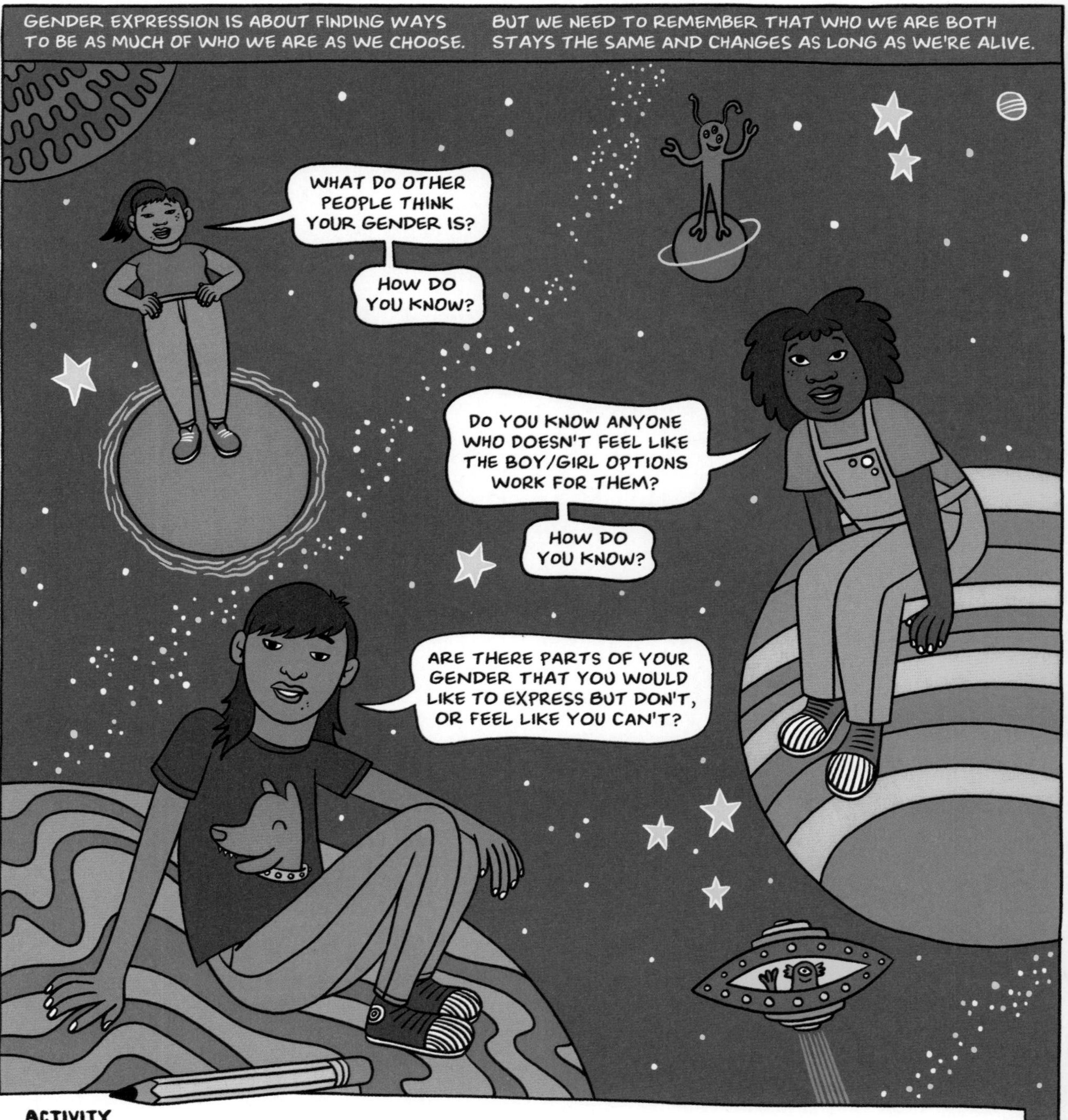
GENDER EXPRESSION IS ABOUT FINDING WAYS TO BE AS MUCH OF WHO WE ARE AS WE CHOOSE.
BUT WE NEED TO REMEMBER THAT WHO WE ARE BOTH STAYS THE SAME AND CHANGES AS LONG AS WE'RE ALIVE.
WHAT DO OTHER PEOPLE THINK YOUR GENDER IS?
HOW DO YOU KNOW?
DO YOU KNOW ANYONE WHO DOESN'T FEEL LIKE THE BOY/GIRL OPTIONS WORK FOR THEM?
HOW DO YOU KNOW?
ARE THERE PARTS OF YOUR GENDER THAT YOU WOULD LIKE TO EXPRESS BUT DON'T, OR FEEL LIKE YOU CAN'T?

ACTIVITY

FIND AN ADULT IN YOUR LIFE WHO YOU TRUST AND ASK THEM IF YOU CAN INTERVIEW THEM ABOUT THEIR GENDER. IF THEY AGREE, START THE INTERVIEW WITH THESE THREE QUESTIONS:

1. WHAT WORD OR WORDS DO YOU USE TO DESCRIBE YOUR GENDER?
2. CAN YOU DESCRIBE A TIME WHEN YOU FELT LIKE YOU DIDN'T MATCH PEOPLE'S EXPECTATIONS OF YOUR GENDER?
3. WHAT DO YOU THINK ABOUT THE IDEA THAT SOME THINGS ARE FOR MEN AND OTHERS ARE FOR WOMEN?

THEN ADD YOUR OWN QUESTIONS!

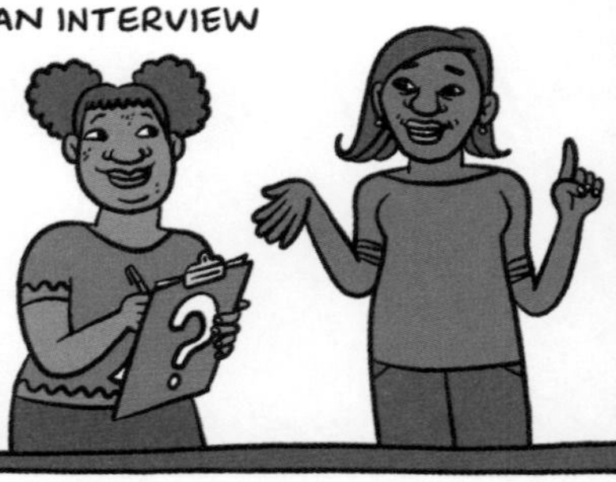

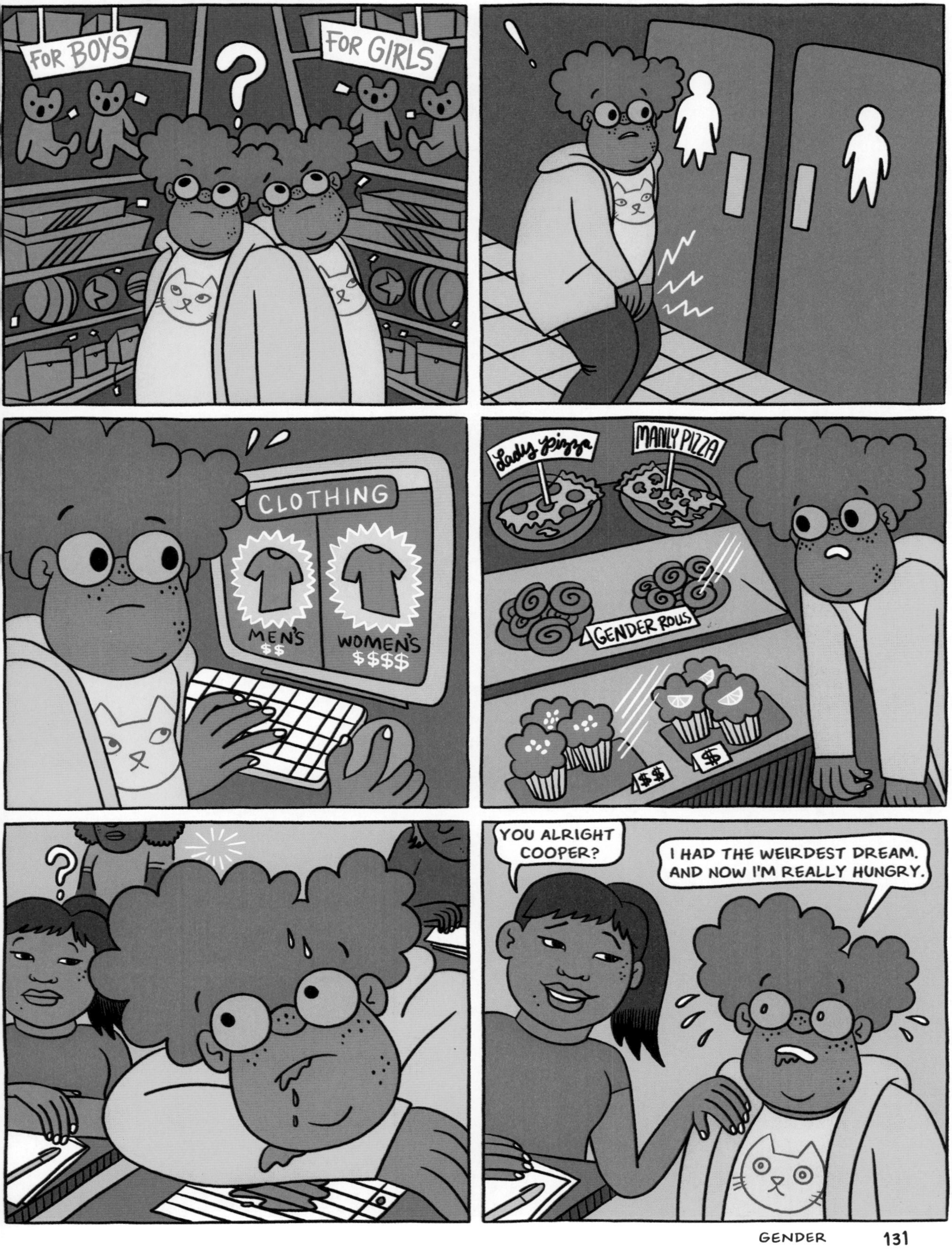
FOR BOYS
FOR GIRLS
CLOTHING
MEN'S $$
WOMEN'S $$$$
Lady pizza
MANLY PIZZA
GENDER ROLLS
$$
$
YOU ALRIGHT COOPER?
I HAD THE WEIRDEST DREAM. AND NOW I'M REALLY HUNGRY.

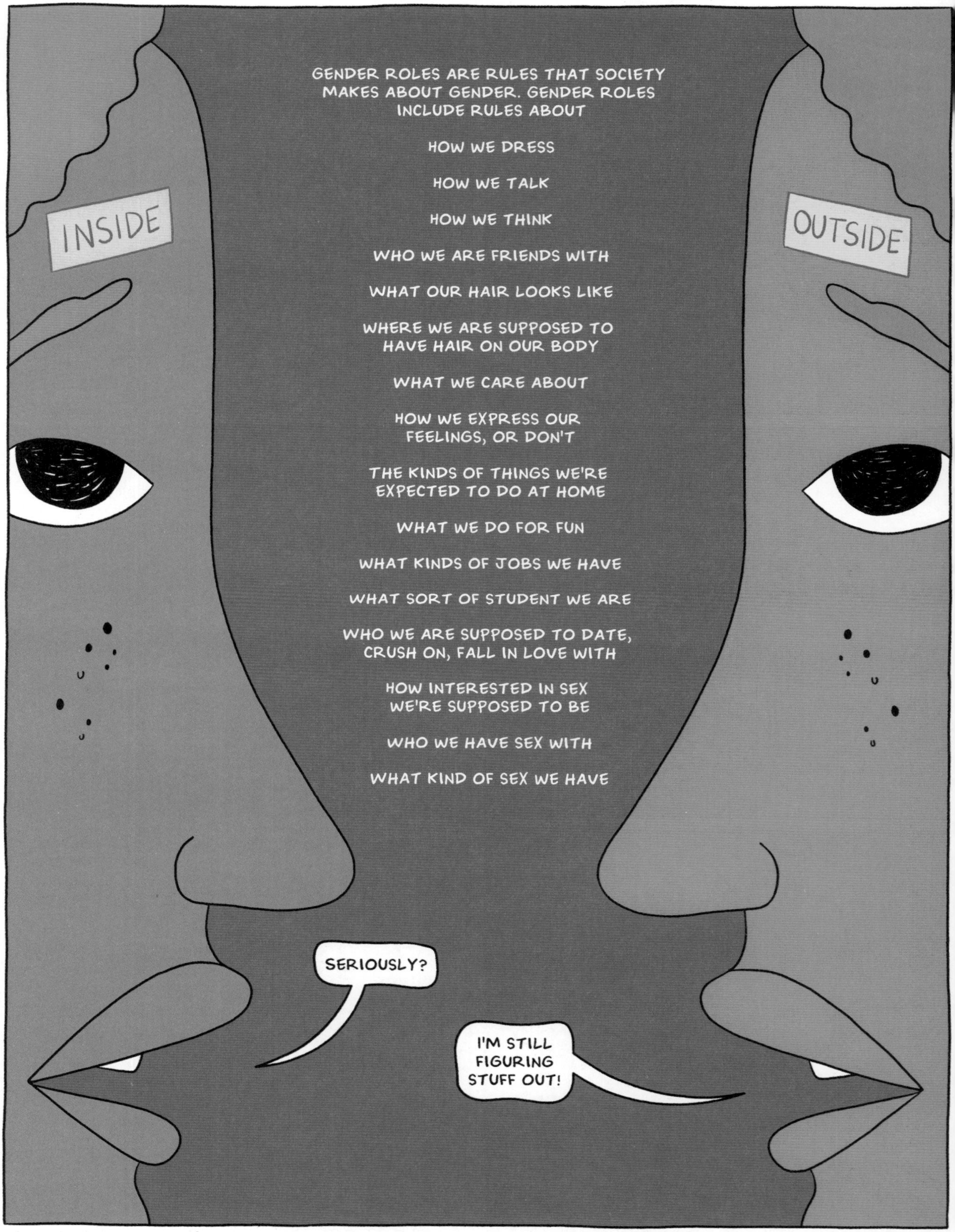
INSIDE
OUTSIDE
GENDER ROLES ARE RULES THAT SOCIETY MAKES ABOUT GENDER. GENDER ROLES INCLUDE RULES ABOUT
HOW WE DRESS
HOW WE TALK
HOW WE THINK
WHO WE ARE FRIENDS WITH
WHAT OUR HAIR LOOKS LIKE
WHERE WE ARE SUPPOSED TO HAVE HAIR ON OUR BODY
WHAT WE CARE ABOUT
HOW WE EXPRESS OUR FEELINGS, OR DON'T
THE KINDS OF THINGS WE'RE EXPECTED TO DO AT HOME
WHAT WE DO FOR FUN
WHAT KINDS OF JOBS WE HAVE
WHAT SORT OF STUDENT WE ARE
WHO WE ARE SUPPOSED TO DATE, CRUSH ON, FALL IN LOVE WITH
HOW INTERESTED IN SEX WE'RE SUPPOSED TO BE
WHO WE HAVE SEX WITH
WHAT KIND OF SEX WE HAVE
SERIOUSLY?
I'M STILL FIGURING STUFF OUT!

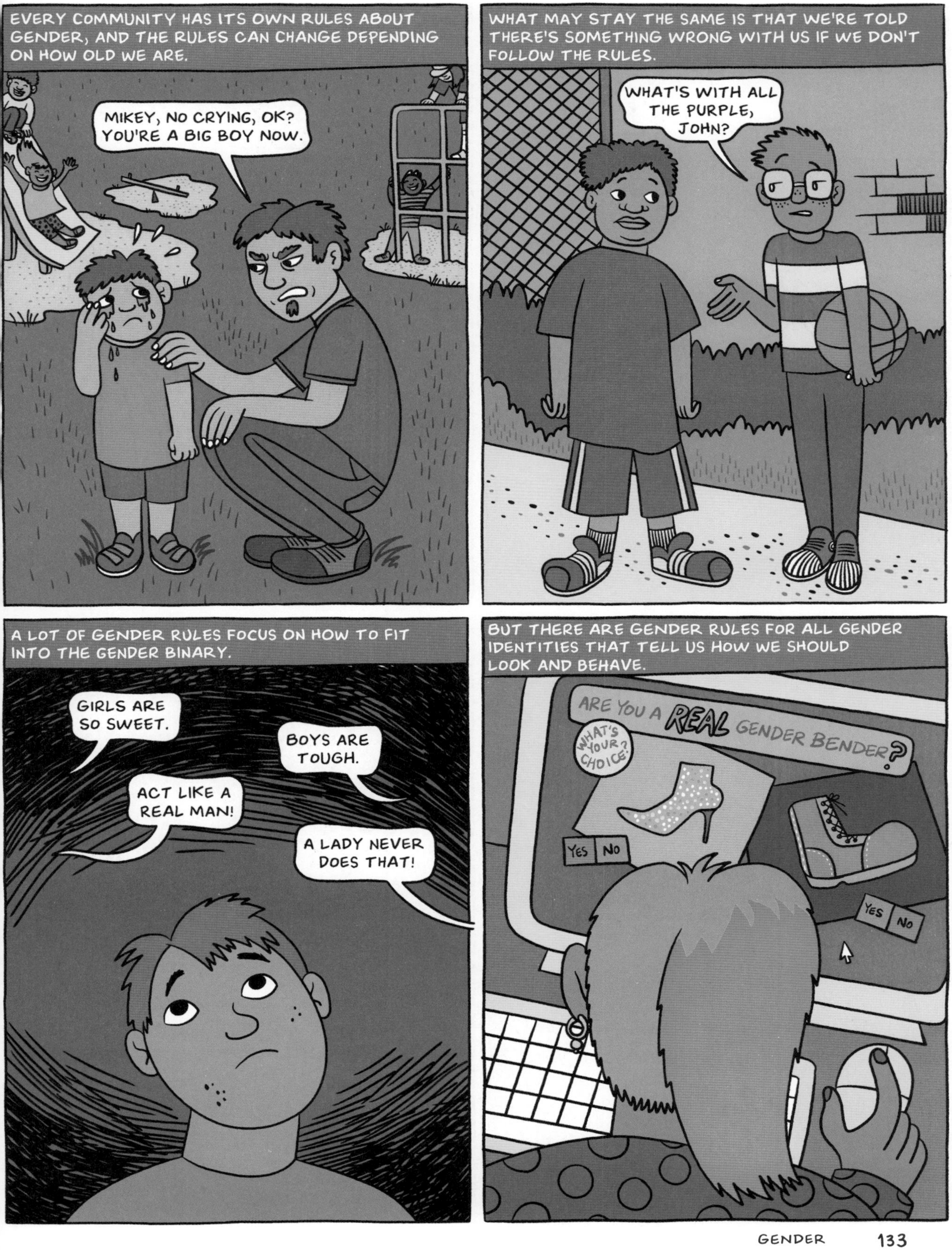
EVERY COMMUNITY HAS ITS OWN RULES ABOUT GENDER, AND THE RULES CAN CHANGE DEPENDING ON HOW OLD WE ARE.
MIKEY, NO CRYING, OK? YOU'RE A BIG BOY NOW.
WHAT MAY STAY THE SAME IS THAT WE'RE TOLD THERE'S SOMETHING WRONG WITH US IF WE DON'T FOLLOW THE RULES.
WHAT'S WITH ALL THE PURPLE, JOHN?
A LOT OF GENDER RULES FOCUS ON HOW TO FIT INTO THE GENDER BINARY.
GIRLS ARE SO SWEET.
BOYS ARE TOUGH.
ACT LIKE A REAL MAN!
A LADY NEVER DOES THAT!
BUT THERE ARE GENDER RULES FOR ALL GENDER IDENTITIES THAT TELL US HOW WE SHOULD LOOK AND BEHAVE.
ARE YOU A REAL GENDER BENDER?
WHAT'S YOUR CHOICE?
YES NO
YES NO

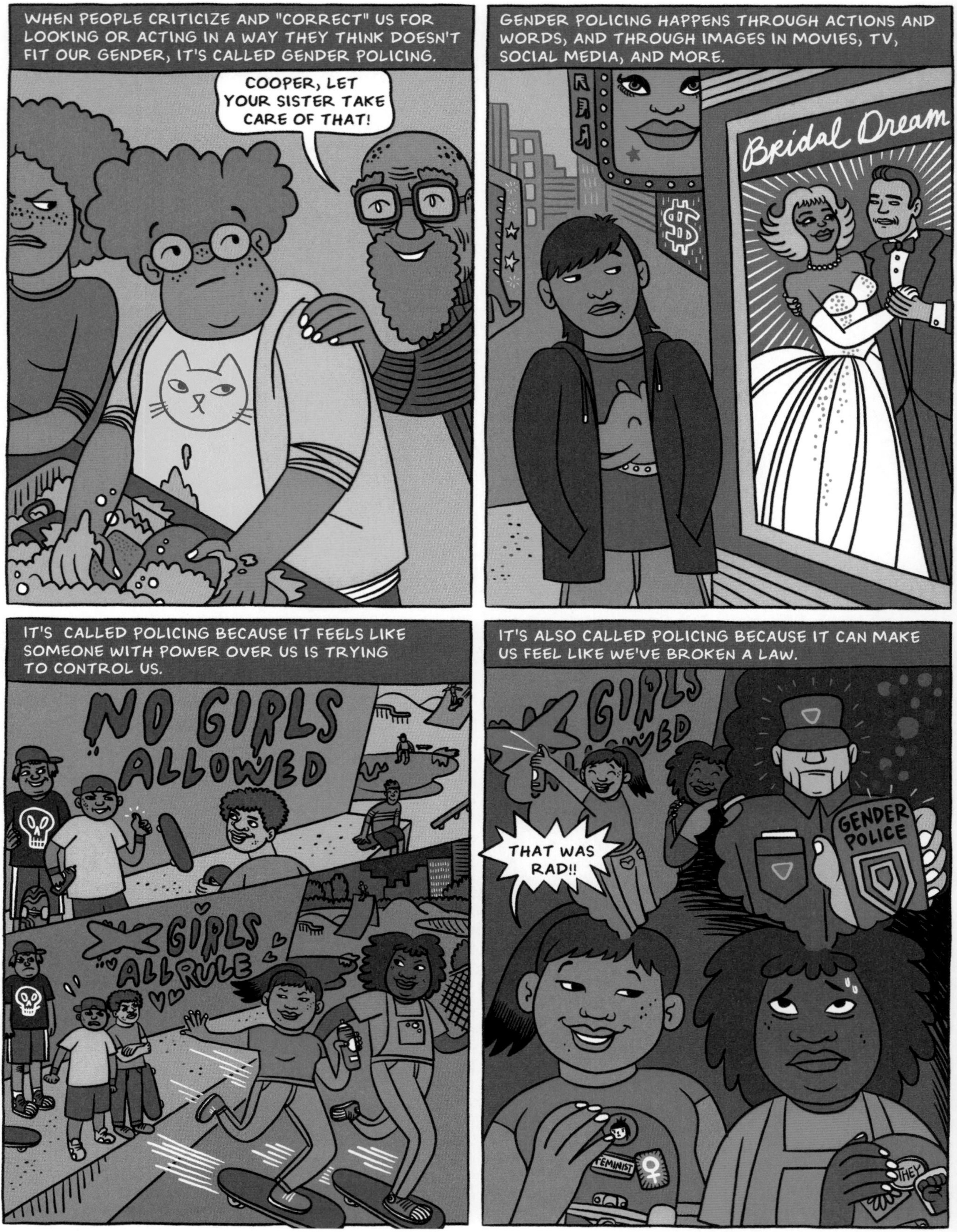
WHEN PEOPLE CRITICIZE AND "CORRECT" US FOR LOOKING OR ACTING IN A WAY THEY THINK DOESN'T FIT OUR GENDER, IT'S CALLED GENDER POLICING.
COOPER, LET YOUR SISTER TAKE CARE OF THAT!
GENDER POLICING HAPPENS THROUGH ACTIONS AND WORDS, AND THROUGH IMAGES IN MOVIES, TV, SOCIAL MEDIA, AND MORE.
Bridal Dream
IT'S CALLED POLICING BECAUSE IT FEELS LIKE SOMEONE WITH POWER OVER US IS TRYING TO CONTROL US.
NO GIRLS ALLOWED
GIRLS ALL RULE
IT'S ALSO CALLED POLICING BECAUSE IT CAN MAKE US FEEL LIKE WE'VE BROKEN A LAW.
THAT WAS RAD!!
GENDER POLICE
FEMINIST
THEY

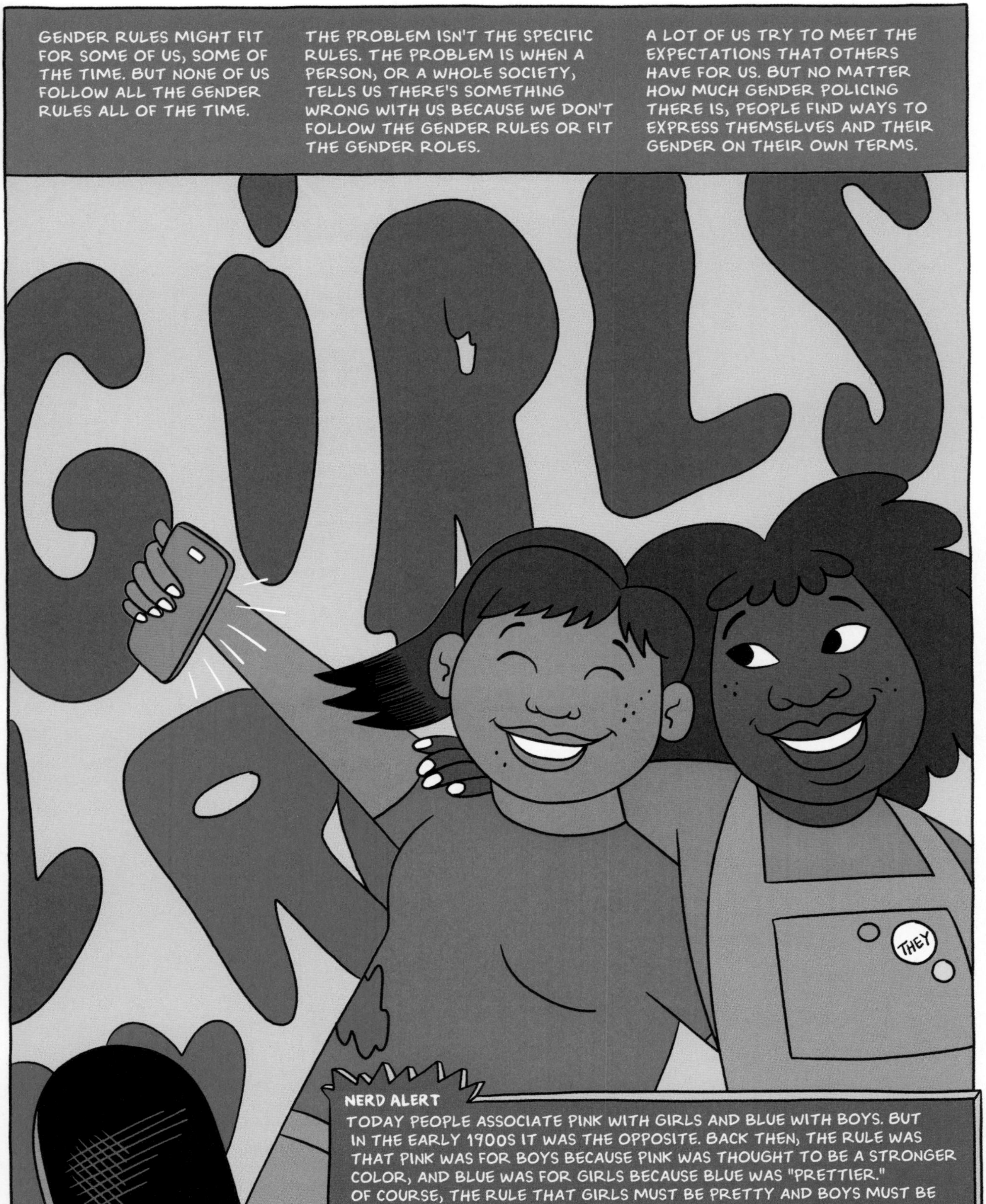
GENDER RULES MIGHT FIT FOR SOME OF US, SOME OF THE TIME. BUT NONE OF US FOLLOW ALL THE GENDER RULES ALL OF THE TIME.
THE PROBLEM ISN'T THE SPECIFIC RULES. THE PROBLEM IS WHEN A PERSON, OR A WHOLE SOCIETY, TELLS US THERE'S SOMETHING WRONG WITH US BECAUSE WE DON'T FOLLOW THE GENDER RULES OR FIT THE GENDER ROLES.
A LOT OF US TRY TO MEET THE EXPECTATIONS THAT OTHERS HAVE FOR US. BUT NO MATTER HOW MUCH GENDER POLICING THERE IS, PEOPLE FIND WAYS TO EXPRESS THEMSELVES AND THEIR GENDER ON THEIR OWN TERMS.
GIRLS
THEY
NERD ALERT
TODAY PEOPLE ASSOCIATE PINK WITH GIRLS AND BLUE WITH BOYS. BUT IN THE EARLY 1900S IT WAS THE OPPOSITE. BACK THEN, THE RULE WAS THAT PINK WAS FOR BOYS BECAUSE PINK WAS THOUGHT TO BE A STRONGER COLOR, AND BLUE WAS FOR GIRLS BECAUSE BLUE WAS "PRETTIER." OF COURSE, THE RULE THAT GIRLS MUST BE PRETTY AND BOYS MUST BE STRONG MAKES NO SENSE. ALL OF US CAN BE PRETTY OR STRONG, AND ALL OF US CAN BE NEITHER. AND WE CAN WEAR WHATEVER COLORS WE WANT.

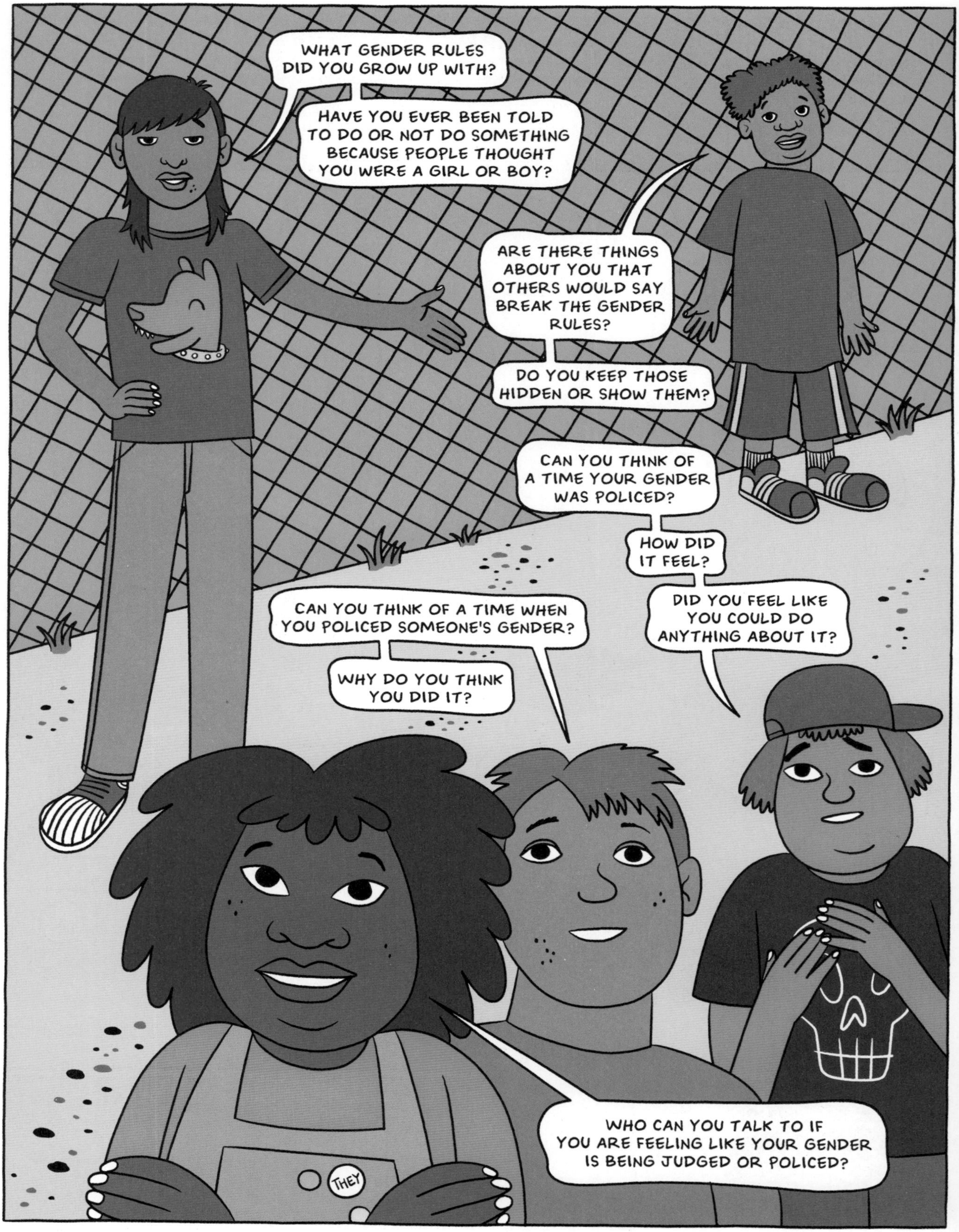
WHAT GENDER RULES DID YOU GROW UP WITH?
HAVE YOU EVER BEEN TOLD TO DO OR NOT DO SOMETHING BECAUSE PEOPLE THOUGHT YOU WERE A GIRL OR BOY?
ARE THERE THINGS ABOUT YOU THAT OTHERS WOULD SAY BREAK THE GENDER RULES?
DO YOU KEEP THOSE HIDDEN OR SHOW THEM?
CAN YOU THINK OF A TIME YOUR GENDER WAS POLICED?
HOW DID IT FEEL?
DID YOU FEEL LIKE YOU COULD DO ANYTHING ABOUT IT?
CAN YOU THINK OF A TIME WHEN YOU POLICED SOMEONE'S GENDER?
WHY DO YOU THINK YOU DID IT?
WHO CAN YOU TALK TO IF YOU ARE FEELING LIKE YOUR GENDER IS BEING JUDGED OR POLICED?
THEY

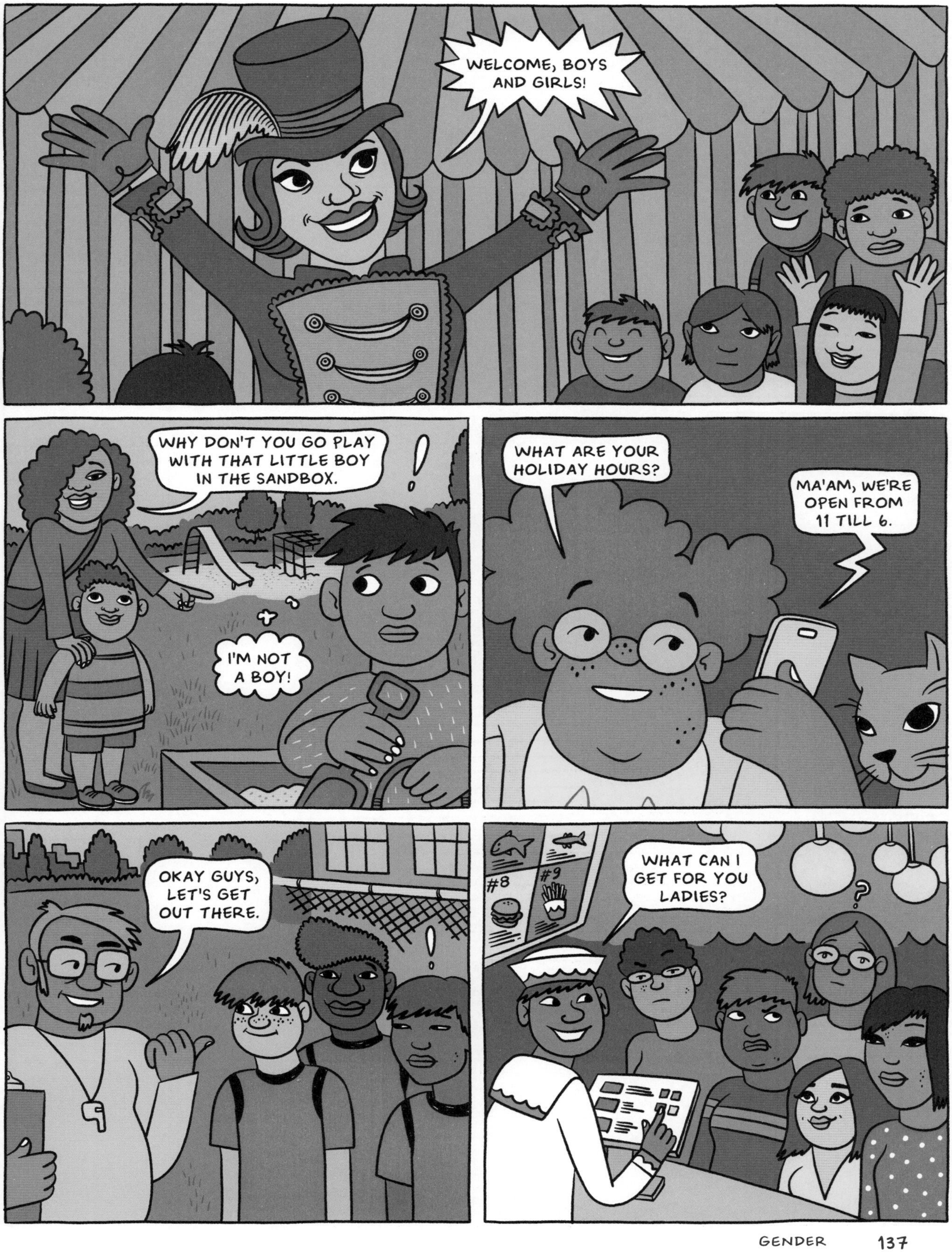
WELCOME, BOYS AND GIRLS!
WHY DON'T YOU GO PLAY WITH THAT LITTLE BOY IN THE SANDBOX.
!
I'M NOT A BOY!
WHAT ARE YOUR HOLIDAY HOURS?
MA'AM, WE'RE OPEN FROM 11 TILL 6.
OKAY GUYS, LET'S GET OUT THERE.
!
#8
#9
WHAT CAN I GET FOR YOU LADIES?
?

PRONOUNS ARE THE SHORT WORDS THAT FILL IN FOR THE NAME OF A PERSON, PLACE, OR THING. IF WE SEE SOMEONE WHO WE THINK LOOKS LIKE A BOY, MOST OF US SAY "HE." IF WE SEE SOMEONE WHO WE THINK LOOKS LIKE A GIRL, MOST OF US SAY "SHE."

WE CHOOSE "HE" OR "SHE" BASED ON WHAT PEOPLE LOOK LIKE ON THE OUTSIDE. WHEN WE CALL SOMEONE "HE" OR "SHE," WE'RE ALSO ASSUMING WE KNOW THEIR GENDER. BUT WE CAN'T KNOW SOMEONE'S GENDER JUST FROM THEIR OUTSIDE. WE CAN'T KNOW UNLESS THEY TELL US.

ZE HIR Mr.

THEM HER

Mx.

WHEN WE GUESS AT SOMEONE'S GENDER, SOMETIMES WE GET IT WRONG. AND WHEN WE ONLY USE "HE" OR "SHE," WE IGNORE EVERYONE ELSE, OR ACT LIKE THEY DON'T EVEN EXIST.

JUST LIKE YOU GET TO CHOOSE WHICH GENDER IDENTITIES FIT YOU BEST, YOU GET TO CHOOSE WHICH PRONOUNS YOU WOULD LIKE PEOPLE TO USE. EVEN IF YOU'VE BEEN CALLED BY ONE PRONOUN YOUR WHOLE LIFE, YOU MAY KNOW THAT IT DOESN'T FIT, AND WANT PEOPLE TO USE A DIFFERENT PRONOUN.

ONE WAY WE CAN SHOW RESPECT IS BY PAYING ATTENTION TO THE WORDS PEOPLE USE FOR THEMSELVES AND USING THOSE WORDS, NOT THE WORDS WE THINK THEY SHOULD USE.

Ms.

THEY Mrs.

HE HIM

SHE

WHEN WE CALL SOMEONE BY A PRONOUN THAT DOESN'T FIT FOR THEM IT'S CALLED MISGENDERING.

WHEN WE DON'T KNOW WHAT PRONOUNS OR WORDS SOMEONE USES FOR THEMSELVES, THE EASIEST WAY TO BE RESPECTFUL IS TO USE THEIR NAME. SOME PEOPLE USE "THEY" AS A GENDER NEUTRAL PRONOUN IF THEY DON'T KNOW WHAT PRONOUNS A PERSON USES.

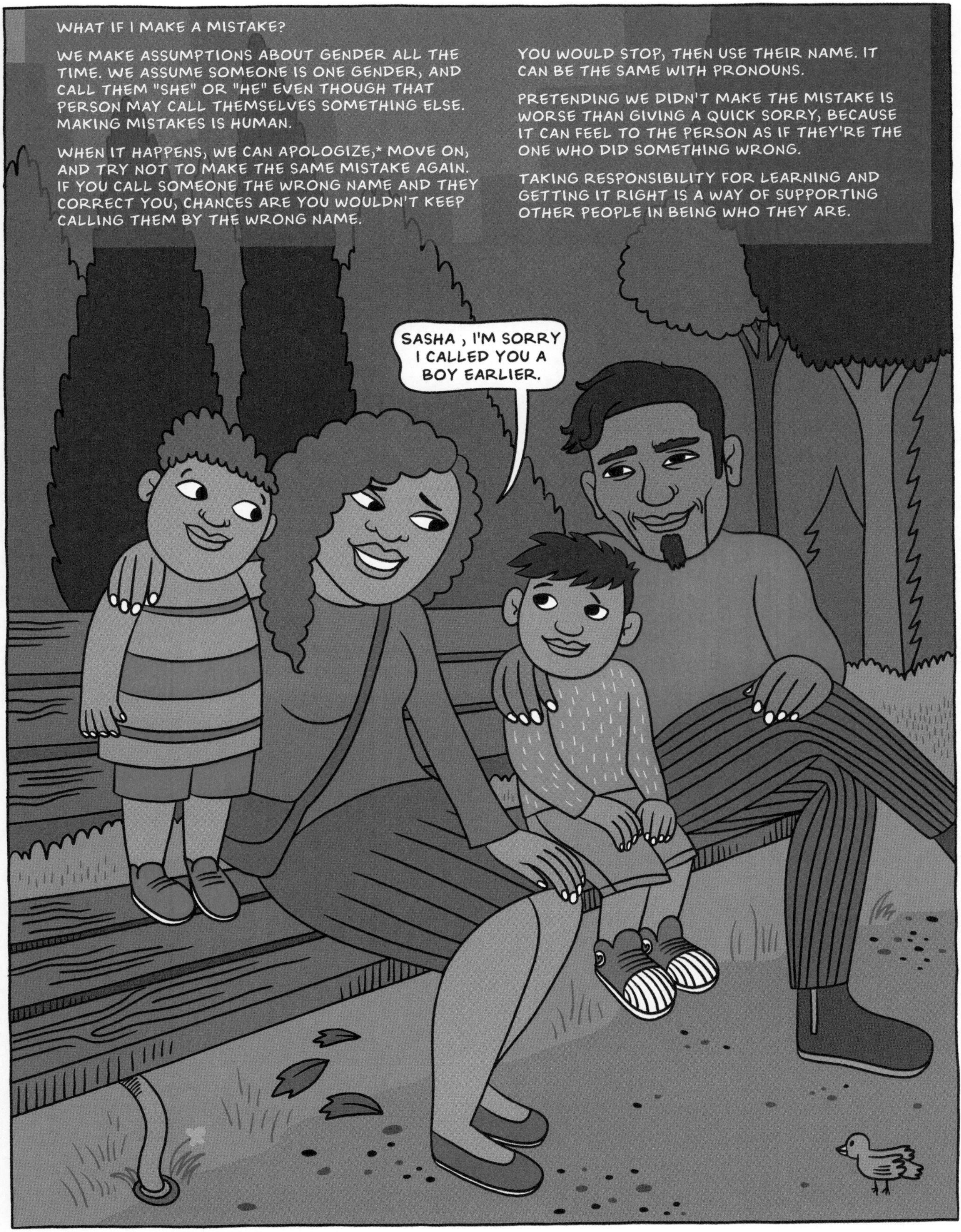
WHAT IF I MAKE A MISTAKE?
WE MAKE ASSUMPTIONS ABOUT GENDER ALL THE TIME. WE ASSUME SOMEONE IS ONE GENDER, AND CALL THEM "SHE" OR "HE" EVEN THOUGH THAT PERSON MAY CALL THEMSELVES SOMETHING ELSE. MAKING MISTAKES IS HUMAN.
WHEN IT HAPPENS, WE CAN APOLOGIZE,* MOVE ON, AND TRY NOT TO MAKE THE SAME MISTAKE AGAIN. IF YOU CALL SOMEONE THE WRONG NAME AND THEY CORRECT YOU, CHANCES ARE YOU WOULDN'T KEEP CALLING THEM BY THE WRONG NAME. YOU WOULD STOP, THEN USE THEIR NAME. IT CAN BE THE SAME WITH PRONOUNS.
PRETENDING WE DIDN'T MAKE THE MISTAKE IS WORSE THAN GIVING A QUICK SORRY, BECAUSE IT CAN FEEL TO THE PERSON AS IF THEY'RE THE ONE WHO DID SOMETHING WRONG.
TAKING RESPONSIBILITY FOR LEARNING AND GETTING IT RIGHT IS A WAY OF SUPPORTING OTHER PEOPLE IN BEING WHO THEY ARE.
SASHA, I'M SORRY I CALLED YOU A BOY EARLIER.

* MORE ABOUT APOLOGIZING ON P. 383

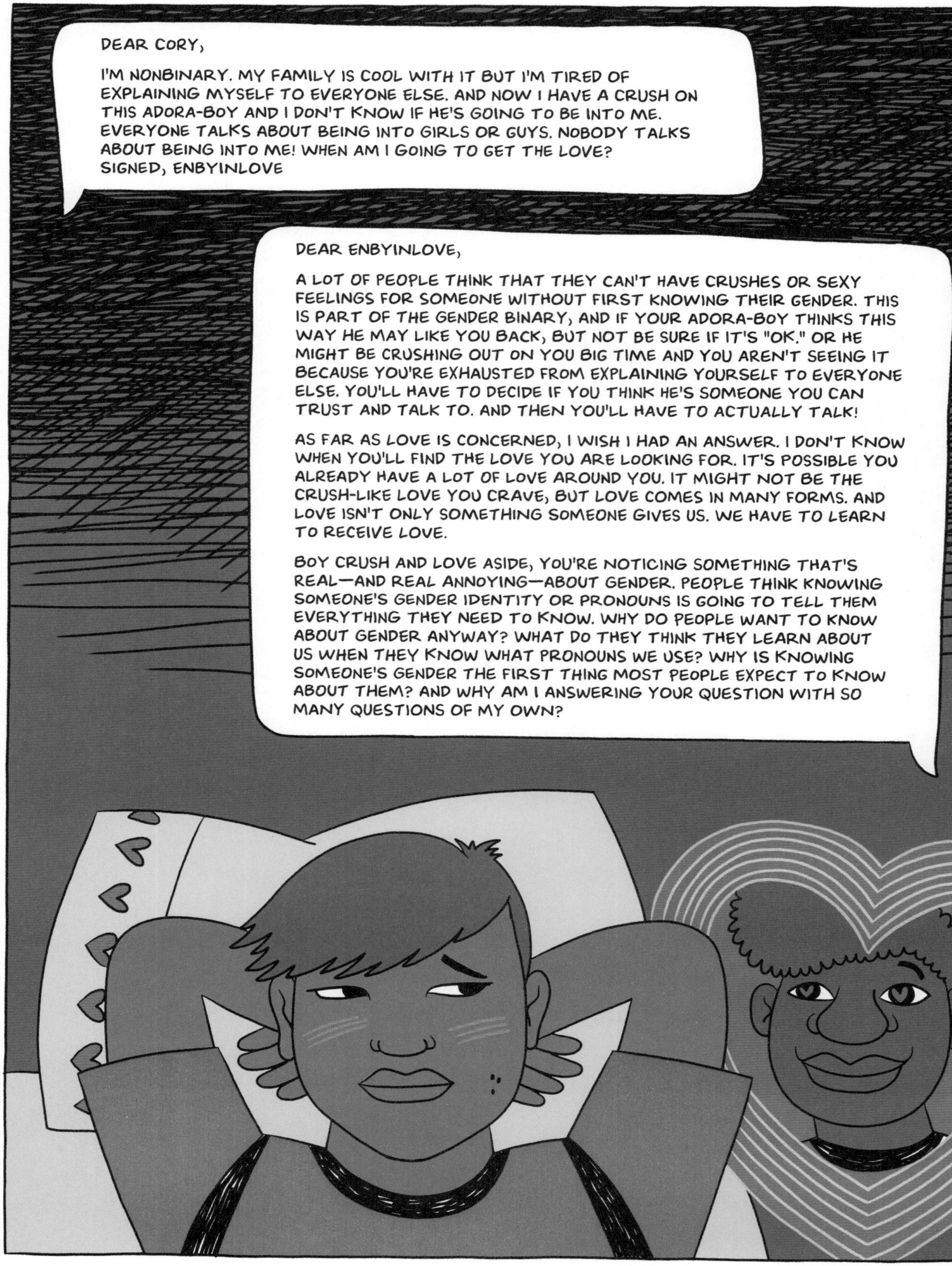

DEAR CORY,

I'M NONBINARY. MY FAMILY IS COOL WITH IT BUT I'M TIRED OF EXPLAINING MYSELF TO EVERYONE ELSE. AND NOW I HAVE A CRUSH ON THIS ADORA-BOY AND I DON'T KNOW IF HE'S GOING TO BE INTO ME. EVERYONE TALKS ABOUT BEING INTO GIRLS OR GUYS. NOBODY TALKS ABOUT BEING INTO ME! WHEN AM I GOING TO GET THE LOVE? SIGNED, ENBYINLOVE

DEAR ENBYINLOVE,

A LOT OF PEOPLE THINK THAT THEY CAN'T HAVE CRUSHES OR SEXY FEELINGS FOR SOMEONE WITHOUT FIRST KNOWING THEIR GENDER. THIS IS PART OF THE GENDER BINARY, AND IF YOUR ADORA-BOY THINKS THIS WAY HE MAY LIKE YOU BACK, BUT NOT BE SURE IF IT'S "OK." OR HE MIGHT BE CRUSHING OUT ON YOU BIG TIME AND YOU AREN'T SEEING IT BECAUSE YOU'RE EXHAUSTED FROM EXPLAINING YOURSELF TO EVERYONE ELSE. YOU'LL HAVE TO DECIDE IF YOU THINK HE'S SOMEONE YOU CAN TRUST AND TALK TO. AND THEN YOU'LL HAVE TO ACTUALLY TALK!

AS FAR AS LOVE IS CONCERNED, I WISH I HAD AN ANSWER. I DON'T KNOW WHEN YOU'LL FIND THE LOVE YOU ARE LOOKING FOR. IT'S POSSIBLE YOU ALREADY HAVE A LOT OF LOVE AROUND YOU. IT MIGHT NOT BE THE CRUSH-LIKE LOVE YOU CRAVE, BUT LOVE COMES IN MANY FORMS. AND LOVE ISN'T ONLY SOMETHING SOMEONE GIVES US. WE HAVE TO LEARN TO RECEIVE LOVE.

BOY CRUSH AND LOVE ASIDE, YOU'RE NOTICING SOMETHING THAT'S REAL—AND REAL ANNOYING—ABOUT GENDER. PEOPLE THINK KNOWING SOMEONE'S GENDER IDENTITY OR PRONOUNS IS GOING TO TELL THEM EVERYTHING THEY NEED TO KNOW. WHY DO PEOPLE WANT TO KNOW ABOUT GENDER ANYWAY? WHAT DO THEY THINK THEY LEARN ABOUT US WHEN THEY KNOW WHAT PRONOUNS WE USE? WHY IS KNOWING SOMEONE'S GENDER THE FIRST THING MOST PEOPLE EXPECT TO KNOW ABOUT THEM? AND WHY AM I ANSWERING YOUR QUESTION WITH SO MANY QUESTIONS OF MY OWN?

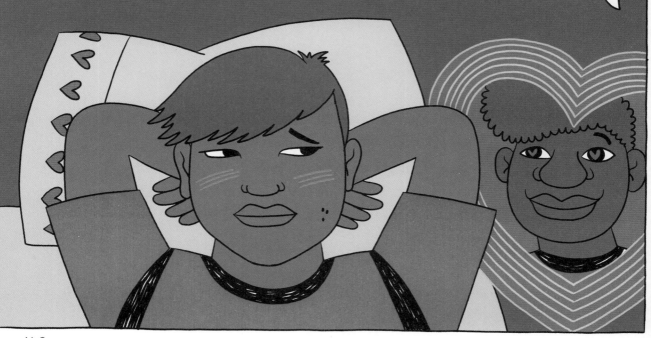

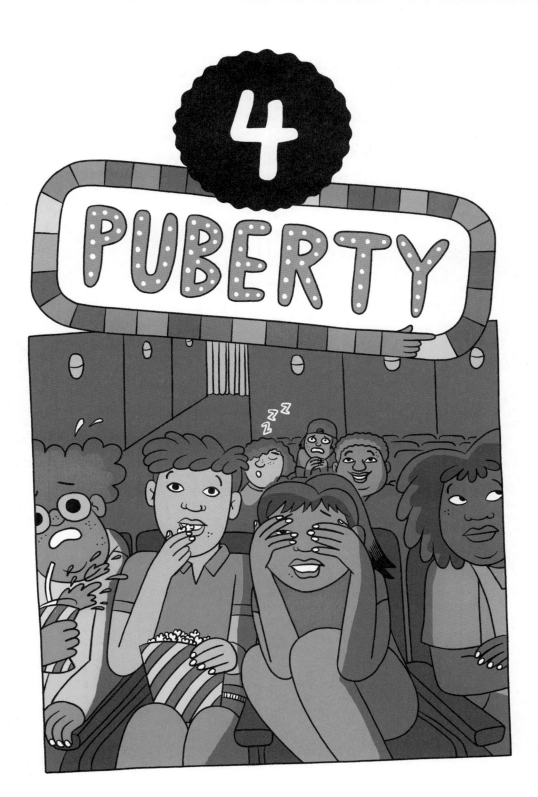

4 PUBERTY

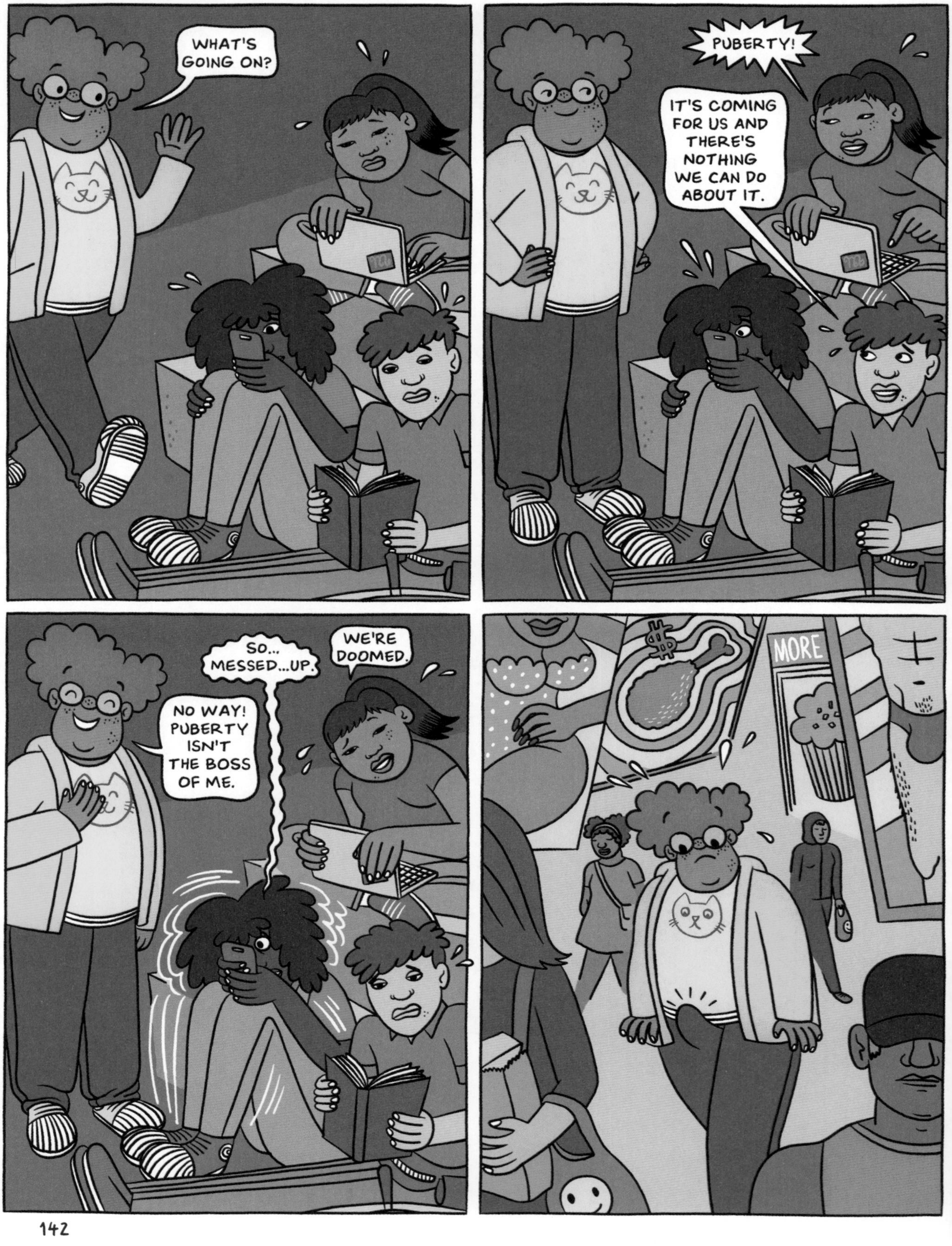
WHAT'S GOING ON?
PUBERTY!
IT'S COMING FOR US AND THERE'S NOTHING WE CAN DO ABOUT IT.
NO WAY! PUBERTY ISN'T THE BOSS OF ME.
SO... MESSED...UP.
WE'RE DOOMED.
MORE

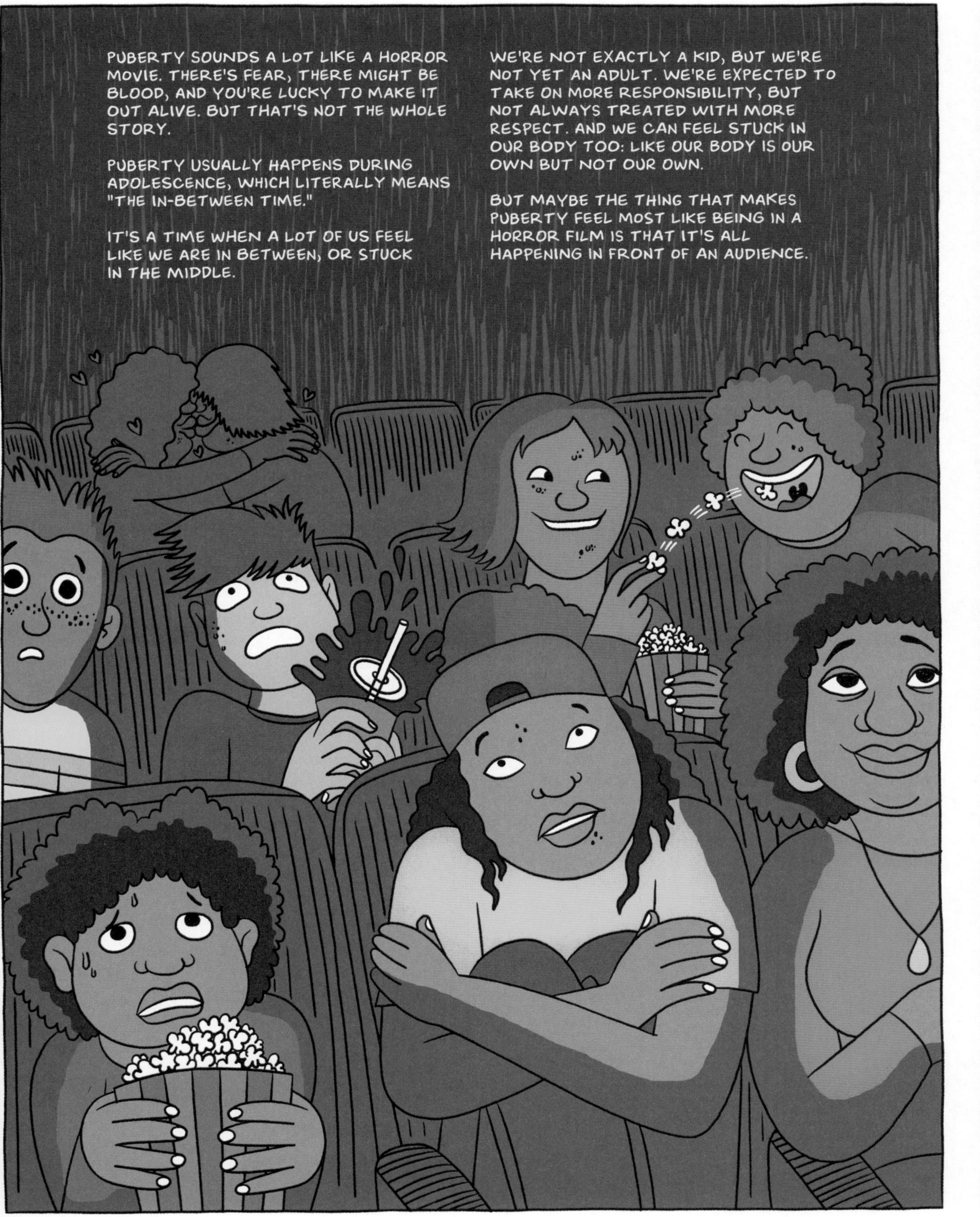
PUBERTY SOUNDS A LOT LIKE A HORROR MOVIE. THERE'S FEAR, THERE MIGHT BE BLOOD, AND YOU'RE LUCKY TO MAKE IT OUT ALIVE. BUT THAT'S NOT THE WHOLE STORY.
PUBERTY USUALLY HAPPENS DURING ADOLESCENCE, WHICH LITERALLY MEANS "THE IN-BETWEEN TIME."
IT'S A TIME WHEN A LOT OF US FEEL LIKE WE ARE IN BETWEEN, OR STUCK IN THE MIDDLE.
WE'RE NOT EXACTLY A KID, BUT WE'RE NOT YET AN ADULT. WE'RE EXPECTED TO TAKE ON MORE RESPONSIBILITY, BUT NOT ALWAYS TREATED WITH MORE RESPECT. AND WE CAN FEEL STUCK IN OUR BODY TOO: LIKE OUR BODY IS OUR OWN BUT NOT OUR OWN.
BUT MAYBE THE THING THAT MAKES PUBERTY FEEL MOST LIKE BEING IN A HORROR FILM IS THAT IT'S ALL HAPPENING IN FRONT OF AN AUDIENCE.

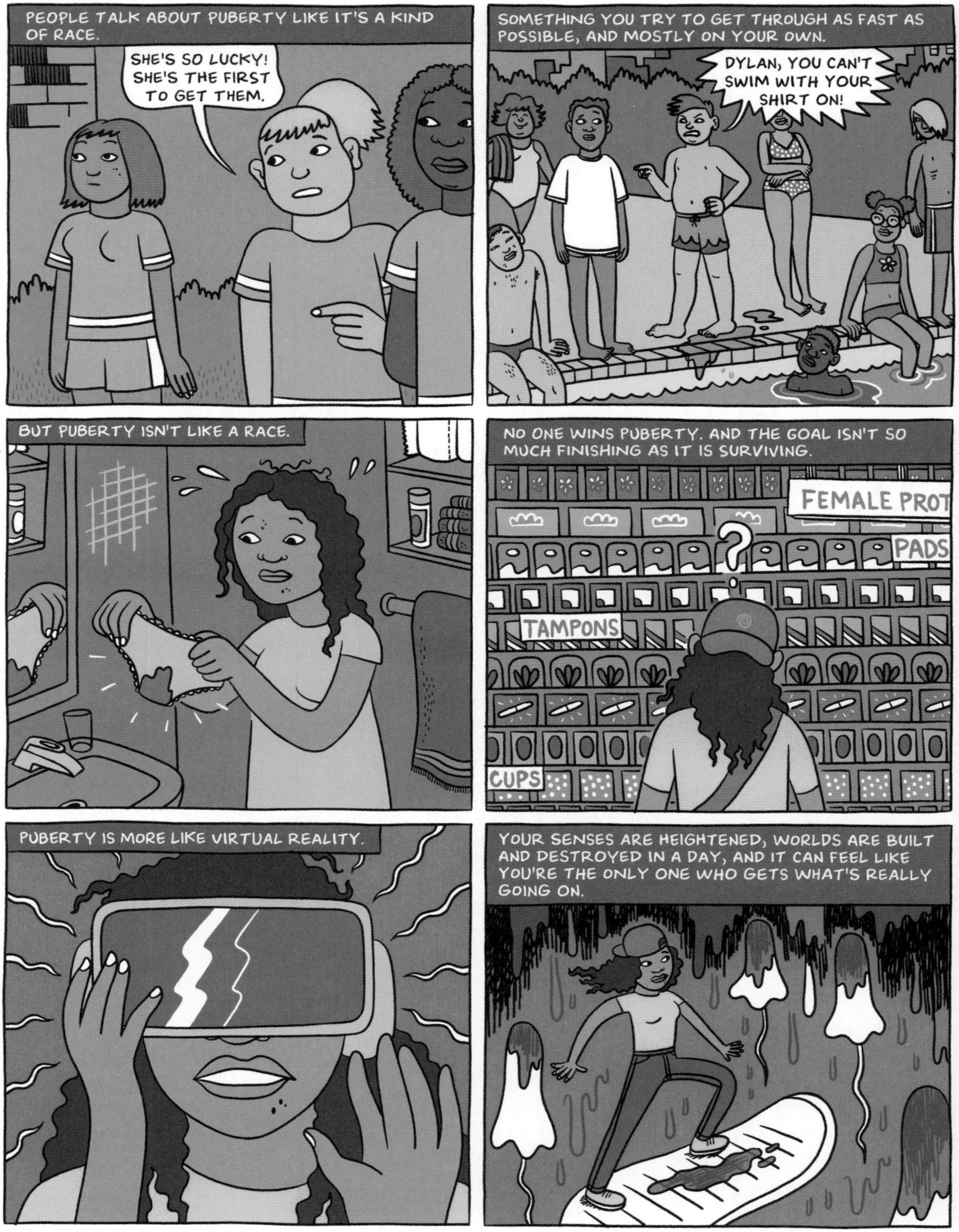
PEOPLE TALK ABOUT PUBERTY LIKE IT'S A KIND OF RACE.
SHE'S SO LUCKY! SHE'S THE FIRST TO GET THEM.
SOMETHING YOU TRY TO GET THROUGH AS FAST AS POSSIBLE, AND MOSTLY ON YOUR OWN.
DYLAN, YOU CAN'T SWIM WITH YOUR SHIRT ON!
BUT PUBERTY ISN'T LIKE A RACE.
NO ONE WINS PUBERTY. AND THE GOAL ISN'T SO MUCH FINISHING AS IT IS SURVIVING.
FEMALE PROT
PADS
?
TAMPONS
CUPS
PUBERTY IS MORE LIKE VIRTUAL REALITY.
YOUR SENSES ARE HEIGHTENED, WORLDS ARE BUILT AND DESTROYED IN A DAY, AND IT CAN FEEL LIKE YOU'RE THE ONLY ONE WHO GETS WHAT'S REALLY GOING ON.

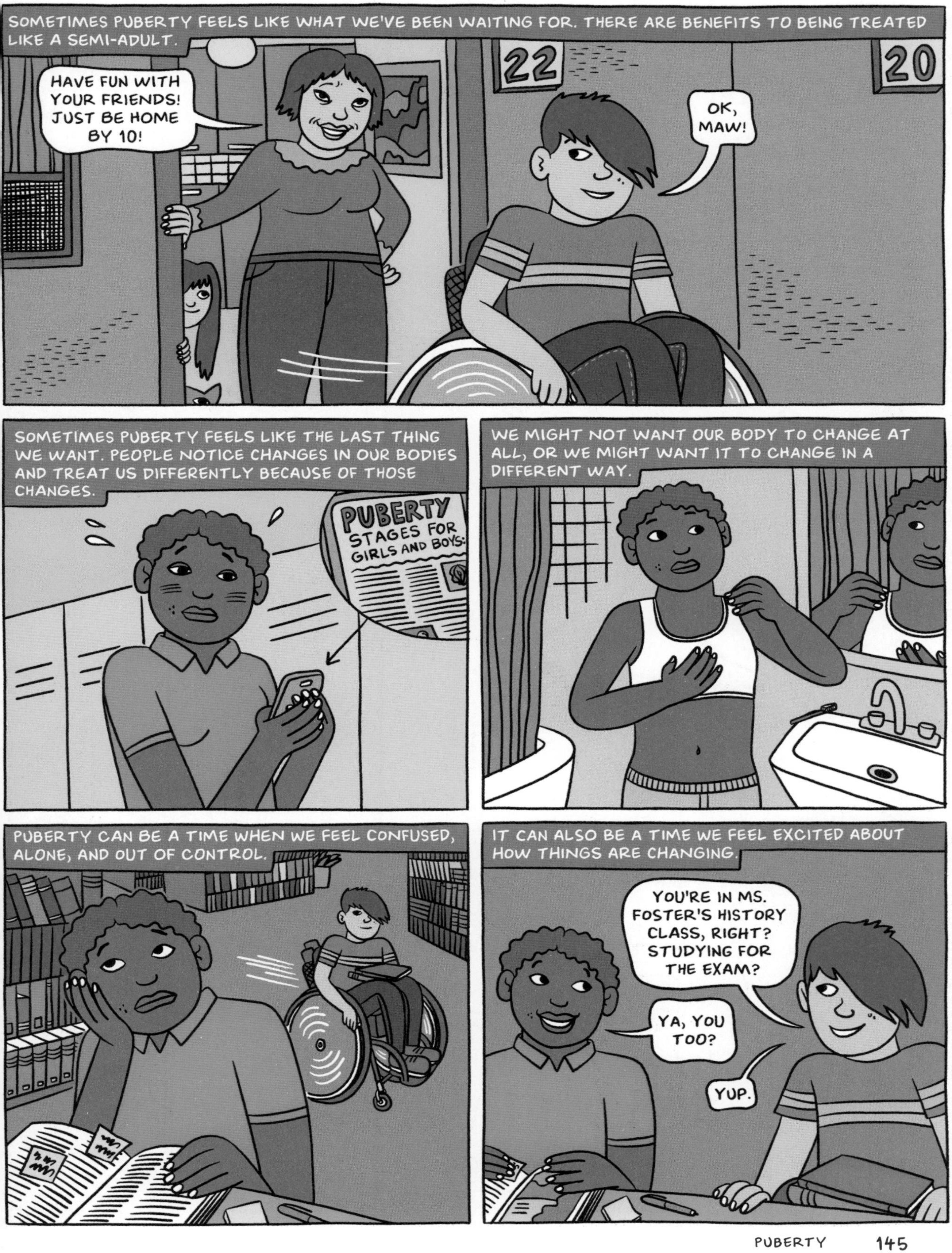
SOMETIMES PUBERTY FEELS LIKE WHAT WE'VE BEEN WAITING FOR. THERE ARE BENEFITS TO BEING TREATED LIKE A SEMI-ADULT.
22
20
HAVE FUN WITH YOUR FRIENDS! JUST BE HOME BY 10!
OK, MAW!
SOMETIMES PUBERTY FEELS LIKE THE LAST THING WE WANT. PEOPLE NOTICE CHANGES IN OUR BODIES AND TREAT US DIFFERENTLY BECAUSE OF THOSE CHANGES.
PUBERTY STAGES FOR GIRLS AND BOYS:
WE MIGHT NOT WANT OUR BODY TO CHANGE AT ALL, OR WE MIGHT WANT IT TO CHANGE IN A DIFFERENT WAY.
PUBERTY CAN BE A TIME WHEN WE FEEL CONFUSED, ALONE, AND OUT OF CONTROL.
IT CAN ALSO BE A TIME WE FEEL EXCITED ABOUT HOW THINGS ARE CHANGING.
YOU'RE IN MS. FOSTER'S HISTORY CLASS, RIGHT? STUDYING FOR THE EXAM?
YA, YOU TOO?
YUP.

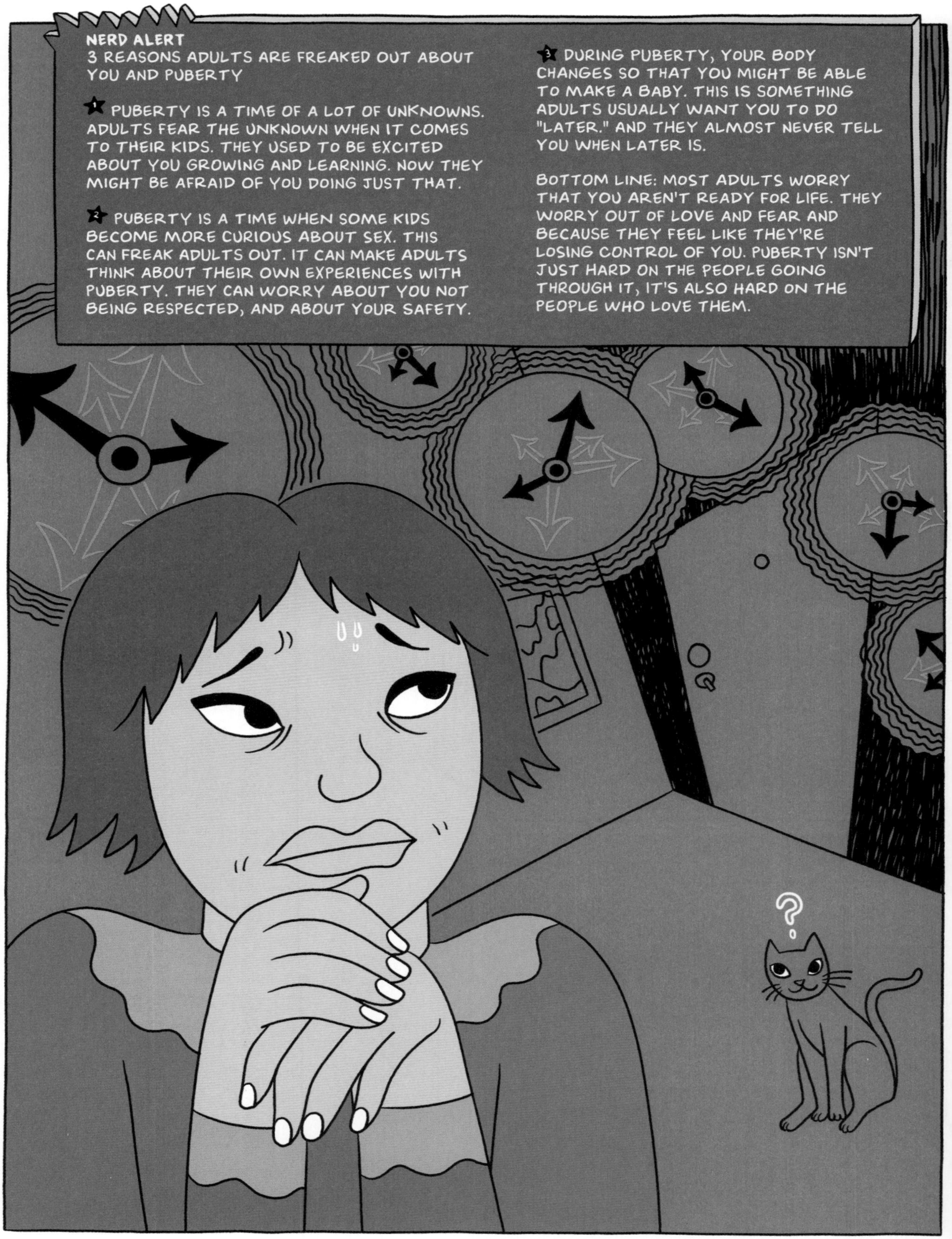
NERD ALERT
3 REASONS ADULTS ARE FREAKED OUT ABOUT YOU AND PUBERTY
1 PUBERTY IS A TIME OF A LOT OF UNKNOWNS. ADULTS FEAR THE UNKNOWN WHEN IT COMES TO THEIR KIDS. THEY USED TO BE EXCITED ABOUT YOU GROWING AND LEARNING. NOW THEY MIGHT BE AFRAID OF YOU DOING JUST THAT.
2 PUBERTY IS A TIME WHEN SOME KIDS BECOME MORE CURIOUS ABOUT SEX. THIS CAN FREAK ADULTS OUT. IT CAN MAKE ADULTS THINK ABOUT THEIR OWN EXPERIENCES WITH PUBERTY. THEY CAN WORRY ABOUT YOU NOT BEING RESPECTED, AND ABOUT YOUR SAFETY.
3 DURING PUBERTY, YOUR BODY CHANGES SO THAT YOU MIGHT BE ABLE TO MAKE A BABY. THIS IS SOMETHING ADULTS USUALLY WANT YOU TO DO "LATER." AND THEY ALMOST NEVER TELL YOU WHEN LATER IS.
BOTTOM LINE: MOST ADULTS WORRY THAT YOU AREN'T READY FOR LIFE. THEY WORRY OUT OF LOVE AND FEAR AND BECAUSE THEY FEEL LIKE THEY'RE LOSING CONTROL OF YOU. PUBERTY ISN'T JUST HARD ON THE PEOPLE GOING THROUGH IT, IT'S ALSO HARD ON THE PEOPLE WHO LOVE THEM.
?

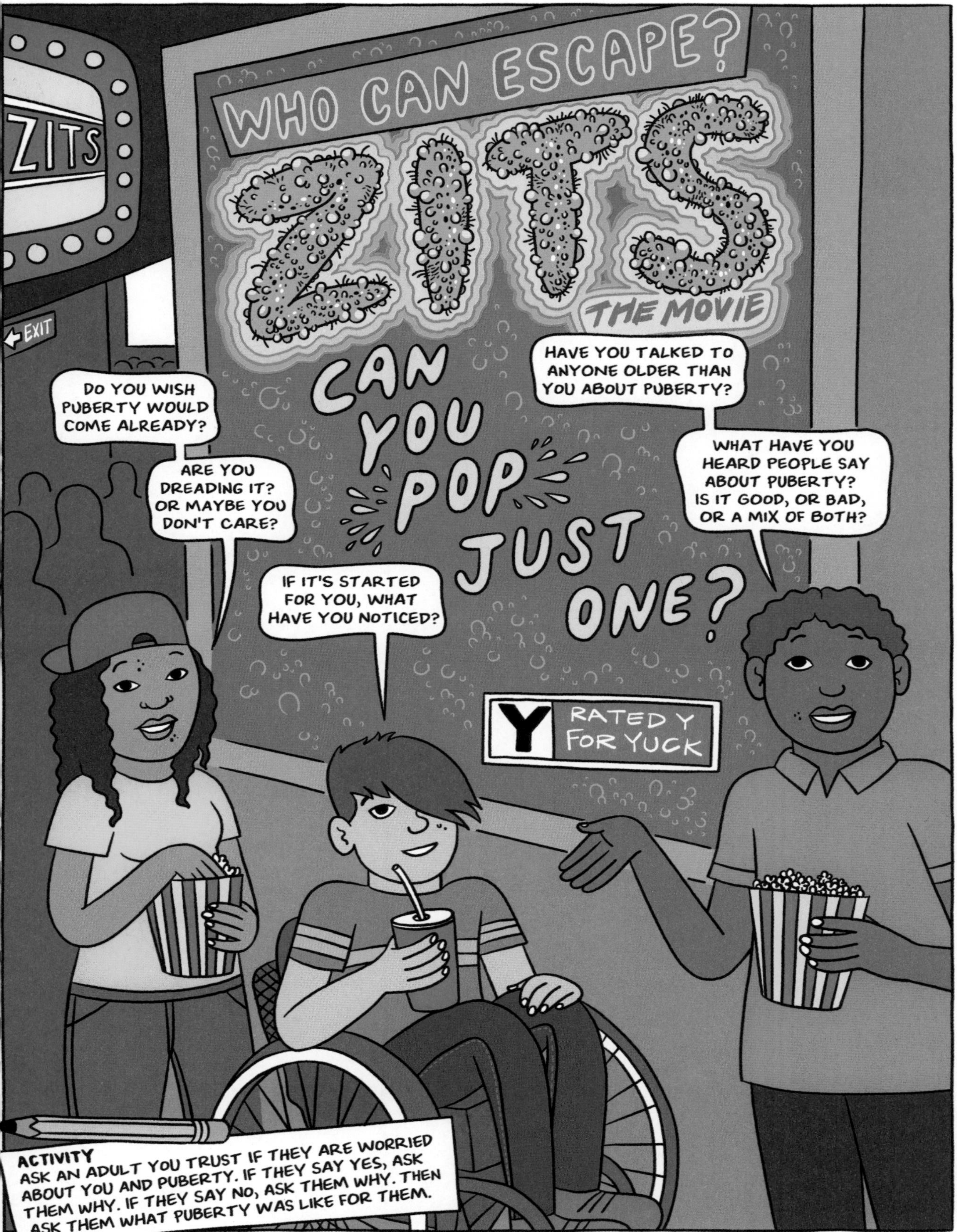
ZITS
EXIT
WHO CAN ESCAPE?
ZITS
THE MOVIE
CAN YOU POP JUST ONE?
Y RATED Y FOR YUCK
DO YOU WISH PUBERTY WOULD COME ALREADY?
ARE YOU DREADING IT? OR MAYBE YOU DON'T CARE?
IF IT'S STARTED FOR YOU, WHAT HAVE YOU NOTICED?
HAVE YOU TALKED TO ANYONE OLDER THAN YOU ABOUT PUBERTY?
WHAT HAVE YOU HEARD PEOPLE SAY ABOUT PUBERTY? IS IT GOOD, OR BAD, OR A MIX OF BOTH?
ACTIVITY
ASK AN ADULT YOU TRUST IF THEY ARE WORRIED ABOUT YOU AND PUBERTY. IF THEY SAY YES, ASK THEM WHY. IF THEY SAY NO, ASK THEM WHY. THEN ASK THEM WHAT PUBERTY WAS LIKE FOR THEM.

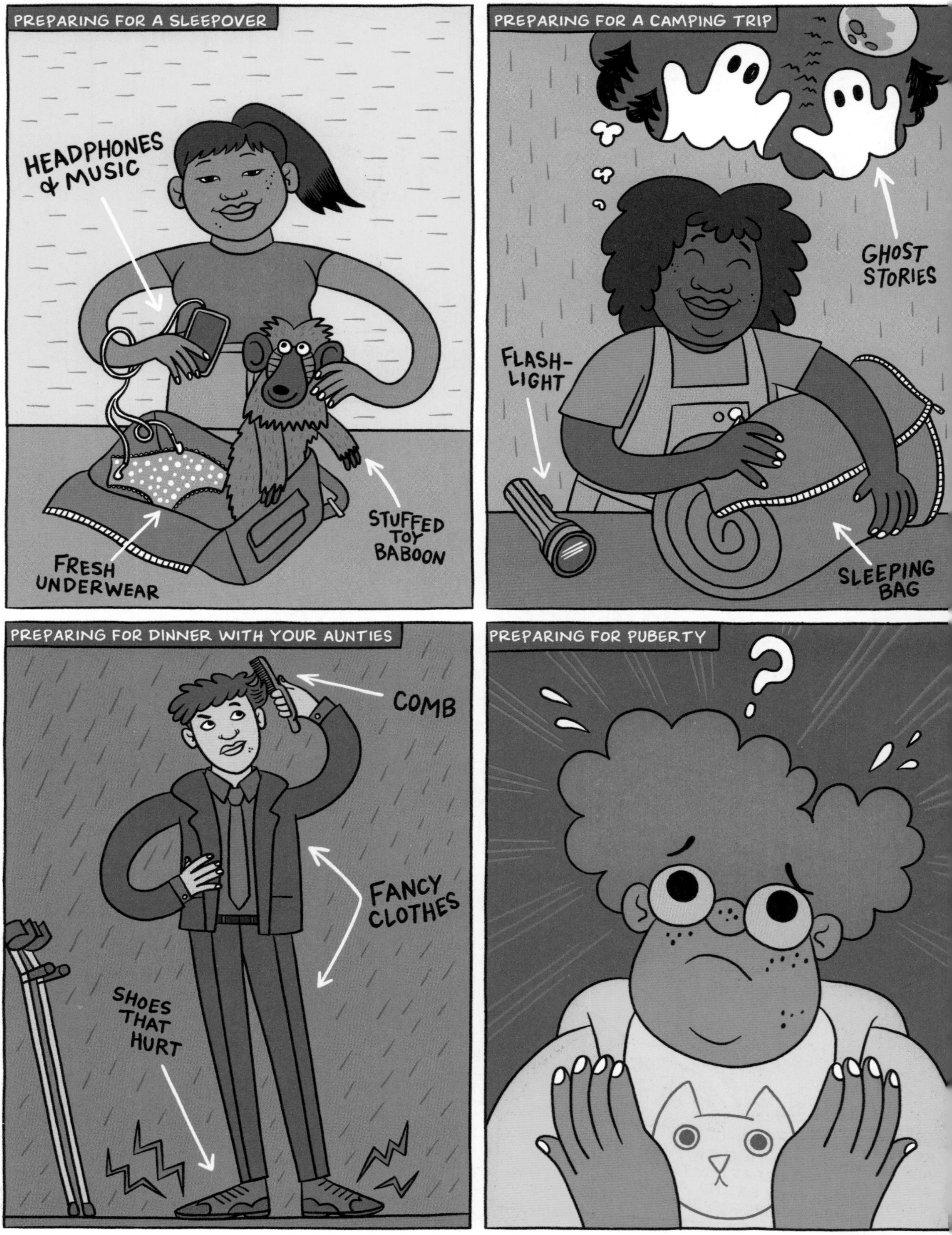
PREPARING FOR A SLEEPOVER
HEADPHONES & MUSIC
STUFFED TOY BABOON
FRESH UNDERWEAR
PREPARING FOR A CAMPING TRIP
GHOST STORIES
FLASH-LIGHT
SLEEPING BAG
PREPARING FOR DINNER WITH YOUR AUNTIES
COMB
FANCY CLOTHES
SHOES THAT HURT
PREPARING FOR PUBERTY
?

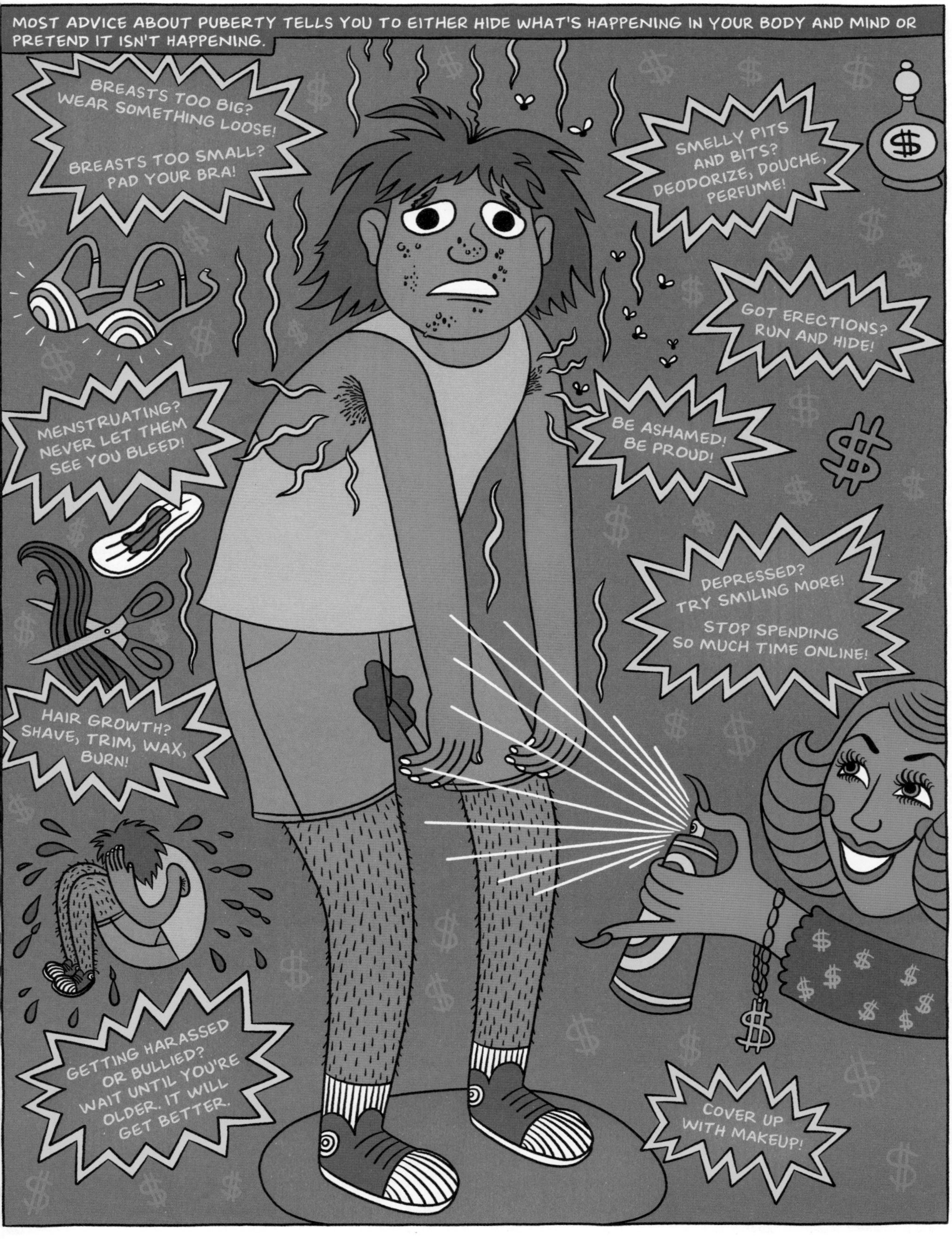
MOST ADVICE ABOUT PUBERTY TELLS YOU TO EITHER HIDE WHAT'S HAPPENING IN YOUR BODY AND MIND OR PRETEND IT ISN'T HAPPENING.
BREASTS TOO BIG? WEAR SOMETHING LOOSE!
BREASTS TOO SMALL? PAD YOUR BRA!
SMELLY PITS AND BITS? DEODORIZE, DOUCHE, PERFUME!
GOT ERECTIONS? RUN AND HIDE!
MENSTRUATING? NEVER LET THEM SEE YOU BLEED!
BE ASHAMED! BE PROUD!
DEPRESSED? TRY SMILING MORE!
STOP SPENDING SO MUCH TIME ONLINE!
HAIR GROWTH? SHAVE, TRIM, WAX, BURN!
GETTING HARASSED OR BULLIED? WAIT UNTIL YOU'RE OLDER. IT WILL GET BETTER.
COVER UP WITH MAKEUP!

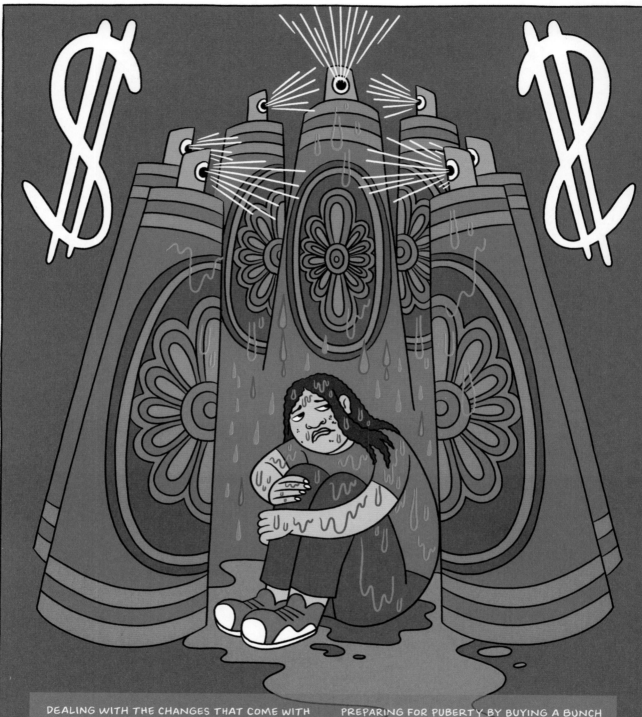

DEALING WITH THE CHANGES THAT COME WITH PUBERTY BY HIDING THEM, OR BY PRETENDING THEY AREN'T HAPPENING, ISN'T A GOOD STRATEGY. IT CAN LEAVE US FEELING ASHAMED, LIKE WE ARE THE PROBLEM.

INSTEAD OF SUFFERING IN SILENCE AND THINKING THERE'S SOMETHING WRONG WITH US, WHAT IF WE FOCUSED ON WHAT'S WRONG WITH THE WORLD AROUND US? WHAT IF WE STARTED IMAGINING HOW TO CHANGE IT?

PREPARING FOR PUBERTY BY BUYING A BUNCH OF STUFF DOESN'T WORK. NOT ALL OF US CAN AFFORD IT, AND NO AMOUNT OF BODY SPRAY AND MAKEUP CAN HIDE THE CHANGES YOU'RE GOING THROUGH.

HERE'S A SHAME-FREE AND PRODUCT-FREE PUBERTY PREPARATION LIST TO HELP WITH SOME OF THE PRESSURE AND EXHAUSTION THAT CAN COME WITH PUBERTY.

SHAME-FREE PUBERTY PREP LIST

★ **FIND SOMEONE WORTHY OF YOUR TRUST**
YOU DESERVE SOMEONE WHO WILL HAVE YOUR BACK, LISTEN TO YOU, KEEP YOUR SECRETS, AND LET YOU BE WHO YOU ARE, EVEN WHEN YOU AREN'T SURE WHO THAT IS. FINDING THAT PERSON ISN'T EASY. SOMETIMES THEY'RE IN OUR LIVES AND WE DON'T EVEN NOTICE THEM.

★ **HAVE A WAY TO ESCAPE**
YOU MIGHT NOT HAVE A ROOM OF YOUR OWN, BUT YOU DESERVE A PLACE WHERE YOU CAN BE ALONE AND FEEL SAFE. WHETHER IT'S CLOSING YOUR EYES, PUTTING ON HEADPHONES, AND HAVING A PLAYLIST THAT FEELS LIKE HOME OR HAVING AN ACTUAL PLACE YOU CAN GO WHERE NO ONE IS GOING TO BOTHER YOU, MAKING YOUR OWN SPACE CAN BE A PUBERTY LIFESAVER.

★ **KNOW WHERE TO FIND MORE INFORMATION**
YOU'RE GOING TO HAVE A LOT OF QUESTIONS. THE INTERNET MAY BE VAST, BUT ALL THE SILENCE ABOUT BODIES, SEX, AND GENDER MEANS IT CAN BE HARD TO FIND THE INFORMATION YOU NEED. AND ONLINE, IT CAN BE HARD TO TELL INACCURATE INFORMATION FROM THE REAL DEAL. IF YOU'RE NOT SURE WHERE TO START, CHECK OUT THE BACK OF THIS BOOK.

★ **PREPARE TO MAKE MISTAKES**
PUBERTY IS FULL OF DRAMA. YOU'RE GOING TO SAY THINGS YOU DON'T MEAN TO PEOPLE YOU LIKE. YOU'RE GOING TO SAY THINGS YOU DO MEAN BUT IN A WAY THAT HURTS OTHERS MORE THAN YOU WANTED. YOU'LL TRY NEW STUFF WITH YOUR BODY AND SOMETIMES WITH OTHER PEOPLE'S BODIES, AND IT MIGHT FEEL GOOD OR BAD OR AWKWARD OR ALL OF THOSE THINGS AT ONCE. YOU'LL PUSH PEOPLE AWAY WHO YOU LOVE, AND MAYBE ATTRACT SOME WHO YOU DON'T. YOU'LL HAVE TO TAKE RESPONSIBILITY FOR YOUR MISTAKES, BUT YOU DON'T NEED TO MAKE IT WORSE BY BEATING YOURSELF UP OVER THEM.

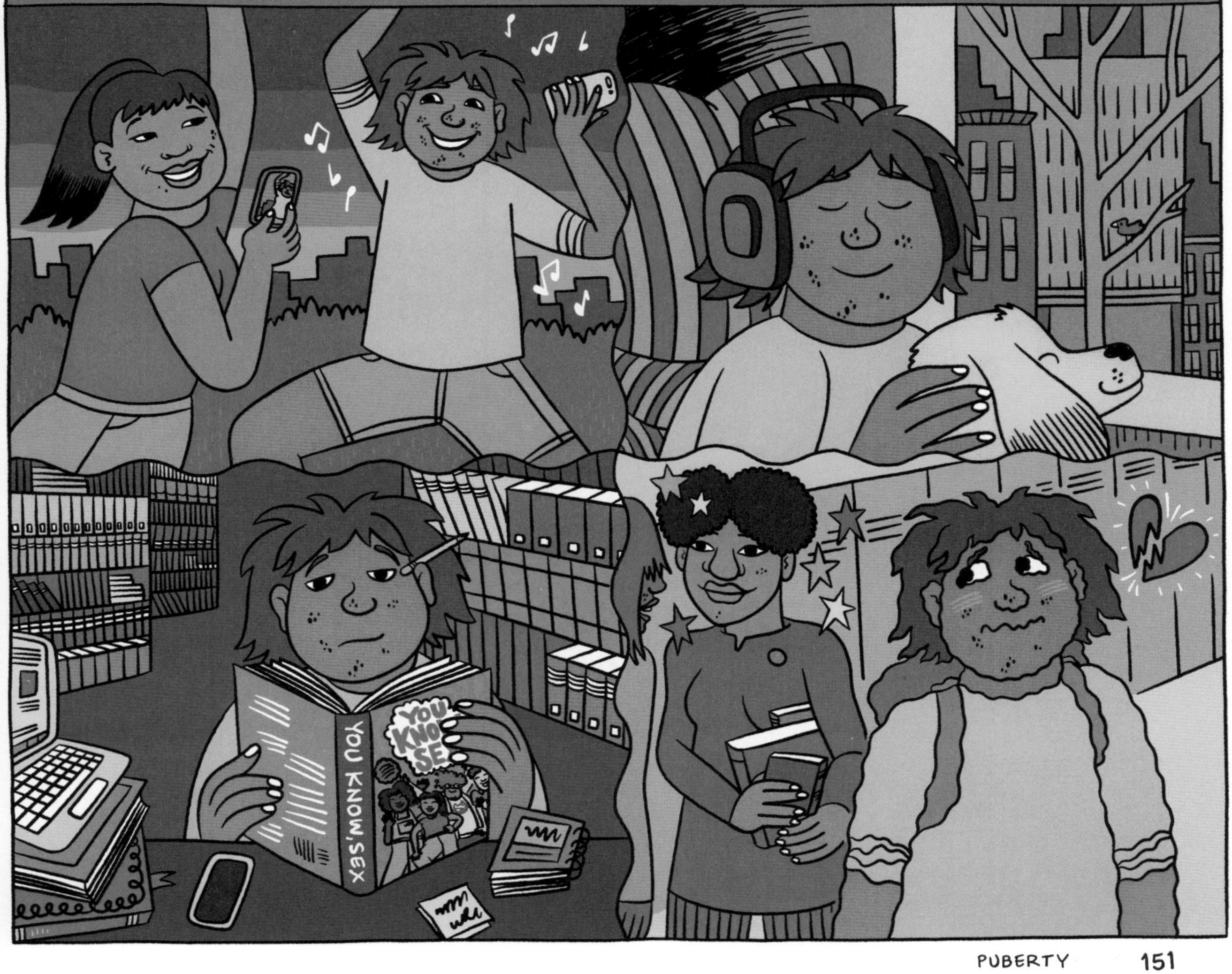
YOU KNOW, SEX

PUBERTY AND GENDER

LOTS OF PEOPLE SAY THAT IF YOU HAVE OVARIES, PUBERTY MEANS YOU'RE A GIRL BECOMING A WOMAN, AND IF YOU HAVE TESTICLES, PUBERTY MEANS YOU'RE A BOY BECOMING A MAN. THAT'S NOT PUBERTY. THAT'S THE GENDER BINARY.* IT LEAVES THE REST OF US, INCLUDING TRANS AND NONBINARY PEOPLE, OUT.

A LOT OF WHAT MAKES PUBERTY FEEL LIKE A BIG PROBLEM IS THE WAY OTHER PEOPLE MAKE IT ABOUT GENDER. IT CAN BE HARD TO BELIEVE, BUT THE PROBLEM ISN'T YOU OR YOUR BODY—THE PROBLEM IS THE GENDER BINARY.

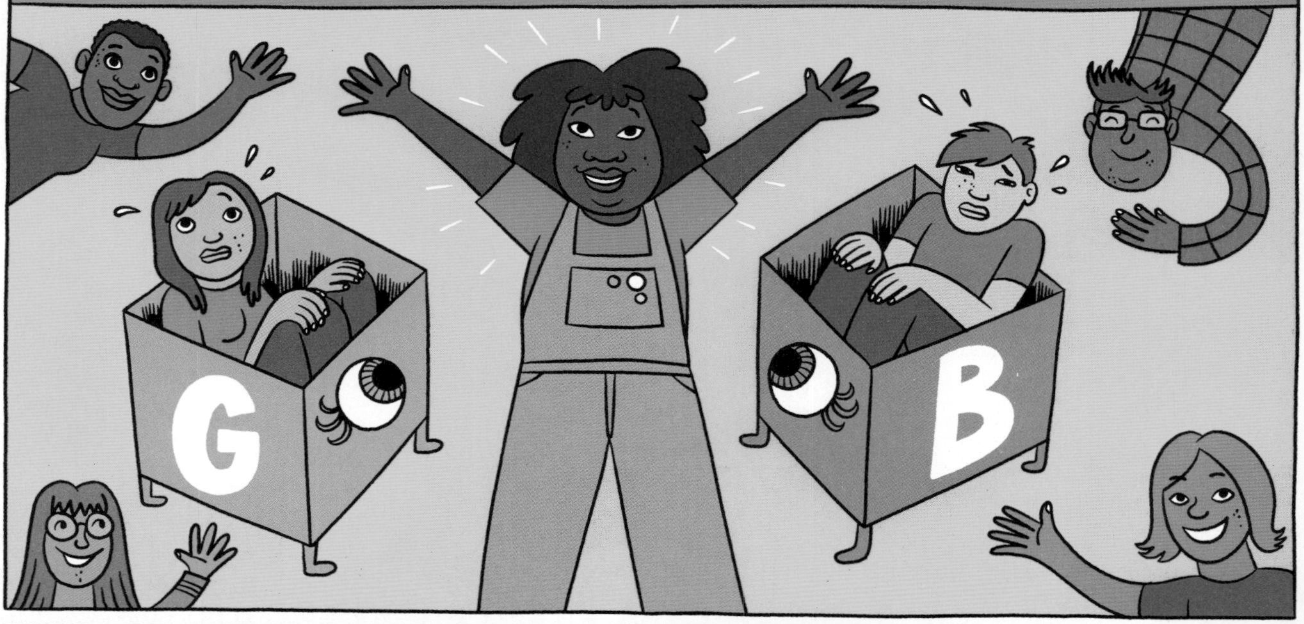
G
B

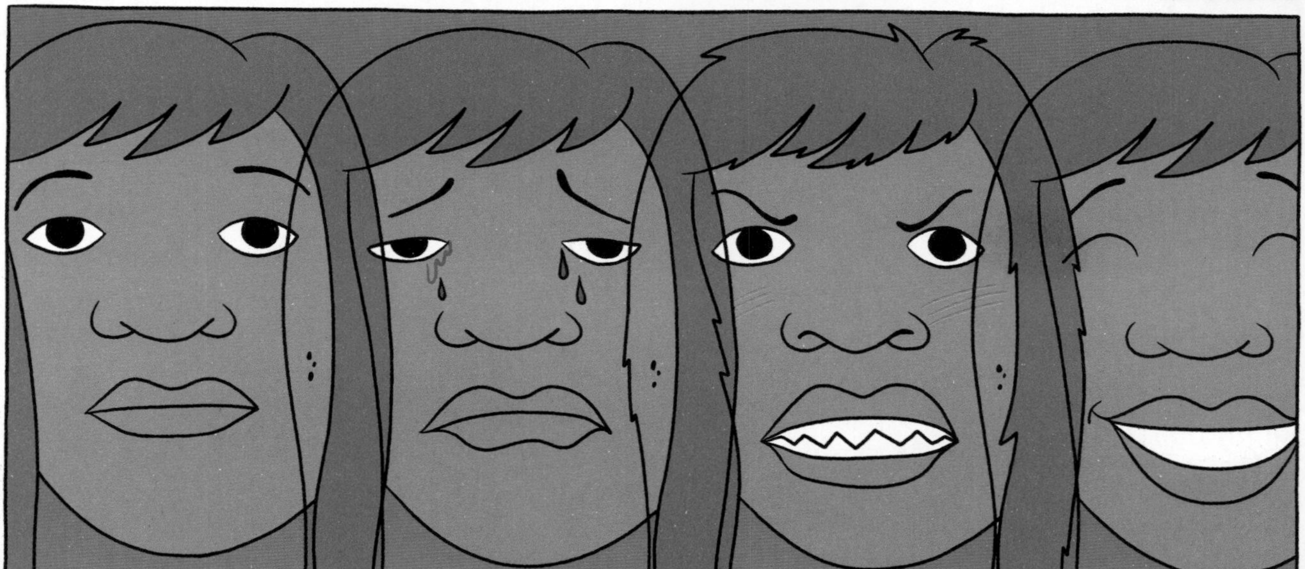

FEELINGS AND MOODS

MOST PEOPLE FOCUS ON THE PHYSICAL CHANGES THAT HAPPEN AT PUBERTY. BUT EVEN BEFORE YOU NOTICE ANY CHANGES IN, AND ON, YOUR BODY, YOU'RE PROBABLY GOING TO START FEELING DIFFERENT.

PART OF THIS COMES AS THE MIX OF HORMONES—CHEMICALS YOUR BODY MAKES—STARTS TO CHANGE. AND PART OF IT HAPPENS BECAUSE BEING IN-BETWEEN IS A LOT. IT CAN FEEL LIKE NO ONE GETS YOU. YOU MAY NOT EVEN GET YOU. YOU CAN HAVE A RUSH OF FEELINGS FOLLOWED BY WHAT FEELS LIKE NOTHING, AND BACK AND FORTH, MANY TIMES A DAY. TAKING CARE OF YOURSELF DURING PUBERTY MEANS TAKING YOUR FEELINGS AND MOODS SERIOUSLY, AND ASKING OTHERS TO DO THE SAME.

* IF YOU SKIPPED THE GENDER CHAPTER, FLIP BACK TO P. 101

FOR MOST OF US, PUBERTY BEGINS SOMETIME BETWEEN 8 AND 14 YEARS OLD, AND ENDS WHEN WE'RE 17 OR 18. IT STARTS WITH CHANGES DEEP IN OUR BODY.

THE CHANGES ARE TRIGGERED BY HORMONES, WHICH ACT LIKE MESSENGERS THROUGHOUT THE BODY, STARTING AND STOPPING CHANGES IN HOW OUR BODIES LOOK AND GROW, AND INFLUENCING HOW WE THINK AND FEEL. TWO HORMONES THAT DO A LOT OF THE WORK DURING PUBERTY ARE ESTROGEN AND TESTOSTERONE.

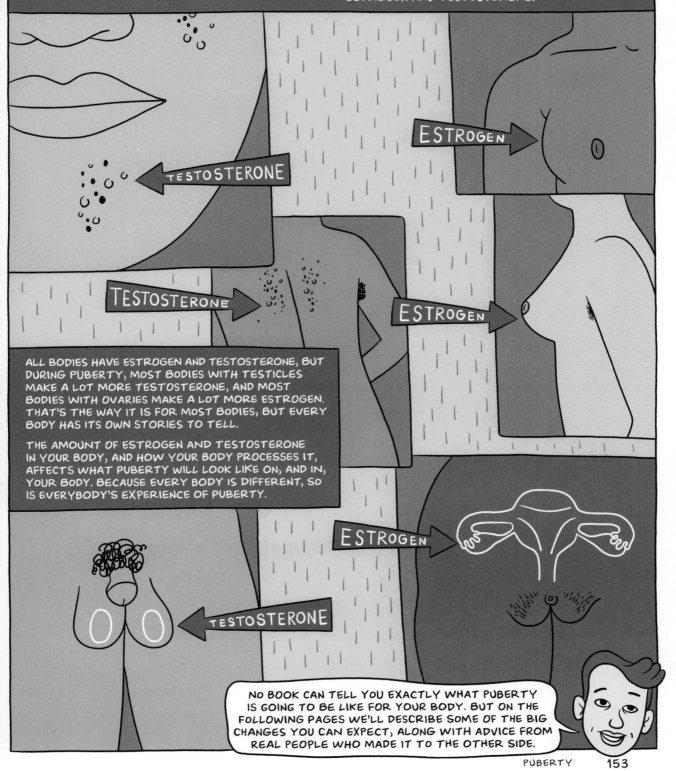

ESTROGEN

TESTOSTERONE

TESTOSTERONE

ESTROGEN

ALL BODIES HAVE ESTROGEN AND TESTOSTERONE, BUT DURING PUBERTY, MOST BODIES WITH TESTICLES MAKE A LOT MORE TESTOSTERONE, AND MOST BODIES WITH OVARIES MAKE A LOT MORE ESTROGEN. THAT'S THE WAY IT IS FOR MOST BODIES, BUT EVERY BODY HAS ITS OWN STORIES TO TELL.

THE AMOUNT OF ESTROGEN AND TESTOSTERONE IN YOUR BODY, AND HOW YOUR BODY PROCESSES IT, AFFECTS WHAT PUBERTY WILL LOOK LIKE ON, AND IN, YOUR BODY. BECAUSE EVERY BODY IS DIFFERENT, SO IS EVERYBODY'S EXPERIENCE OF PUBERTY.

ESTROGEN

TESTOSTERONE

NO BOOK CAN TELL YOU EXACTLY WHAT PUBERTY IS GOING TO BE LIKE FOR YOUR BODY. BUT ON THE FOLLOWING PAGES WE'LL DESCRIBE SOME OF THE BIG CHANGES YOU CAN EXPECT, ALONG WITH ADVICE FROM REAL PEOPLE WHO MADE IT TO THE OTHER SIDE.

DURING PUBERTY, EVERY PART OF YOUR BODY CAN GROW: BONES AND ORGANS, ARMS AND LEGS, PENISES, LABIA, AND MORE.

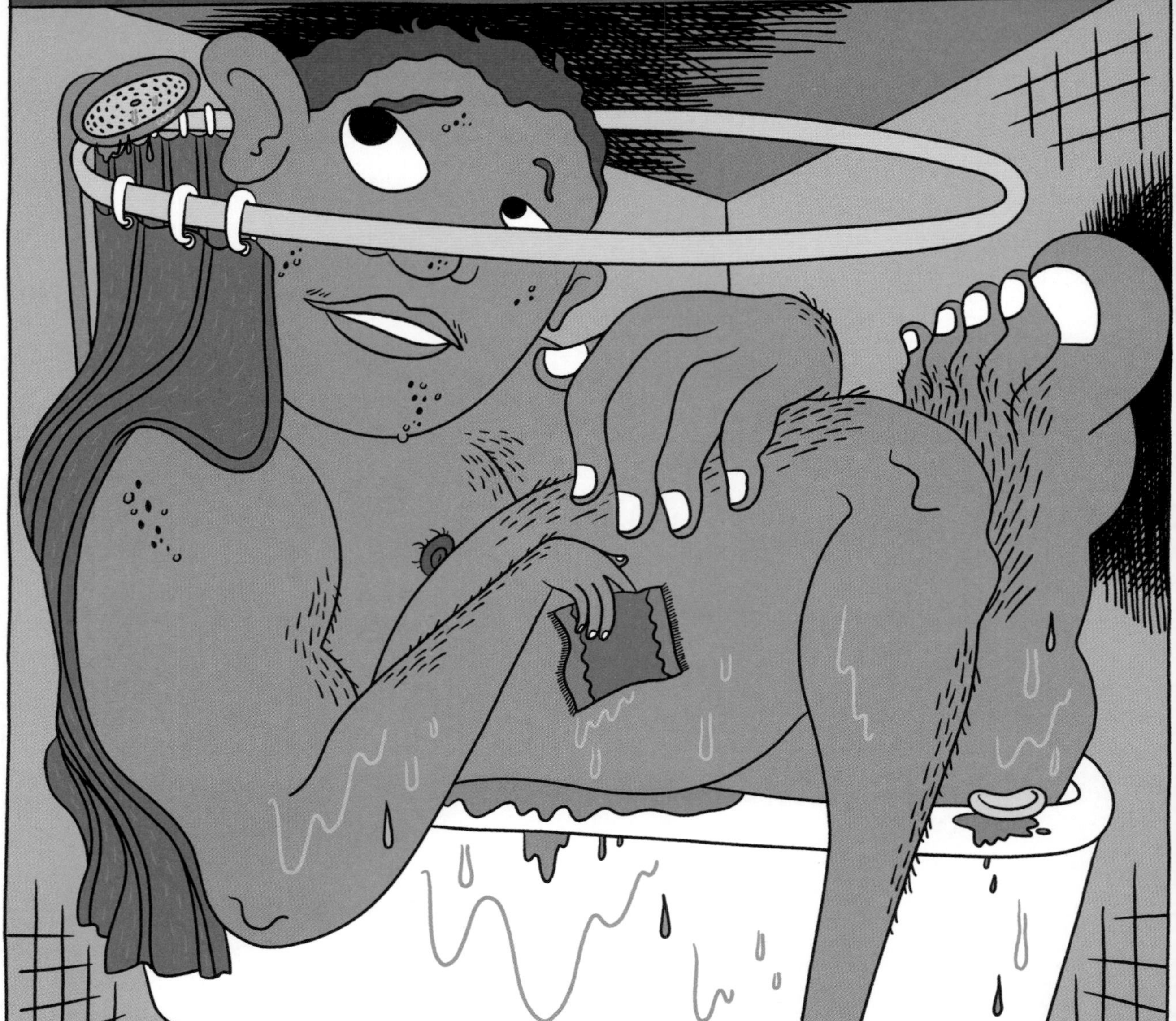

SOMETIMES BODIES GROW SO QUICKLY THAT IT HURTS. THESE ARE CALLED GROWING PAINS. ADULTS AND OTHER KIDS MIGHT SAY, "IT'S IN YOUR HEAD." BUT PAIN IS PAIN, AND IGNORING IT USUALLY DOESN'T HELP. NEITHER DOES BEING TOLD IT'S NOT REAL.

WHEN YOUR BODY GROWS SO MUCH IN SUCH A SHORT TIME, IT CAN FEEL LIKE YOU'RE LEARNING TO LIVE IN A NEW BODY FROM ONE WEEK TO THE NEXT. IT MIGHT SEEM LIKE NOTHING FITS OR FEELS RIGHT.

THERE IS NO RIGHT OR WRONG WAY TO HAVE A BODY, AND NONE OF US ARE ONE SIZE OUR WHOLE LIVES. AS YOUR BODY GROWS, ASK YOURSELF HOW YOU FEEL ABOUT THOSE CHANGES. WHAT FEELS RIGHT FOR YOU? WHAT CLOTHES FEEL RIGHT? WHAT KIND OF PEOPLE FEEL RIGHT TO BE AROUND? IT CAN BE HARD TO TRUST WHAT YOU FEEL WITH ALL THESE CHANGES. WHICH IS OKAY. YOU DON'T HAVE TO HAVE IT ALL FIGURED OUT.

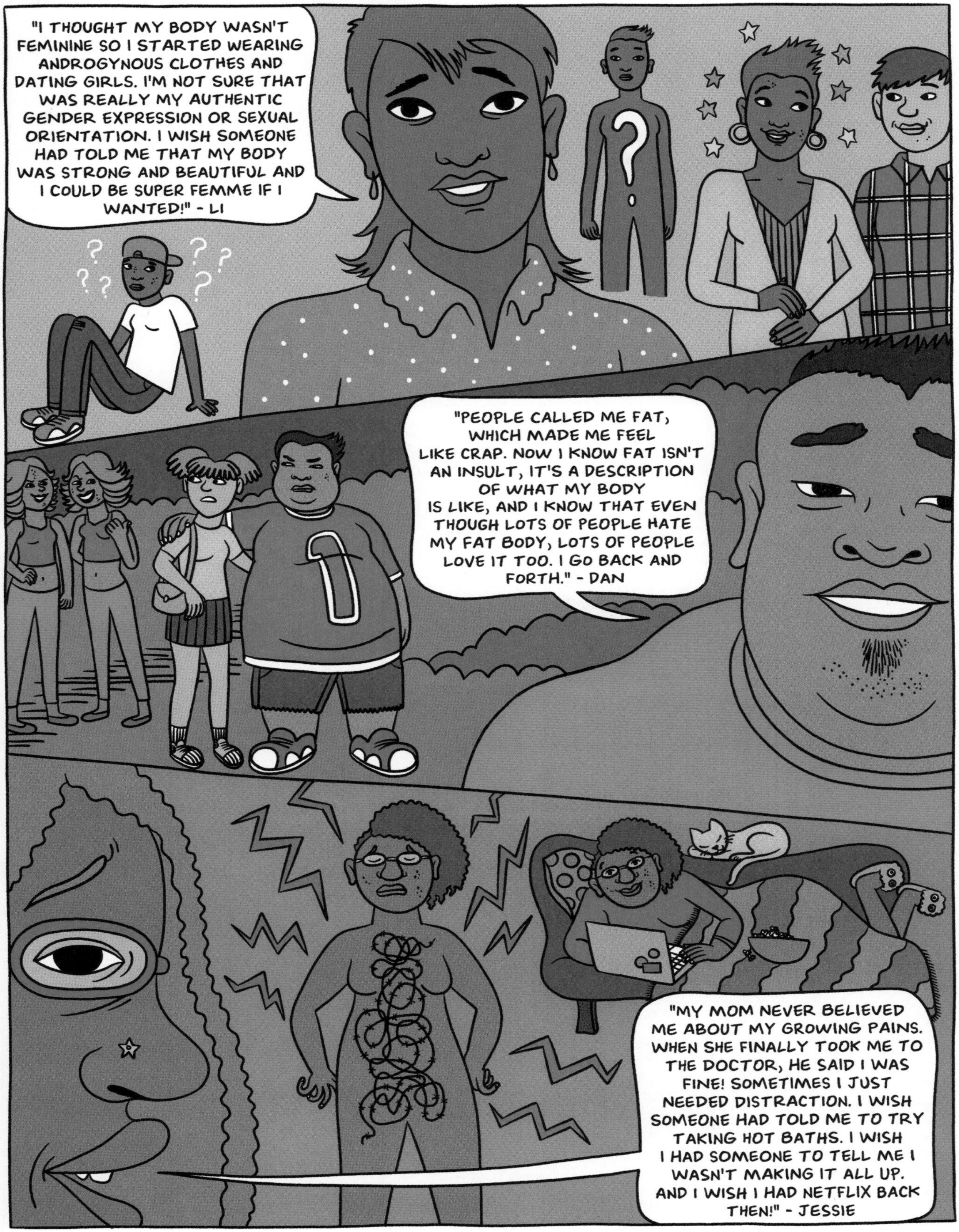
"I THOUGHT MY BODY WASN'T FEMININE SO I STARTED WEARING ANDROGYNOUS CLOTHES AND DATING GIRLS. I'M NOT SURE THAT WAS REALLY MY AUTHENTIC GENDER EXPRESSION OR SEXUAL ORIENTATION. I WISH SOMEONE HAD TOLD ME THAT MY BODY WAS STRONG AND BEAUTIFUL AND I COULD BE SUPER FEMME IF I WANTED!" - LI
"PEOPLE CALLED ME FAT, WHICH MADE ME FEEL LIKE CRAP. NOW I KNOW FAT ISN'T AN INSULT, IT'S A DESCRIPTION OF WHAT MY BODY IS LIKE, AND I KNOW THAT EVEN THOUGH LOTS OF PEOPLE HATE MY FAT BODY, LOTS OF PEOPLE LOVE IT TOO. I GO BACK AND FORTH." - DAN
"MY MOM NEVER BELIEVED ME ABOUT MY GROWING PAINS. WHEN SHE FINALLY TOOK ME TO THE DOCTOR, HE SAID I WAS FINE! SOMETIMES I JUST NEEDED DISTRACTION. I WISH SOMEONE HAD TOLD ME TO TRY TAKING HOT BATHS. I WISH I HAD SOMEONE TO TELL ME I WASN'T MAKING IT ALL UP. AND I WISH I HAD NETFLIX BACK THEN!" - JESSIE

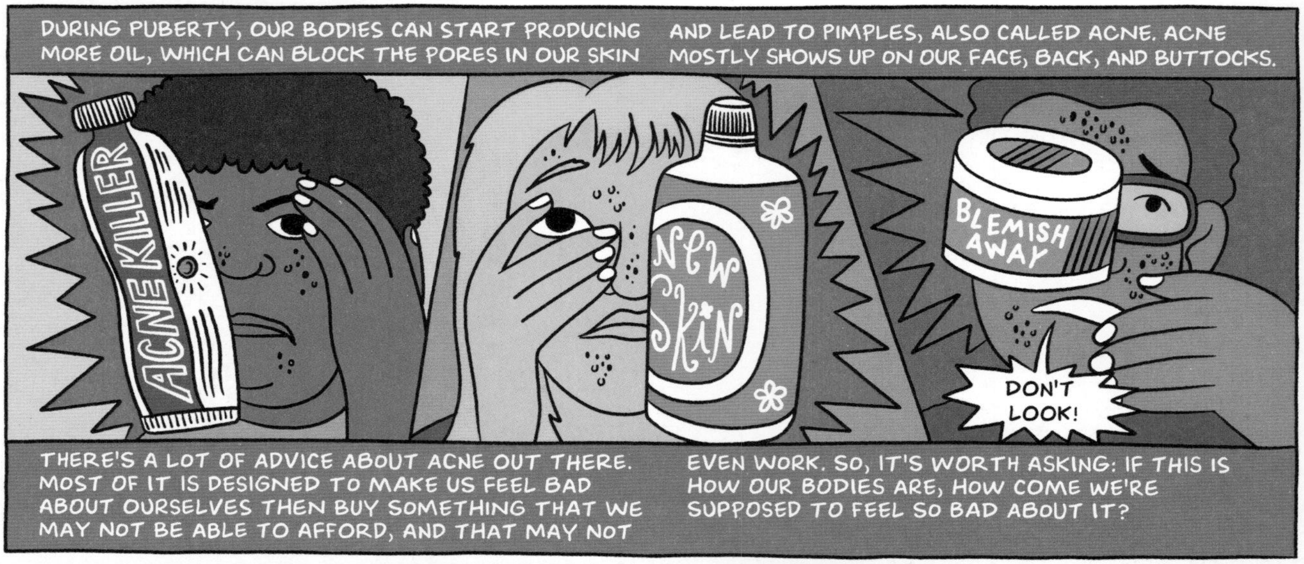
DURING PUBERTY, OUR BODIES CAN START PRODUCING MORE OIL, WHICH CAN BLOCK THE PORES IN OUR SKIN AND LEAD TO PIMPLES, ALSO CALLED ACNE. ACNE MOSTLY SHOWS UP ON OUR FACE, BACK, AND BUTTOCKS.
ACNE KILLER
NEW SKIN
BLEMISH AWAY
DON'T LOOK!
THERE'S A LOT OF ADVICE ABOUT ACNE OUT THERE. MOST OF IT IS DESIGNED TO MAKE US FEEL BAD ABOUT OURSELVES THEN BUY SOMETHING THAT WE MAY NOT BE ABLE TO AFFORD, AND THAT MAY NOT EVEN WORK. SO, IT'S WORTH ASKING: IF THIS IS HOW OUR BODIES ARE, HOW COME WE'RE SUPPOSED TO FEEL SO BAD ABOUT IT?

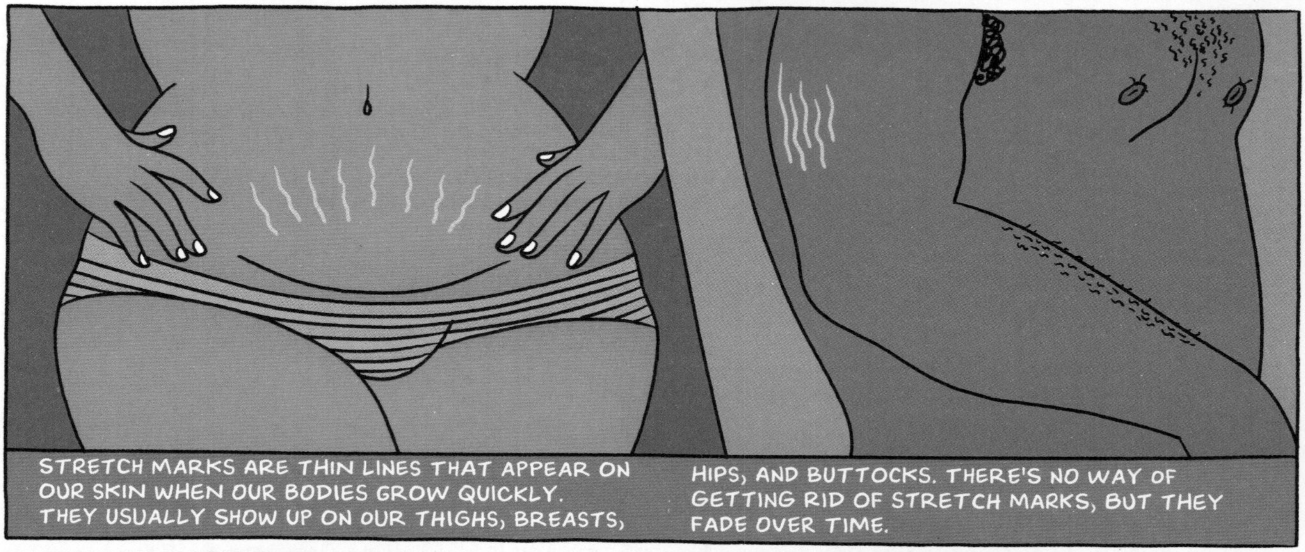
STRETCH MARKS ARE THIN LINES THAT APPEAR ON OUR SKIN WHEN OUR BODIES GROW QUICKLY. THEY USUALLY SHOW UP ON OUR THIGHS, BREASTS, HIPS, AND BUTTOCKS. THERE'S NO WAY OF GETTING RID OF STRETCH MARKS, BUT THEY FADE OVER TIME.

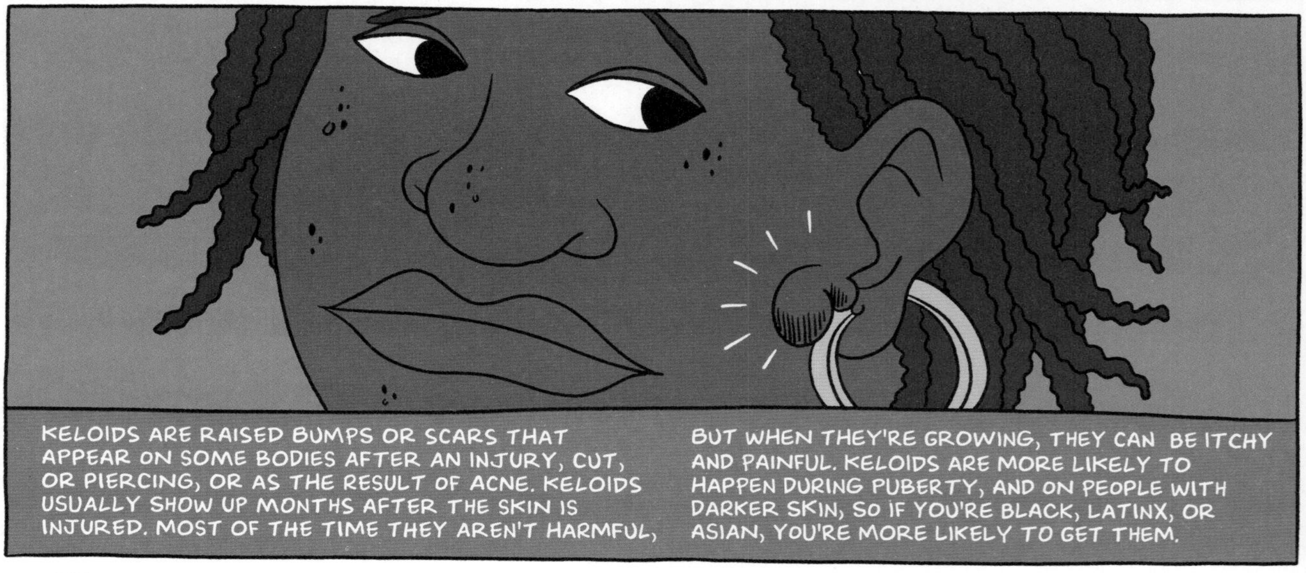
KELOIDS ARE RAISED BUMPS OR SCARS THAT APPEAR ON SOME BODIES AFTER AN INJURY, CUT, OR PIERCING, OR AS THE RESULT OF ACNE. KELOIDS USUALLY SHOW UP MONTHS AFTER THE SKIN IS INJURED. MOST OF THE TIME THEY AREN'T HARMFUL, BUT WHEN THEY'RE GROWING, THEY CAN BE ITCHY AND PAINFUL. KELOIDS ARE MORE LIKELY TO HAPPEN DURING PUBERTY, AND ON PEOPLE WITH DARKER SKIN, SO IF YOU'RE BLACK, LATINX, OR ASIAN, YOU'RE MORE LIKELY TO GET THEM.

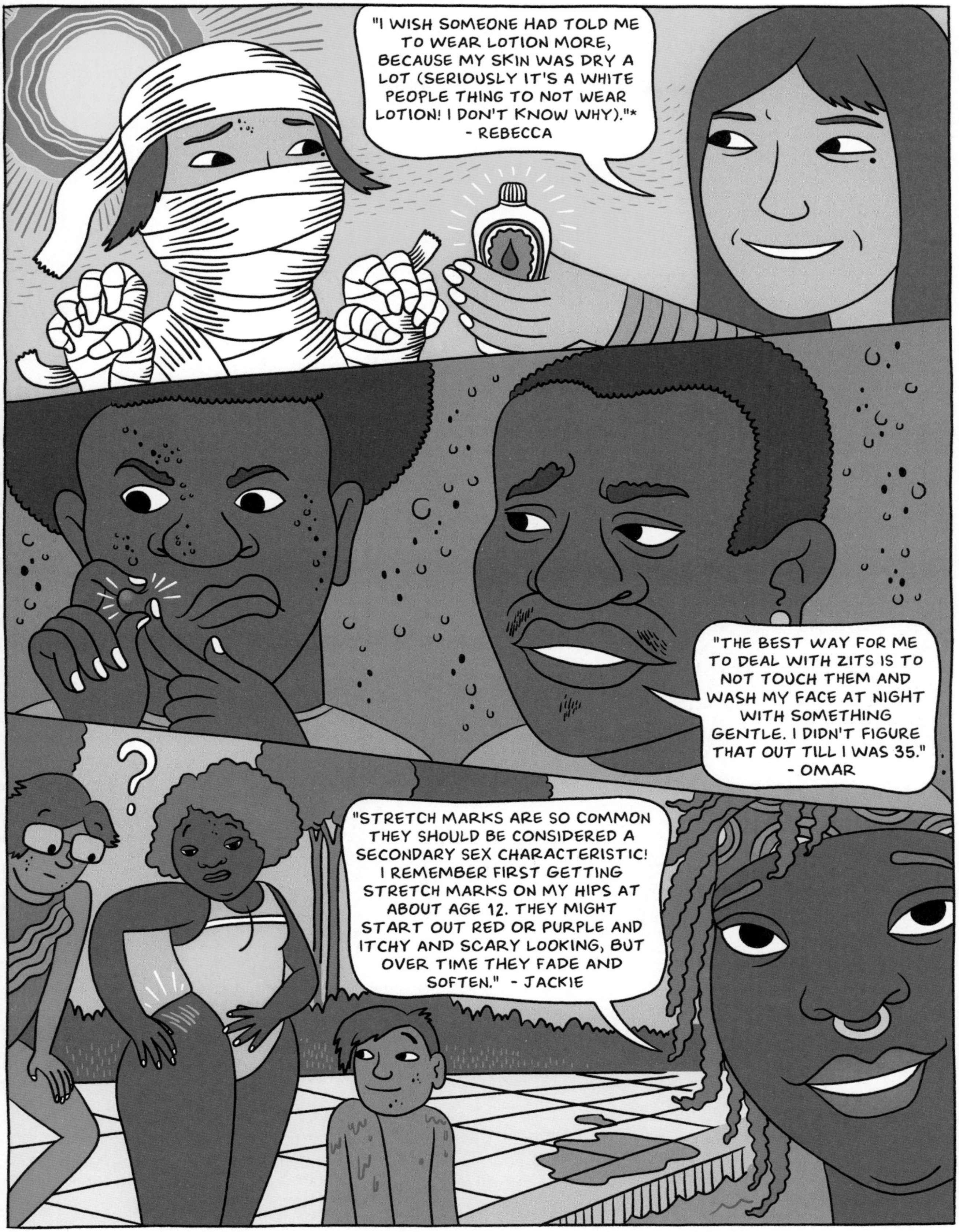
"I WISH SOMEONE HAD TOLD ME TO WEAR LOTION MORE, BECAUSE MY SKIN WAS DRY A LOT (SERIOUSLY IT'S A WHITE PEOPLE THING TO NOT WEAR LOTION! I DON'T KNOW WHY)."* - REBECCA
"THE BEST WAY FOR ME TO DEAL WITH ZITS IS TO NOT TOUCH THEM AND WASH MY FACE AT NIGHT WITH SOMETHING GENTLE. I DIDN'T FIGURE THAT OUT TILL I WAS 35." - OMAR
?
"STRETCH MARKS ARE SO COMMON THEY SHOULD BE CONSIDERED A SECONDARY SEX CHARACTERISTIC! I REMEMBER FIRST GETTING STRETCH MARKS ON MY HIPS AT ABOUT AGE 12. THEY MIGHT START OUT RED OR PURPLE AND ITCHY AND SCARY LOOKING, BUT OVER TIME THEY FADE AND SOFTEN." - JACKIE

* LOTION IS GREAT TO HYDRATE THE SKIN, BUT EVERYONE NEEDS SUNSCREEN, NOT JUST WHITE PEOPLE!

DURING PUBERTY, THE WAY OUR HAIR LOOKS AND FEELS CAN CHANGE, IN PART BECAUSE OF THE SAME OILS THAT ARE CHANGING OUR SKIN.

FOR MOST OF US, HAIR WILL START TO GROW PLACES IT HADN'T BEFORE: ON THE UPPER LIP, FACE, CHEST, ARMS, LEGS, UNDERARMS, AND AROUND NIPPLES AND GENITALS.

PUBIC HAIR—THE HAIR AROUND OUR GENITALS— LOOKS AND FEELS DIFFERENT FROM THE HAIR THAT GROWS ON OUR HEAD AND UNDER OUR ARMS. IT'S SHORTER AND COARSER. PUBIC HAIR

GROWS AROUND THE BASE OF THE PENIS AND ON THE TESTICLES, ABOVE THE VULVA ON THE PUBIC MOUND, ON THE LABIA, AND SOMETIMES AROUND THE ANUS. PUBIC HAIR CAN GROW UP TOWARD THE STOMACH AND DOWN THE THIGHS.

HOW MUCH HAIR GROWS AND HOW DARK OR THICK IT IS DEPENDS ON THE BLEND OF HORMONES IN OUR BODIES. BODIES WITH MORE TESTOSTERONE TEND TO DEVELOP MORE NOTICEABLE HAIR ON THE FACE, ARMS, AND LEGS. BUT ALMOST EVERYONE GETS MORE HAIR DURING PUBERTY.

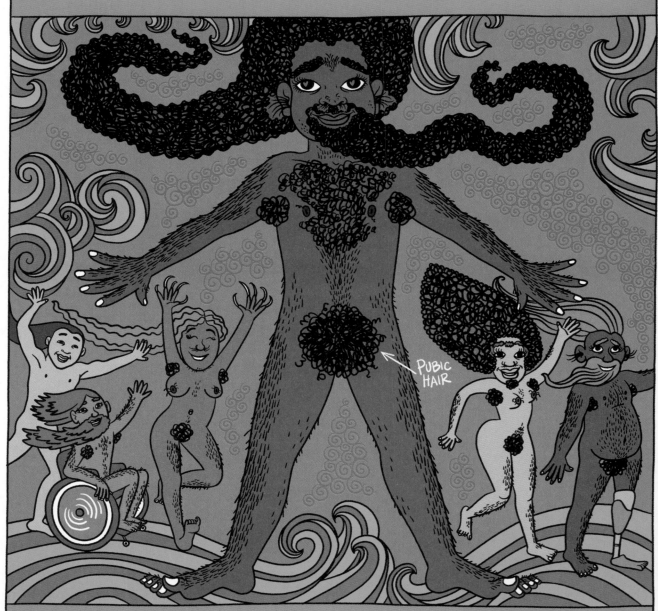

PUBIC HAIR

EVERYONE HAS AN OPINION ABOUT BODY HAIR— WHO SHOULD AND SHOULDN'T HAVE IT, WHERE IT SHOULD BE, AND WHETHER YOU SHOULD CELEBRATE IT OR GET RID OF IT. YOU MAY HAVE RULES YOU HAVE TO FOLLOW AT HOME, BUT BODY AUTONOMY MEANS THAT ULTIMATELY THE ONLY ONE WHO SHOULD BE DECIDING WHAT YOU DO WITH YOUR BODY IS YOU.

158

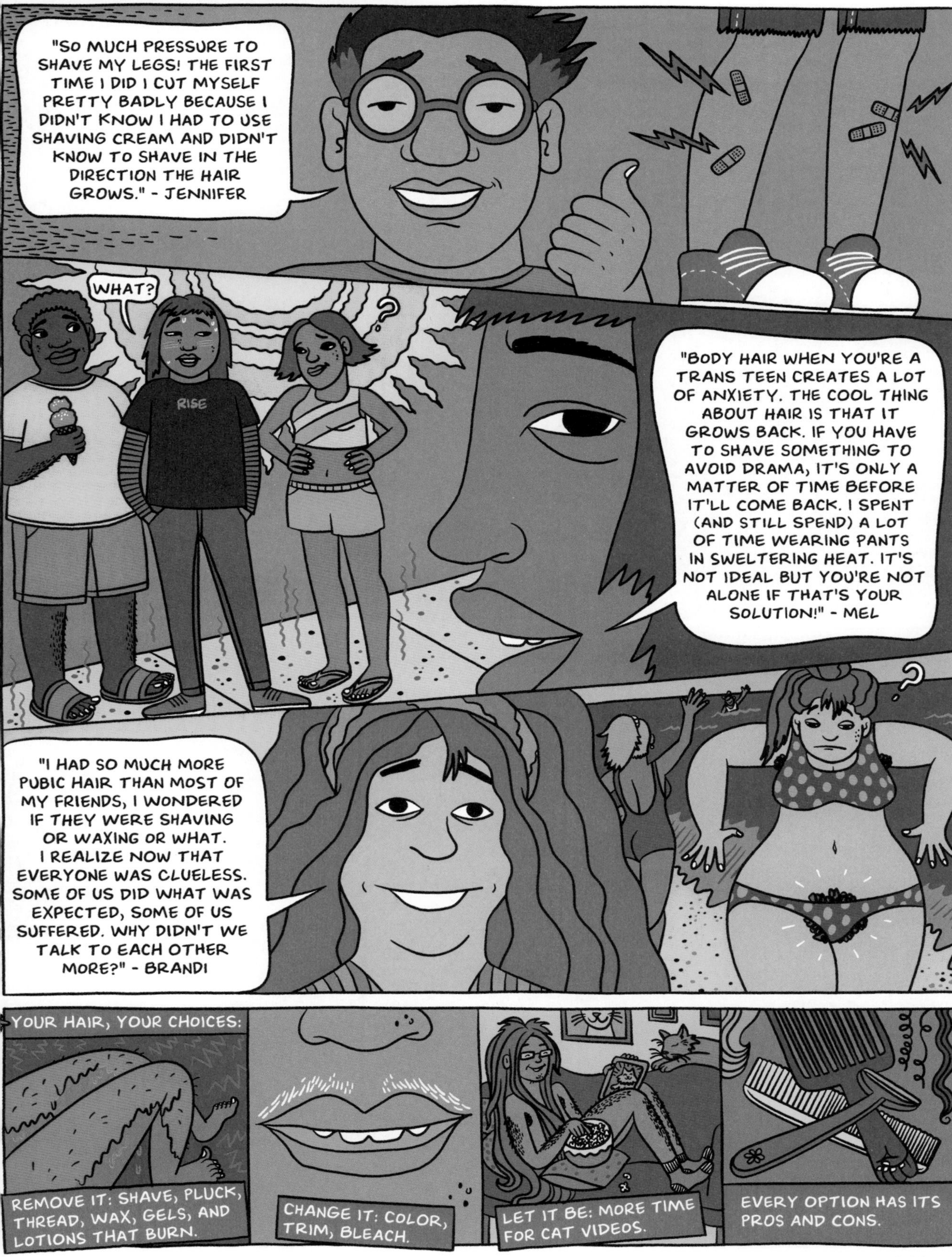
"SO MUCH PRESSURE TO SHAVE MY LEGS! THE FIRST TIME I DID I CUT MYSELF PRETTY BADLY BECAUSE I DIDN'T KNOW I HAD TO USE SHAVING CREAM AND DIDN'T KNOW TO SHAVE IN THE DIRECTION THE HAIR GROWS." - JENNIFER
WHAT?
RISE
"BODY HAIR WHEN YOU'RE A TRANS TEEN CREATES A LOT OF ANXIETY. THE COOL THING ABOUT HAIR IS THAT IT GROWS BACK. IF YOU HAVE TO SHAVE SOMETHING TO AVOID DRAMA, IT'S ONLY A MATTER OF TIME BEFORE IT'LL COME BACK. I SPENT (AND STILL SPEND) A LOT OF TIME WEARING PANTS IN SWELTERING HEAT. IT'S NOT IDEAL BUT YOU'RE NOT ALONE IF THAT'S YOUR SOLUTION!" - MEL
"I HAD SO MUCH MORE PUBIC HAIR THAN MOST OF MY FRIENDS, I WONDERED IF THEY WERE SHAVING OR WAXING OR WHAT. I REALIZE NOW THAT EVERYONE WAS CLUELESS. SOME OF US DID WHAT WAS EXPECTED, SOME OF US SUFFERED. WHY DIDN'T WE TALK TO EACH OTHER MORE?" - BRANDI
YOUR HAIR, YOUR CHOICES:
REMOVE IT: SHAVE, PLUCK, THREAD, WAX, GELS, AND LOTIONS THAT BURN.
CHANGE IT: COLOR, TRIM, BLEACH.
LET IT BE: MORE TIME FOR CAT VIDEOS.
EVERY OPTION HAS ITS PROS AND CONS.

DURING PUBERTY, AS SWEAT GLANDS DEVELOP AND GROW, MOST BODIES START SWEATING MORE. MORE SWEAT—COMBINED WITH MORE HAIR ON THE BODY AND OTHER NEW FLUIDS YOUR BODY STARTS MAKING—MEANS PUBERTY IS A TIME WHEN YOUR BODY SMELL EMERGES, AND BECOMES MORE NOTICEABLE. EVERY BODY HAS A SMELL. BODY ODOR ISN'T A RESULT OF NOT BEING CLEAN—IT'S A RESULT OF HAVING A BODY.

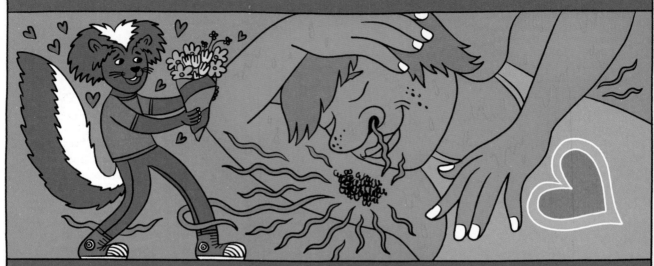

SOME PEOPLE FIND REGULAR SHOWERS OR BATHS LEAVE THEM FEELING AND SMELLING THE WAY THEY WANT. SOME PEOPLE CHOOSE TO COVER UP HOW THEY SMELL WITH DEODORANT OR PERFUMES. OTHER PEOPLE DON'T LIKE THOSE SCENTS. AND SOME OF US CAN'T WEAR THEM BECAUSE THEY HURT OUR BODIES OR MAKE US SICK.

WHAT YOU DO WITH YOUR BODY IS YOUR CHOICE. BUT IF YOU'RE WEARING A STRONG SCENT BECAUSE SOMEONE MADE YOU FEEL ASHAMED OF YOUR BODY, THINK ABOUT THE FACT THAT DEODORANTS AND PERFUMES ATTRACT SOME AND REPEL OTHERS.

VOICE CHANGES

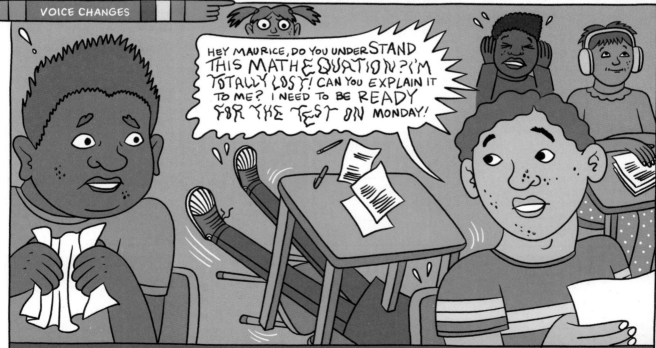

HEY MAURICE, DO YOU UNDERSTAND THIS MATH EQUATION? I'M TOTALLY LOST! CAN YOU EXPLAIN IT TO ME? I NEED TO BE READY FOR THE TEST ON MONDAY!

YOU MAY HEAR OR FEEL YOUR VOICE GETTING LOWER DURING PUBERTY. AS THE VOICE BOX AND VOCAL CORDS GROW, THE VOICE DEEPENS. BODIES WITH TESTICLES AND MORE TESTOSTERONE USUALLY END UP WITH LOWER VOICES, WHICH MAY GO THROUGH A FEW MONTHS OF CRACKING BEFORE THEY SETTLE. BODIES WITH OVARIES AND MORE ESTROGEN WILL ALSO GO THROUGH VOICE CHANGES, BUT USUALLY IT'S NOT AS LOW, AND DOESN'T COME WITH AS MUCH CRACKING.

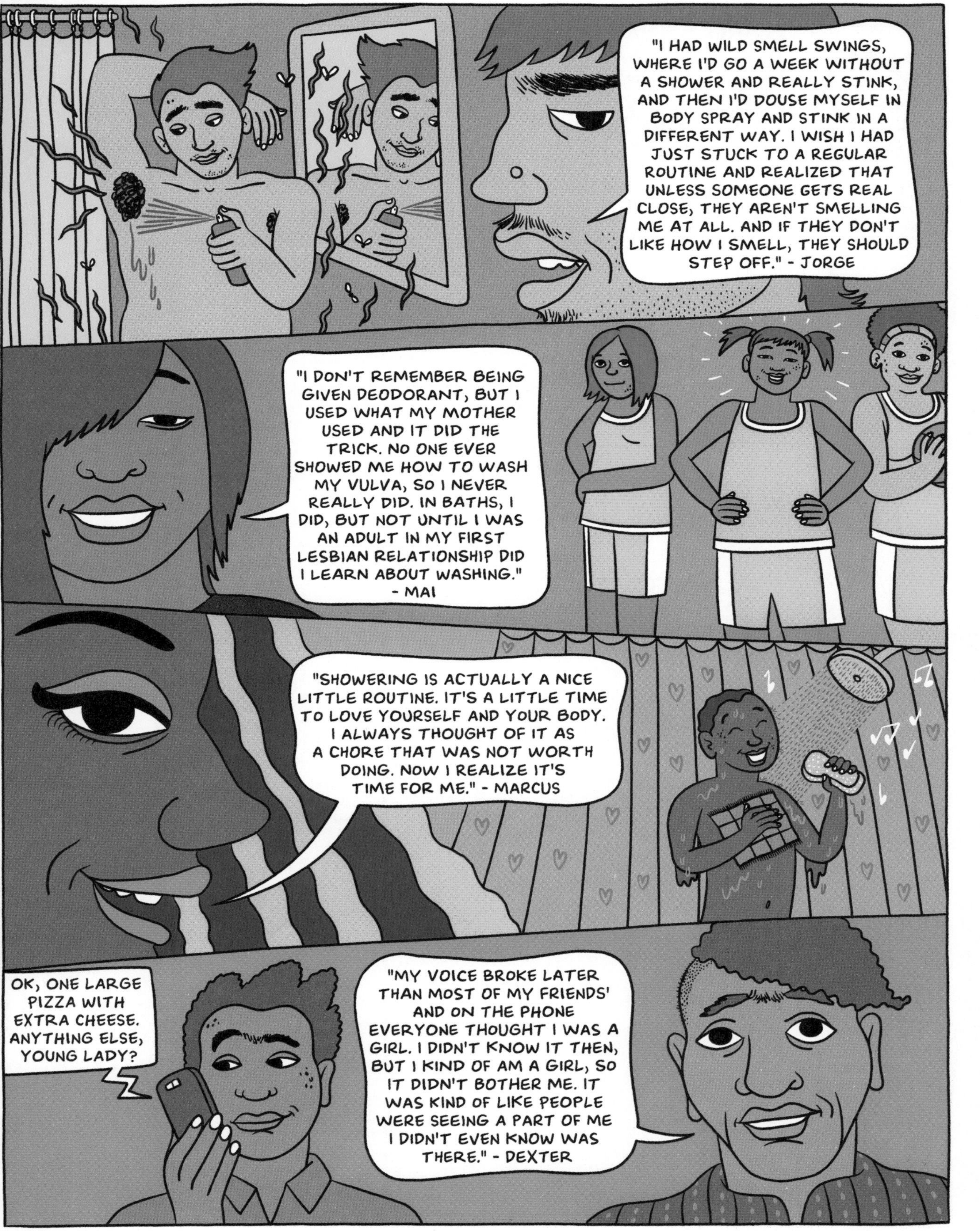
"I HAD WILD SMELL SWINGS, WHERE I'D GO A WEEK WITHOUT A SHOWER AND REALLY STINK, AND THEN I'D DOUSE MYSELF IN BODY SPRAY AND STINK IN A DIFFERENT WAY. I WISH I HAD JUST STUCK TO A REGULAR ROUTINE AND REALIZED THAT UNLESS SOMEONE GETS REAL CLOSE, THEY AREN'T SMELLING ME AT ALL. AND IF THEY DON'T LIKE HOW I SMELL, THEY SHOULD STEP OFF." - JORGE
"I DON'T REMEMBER BEING GIVEN DEODORANT, BUT I USED WHAT MY MOTHER USED AND IT DID THE TRICK. NO ONE EVER SHOWED ME HOW TO WASH MY VULVA, SO I NEVER REALLY DID. IN BATHS, I DID, BUT NOT UNTIL I WAS AN ADULT IN MY FIRST LESBIAN RELATIONSHIP DID I LEARN ABOUT WASHING." - MAI
"SHOWERING IS ACTUALLY A NICE LITTLE ROUTINE. IT'S A LITTLE TIME TO LOVE YOURSELF AND YOUR BODY. I ALWAYS THOUGHT OF IT AS A CHORE THAT WAS NOT WORTH DOING. NOW I REALIZE IT'S TIME FOR ME." - MARCUS
OK, ONE LARGE PIZZA WITH EXTRA CHEESE. ANYTHING ELSE, YOUNG LADY?
"MY VOICE BROKE LATER THAN MOST OF MY FRIENDS' AND ON THE PHONE EVERYONE THOUGHT I WAS A GIRL. I DIDN'T KNOW IT THEN, BUT I KIND OF AM A GIRL, SO IT DIDN'T BOTHER ME. IT WAS KIND OF LIKE PEOPLE WERE SEEING A PART OF ME I DIDN'T EVEN KNOW WAS THERE." - DEXTER

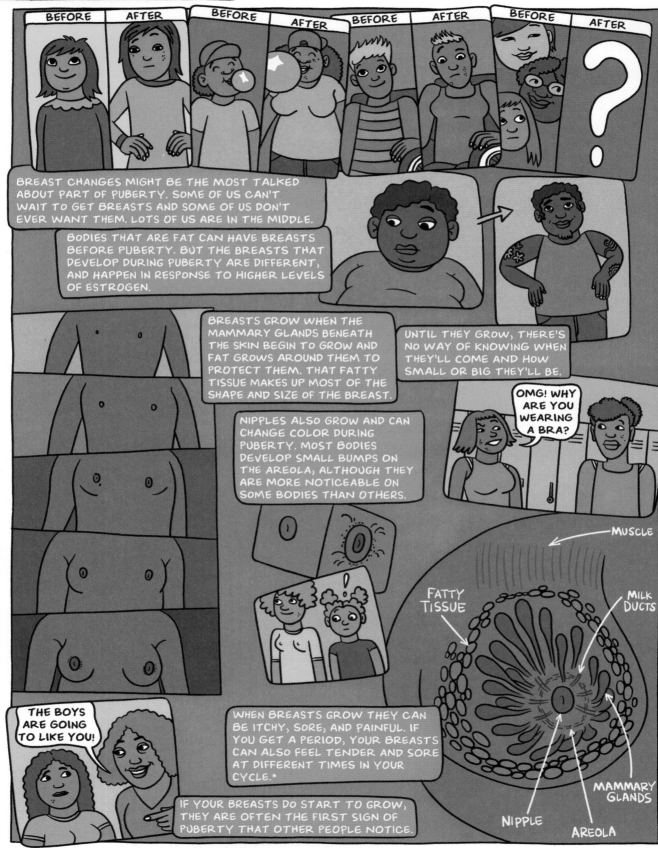

BEFORE | AFTER | BEFORE | AFTER | BEFORE | AFTER | BEFORE | AFTER

BREAST CHANGES MIGHT BE THE MOST TALKED ABOUT PART OF PUBERTY. SOME OF US CAN'T WAIT TO GET BREASTS AND SOME OF US DON'T EVER WANT THEM. LOTS OF US ARE IN THE MIDDLE.

BODIES THAT ARE FAT CAN HAVE BREASTS BEFORE PUBERTY. BUT THE BREASTS THAT DEVELOP DURING PUBERTY ARE DIFFERENT, AND HAPPEN IN RESPONSE TO HIGHER LEVELS OF ESTROGEN.

BREASTS GROW WHEN THE MAMMARY GLANDS BENEATH THE SKIN BEGIN TO GROW AND FAT GROWS AROUND THEM TO PROTECT THEM. THAT FATTY TISSUE MAKES UP MOST OF THE SHAPE AND SIZE OF THE BREAST.

UNTIL THEY GROW, THERE'S NO WAY OF KNOWING WHEN THEY'LL COME AND HOW SMALL OR BIG THEY'LL BE.

NIPPLES ALSO GROW AND CAN CHANGE COLOR DURING PUBERTY. MOST BODIES DEVELOP SMALL BUMPS ON THE AREOLA, ALTHOUGH THEY ARE MORE NOTICEABLE ON SOME BODIES THAN OTHERS.

OMG! WHY ARE YOU WEARING A BRA?

MUSCLE

FATTY TISSUE

MILK DUCTS

THE BOYS ARE GOING TO LIKE YOU!

WHEN BREASTS GROW THEY CAN BE ITCHY, SORE, AND PAINFUL. IF YOU GET A PERIOD, YOUR BREASTS CAN ALSO FEEL TENDER AND SORE AT DIFFERENT TIMES IN YOUR CYCLE.*

IF YOUR BREASTS DO START TO GROW, THEY ARE OFTEN THE FIRST SIGN OF PUBERTY THAT OTHER PEOPLE NOTICE.

MAMMARY GLANDS

NIPPLE

AREOLA

* READ MORE ABOUT PERIODS AND CYCLES ON P. 172

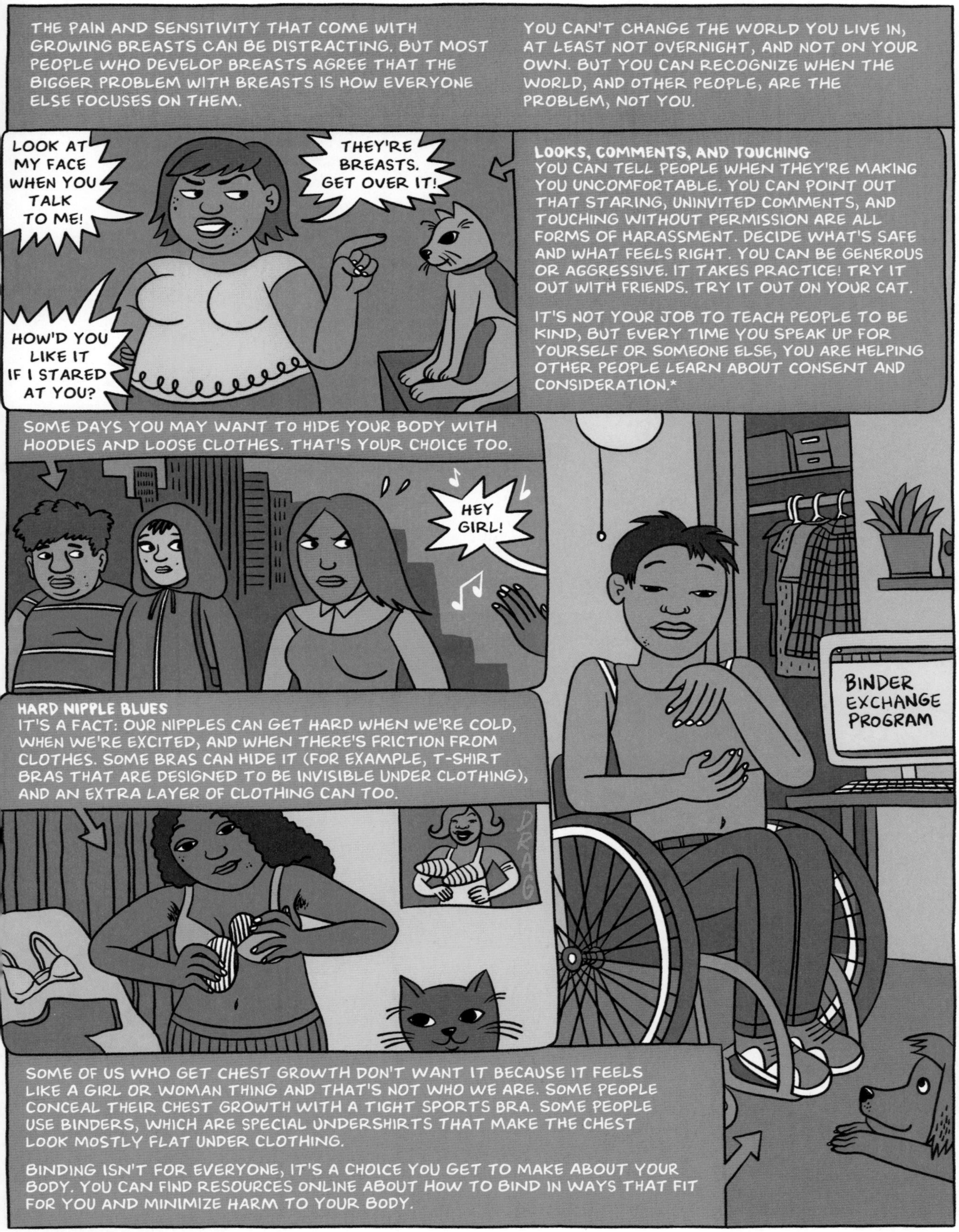
THE PAIN AND SENSITIVITY THAT COME WITH GROWING BREASTS CAN BE DISTRACTING. BUT MOST PEOPLE WHO DEVELOP BREASTS AGREE THAT THE BIGGER PROBLEM WITH BREASTS IS HOW EVERYONE ELSE FOCUSES ON THEM.
YOU CAN'T CHANGE THE WORLD YOU LIVE IN, AT LEAST NOT OVERNIGHT, AND NOT ON YOUR OWN. BUT YOU CAN RECOGNIZE WHEN THE WORLD, AND OTHER PEOPLE, ARE THE PROBLEM, NOT YOU.
LOOK AT MY FACE WHEN YOU TALK TO ME!
THEY'RE BREASTS. GET OVER IT!
HOW'D YOU LIKE IT IF I STARED AT YOU?
LOOKS, COMMENTS, AND TOUCHING
YOU CAN TELL PEOPLE WHEN THEY'RE MAKING YOU UNCOMFORTABLE. YOU CAN POINT OUT THAT STARING, UNINVITED COMMENTS, AND TOUCHING WITHOUT PERMISSION ARE ALL FORMS OF HARASSMENT. DECIDE WHAT'S SAFE AND WHAT FEELS RIGHT. YOU CAN BE GENEROUS OR AGGRESSIVE. IT TAKES PRACTICE! TRY IT OUT WITH FRIENDS. TRY IT OUT ON YOUR CAT.
IT'S NOT YOUR JOB TO TEACH PEOPLE TO BE KIND, BUT EVERY TIME YOU SPEAK UP FOR YOURSELF OR SOMEONE ELSE, YOU ARE HELPING OTHER PEOPLE LEARN ABOUT CONSENT AND CONSIDERATION.*
SOME DAYS YOU MAY WANT TO HIDE YOUR BODY WITH HOODIES AND LOOSE CLOTHES. THAT'S YOUR CHOICE TOO.
HEY GIRL!
BINDER EXCHANGE PROGRAM
HARD NIPPLE BLUES
IT'S A FACT: OUR NIPPLES CAN GET HARD WHEN WE'RE COLD, WHEN WE'RE EXCITED, AND WHEN THERE'S FRICTION FROM CLOTHES. SOME BRAS CAN HIDE IT (FOR EXAMPLE, T-SHIRT BRAS THAT ARE DESIGNED TO BE INVISIBLE UNDER CLOTHING), AND AN EXTRA LAYER OF CLOTHING CAN TOO.
DRAG
SOME OF US WHO GET CHEST GROWTH DON'T WANT IT BECAUSE IT FEELS LIKE A GIRL OR WOMAN THING AND THAT'S NOT WHO WE ARE. SOME PEOPLE CONCEAL THEIR CHEST GROWTH WITH A TIGHT SPORTS BRA. SOME PEOPLE USE BINDERS, WHICH ARE SPECIAL UNDERSHIRTS THAT MAKE THE CHEST LOOK MOSTLY FLAT UNDER CLOTHING.
BINDING ISN'T FOR EVERYONE, IT'S A CHOICE YOU GET TO MAKE ABOUT YOUR BODY. YOU CAN FIND RESOURCES ONLINE ABOUT HOW TO BIND IN WAYS THAT FIT FOR YOU AND MINIMIZE HARM TO YOUR BODY.

* MORE ON CONSENT ON P. 205

THE PURPOSE OF A BRA IS TO PROVIDE SUPPORT, COMFORT, AND SOMETIMES SHAPE. SOME PEOPLE WEAR BRAS, SOME PEOPLE DON'T; IT'S A PERSONAL CHOICE. GETTING A FIRST BRA CAN BE A BIG DEAL, AND THERE'S NO RIGHT TIME TO DO IT. IF YOU FEEL LIKE YOU WANT ONE, EVEN IF OTHERS DISAGREE, YOU CAN ASK FOR ONE. TRYING OUT BRAS BEFORE OTHER PEOPLE THINK YOU "NEED" THEM MAY BE ONE WAY OF TAKING CONTROL OF A SITUATION WHERE IT FEELS LIKE EVERYONE ELSE HAS THE POWER.

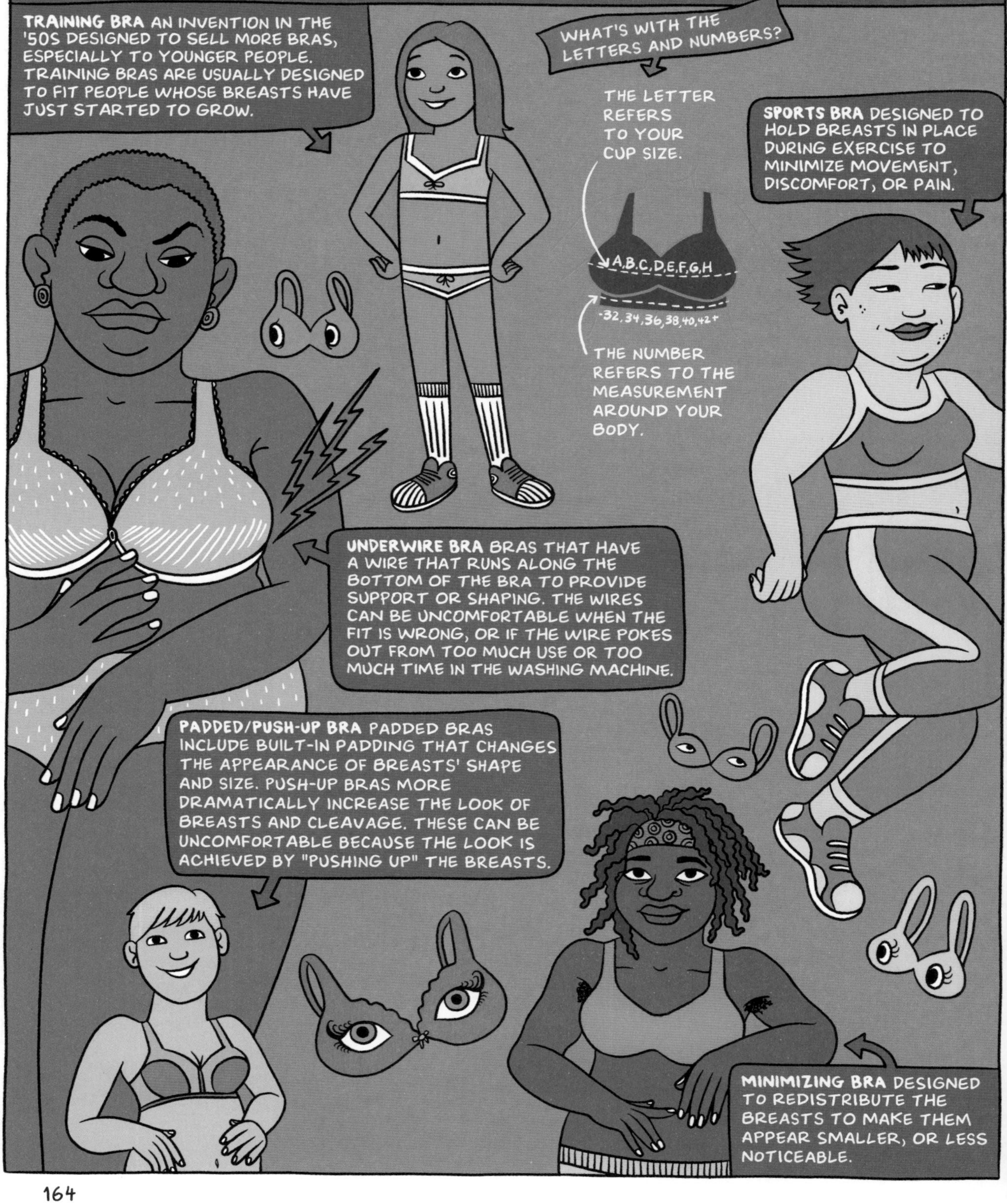
TRAINING BRA AN INVENTION IN THE '50S DESIGNED TO SELL MORE BRAS, ESPECIALLY TO YOUNGER PEOPLE. TRAINING BRAS ARE USUALLY DESIGNED TO FIT PEOPLE WHOSE BREASTS HAVE JUST STARTED TO GROW.
WHAT'S WITH THE LETTERS AND NUMBERS?
THE LETTER REFERS TO YOUR CUP SIZE.
A,B,C,D,E,F,G,H
32,34,36,38,40,42+
THE NUMBER REFERS TO THE MEASUREMENT AROUND YOUR BODY.
SPORTS BRA DESIGNED TO HOLD BREASTS IN PLACE DURING EXERCISE TO MINIMIZE MOVEMENT, DISCOMFORT, OR PAIN.
UNDERWIRE BRA BRAS THAT HAVE A WIRE THAT RUNS ALONG THE BOTTOM OF THE BRA TO PROVIDE SUPPORT OR SHAPING. THE WIRES CAN BE UNCOMFORTABLE WHEN THE FIT IS WRONG, OR IF THE WIRE POKES OUT FROM TOO MUCH USE OR TOO MUCH TIME IN THE WASHING MACHINE.
PADDED/PUSH-UP BRA PADDED BRAS INCLUDE BUILT-IN PADDING THAT CHANGES THE APPEARANCE OF BREASTS' SHAPE AND SIZE. PUSH-UP BRAS MORE DRAMATICALLY INCREASE THE LOOK OF BREASTS AND CLEAVAGE. THESE CAN BE UNCOMFORTABLE BECAUSE THE LOOK IS ACHIEVED BY "PUSHING UP" THE BREASTS.
MINIMIZING BRA DESIGNED TO REDISTRIBUTE THE BREASTS TO MAKE THEM APPEAR SMALLER, OR LESS NOTICEABLE.

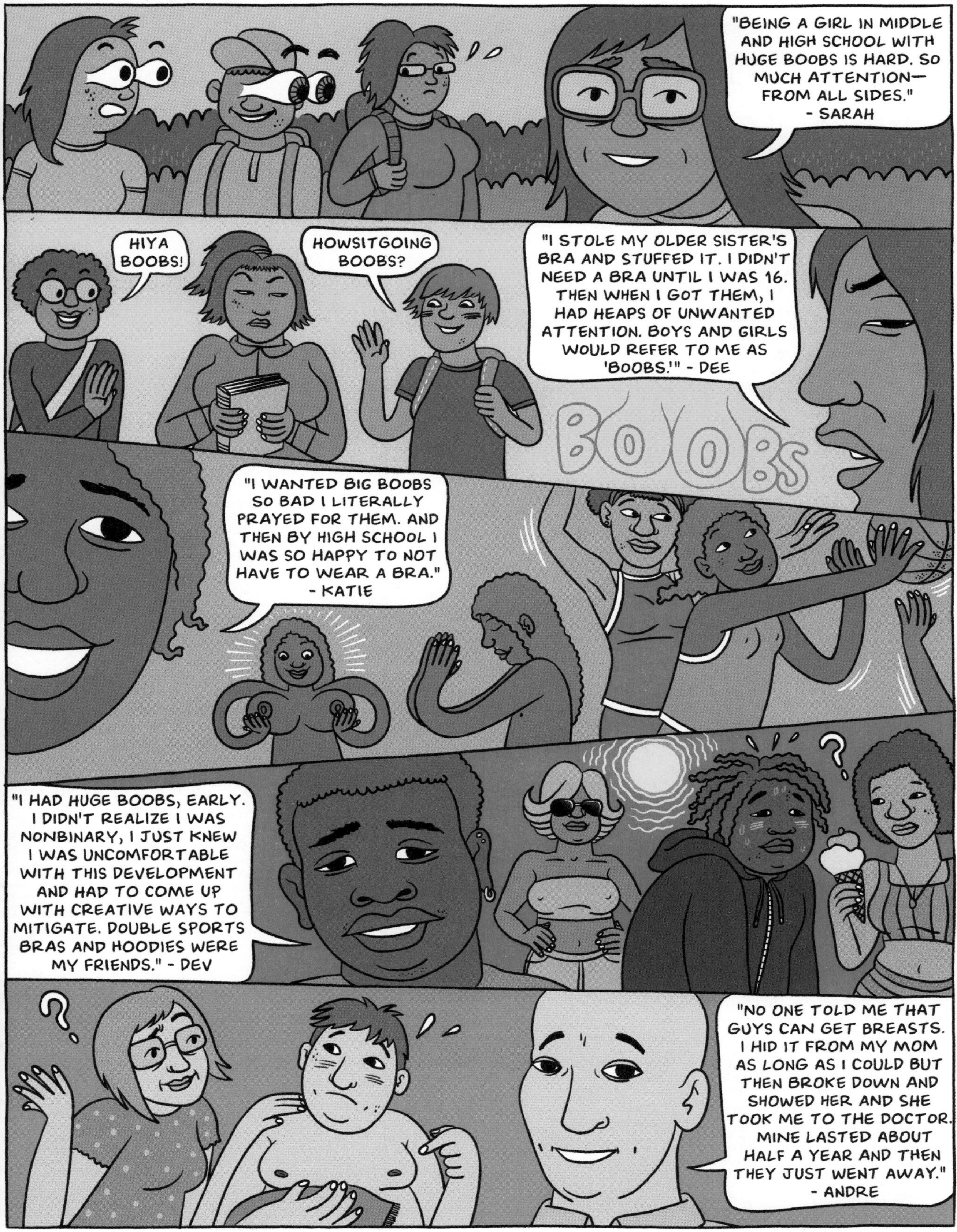
"BEING A GIRL IN MIDDLE AND HIGH SCHOOL WITH HUGE BOOBS IS HARD. SO MUCH ATTENTION—FROM ALL SIDES." - SARAH
HIYA BOOBS!
HOWSITGOING BOOBS?
"I STOLE MY OLDER SISTER'S BRA AND STUFFED IT. I DIDN'T NEED A BRA UNTIL I WAS 16. THEN WHEN I GOT THEM, I HAD HEAPS OF UNWANTED ATTENTION. BOYS AND GIRLS WOULD REFER TO ME AS 'BOOBS.'" - DEE
BOOBS
"I WANTED BIG BOOBS SO BAD I LITERALLY PRAYED FOR THEM. AND THEN BY HIGH SCHOOL I WAS SO HAPPY TO NOT HAVE TO WEAR A BRA." - KATIE
"I HAD HUGE BOOBS, EARLY. I DIDN'T REALIZE I WAS NONBINARY, I JUST KNEW I WAS UNCOMFORTABLE WITH THIS DEVELOPMENT AND HAD TO COME UP WITH CREATIVE WAYS TO MITIGATE. DOUBLE SPORTS BRAS AND HOODIES WERE MY FRIENDS." - DEV
"NO ONE TOLD ME THAT GUYS CAN GET BREASTS. I HID IT FROM MY MOM AS LONG AS I COULD BUT THEN BROKE DOWN AND SHOWED HER AND SHE TOOK ME TO THE DOCTOR. MINE LASTED ABOUT HALF A YEAR AND THEN THEY JUST WENT AWAY." - ANDRE

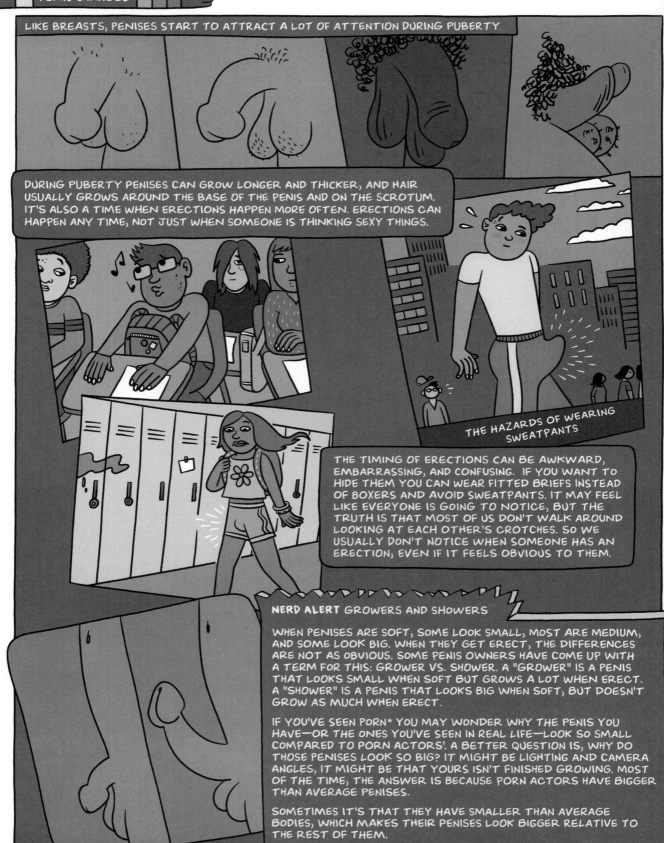

LIKE BREASTS, PENISES START TO ATTRACT A LOT OF ATTENTION DURING PUBERTY.

DURING PUBERTY PENISES CAN GROW LONGER AND THICKER, AND HAIR USUALLY GROWS AROUND THE BASE OF THE PENIS AND ON THE SCROTUM. IT'S ALSO A TIME WHEN ERECTIONS HAPPEN MORE OFTEN. ERECTIONS CAN HAPPEN ANY TIME, NOT JUST WHEN SOMEONE IS THINKING SEXY THINGS.

THE HAZARDS OF WEARING SWEATPANTS

THE TIMING OF ERECTIONS CAN BE AWKWARD, EMBARRASSING, AND CONFUSING. IF YOU WANT TO HIDE THEM YOU CAN WEAR FITTED BRIEFS INSTEAD OF BOXERS AND AVOID SWEATPANTS. IT MAY FEEL LIKE EVERYONE IS GOING TO NOTICE, BUT THE TRUTH IS THAT MOST OF US DON'T WALK AROUND LOOKING AT EACH OTHER'S CROTCHES. SO WE USUALLY DON'T NOTICE WHEN SOMEONE HAS AN ERECTION, EVEN IF IT FEELS OBVIOUS TO THEM.

NERD ALERT GROWERS AND SHOWERS

WHEN PENISES ARE SOFT, SOME LOOK SMALL, MOST ARE MEDIUM, AND SOME LOOK BIG. WHEN THEY GET ERECT, THE DIFFERENCES ARE NOT AS OBVIOUS. SOME PENIS OWNERS HAVE COME UP WITH A TERM FOR THIS: GROWER VS. SHOWER. A "GROWER" IS A PENIS THAT LOOKS SMALL WHEN SOFT BUT GROWS A LOT WHEN ERECT. A "SHOWER" IS A PENIS THAT LOOKS BIG WHEN SOFT, BUT DOESN'T GROW AS MUCH WHEN ERECT.

IF YOU'VE SEEN PORN* YOU MAY WONDER WHY THE PENIS YOU HAVE—OR THE ONES YOU'VE SEEN IN REAL LIFE—LOOK SO SMALL COMPARED TO PORN ACTORS'. A BETTER QUESTION IS, WHY DO THOSE PENISES LOOK SO BIG? IT MIGHT BE LIGHTING AND CAMERA ANGLES, IT MIGHT BE THAT YOURS ISN'T FINISHED GROWING. MOST OF THE TIME, THE ANSWER IS BECAUSE PORN ACTORS HAVE BIGGER THAN AVERAGE PENISES.

SOMETIMES IT'S THAT THEY HAVE SMALLER THAN AVERAGE BODIES, WHICH MAKES THEIR PENISES LOOK BIGGER RELATIVE TO THE REST OF THEM.

 * READ MORE ABOUT PORNOGRAPHY ON P. 357

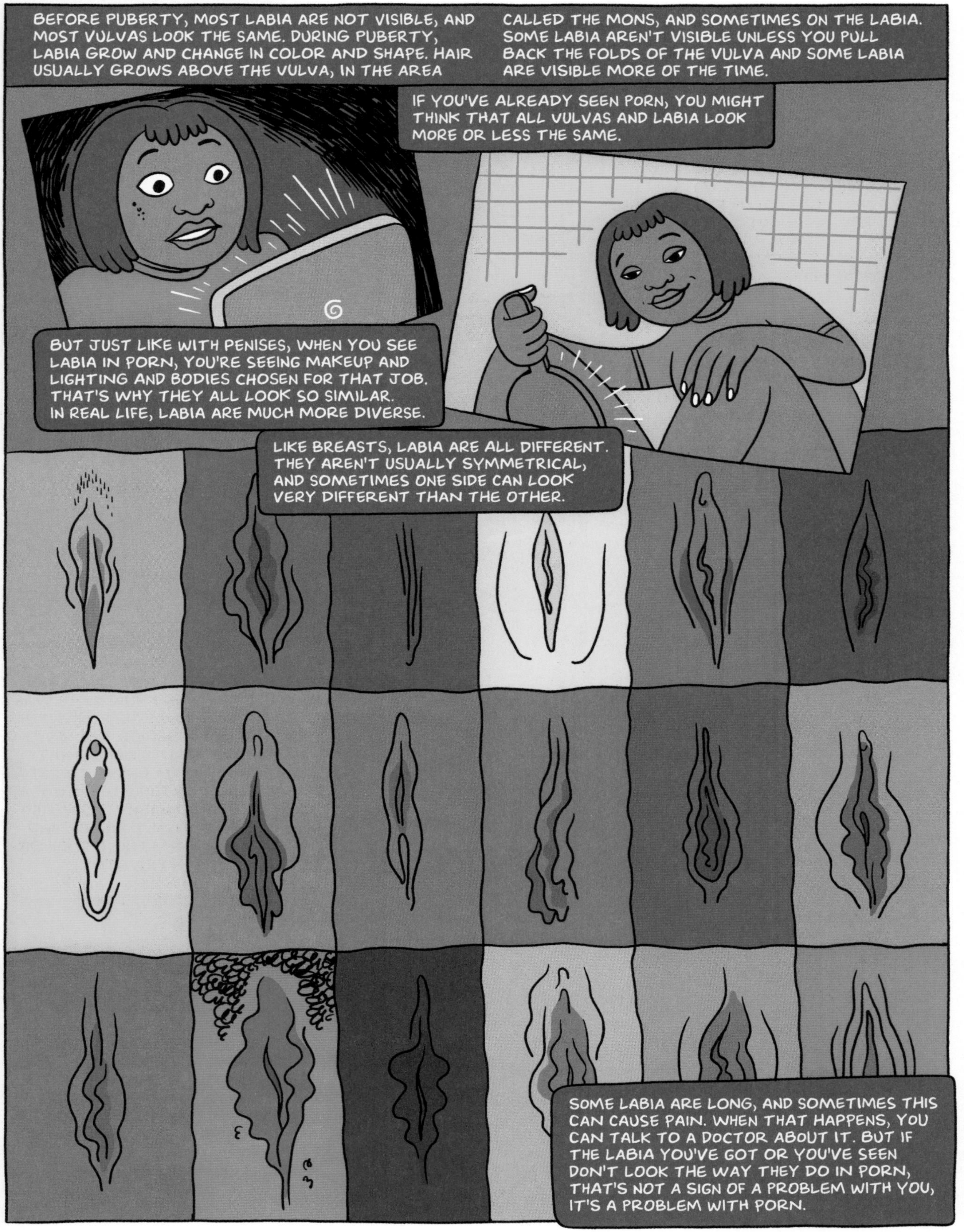
BEFORE PUBERTY, MOST LABIA ARE NOT VISIBLE, AND MOST VULVAS LOOK THE SAME. DURING PUBERTY, LABIA GROW AND CHANGE IN COLOR AND SHAPE. HAIR USUALLY GROWS ABOVE THE VULVA, IN THE AREA CALLED THE MONS, AND SOMETIMES ON THE LABIA. SOME LABIA AREN'T VISIBLE UNLESS YOU PULL BACK THE FOLDS OF THE VULVA AND SOME LABIA ARE VISIBLE MORE OF THE TIME.
IF YOU'VE ALREADY SEEN PORN, YOU MIGHT THINK THAT ALL VULVAS AND LABIA LOOK MORE OR LESS THE SAME.
BUT JUST LIKE WITH PENISES, WHEN YOU SEE LABIA IN PORN, YOU'RE SEEING MAKEUP AND LIGHTING AND BODIES CHOSEN FOR THAT JOB. THAT'S WHY THEY ALL LOOK SO SIMILAR. IN REAL LIFE, LABIA ARE MUCH MORE DIVERSE.
LIKE BREASTS, LABIA ARE ALL DIFFERENT. THEY AREN'T USUALLY SYMMETRICAL, AND SOMETIMES ONE SIDE CAN LOOK VERY DIFFERENT THAN THE OTHER.
SOME LABIA ARE LONG, AND SOMETIMES THIS CAN CAUSE PAIN. WHEN THAT HAPPENS, YOU CAN TALK TO A DOCTOR ABOUT IT. BUT IF THE LABIA YOU'VE GOT OR YOU'VE SEEN DON'T LOOK THE WAY THEY DO IN PORN, THAT'S NOT A SIGN OF A PROBLEM WITH YOU, IT'S A PROBLEM WITH PORN.

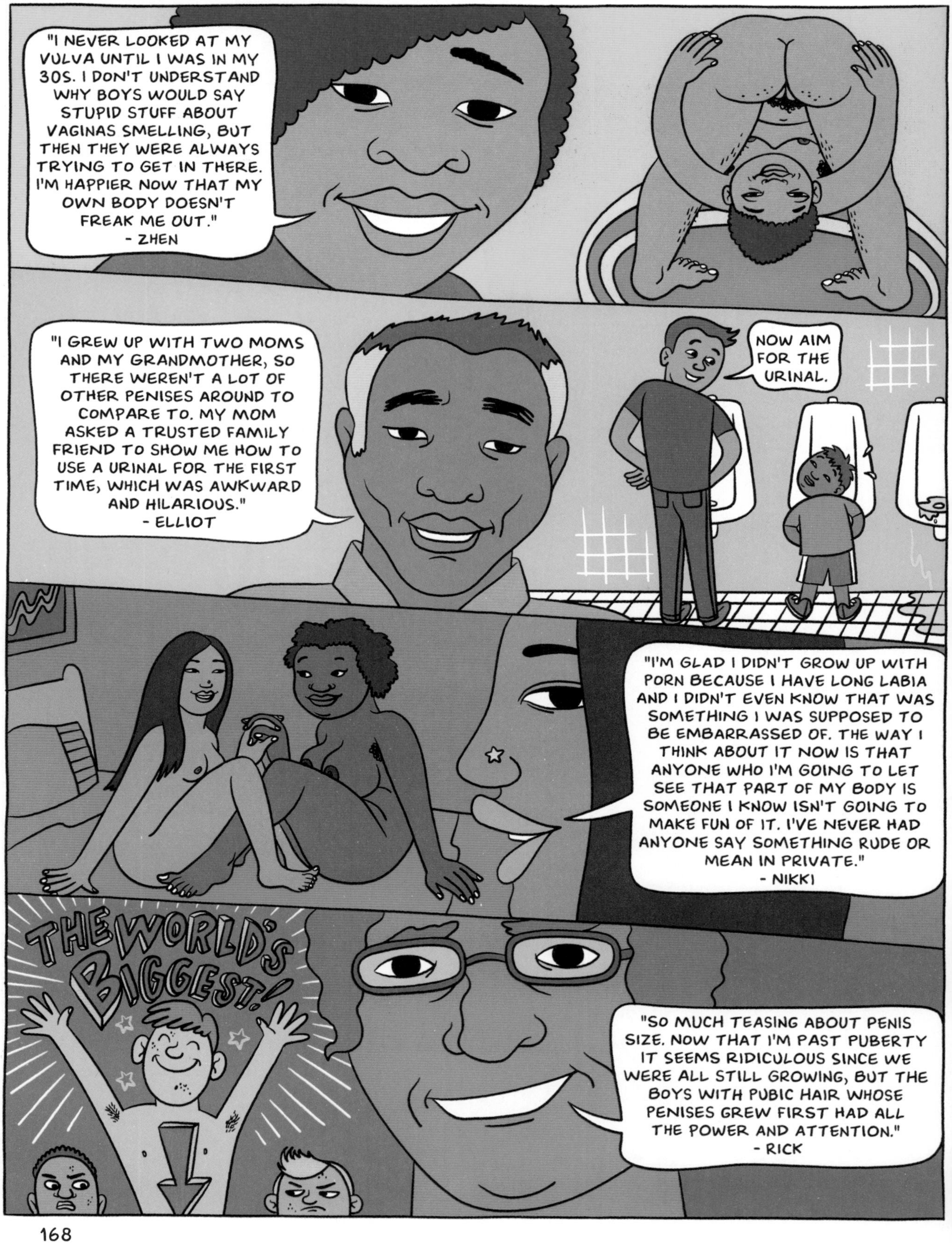
"I NEVER LOOKED AT MY VULVA UNTIL I WAS IN MY 30S. I DON'T UNDERSTAND WHY BOYS WOULD SAY STUPID STUFF ABOUT VAGINAS SMELLING, BUT THEN THEY WERE ALWAYS TRYING TO GET IN THERE. I'M HAPPIER NOW THAT MY OWN BODY DOESN'T FREAK ME OUT." - ZHEN
"I GREW UP WITH TWO MOMS AND MY GRANDMOTHER, SO THERE WEREN'T A LOT OF OTHER PENISES AROUND TO COMPARE TO. MY MOM ASKED A TRUSTED FAMILY FRIEND TO SHOW ME HOW TO USE A URINAL FOR THE FIRST TIME, WHICH WAS AWKWARD AND HILARIOUS." - ELLIOT
NOW AIM FOR THE URINAL.
"I'M GLAD I DIDN'T GROW UP WITH PORN BECAUSE I HAVE LONG LABIA AND I DIDN'T EVEN KNOW THAT WAS SOMETHING I WAS SUPPOSED TO BE EMBARRASSED OF. THE WAY I THINK ABOUT IT NOW IS THAT ANYONE WHO I'M GOING TO LET SEE THAT PART OF MY BODY IS SOMEONE I KNOW ISN'T GOING TO MAKE FUN OF IT. I'VE NEVER HAD ANYONE SAY SOMETHING RUDE OR MEAN IN PRIVATE." - NIKKI
THE WORLD'S BIGGEST!
"SO MUCH TEASING ABOUT PENIS SIZE. NOW THAT I'M PAST PUBERTY IT SEEMS RIDICULOUS SINCE WE WERE ALL STILL GROWING, BUT THE BOYS WITH PUBIC HAIR WHOSE PENISES GREW FIRST HAD ALL THE POWER AND ATTENTION." - RICK

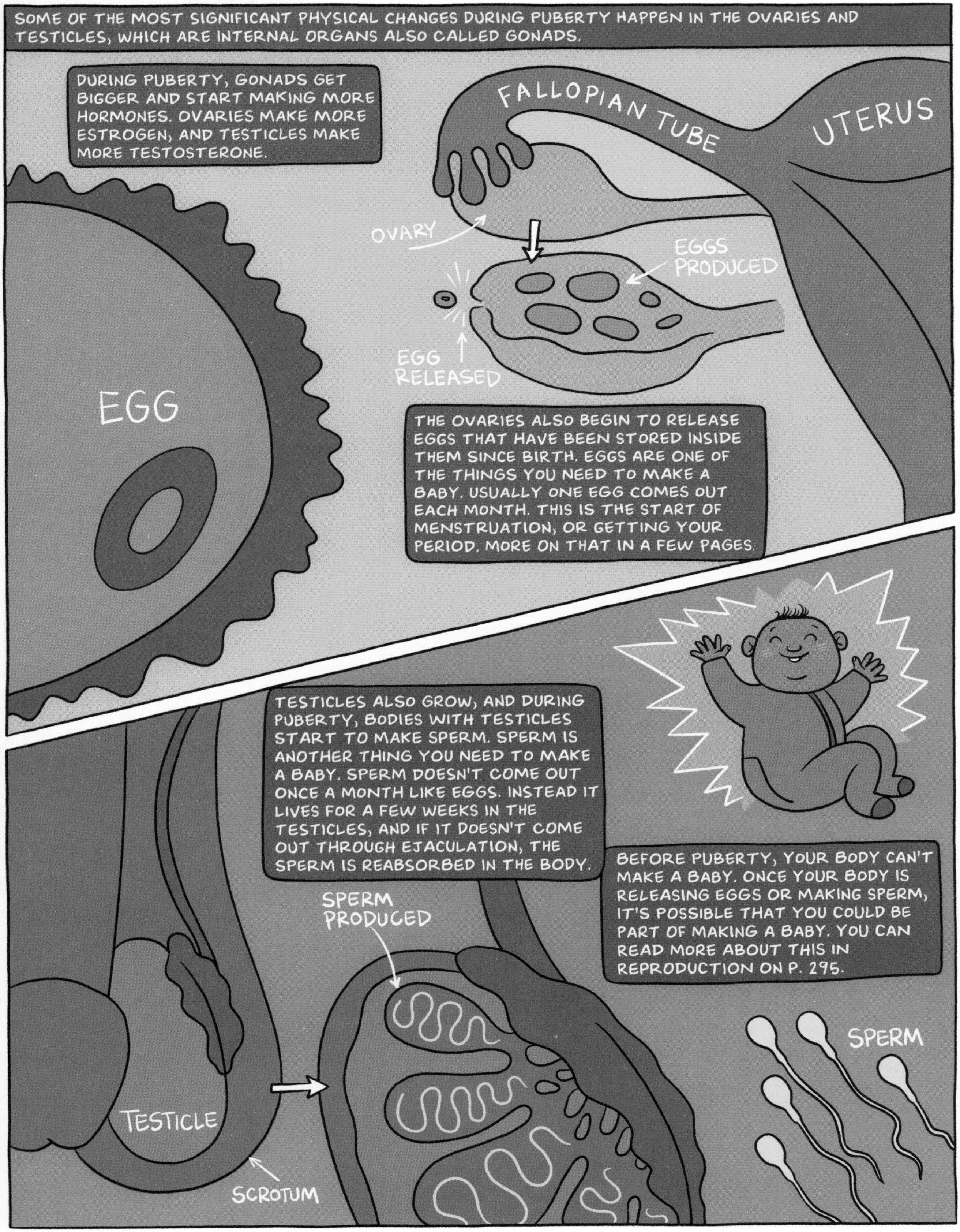
SOME OF THE MOST SIGNIFICANT PHYSICAL CHANGES DURING PUBERTY HAPPEN IN THE OVARIES AND TESTICLES, WHICH ARE INTERNAL ORGANS ALSO CALLED GONADS.
DURING PUBERTY, GONADS GET BIGGER AND START MAKING MORE HORMONES. OVARIES MAKE MORE ESTROGEN, AND TESTICLES MAKE MORE TESTOSTERONE.
FALLOPIAN TUBE
UTERUS
OVARY
EGGS PRODUCED
EGG RELEASED
EGG
THE OVARIES ALSO BEGIN TO RELEASE EGGS THAT HAVE BEEN STORED INSIDE THEM SINCE BIRTH. EGGS ARE ONE OF THE THINGS YOU NEED TO MAKE A BABY. USUALLY ONE EGG COMES OUT EACH MONTH. THIS IS THE START OF MENSTRUATION, OR GETTING YOUR PERIOD. MORE ON THAT IN A FEW PAGES.
TESTICLES ALSO GROW, AND DURING PUBERTY, BODIES WITH TESTICLES START TO MAKE SPERM. SPERM IS ANOTHER THING YOU NEED TO MAKE A BABY. SPERM DOESN'T COME OUT ONCE A MONTH LIKE EGGS. INSTEAD IT LIVES FOR A FEW WEEKS IN THE TESTICLES, AND IF IT DOESN'T COME OUT THROUGH EJACULATION, THE SPERM IS REABSORBED IN THE BODY.
BEFORE PUBERTY, YOUR BODY CAN'T MAKE A BABY. ONCE YOUR BODY IS RELEASING EGGS OR MAKING SPERM, IT'S POSSIBLE THAT YOU COULD BE PART OF MAKING A BABY. YOU CAN READ MORE ABOUT THIS IN REPRODUCTION ON P. 295.
SPERM PRODUCED
TESTICLE
SCROTUM
SPERM

BEFORE PUBERTY, NO BODY EJACULATES, BUT DURING AND AFTER PUBERTY, MANY BODIES ARE ABLE TO EJACULATE. FOR BODIES WITH PENISES, EJACULATION HAPPENS WHEN THE MUSCLES AROUND THE BASE OF THE PENIS BEGIN TO SQUEEZE, AND FLUID (CALLED SEMEN) IS PUSHED UP THROUGH THE URETHRA AND OUT THE TIP OF THE PENIS. THIS USUALLY HAPPENS BECAUSE THE PENIS IS BEING STIMULATED. MOST OF THE TIME, EJACULATION FEELS GOOD.

BODIES WITH A VULVA, VAGINA, AND CLITORIS CAN ALSO RELEASE FLUID IN RESPONSE TO STIMULATION. IT'S USUALLY NOT AS NOTICEABLE, OR AS STICKY, BUT IT'S WET AND IT CAN FEEL GOOD WHEN IT HAPPENS.

SOME BODIES CAN EJACULATE AND SOME BODIES CAN'T. WHETHER YOU CAN OR CAN'T MAY CHANGE OVER TIME. BUT ALL BODIES CAN FEEL GOOD, WHETHER OR NOT THEY EJACULATE.

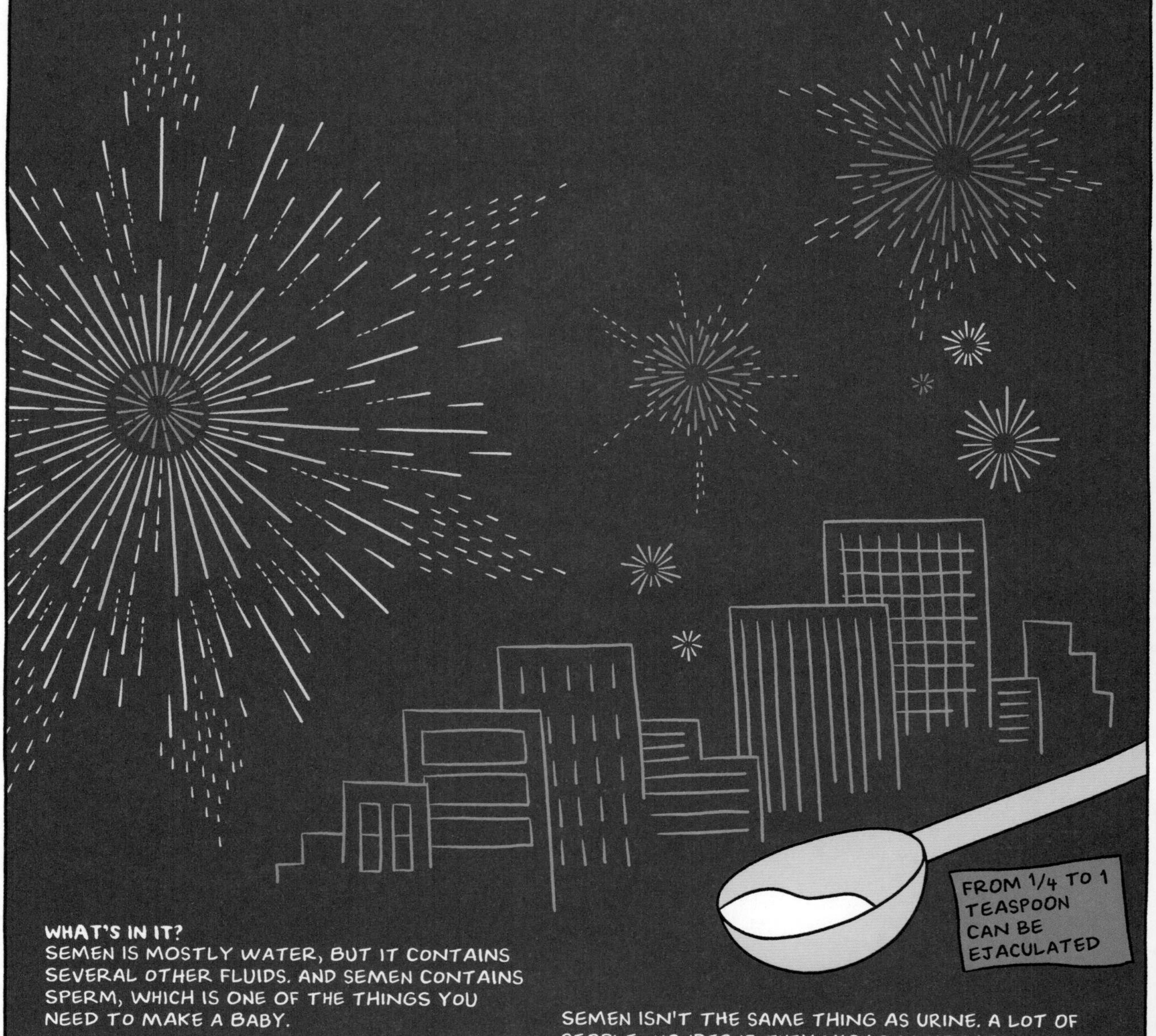
FROM 1/4 TO 1 TEASPOON CAN BE EJACULATED

WHAT'S IN IT?

SEMEN IS MOSTLY WATER, BUT IT CONTAINS SEVERAL OTHER FLUIDS. AND SEMEN CONTAINS SPERM, WHICH IS ONE OF THE THINGS YOU NEED TO MAKE A BABY.

WHEN IT COMES OUT OF THE PENIS, SEMEN IS USUALLY WHITISH AND A BIT STICKY. WHEN IT DRIES, IT'S CLEAR AND IT LEAVES A KIND OF CRUNCHY FEELING ON YOUR SKIN AND ON CLOTHING OR SHEETS. IT WASHES OFF WITH WATER.

SEMEN ISN'T THE SAME THING AS URINE. A LOT OF PEOPLE WONDER IF THEY MIGHT ACCIDENTALLY PEE INSTEAD OF EJACULATE, BUT BODIES WITH PENISES WORK IN A WAY THAT PREVENTS THAT FROM HAPPENING.

BODIES WITH VULVAS CAN ALSO RELEASE FLUID, WHICH IS DIFFERENT FROM SEMEN AND DOESN'T CONTAIN SPERM.

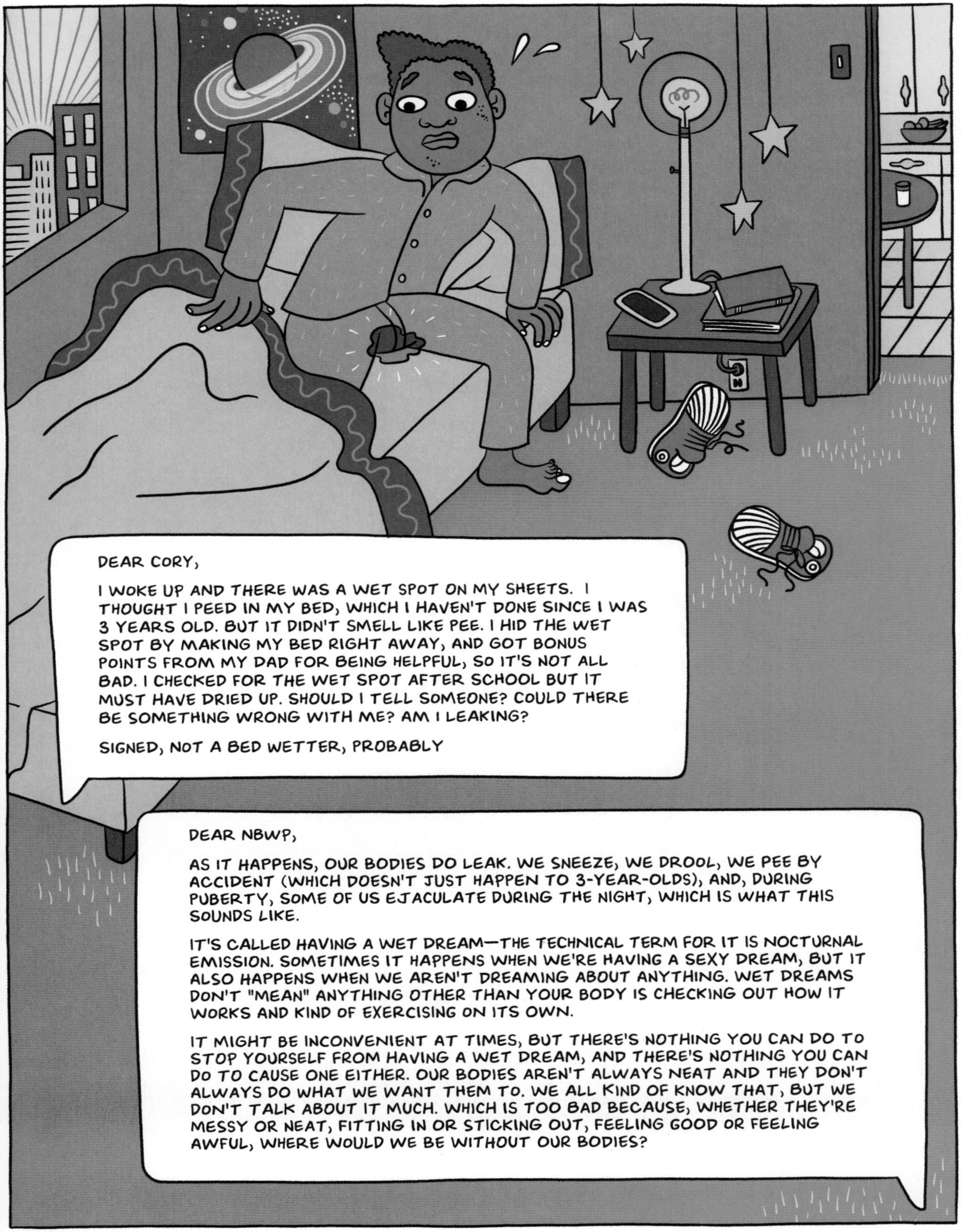
DEAR CORY,
I WOKE UP AND THERE WAS A WET SPOT ON MY SHEETS. I THOUGHT I PEED IN MY BED, WHICH I HAVEN'T DONE SINCE I WAS 3 YEARS OLD. BUT IT DIDN'T SMELL LIKE PEE. I HID THE WET SPOT BY MAKING MY BED RIGHT AWAY, AND GOT BONUS POINTS FROM MY DAD FOR BEING HELPFUL, SO IT'S NOT ALL BAD. I CHECKED FOR THE WET SPOT AFTER SCHOOL BUT IT MUST HAVE DRIED UP. SHOULD I TELL SOMEONE? COULD THERE BE SOMETHING WRONG WITH ME? AM I LEAKING?
SIGNED, NOT A BED WETTER, PROBABLY
DEAR NBWP,
AS IT HAPPENS, OUR BODIES DO LEAK. WE SNEEZE, WE DROOL, WE PEE BY ACCIDENT (WHICH DOESN'T JUST HAPPEN TO 3-YEAR-OLDS), AND, DURING PUBERTY, SOME OF US EJACULATE DURING THE NIGHT, WHICH IS WHAT THIS SOUNDS LIKE.
IT'S CALLED HAVING A WET DREAM—THE TECHNICAL TERM FOR IT IS NOCTURNAL EMISSION. SOMETIMES IT HAPPENS WHEN WE'RE HAVING A SEXY DREAM, BUT IT ALSO HAPPENS WHEN WE AREN'T DREAMING ABOUT ANYTHING. WET DREAMS DON'T "MEAN" ANYTHING OTHER THAN YOUR BODY IS CHECKING OUT HOW IT WORKS AND KIND OF EXERCISING ON ITS OWN.
IT MIGHT BE INCONVENIENT AT TIMES, BUT THERE'S NOTHING YOU CAN DO TO STOP YOURSELF FROM HAVING A WET DREAM, AND THERE'S NOTHING YOU CAN DO TO CAUSE ONE EITHER. OUR BODIES AREN'T ALWAYS NEAT AND THEY DON'T ALWAYS DO WHAT WE WANT THEM TO. WE ALL KIND OF KNOW THAT, BUT WE DON'T TALK ABOUT IT MUCH. WHICH IS TOO BAD BECAUSE, WHETHER THEY'RE MESSY OR NEAT, FITTING IN OR STICKING OUT, FEELING GOOD OR FEELING AWFUL, WHERE WOULD WE BE WITHOUT OUR BODIES?

IF A BODY HAS OVARIES AND A UTERUS, ONE OF THE BIGGEST CHANGES DURING PUBERTY IS THAT IT CAN START TO RELEASE EGGS, ABOUT ONCE PER MONTH, AS PART OF THE MENSTRUAL CYCLE.

PERIODS CAN SEEM LIKE A STRANGE OR SCARY PART OF PUBERTY BECAUSE THEY COMBINE TWO THINGS PEOPLE DON'T TALK ABOUT MUCH: VAGINAS AND BLOOD.

BUT JUST BECAUSE PEOPLE DON'T TALK ABOUT SOMETHING DOESN'T MEAN WE SHOULDN'T OR CAN'T. AND IT DOESN'T MEAN WE NEED TO FEEL EMBARRASSED OR ASHAMED OF IT. A LOT OF PEOPLE FIND PERIODS AND MENSTRUATION COOL AND FASCINATING, NOT SCARY.

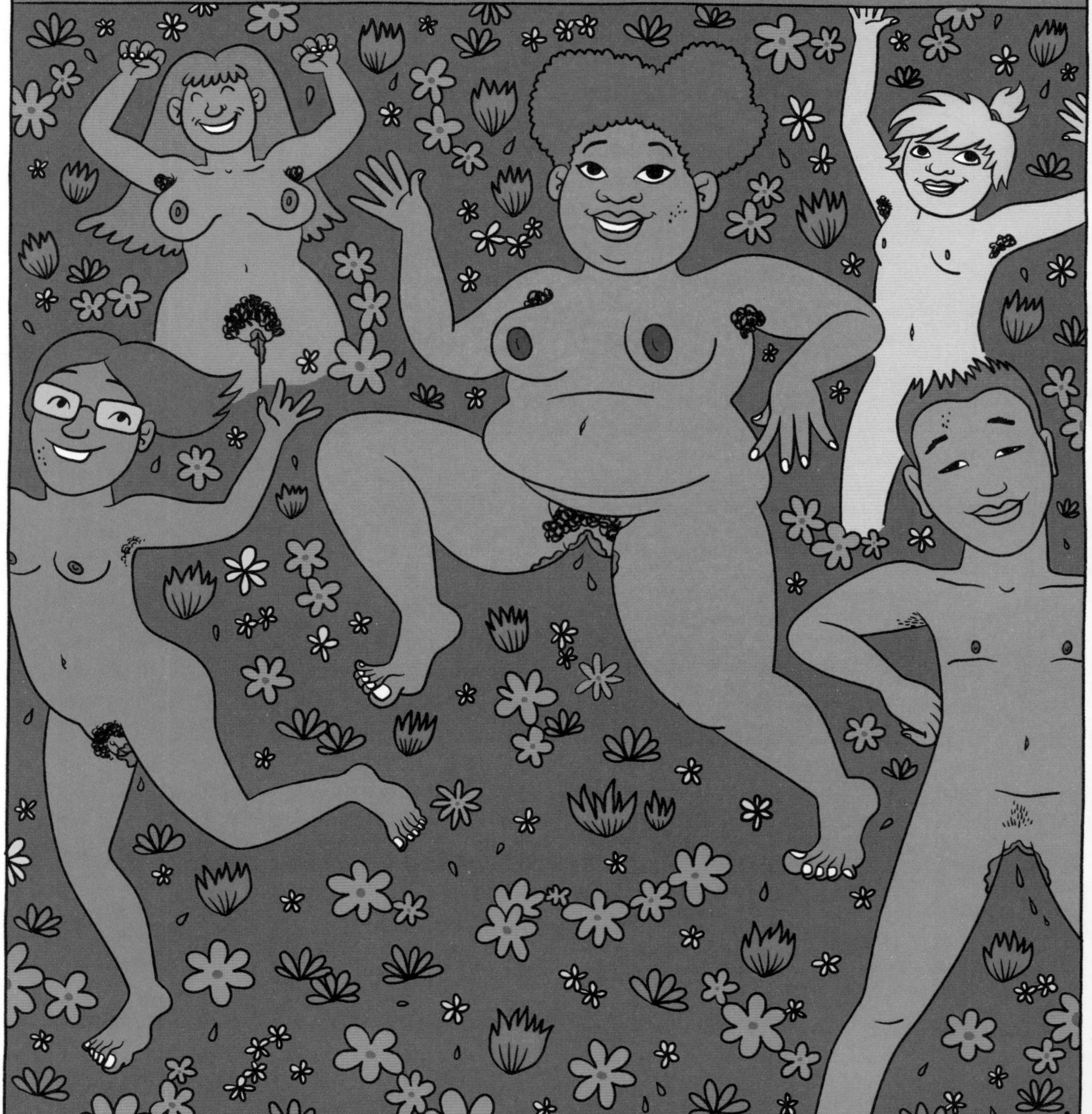

MOST BODIES WITH OVARIES AND A UTERUS WILL HAVE A MENSTRUAL CYCLE EVERY MONTH OR SO. BUT EVERY BODY IS DIFFERENT. SOME MAY BLEED LESS OFTEN OR ALMOST NEVER, BUT STILL EXPERIENCE OTHER PARTS OF WHAT GETS CALLED A PERIOD. REMEMBER, THERE ISN'T ONE WAY TO HAVE A BODY OR A PERIOD.

HERE'S HOW IT USUALLY WORKS.

ABOUT ONCE A MONTH AN EGG PUSHES OUT FROM THE OVARY AND IS PULLED INTO THE FALLOPIAN

TUBE (ALSO CALLED A UTERINE TUBE), WHERE IT BEGINS TO MOVE TOWARD THE UTERUS.

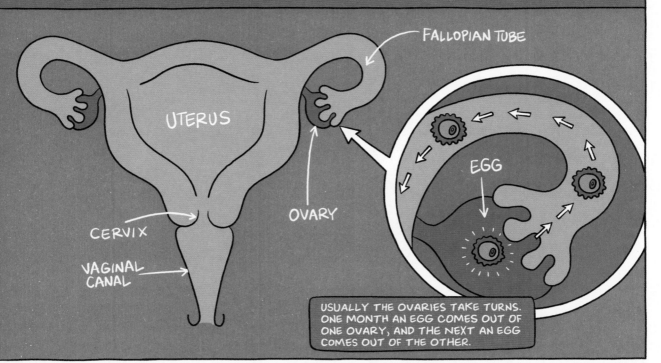

FALLOPIAN TUBE

UTERUS

CERVIX

VAGINAL CANAL

OVARY

EGG

USUALLY THE OVARIES TAKE TURNS. ONE MONTH AN EGG COMES OUT OF ONE OVARY, AND THE NEXT AN EGG COMES OUT OF THE OTHER.

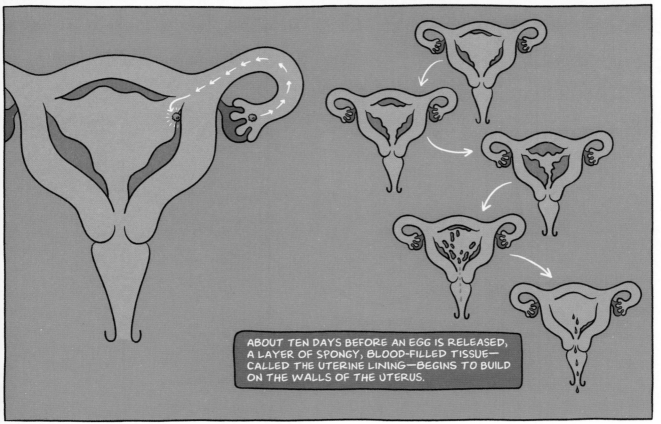

ABOUT TEN DAYS BEFORE AN EGG IS RELEASED, A LAYER OF SPONGY, BLOOD-FILLED TISSUE—CALLED THE UTERINE LINING—BEGINS TO BUILD ON THE WALLS OF THE UTERUS.

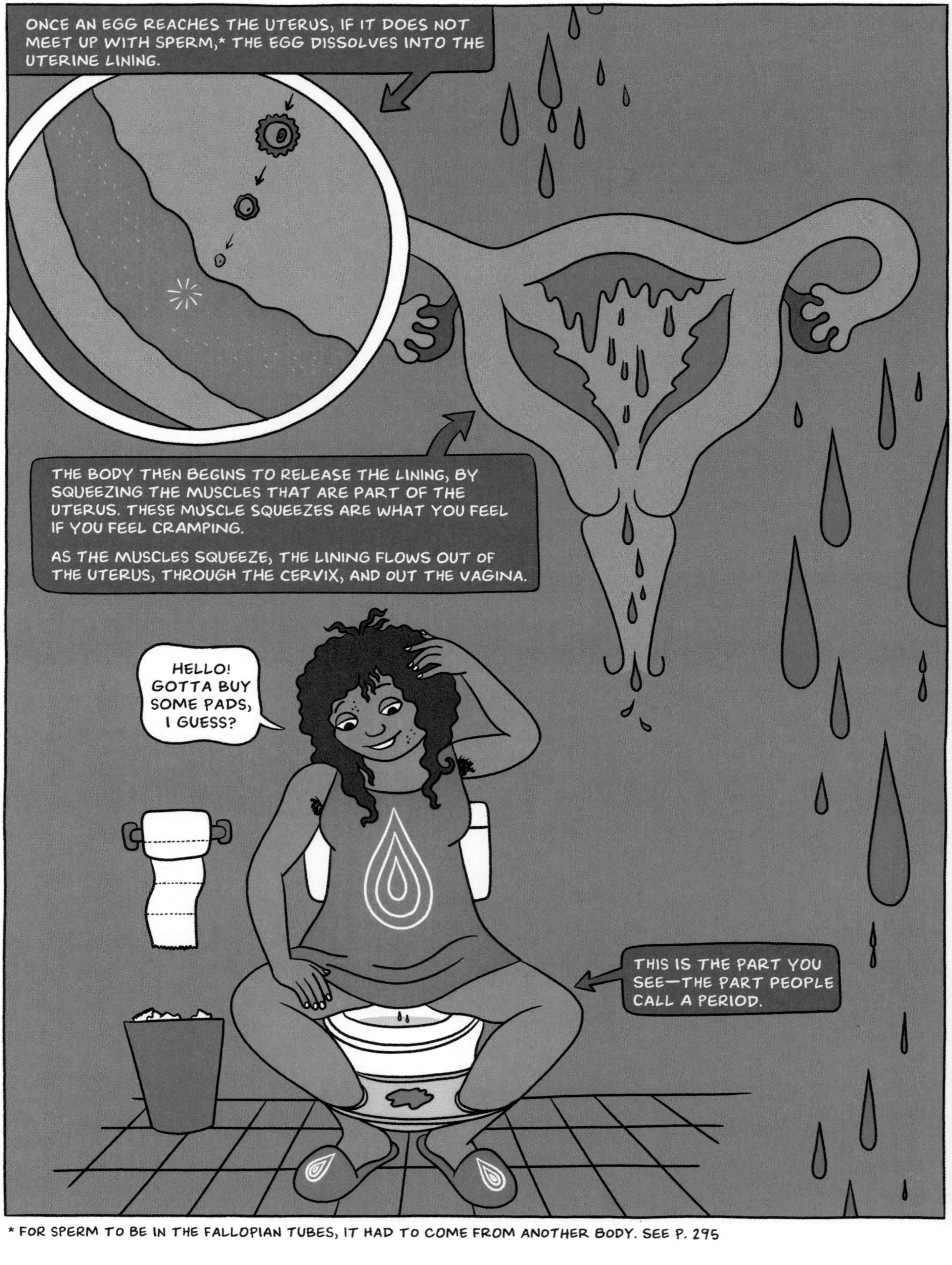
ONCE AN EGG REACHES THE UTERUS, IF IT DOES NOT MEET UP WITH SPERM,* THE EGG DISSOLVES INTO THE UTERINE LINING.
THE BODY THEN BEGINS TO RELEASE THE LINING, BY SQUEEZING THE MUSCLES THAT ARE PART OF THE UTERUS. THESE MUSCLE SQUEEZES ARE WHAT YOU FEEL IF YOU FEEL CRAMPING.
AS THE MUSCLES SQUEEZE, THE LINING FLOWS OUT OF THE UTERUS, THROUGH THE CERVIX, AND OUT THE VAGINA.
HELLO! GOTTA BUY SOME PADS, I GUESS?
THIS IS THE PART YOU SEE—THE PART PEOPLE CALL A PERIOD.

* FOR SPERM TO BE IN THE FALLOPIAN TUBES, IT HAD TO COME FROM ANOTHER BODY. SEE P. 295

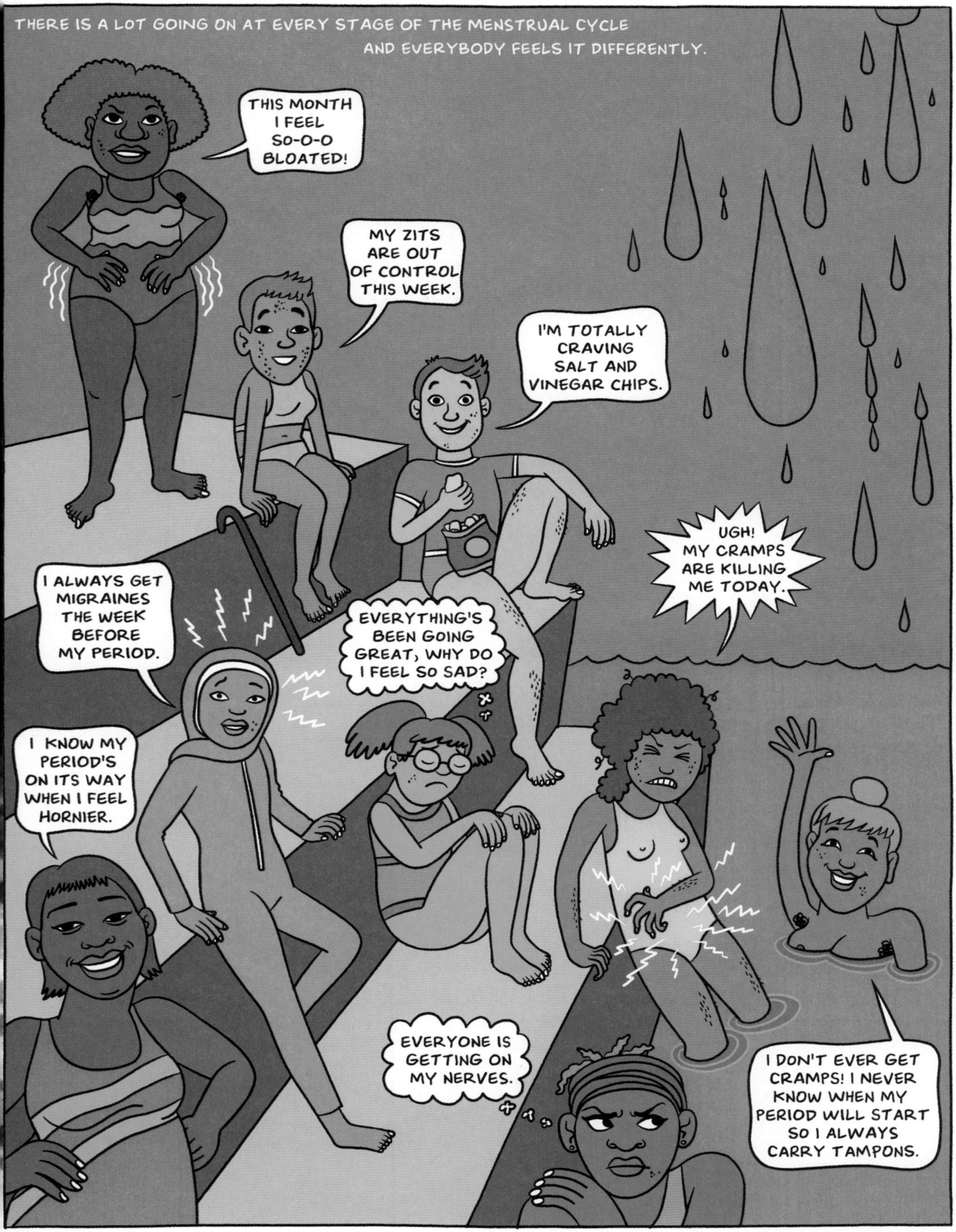

THERE IS A LOT GOING ON AT EVERY STAGE OF THE MENSTRUAL CYCLE
AND EVERYBODY FEELS IT DIFFERENTLY.
THIS MONTH I FEEL SO-O-O BLOATED!
MY ZITS ARE OUT OF CONTROL THIS WEEK.
I'M TOTALLY CRAVING SALT AND VINEGAR CHIPS.
UGH! MY CRAMPS ARE KILLING ME TODAY.
I ALWAYS GET MIGRAINES THE WEEK BEFORE MY PERIOD.
EVERYTHING'S BEEN GOING GREAT, WHY DO I FEEL SO SAD?
I KNOW MY PERIOD'S ON ITS WAY WHEN I FEEL HORNIER.
EVERYONE IS GETTING ON MY NERVES.
I DON'T EVER GET CRAMPS! I NEVER KNOW WHEN MY PERIOD WILL START SO I ALWAYS CARRY TAMPONS.

WHEN IT COMES OUT, MENSTRUAL BLOOD CAN LOOK BROWN OR PINK OR RED. IT DOESN'T FLOW OUT OF THE BODY LIKE WHEN YOU HAVE A CUT. SOMETIMES IT COMES OUT IN CLUMPS. AND IT NEVER COMES OUT ALL AT ONCE. IT USUALLY TAKES BETWEEN THREE AND FIVE DAYS FOR ALL THE BLOOD TO FLOW OUT OF THE UTERUS.

WHEN SOMEONE FIRST GETS A PERIOD, THEIR FLOW MIGHT BE DIFFERENT EACH MONTH. FOR SOME PEOPLE IT EVENS OUT AND A PATTERN EMERGES. SOME PEOPLE START GETTING A PERIOD AND THEN GO THROUGH A TIME WHEN THEY DON'T GET IT. THIS CAN BE RELATED TO STRESS, HOW AND WHAT THEY'RE EATING, MEDICATIONS THEY TAKE, AND MORE.

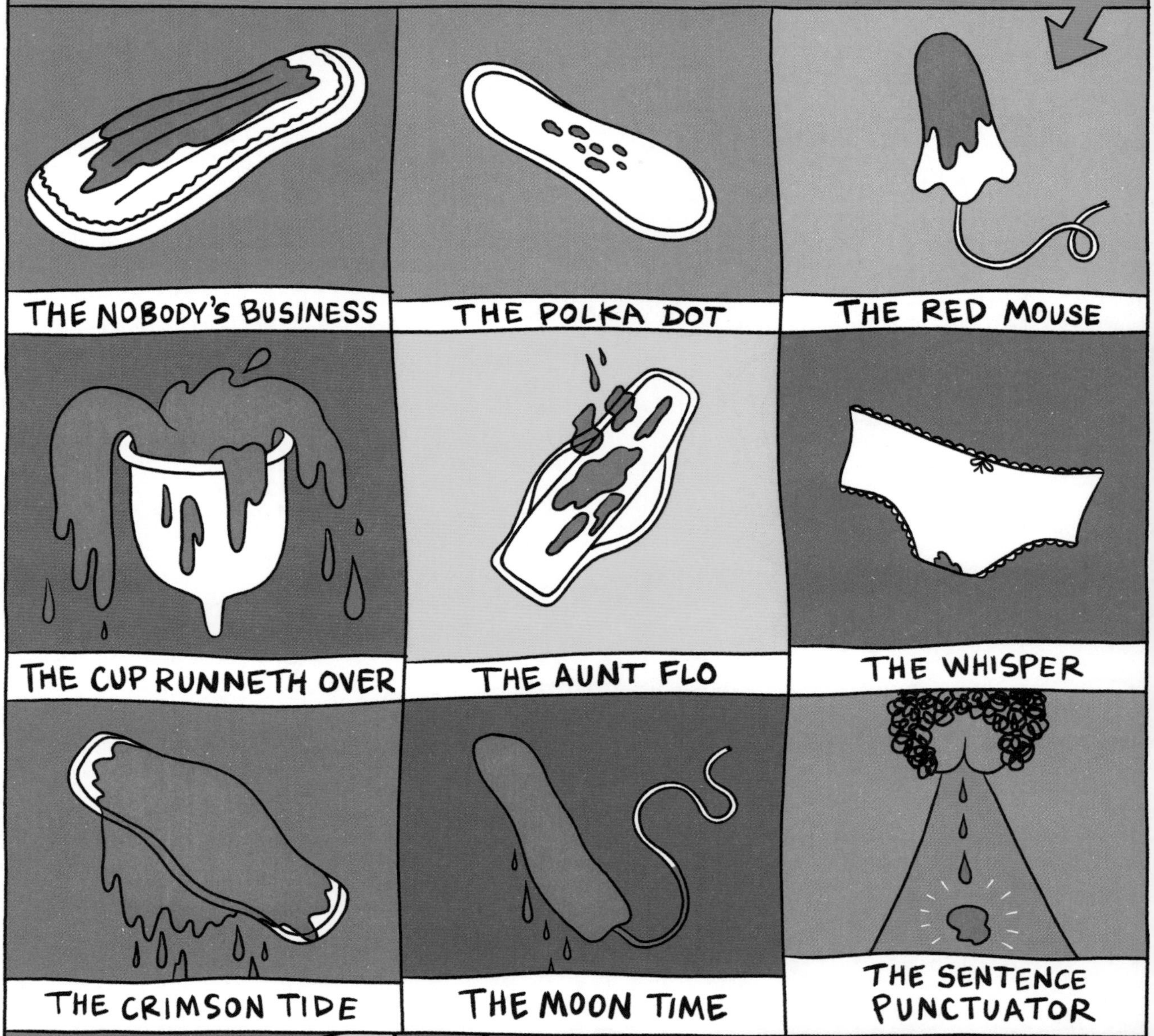
THE NOBODY'S BUSINESS
THE POLKA DOT
THE RED MOUSE
THE CUP RUNNETH OVER
THE AUNT FLO
THE WHISPER
THE CRIMSON TIDE
THE MOON TIME
THE SENTENCE PUNCTUATOR

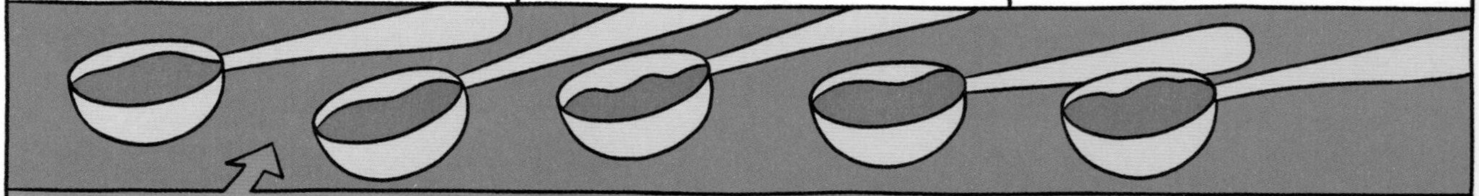

THE FLOW

HOW MUCH BLOOD COMES OUT IS DIFFERENT FOR EVERYONE. FOR MOST PEOPLE, IT'S BETWEEN TWO TO FIVE TABLESPOONS, BUT IT CAN SEEM LIKE A LOT MORE. IT'S COMMON FOR THERE TO BE A HEAVIER FLOW ON THE FIRST FEW DAYS.

THERE ARE LOTS OF PRODUCTS DESIGNED TO DEAL WITH MENSTRUAL BLOOD. IF YOU NEED THEM, YOU'LL HAVE YEARS TO TRY THEM OUT AND FIND THE ONES THAT WORK BEST FOR YOU. WHAT WORKS MAY CHANGE OVER TIME. MANY MENSTRUAL PRODUCTS ARE FULL OF CHEMICALS AND PERFUMES. THESE MAKE SOME OF US SICK OR UNCOMFORTABLE, AND ARE NOT GREAT FOR OUR PLANET. THERE ARE OTHER OPTIONS. ALL OF THEM TAKE A WHILE TO GET USED TO, AND SOMETIMES YOU'LL USE MORE THAN ONE DURING THE SAME PERIOD.

MENSTRUAL PADS

A PAD OF ABSORBENT MATERIAL WORN IN UNDERWEAR TO ABSORB BLOOD. THE DISPOSABLE KINDS USUALLY HAVE A STICKY SIDE THAT ADHERES TO UNDERWEAR TO PREVENT SLIPPAGE. REUSABLE PADS ARE NICER FOR THE BODY —NO CHEMICALS OR PERFUMES—AND BETTER FOR THE PLANET, BUT REQUIRE WASHING. REUSABLE PADS ALSO MEAN ONE SEES MORE OF WHAT'S HAPPENING IN THE BODY, WHICH FOR SOME PEOPLE IS A PLUS AND FOR OTHERS A MINUS!

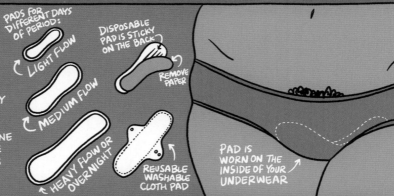

PADS FOR DIFFERENT DAYS OF PERIOD:

LIGHT FLOW

MEDIUM FLOW

HEAVY FLOW OR OVERNIGHT

DISPOSABLE PAD IS STICKY ON THE BACK

REMOVE PAPER

REUSABLE WASHABLE CLOTH PAD

PAD IS WORN ON THE INSIDE OF YOUR UNDERWEAR

TAMPONS

SIMILAR ABSORBENT MATERIAL AS PADS, BUT IN A SMALL CYLINDER SHAPE THAT CAN BE INSERTED INTO THE VAGINA TO ABSORB BLOOD BEFORE IT LEAVES THE BODY. TAMPONS ARE AN OPTION IF ONE CAN GET COMFORTABLE WITH SOMETHING INSERTED IN THEIR VAGINA. TAMPONS MUST BE CHANGED EVERY EIGHT HOURS, AND DURING HEAVY FLOW DAYS THEY MAY HAVE TO BE CHANGED MORE OFTEN. IT'S RARE, BUT LEAVING A TAMPON IN FOR MORE THAN EIGHT HOURS CAN LEAD TO TOXIC SHOCK SYNDROME (TSS), WHICH IS DANGEROUS. YOU CAN READ MORE ABOUT TSS IN THE BACK OF THE BOOK.

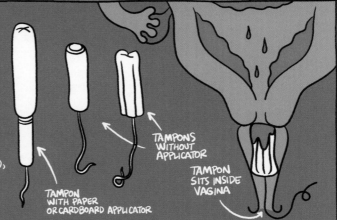

TAMPON WITH PAPER OR CARDBOARD APPLICATOR

TAMPONS WITHOUT APPLICATOR

TAMPON SITS INSIDE VAGINA

MENSTRUAL CUPS

A SMALL CUP THAT IS INSERTED INTO THE VAGINA THAT CATCHES THE BLOOD. MADE OF REUSABLE SILICONE, OR DISPOSABLE MATERIAL, THE CUP NEEDS TO BE TAKEN OUT AND EMPTIED MORE OR LESS OFTEN, DEPENDING ON ONE'S FLOW. LIKE TAMPONS, THIS METHOD MEANS INSERTING SOMETHING INTO THE VAGINA. IT TAKES A WHILE TO GET USED TO. CUPS ARE MUCH LESS EXPENSIVE IN THE LONG RUN, AND LIKE CLOTH PADS THEY ALLOW ONE TO SEE MORE OF WHAT'S HAPPENING. IN RARE CASES, TSS CAN HAPPEN WITH MENSTRUAL CUPS TOO.

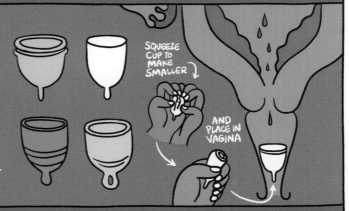

SQUEEZE CUP TO MAKE SMALLER

AND PLACE IN VAGINA

HOW TO CHOOSE

IT DEPENDS ON WHAT YOU CAN AFFORD AND WHAT YOU NEED. IF YOU DON'T WANT TO DEAL WITH WHAT'S HAPPENING INSIDE YOUR BODY, TAMPONS PRODUCE THE LEAST MESS. BUT YOU HAVE TO CHANGE THEM, AND IF YOU HAVE A VERY HEAVY FLOW YOU MAY HAVE TO CHANGE THEM A LOT. SO A PAD, OR PAD IN COMBINATION WITH A TAMPON, MIGHT BE BETTER FOR SOME DAYS.

IF YOU WANT TO KNOW EVERYTHING ABOUT WHAT'S HAPPENING, CLOTH PADS OR MENSTRUAL CUPS ARE A BETTER CHOICE. BUT NEITHER MAY WORK FOR YOU IF YOU HAVE HEAVY FLOW AND CAN'T BE STEPPING OUT OF CLASS ALL THE TIME TO CHANGE THEM. MENSTRUAL CUPS CAN ALSO TAKE A WHILE TO GET USED TO, AND REUSABLE ONES NEED TO BE KEPT CLEAN AND SANITIZED IN BOILING WATER EVERY MONTH OR SO.

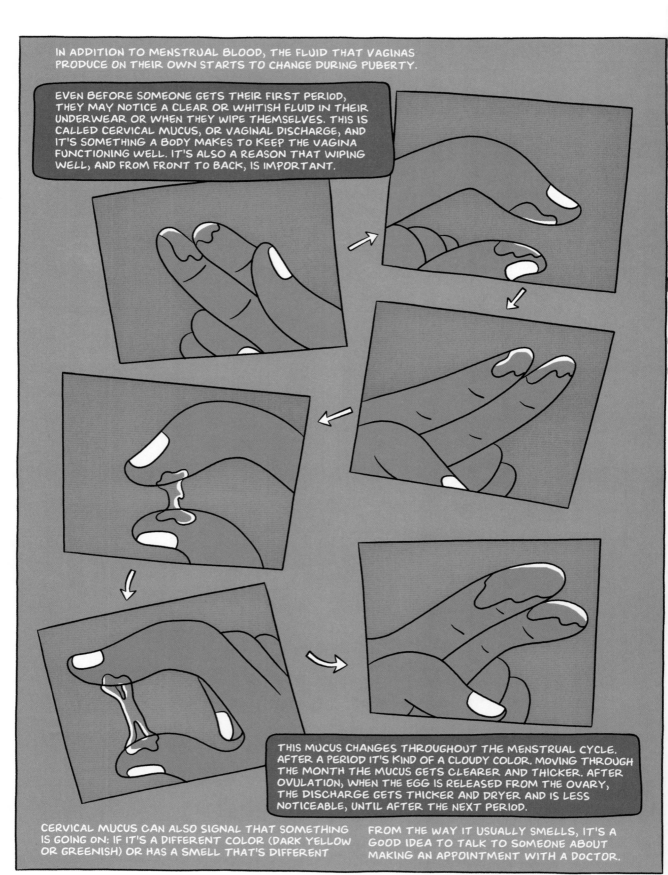

IN ADDITION TO MENSTRUAL BLOOD, THE FLUID THAT VAGINAS PRODUCE ON THEIR OWN STARTS TO CHANGE DURING PUBERTY.

EVEN BEFORE SOMEONE GETS THEIR FIRST PERIOD, THEY MAY NOTICE A CLEAR OR WHITISH FLUID IN THEIR UNDERWEAR OR WHEN THEY WIPE THEMSELVES. THIS IS CALLED CERVICAL MUCUS, OR VAGINAL DISCHARGE, AND IT'S SOMETHING A BODY MAKES TO KEEP THE VAGINA FUNCTIONING WELL. IT'S ALSO A REASON THAT WIPING WELL, AND FROM FRONT TO BACK, IS IMPORTANT.

THIS MUCUS CHANGES THROUGHOUT THE MENSTRUAL CYCLE. AFTER A PERIOD IT'S KIND OF A CLOUDY COLOR. MOVING THROUGH THE MONTH THE MUCUS GETS CLEARER AND THICKER. AFTER OVULATION, WHEN THE EGG IS RELEASED FROM THE OVARY, THE DISCHARGE GETS THICKER AND DRYER AND IS LESS NOTICEABLE, UNTIL AFTER THE NEXT PERIOD.

CERVICAL MUCUS CAN ALSO SIGNAL THAT SOMETHING IS GOING ON: IF IT'S A DIFFERENT COLOR (DARK YELLOW OR GREENISH) OR HAS A SMELL THAT'S DIFFERENT FROM THE WAY IT USUALLY SMELLS, IT'S A GOOD IDEA TO TALK TO SOMEONE ABOUT MAKING AN APPOINTMENT WITH A DOCTOR.

SO MUCH IS HAPPENING IN A BODY DURING MENSTRUATION. AT DIFFERENT TIMES IN THEIR CYCLE PEOPLE DESCRIBE HAVING LESS ENERGY AND PATIENCE. THEY CAN BE MORE SENSITIVE, OR FEEL LIKE THEY NEED MORE FROM OTHERS BUT HAVE LESS TO GIVE. THEY CAN FEEL WILDLY DIFFERENT FROM ONE DAY TO THE NEXT, AND FROM ONE HOUR TO THE NEXT. SOME PEOPLE DESCRIBE FEELING AS IF THEY AREN'T THEMSELVES, WHICH CAN BE KIND OF SCARY.

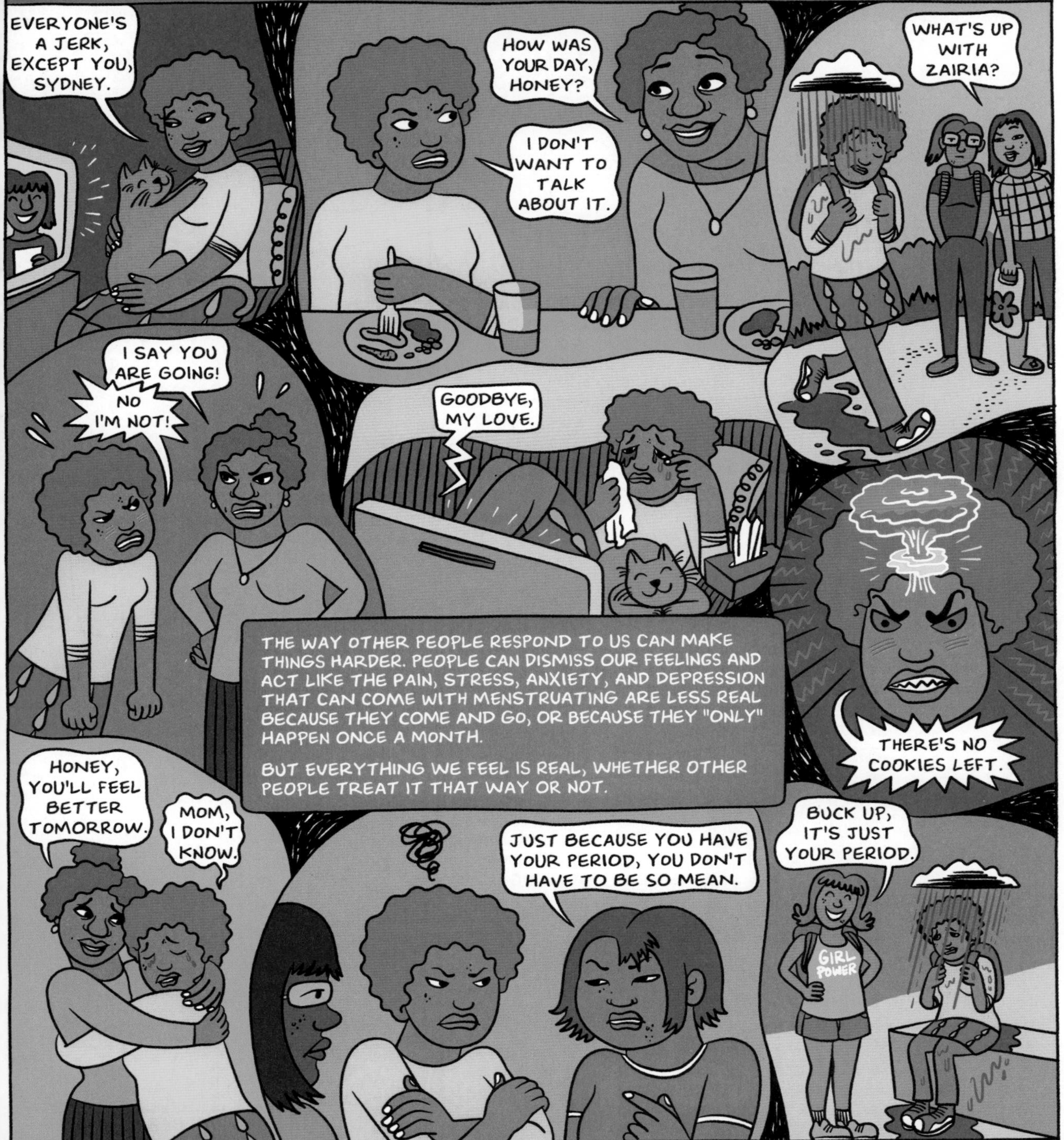
EVERYONE'S A JERK, EXCEPT YOU, SYDNEY.
HOW WAS YOUR DAY, HONEY?
I DON'T WANT TO TALK ABOUT IT.
WHAT'S UP WITH ZAIRIA?
I SAY YOU ARE GOING!
NO I'M NOT!
GOODBYE, MY LOVE.
THERE'S NO COOKIES LEFT.
HONEY, YOU'LL FEEL BETTER TOMORROW.
MOM, I DON'T KNOW.
JUST BECAUSE YOU HAVE YOUR PERIOD, YOU DON'T HAVE TO BE SO MEAN.
BUCK UP, IT'S JUST YOUR PERIOD.
GIRL POWER

THE WAY OTHER PEOPLE RESPOND TO US CAN MAKE THINGS HARDER. PEOPLE CAN DISMISS OUR FEELINGS AND ACT LIKE THE PAIN, STRESS, ANXIETY, AND DEPRESSION THAT CAN COME WITH MENSTRUATING ARE LESS REAL BECAUSE THEY COME AND GO, OR BECAUSE THEY "ONLY" HAPPEN ONCE A MONTH.

BUT EVERYTHING WE FEEL IS REAL, WHETHER OTHER PEOPLE TREAT IT THAT WAY OR NOT.

BODIES THAT GET PERIODS WILL EVENTUALLY STOP GETTING THEM WHEN THE AMOUNT OF ESTROGEN A BODY MAKES STARTS TO DROP. THIS IS CALLED MENOPAUSE, AND IT USUALLY STARTS WHEN PEOPLE ARE IN THEIR 40S, ALTHOUGH IT CAN START EARLIER OR LATER THAN THAT. THERE ARE ALSO FORMS OF BIRTH CONTROL THAT STOP A BODY FROM GETTING A PERIOD.

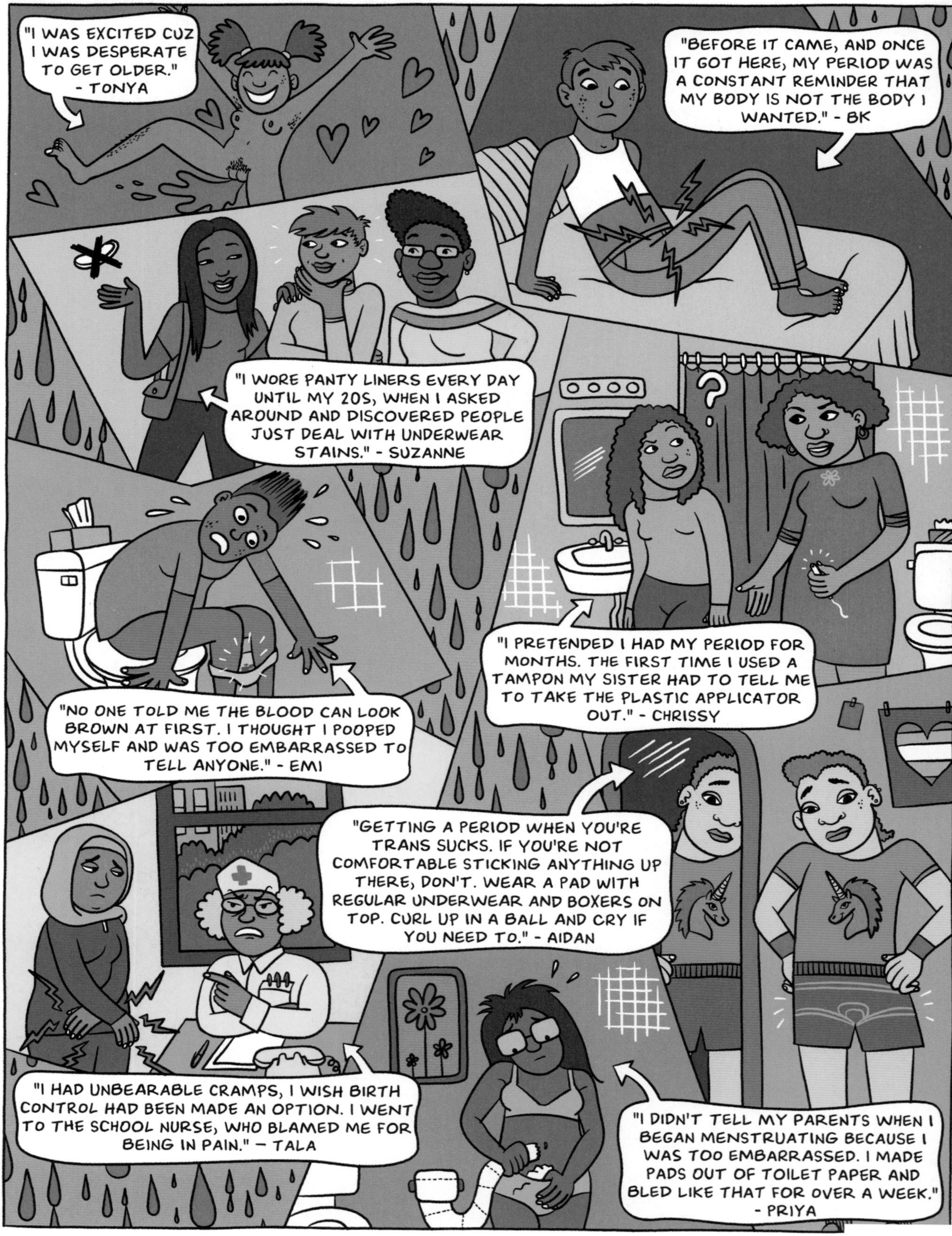
"I WAS EXCITED CUZ I WAS DESPERATE TO GET OLDER." - TONYA
"BEFORE IT CAME, AND ONCE IT GOT HERE, MY PERIOD WAS A CONSTANT REMINDER THAT MY BODY IS NOT THE BODY I WANTED." - BK
"I WORE PANTY LINERS EVERY DAY UNTIL MY 20S, WHEN I ASKED AROUND AND DISCOVERED PEOPLE JUST DEAL WITH UNDERWEAR STAINS." - SUZANNE
"NO ONE TOLD ME THE BLOOD CAN LOOK BROWN AT FIRST. I THOUGHT I POOPED MYSELF AND WAS TOO EMBARRASSED TO TELL ANYONE." - EMI
"I PRETENDED I HAD MY PERIOD FOR MONTHS. THE FIRST TIME I USED A TAMPON MY SISTER HAD TO TELL ME TO TAKE THE PLASTIC APPLICATOR OUT." - CHRISSY
"GETTING A PERIOD WHEN YOU'RE TRANS SUCKS. IF YOU'RE NOT COMFORTABLE STICKING ANYTHING UP THERE, DON'T. WEAR A PAD WITH REGULAR UNDERWEAR AND BOXERS ON TOP. CURL UP IN A BALL AND CRY IF YOU NEED TO." - AIDAN
"I HAD UNBEARABLE CRAMPS, I WISH BIRTH CONTROL HAD BEEN MADE AN OPTION. I WENT TO THE SCHOOL NURSE, WHO BLAMED ME FOR BEING IN PAIN." – TALA
"I DIDN'T TELL MY PARENTS WHEN I BEGAN MENSTRUATING BECAUSE I WAS TOO EMBARRASSED. I MADE PADS OUT OF TOILET PAPER AND BLED LIKE THAT FOR OVER A WEEK." - PRIYA

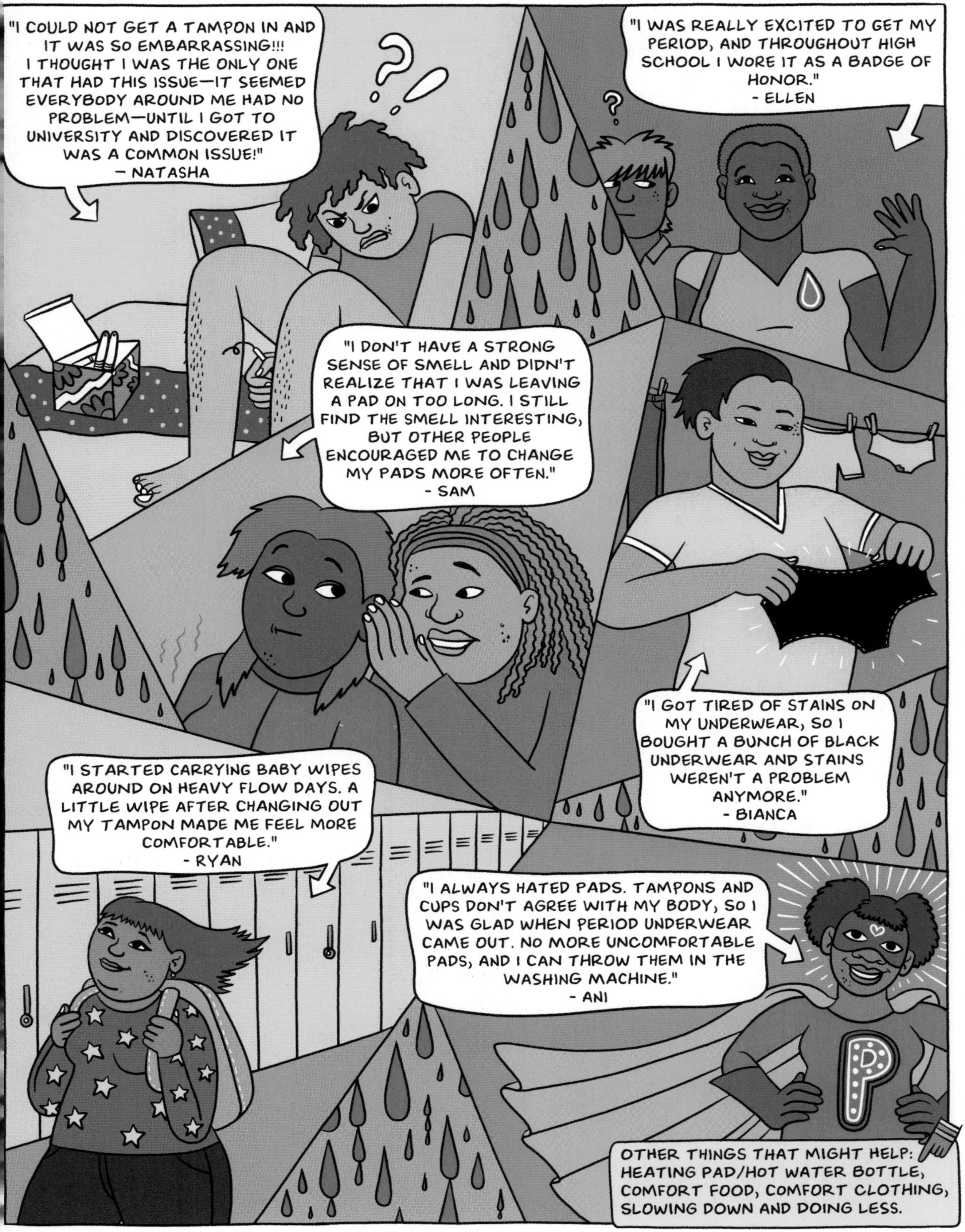
"I COULD NOT GET A TAMPON IN AND IT WAS SO EMBARRASSING!!! I THOUGHT I WAS THE ONLY ONE THAT HAD THIS ISSUE—IT SEEMED EVERYBODY AROUND ME HAD NO PROBLEM—UNTIL I GOT TO UNIVERSITY AND DISCOVERED IT WAS A COMMON ISSUE!" – NATASHA
?
!
?
"I WAS REALLY EXCITED TO GET MY PERIOD, AND THROUGHOUT HIGH SCHOOL I WORE IT AS A BADGE OF HONOR." - ELLEN
"I DON'T HAVE A STRONG SENSE OF SMELL AND DIDN'T REALIZE THAT I WAS LEAVING A PAD ON TOO LONG. I STILL FIND THE SMELL INTERESTING, BUT OTHER PEOPLE ENCOURAGED ME TO CHANGE MY PADS MORE OFTEN." - SAM
"I GOT TIRED OF STAINS ON MY UNDERWEAR, SO I BOUGHT A BUNCH OF BLACK UNDERWEAR AND STAINS WEREN'T A PROBLEM ANYMORE." - BIANCA
"I STARTED CARRYING BABY WIPES AROUND ON HEAVY FLOW DAYS. A LITTLE WIPE AFTER CHANGING OUT MY TAMPON MADE ME FEEL MORE COMFORTABLE." - RYAN
"I ALWAYS HATED PADS. TAMPONS AND CUPS DON'T AGREE WITH MY BODY, SO I WAS GLAD WHEN PERIOD UNDERWEAR CAME OUT. NO MORE UNCOMFORTABLE PADS, AND I CAN THROW THEM IN THE WASHING MACHINE." - ANI
P
OTHER THINGS THAT MIGHT HELP: HEATING PAD/HOT WATER BOTTLE, COMFORT FOOD, COMFORT CLOTHING, SLOWING DOWN AND DOING LESS.

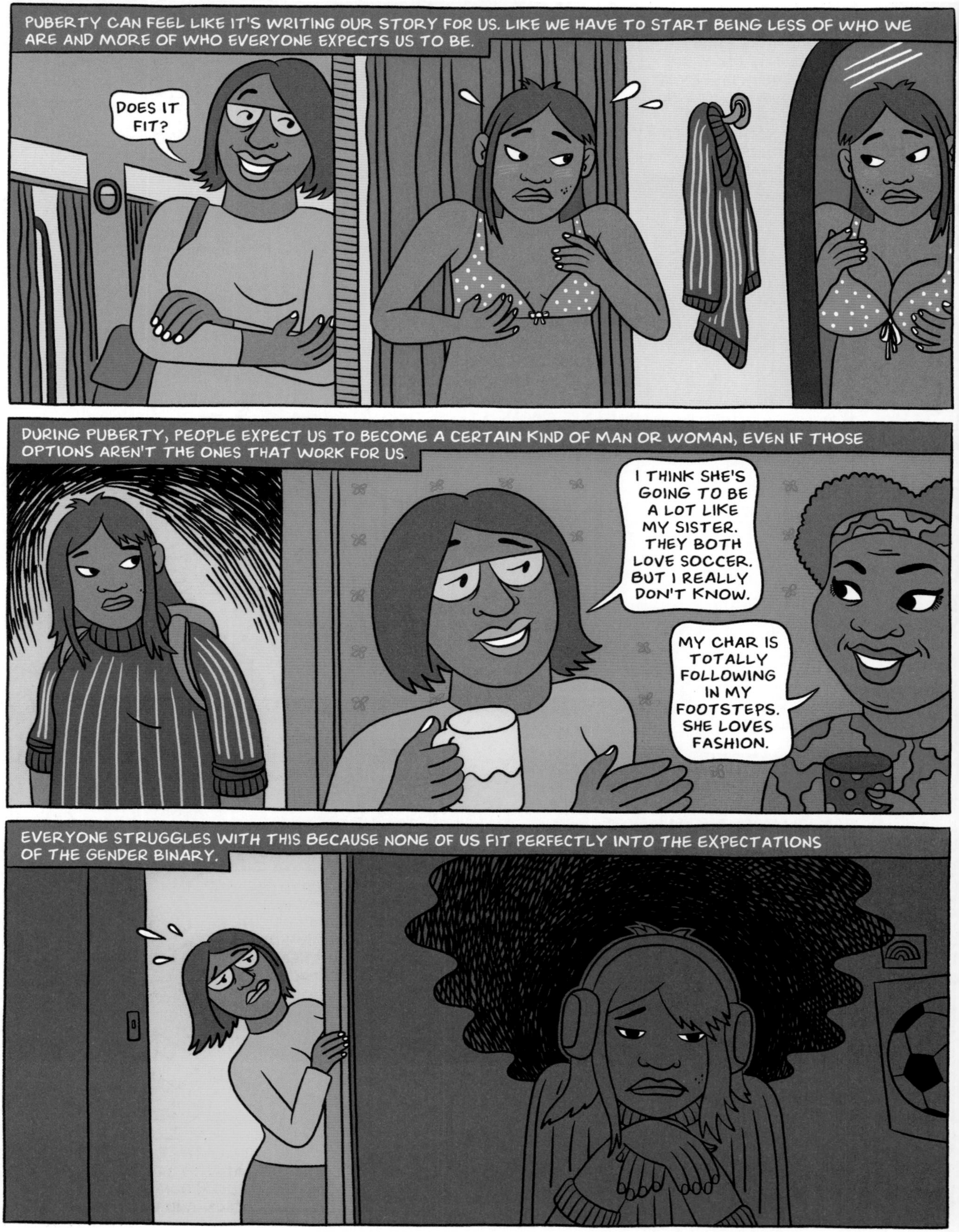
PUBERTY CAN FEEL LIKE IT'S WRITING OUR STORY FOR US. LIKE WE HAVE TO START BEING LESS OF WHO WE ARE AND MORE OF WHO EVERYONE EXPECTS US TO BE.
DOES IT FIT?
DURING PUBERTY, PEOPLE EXPECT US TO BECOME A CERTAIN KIND OF MAN OR WOMAN, EVEN IF THOSE OPTIONS AREN'T THE ONES THAT WORK FOR US.
I THINK SHE'S GOING TO BE A LOT LIKE MY SISTER. THEY BOTH LOVE SOCCER. BUT I REALLY DON'T KNOW.
MY CHAR IS TOTALLY FOLLOWING IN MY FOOTSTEPS. SHE LOVES FASHION.
EVERYONE STRUGGLES WITH THIS BECAUSE NONE OF US FIT PERFECTLY INTO THE EXPECTATIONS OF THE GENDER BINARY.

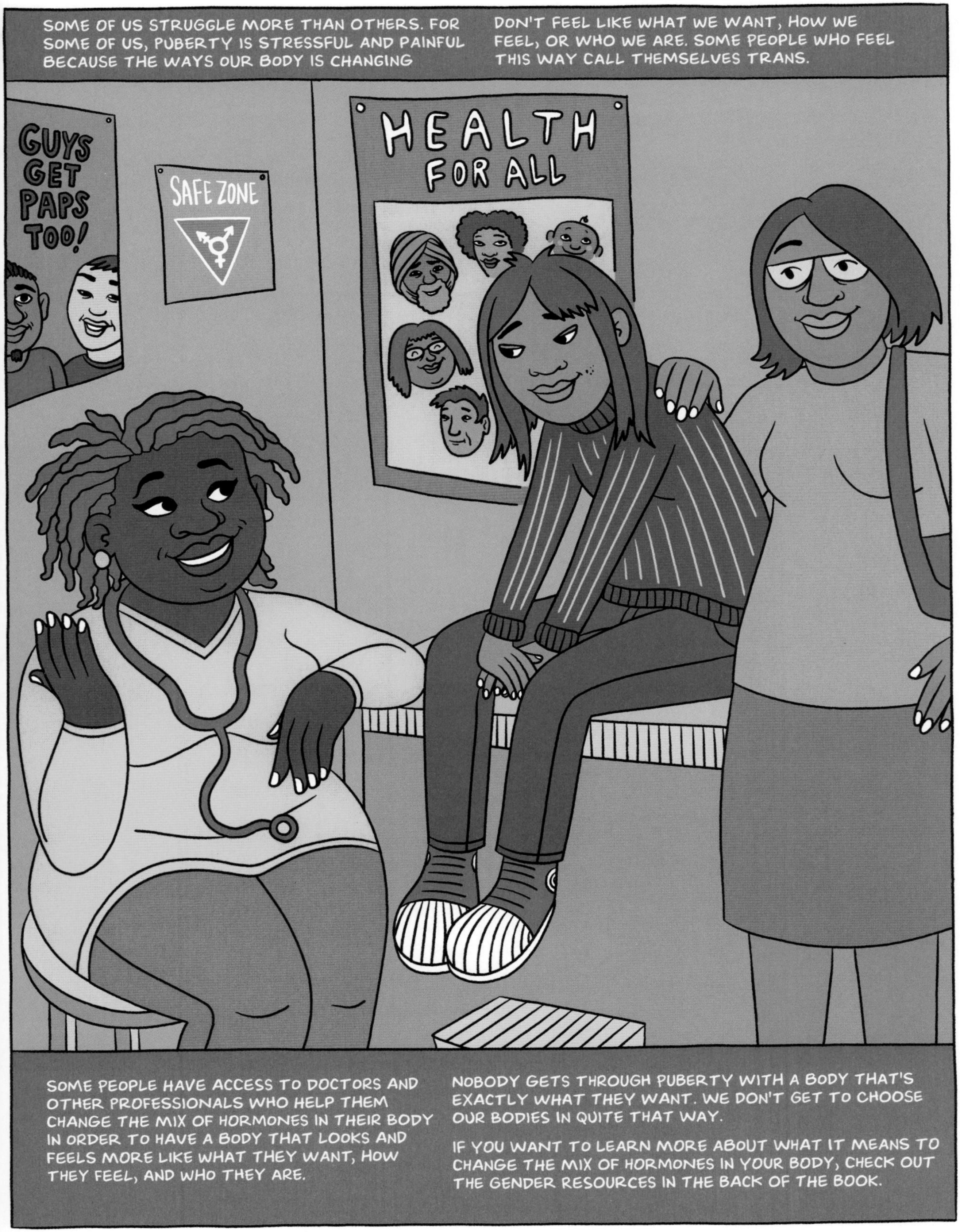
SOME OF US STRUGGLE MORE THAN OTHERS. FOR SOME OF US, PUBERTY IS STRESSFUL AND PAINFUL BECAUSE THE WAYS OUR BODY IS CHANGING DON'T FEEL LIKE WHAT WE WANT, HOW WE FEEL, OR WHO WE ARE. SOME PEOPLE WHO FEEL THIS WAY CALL THEMSELVES TRANS.
GUYS GET PAPS TOO!
SAFE ZONE
HEALTH FOR ALL
SOME PEOPLE HAVE ACCESS TO DOCTORS AND OTHER PROFESSIONALS WHO HELP THEM CHANGE THE MIX OF HORMONES IN THEIR BODY IN ORDER TO HAVE A BODY THAT LOOKS AND FEELS MORE LIKE WHAT THEY WANT, HOW THEY FEEL, AND WHO THEY ARE.
NOBODY GETS THROUGH PUBERTY WITH A BODY THAT'S EXACTLY WHAT THEY WANT. WE DON'T GET TO CHOOSE OUR BODIES IN QUITE THAT WAY.
IF YOU WANT TO LEARN MORE ABOUT WHAT IT MEANS TO CHANGE THE MIX OF HORMONES IN YOUR BODY, CHECK OUT THE GENDER RESOURCES IN THE BACK OF THE BOOK.

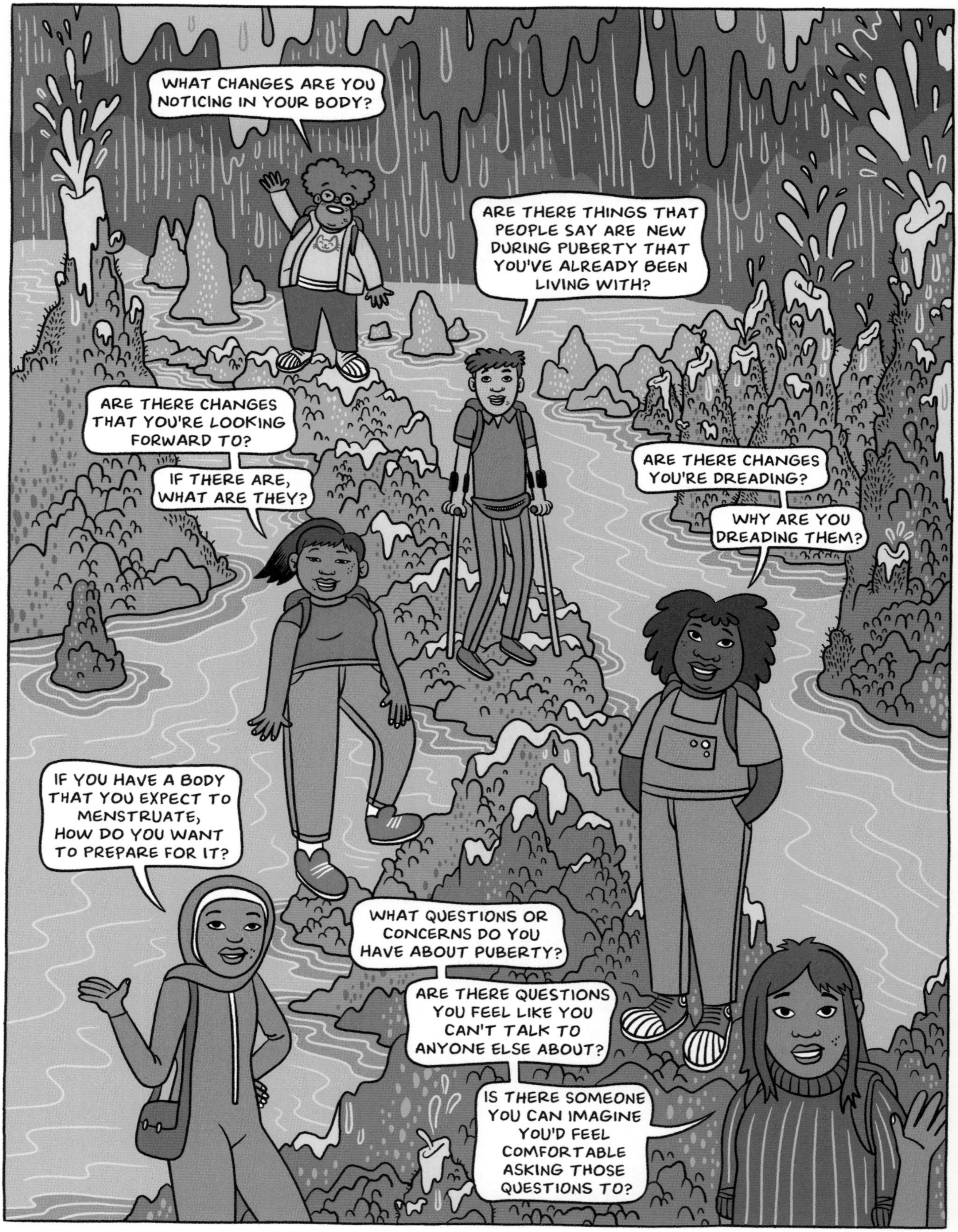
WHAT CHANGES ARE YOU NOTICING IN YOUR BODY?
ARE THERE THINGS THAT PEOPLE SAY ARE NEW DURING PUBERTY THAT YOU'VE ALREADY BEEN LIVING WITH?
ARE THERE CHANGES THAT YOU'RE LOOKING FORWARD TO?
IF THERE ARE, WHAT ARE THEY?
ARE THERE CHANGES YOU'RE DREADING?
WHY ARE YOU DREADING THEM?
IF YOU HAVE A BODY THAT YOU EXPECT TO MENSTRUATE, HOW DO YOU WANT TO PREPARE FOR IT?
WHAT QUESTIONS OR CONCERNS DO YOU HAVE ABOUT PUBERTY?
ARE THERE QUESTIONS YOU FEEL LIKE YOU CAN'T TALK TO ANYONE ELSE ABOUT?
IS THERE SOMEONE YOU CAN IMAGINE YOU'D FEEL COMFORTABLE ASKING THOSE QUESTIONS TO?

5 FEELINGS

SOMEONE ON YOUR MIND, ZAI?

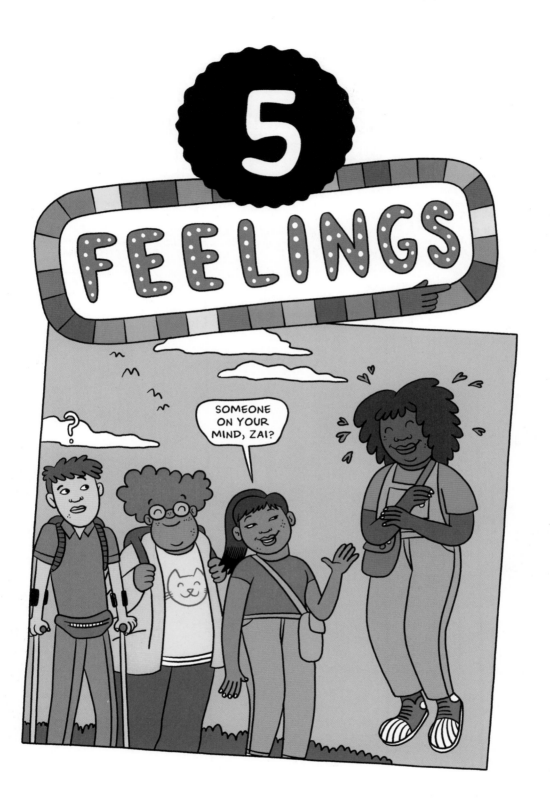

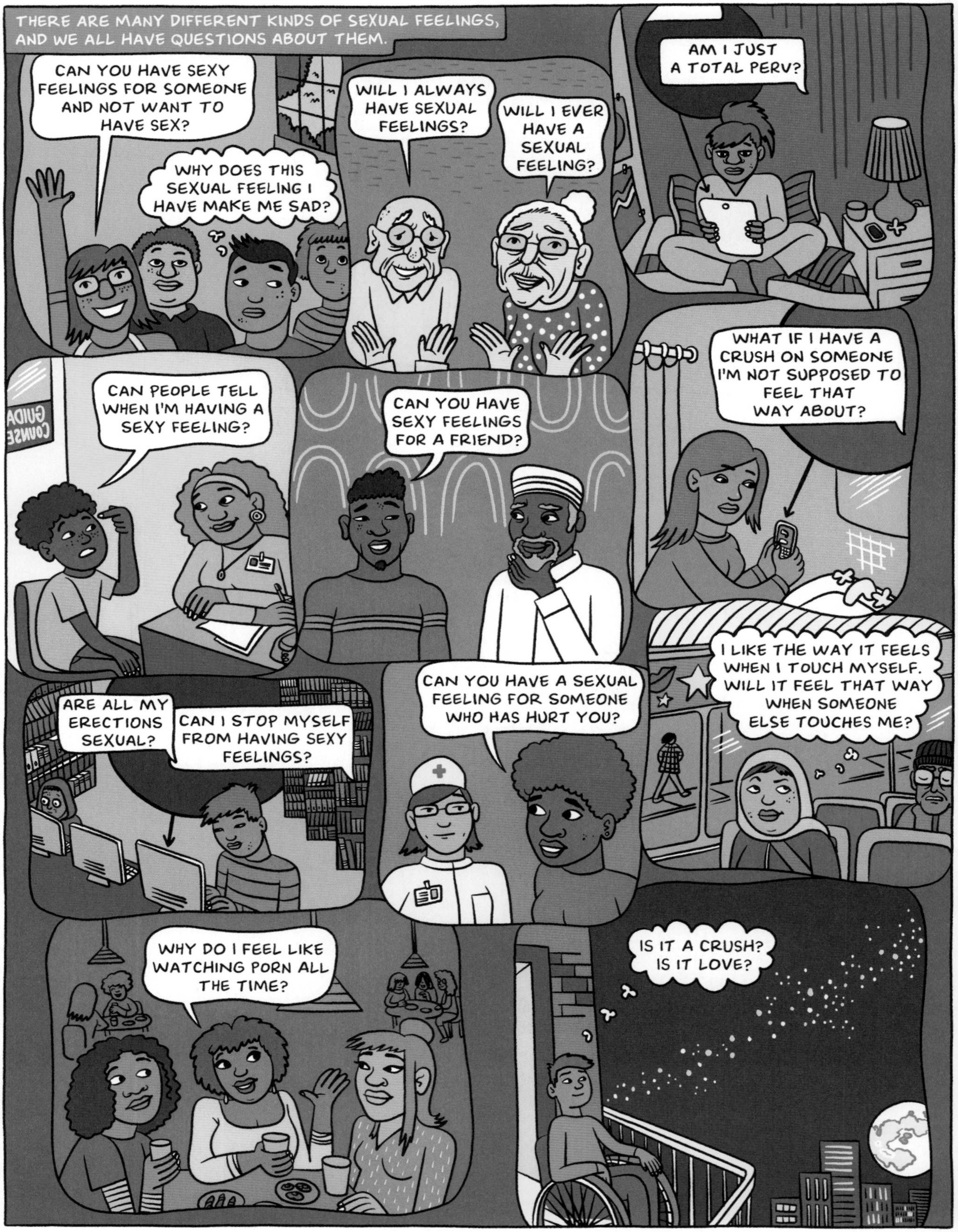
THERE ARE MANY DIFFERENT KINDS OF SEXUAL FEELINGS, AND WE ALL HAVE QUESTIONS ABOUT THEM.
CAN YOU HAVE SEXY FEELINGS FOR SOMEONE AND NOT WANT TO HAVE SEX?
WHY DOES THIS SEXUAL FEELING I HAVE MAKE ME SAD?
WILL I ALWAYS HAVE SEXUAL FEELINGS?
WILL I EVER HAVE A SEXUAL FEELING?
AM I JUST A TOTAL PERV?
CAN PEOPLE TELL WHEN I'M HAVING A SEXY FEELING?
CAN YOU HAVE SEXY FEELINGS FOR A FRIEND?
WHAT IF I HAVE A CRUSH ON SOMEONE I'M NOT SUPPOSED TO FEEL THAT WAY ABOUT?
ARE ALL MY ERECTIONS SEXUAL?
CAN I STOP MYSELF FROM HAVING SEXY FEELINGS?
CAN YOU HAVE A SEXUAL FEELING FOR SOMEONE WHO HAS HURT YOU?
I LIKE THE WAY IT FEELS WHEN I TOUCH MYSELF. WILL IT FEEL THAT WAY WHEN SOMEONE ELSE TOUCHES ME?
WHY DO I FEEL LIKE WATCHING PORN ALL THE TIME?
IS IT A CRUSH? IS IT LOVE?

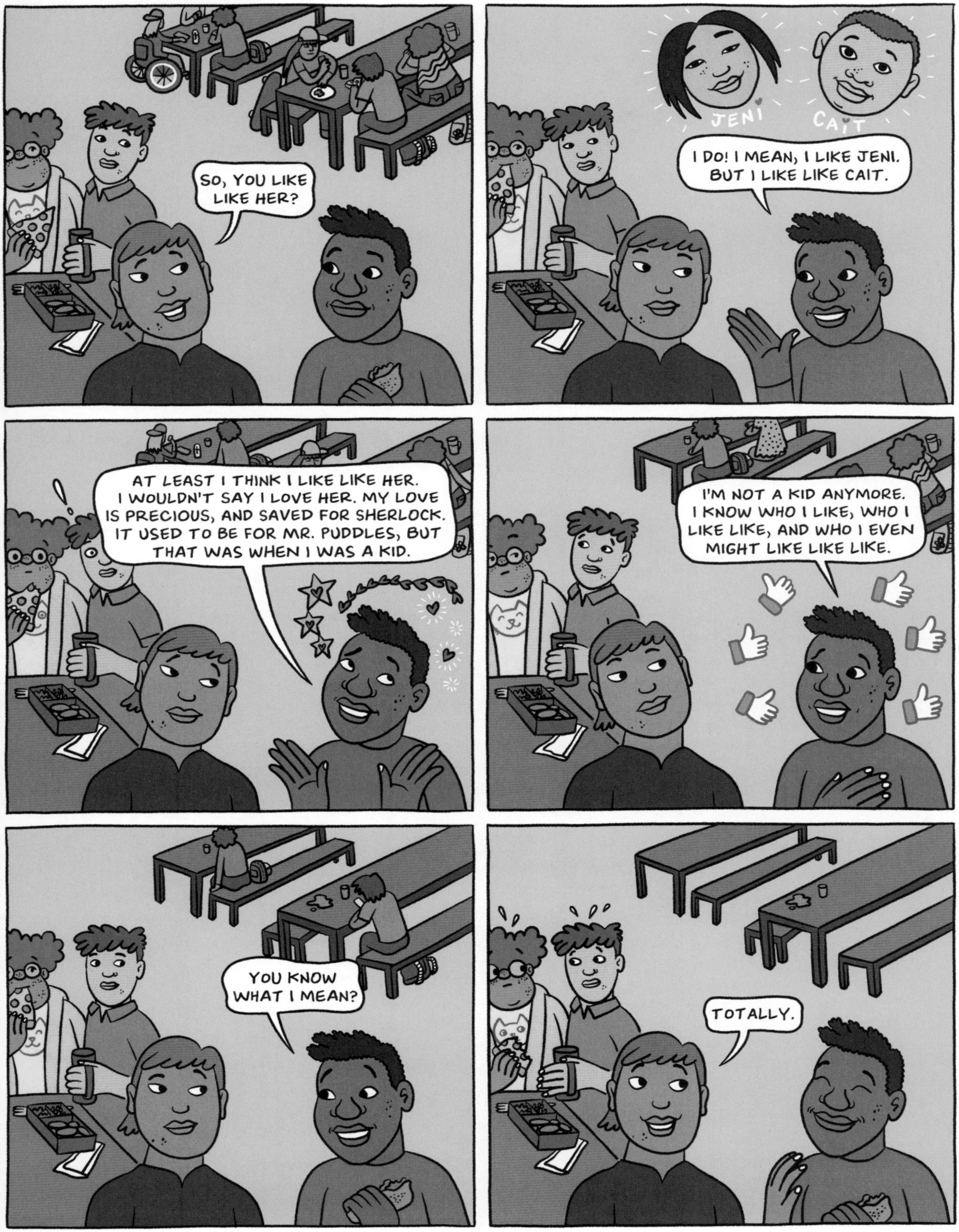
SO, YOU LIKE LIKE HER?
JENI
CAIT
I DO! I MEAN, I LIKE JENI. BUT I LIKE LIKE CAIT.
AT LEAST I THINK I LIKE LIKE HER. I WOULDN'T SAY I LOVE HER. MY LOVE IS PRECIOUS, AND SAVED FOR SHERLOCK. IT USED TO BE FOR MR. PUDDLES, BUT THAT WAS WHEN I WAS A KID.
I'M NOT A KID ANYMORE. I KNOW WHO I LIKE, WHO I LIKE LIKE, AND WHO I EVEN MIGHT LIKE LIKE LIKE.
YOU KNOW WHAT I MEAN?
TOTALLY.

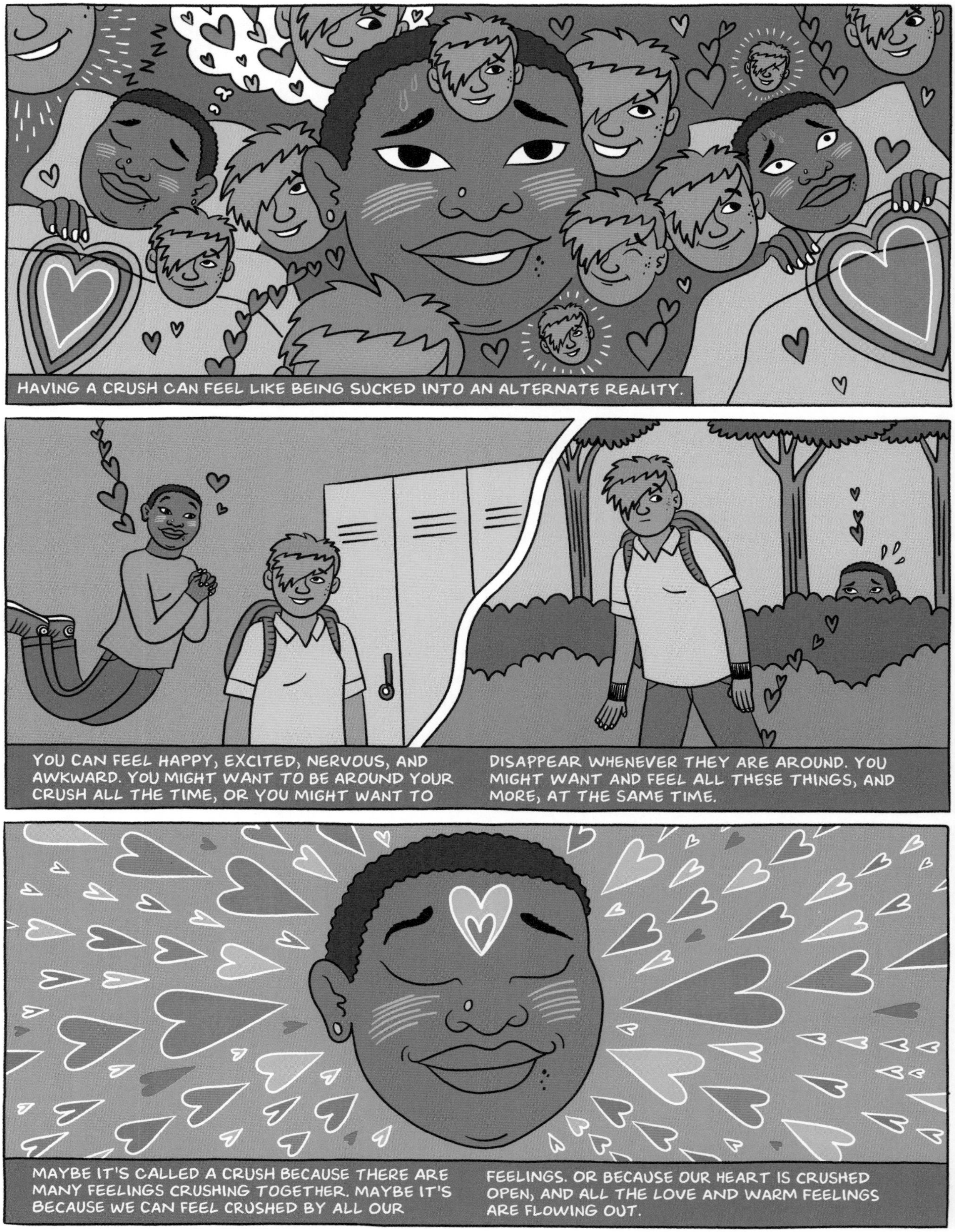
HAVING A CRUSH CAN FEEL LIKE BEING SUCKED INTO AN ALTERNATE REALITY.
YOU CAN FEEL HAPPY, EXCITED, NERVOUS, AND AWKWARD. YOU MIGHT WANT TO BE AROUND YOUR CRUSH ALL THE TIME, OR YOU MIGHT WANT TO DISAPPEAR WHENEVER THEY ARE AROUND. YOU MIGHT WANT AND FEEL ALL THESE THINGS, AND MORE, AT THE SAME TIME.
MAYBE IT'S CALLED A CRUSH BECAUSE THERE ARE MANY FEELINGS CRUSHING TOGETHER. MAYBE IT'S BECAUSE WE CAN FEEL CRUSHED BY ALL OUR FEELINGS. OR BECAUSE OUR HEART IS CRUSHED OPEN, AND ALL THE LOVE AND WARM FEELINGS ARE FLOWING OUT.

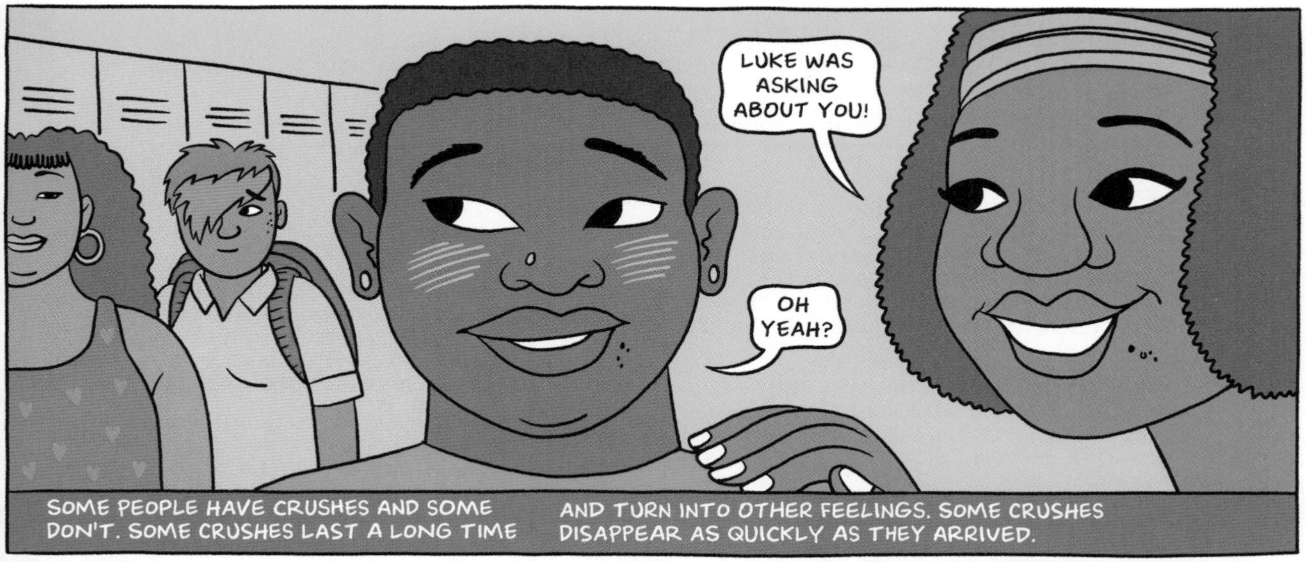
LUKE WAS ASKING ABOUT YOU!
OH YEAH?
SOME PEOPLE HAVE CRUSHES AND SOME DON'T. SOME CRUSHES LAST A LONG TIME AND TURN INTO OTHER FEELINGS. SOME CRUSHES DISAPPEAR AS QUICKLY AS THEY ARRIVED.

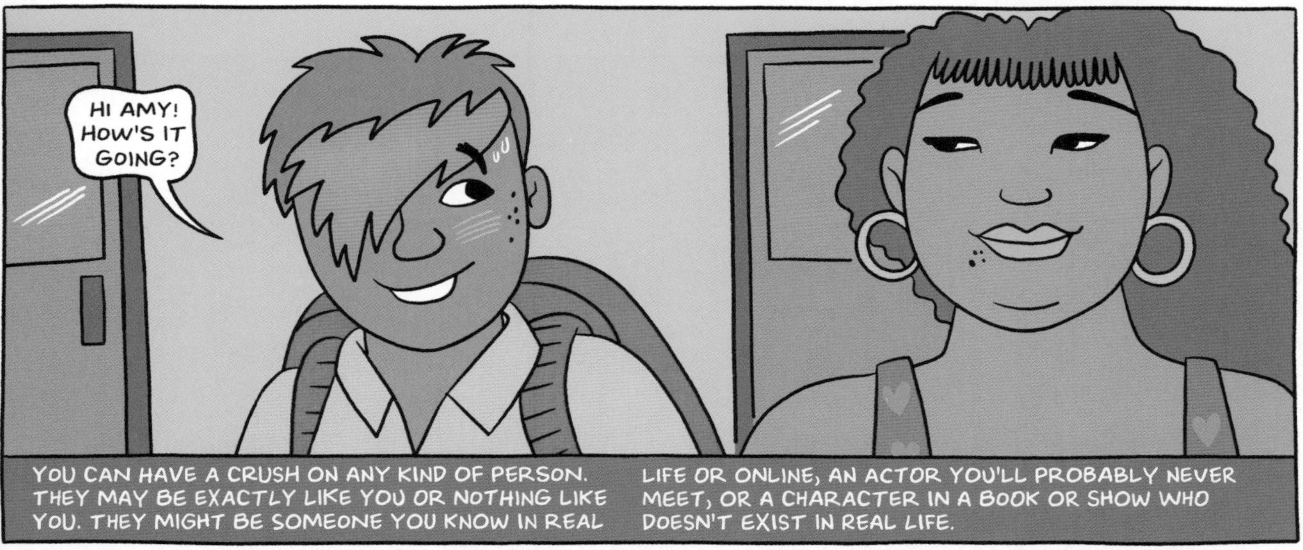
HI AMY! HOW'S IT GOING?
YOU CAN HAVE A CRUSH ON ANY KIND OF PERSON. THEY MAY BE EXACTLY LIKE YOU OR NOTHING LIKE YOU. THEY MIGHT BE SOMEONE YOU KNOW IN REAL LIFE OR ONLINE, AN ACTOR YOU'LL PROBABLY NEVER MEET, OR A CHARACTER IN A BOOK OR SHOW WHO DOESN'T EXIST IN REAL LIFE.

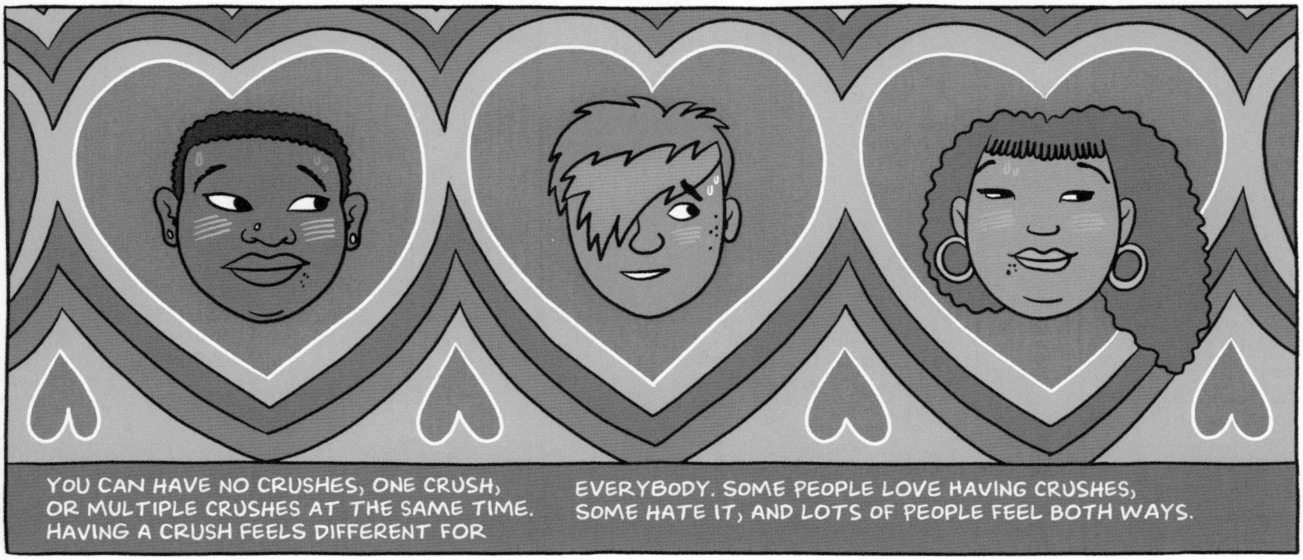
YOU CAN HAVE NO CRUSHES, ONE CRUSH, OR MULTIPLE CRUSHES AT THE SAME TIME. HAVING A CRUSH FEELS DIFFERENT FOR EVERYBODY. SOME PEOPLE LOVE HAVING CRUSHES, SOME HATE IT, AND LOTS OF PEOPLE FEEL BOTH WAYS.

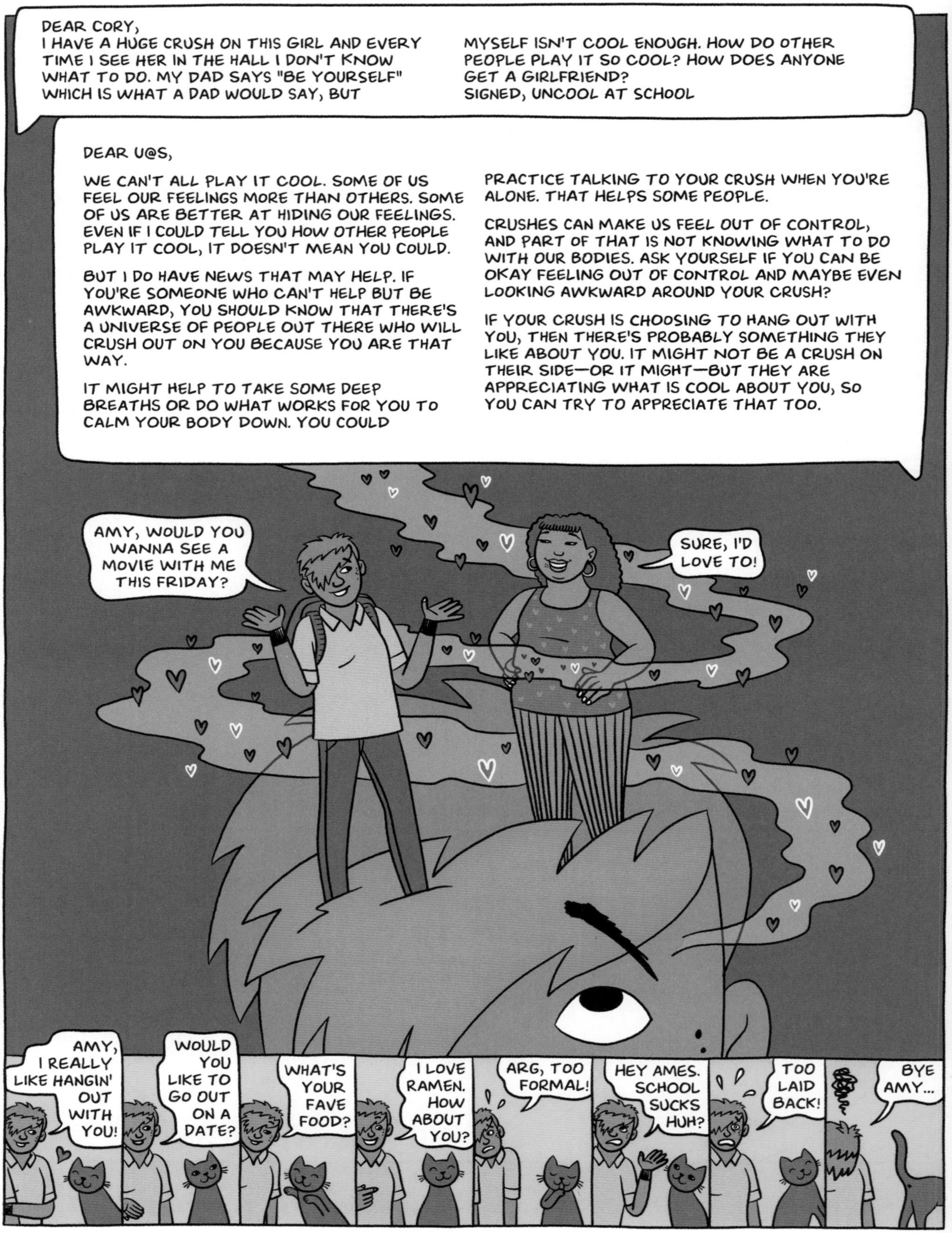
DEAR CORY,
I HAVE A HUGE CRUSH ON THIS GIRL AND EVERY TIME I SEE HER IN THE HALL I DON'T KNOW WHAT TO DO. MY DAD SAYS "BE YOURSELF" WHICH IS WHAT A DAD WOULD SAY, BUT MYSELF ISN'T COOL ENOUGH. HOW DO OTHER PEOPLE PLAY IT SO COOL? HOW DOES ANYONE GET A GIRLFRIEND?
SIGNED, UNCOOL AT SCHOOL
DEAR U@S,
WE CAN'T ALL PLAY IT COOL. SOME OF US FEEL OUR FEELINGS MORE THAN OTHERS. SOME OF US ARE BETTER AT HIDING OUR FEELINGS. EVEN IF I COULD TELL YOU HOW OTHER PEOPLE PLAY IT COOL, IT DOESN'T MEAN YOU COULD.
BUT I DO HAVE NEWS THAT MAY HELP. IF YOU'RE SOMEONE WHO CAN'T HELP BUT BE AWKWARD, YOU SHOULD KNOW THAT THERE'S A UNIVERSE OF PEOPLE OUT THERE WHO WILL CRUSH OUT ON YOU BECAUSE YOU ARE THAT WAY.
IT MIGHT HELP TO TAKE SOME DEEP BREATHS OR DO WHAT WORKS FOR YOU TO CALM YOUR BODY DOWN. YOU COULD PRACTICE TALKING TO YOUR CRUSH WHEN YOU'RE ALONE. THAT HELPS SOME PEOPLE.
CRUSHES CAN MAKE US FEEL OUT OF CONTROL, AND PART OF THAT IS NOT KNOWING WHAT TO DO WITH OUR BODIES. ASK YOURSELF IF YOU CAN BE OKAY FEELING OUT OF CONTROL AND MAYBE EVEN LOOKING AWKWARD AROUND YOUR CRUSH?
IF YOUR CRUSH IS CHOOSING TO HANG OUT WITH YOU, THEN THERE'S PROBABLY SOMETHING THEY LIKE ABOUT YOU. IT MIGHT NOT BE A CRUSH ON THEIR SIDE—OR IT MIGHT—BUT THEY ARE APPRECIATING WHAT IS COOL ABOUT YOU, SO YOU CAN TRY TO APPRECIATE THAT TOO.
AMY, WOULD YOU WANNA SEE A MOVIE WITH ME THIS FRIDAY?
SURE, I'D LOVE TO!
AMY, I REALLY LIKE HANGIN' OUT WITH YOU!
WOULD YOU LIKE TO GO OUT ON A DATE?
WHAT'S YOUR FAVE FOOD?
I LOVE RAMEN. HOW ABOUT YOU?
ARG, TOO FORMAL!
HEY AMES. SCHOOL SUCKS HUH?
TOO LAID BACK!
BYE AMY...

NERD ALERT FRIEND CRUSHES

A FRIEND CRUSH IS A CRUSH THAT DOESN'T COME WITH SEXY FEELINGS. YOU FEEL EVERYTHING ELSE—EXCITED, CONFUSED, OVERWHELMED, LIKE YOU WANT TO SPEND ALL YOUR TIME WITH THEM—BUT IT DOESN'T COME WITH WANTING ANYTHING MORE THAN BEING REALLY CLOSE FRIENDS.

FRIEND CRUSHES AREN'T CRUSH-LITE, THEY ARE REAL AND AMAZING, AND SOMETIMES THEY'RE ALL WE NEED AND WANT.

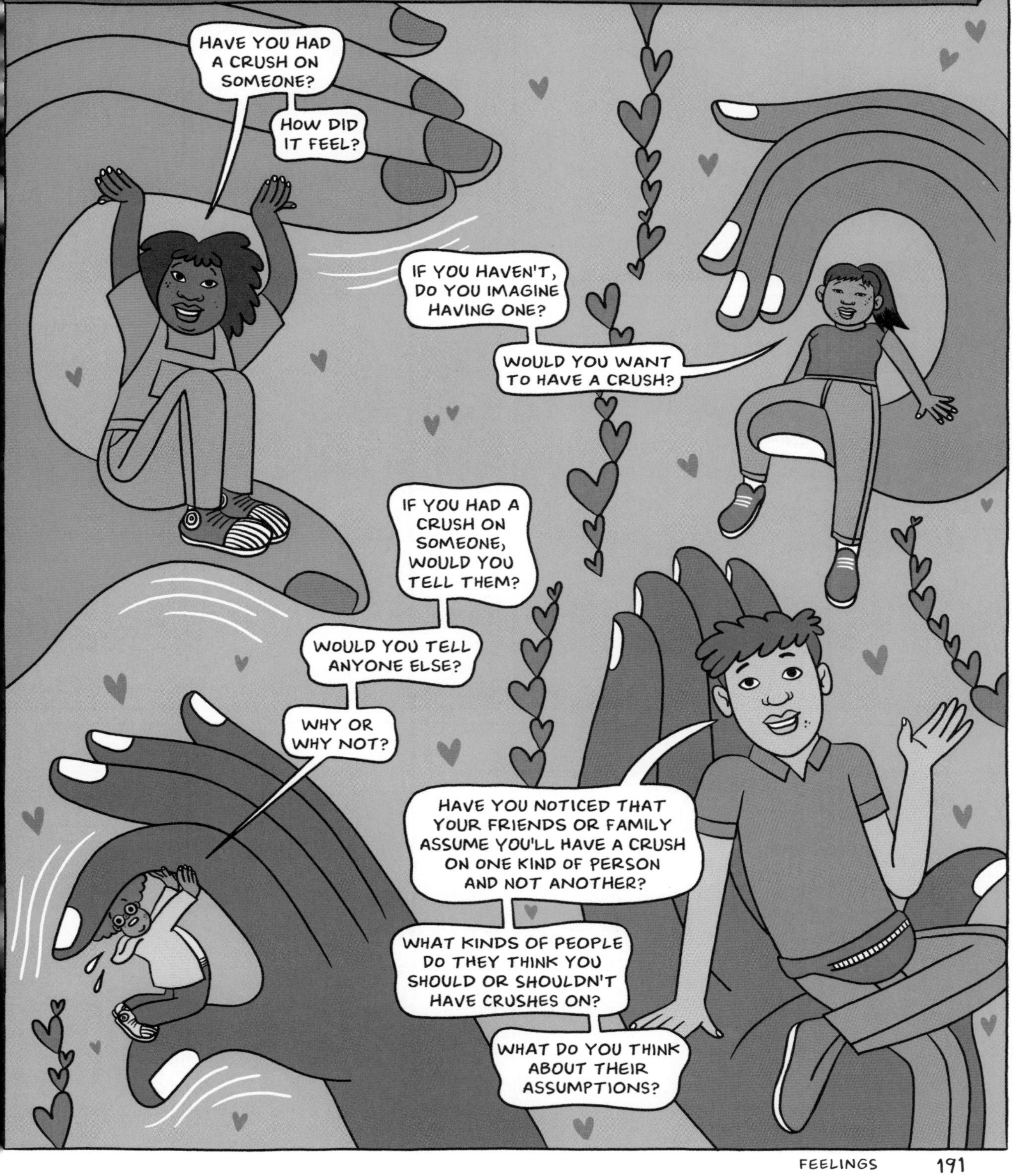
HAVE YOU HAD A CRUSH ON SOMEONE?
HOW DID IT FEEL?
IF YOU HAVEN'T, DO YOU IMAGINE HAVING ONE?
WOULD YOU WANT TO HAVE A CRUSH?
IF YOU HAD A CRUSH ON SOMEONE, WOULD YOU TELL THEM?
WOULD YOU TELL ANYONE ELSE?
WHY OR WHY NOT?
HAVE YOU NOTICED THAT YOUR FRIENDS OR FAMILY ASSUME YOU'LL HAVE A CRUSH ON ONE KIND OF PERSON AND NOT ANOTHER?
WHAT KINDS OF PEOPLE DO THEY THINK YOU SHOULD OR SHOULDN'T HAVE CRUSHES ON?
WHAT DO YOU THINK ABOUT THEIR ASSUMPTIONS?

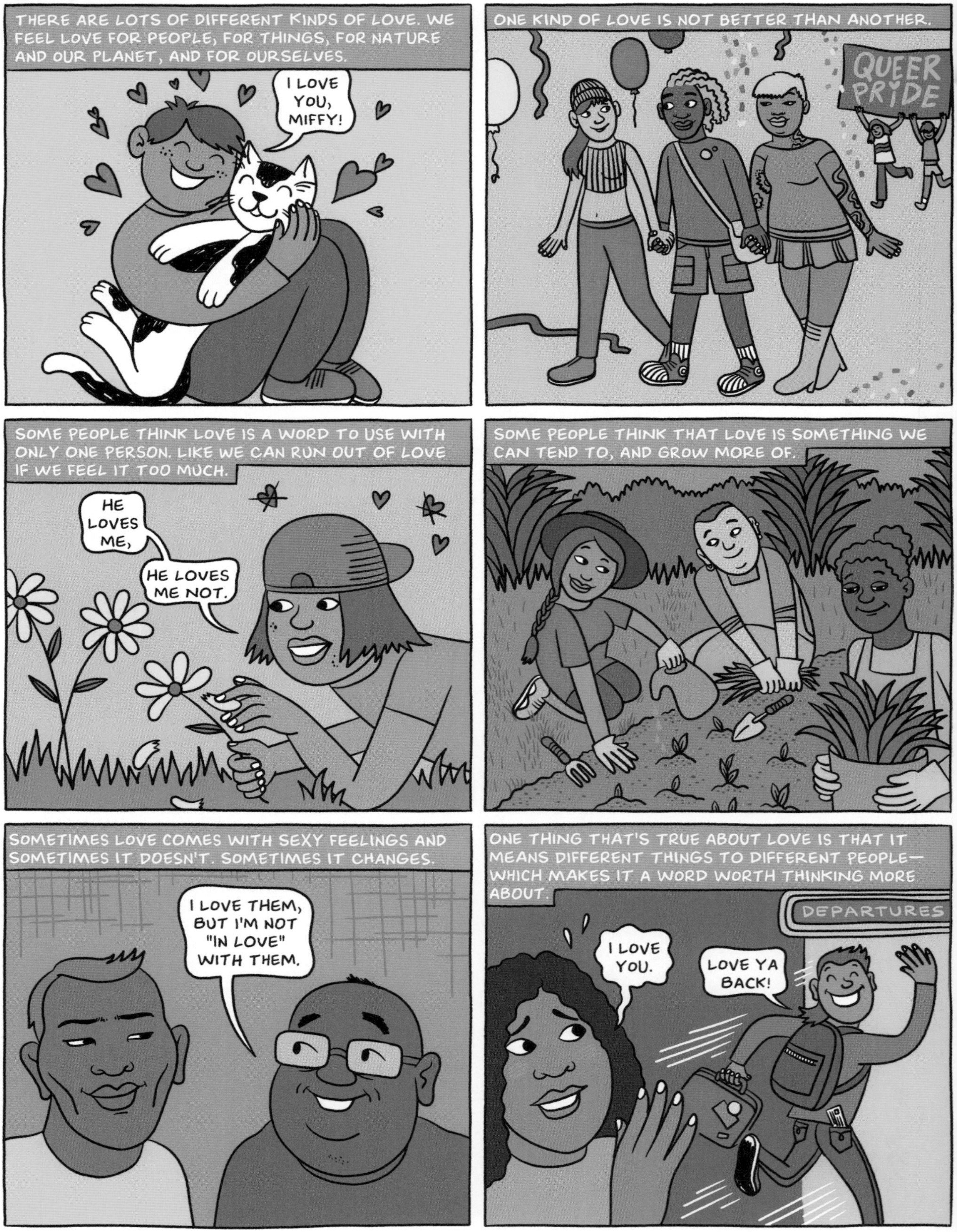
THERE ARE LOTS OF DIFFERENT KINDS OF LOVE. WE FEEL LOVE FOR PEOPLE, FOR THINGS, FOR NATURE AND OUR PLANET, AND FOR OURSELVES.
I LOVE YOU, MIFFY!
ONE KIND OF LOVE IS NOT BETTER THAN ANOTHER.
QUEER PRIDE
SOME PEOPLE THINK LOVE IS A WORD TO USE WITH ONLY ONE PERSON. LIKE WE CAN RUN OUT OF LOVE IF WE FEEL IT TOO MUCH.
HE LOVES ME,
HE LOVES ME NOT.
SOME PEOPLE THINK THAT LOVE IS SOMETHING WE CAN TEND TO, AND GROW MORE OF.
SOMETIMES LOVE COMES WITH SEXY FEELINGS AND SOMETIMES IT DOESN'T. SOMETIMES IT CHANGES.
I LOVE THEM, BUT I'M NOT "IN LOVE" WITH THEM.
ONE THING THAT'S TRUE ABOUT LOVE IS THAT IT MEANS DIFFERENT THINGS TO DIFFERENT PEOPLE—WHICH MAKES IT A WORD WORTH THINKING MORE ABOUT.
DEPARTURES
I LOVE YOU.
LOVE YA BACK!

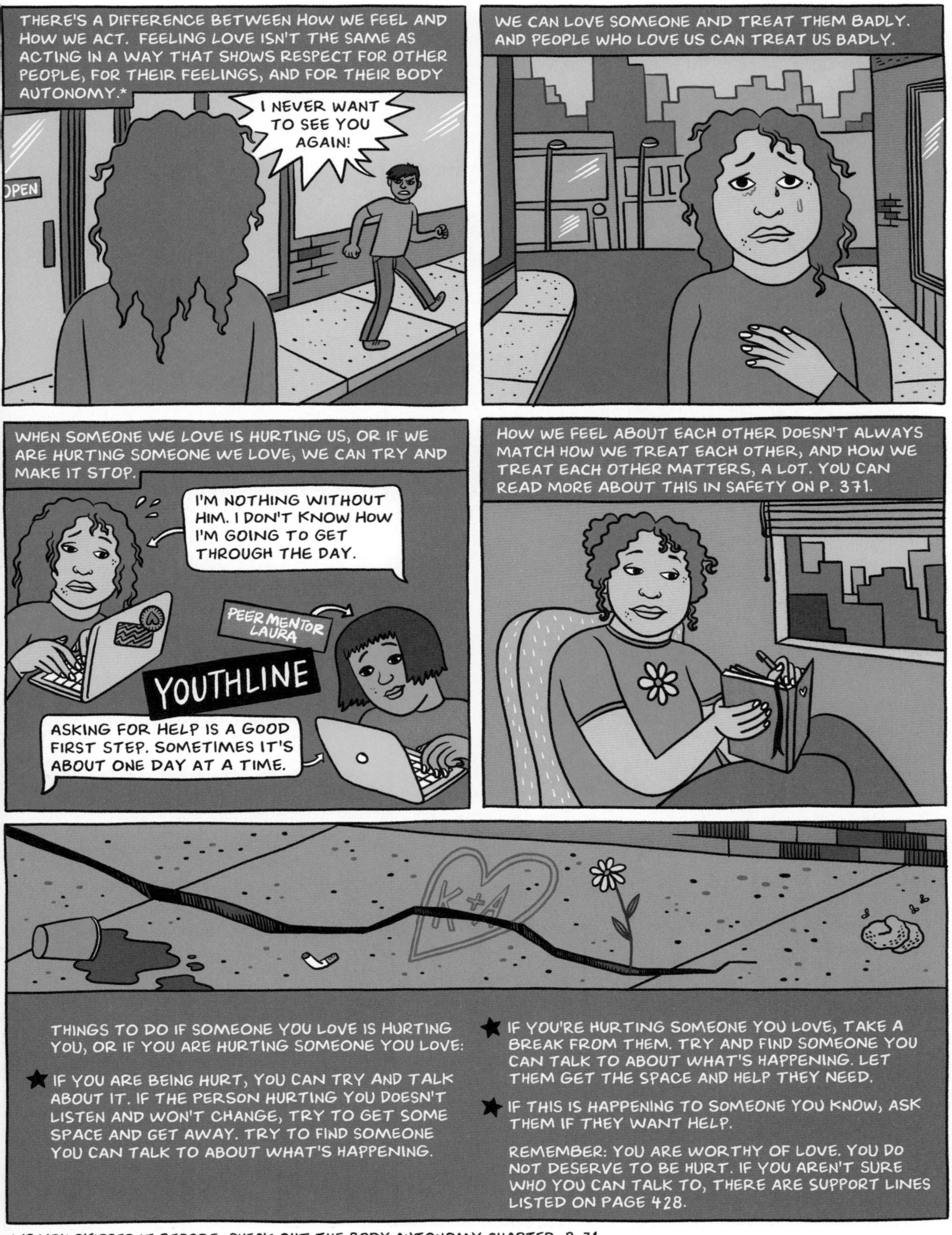
THERE'S A DIFFERENCE BETWEEN HOW WE FEEL AND HOW WE ACT. FEELING LOVE ISN'T THE SAME AS ACTING IN A WAY THAT SHOWS RESPECT FOR OTHER PEOPLE, FOR THEIR FEELINGS, AND FOR THEIR BODY AUTONOMY.*
I NEVER WANT TO SEE YOU AGAIN!
OPEN
WE CAN LOVE SOMEONE AND TREAT THEM BADLY. AND PEOPLE WHO LOVE US CAN TREAT US BADLY.
WHEN SOMEONE WE LOVE IS HURTING US, OR IF WE ARE HURTING SOMEONE WE LOVE, WE CAN TRY AND MAKE IT STOP.
I'M NOTHING WITHOUT HIM. I DON'T KNOW HOW I'M GOING TO GET THROUGH THE DAY.
PEER MENTOR LAURA
YOUTHLINE
ASKING FOR HELP IS A GOOD FIRST STEP. SOMETIMES IT'S ABOUT ONE DAY AT A TIME.
HOW WE FEEL ABOUT EACH OTHER DOESN'T ALWAYS MATCH HOW WE TREAT EACH OTHER, AND HOW WE TREAT EACH OTHER MATTERS, A LOT. YOU CAN READ MORE ABOUT THIS IN SAFETY ON P. 371.
K+A
THINGS TO DO IF SOMEONE YOU LOVE IS HURTING YOU, OR IF YOU ARE HURTING SOMEONE YOU LOVE:
★ IF YOU ARE BEING HURT, YOU CAN TRY AND TALK ABOUT IT. IF THE PERSON HURTING YOU DOESN'T LISTEN AND WON'T CHANGE, TRY TO GET SOME SPACE AND GET AWAY. TRY TO FIND SOMEONE YOU CAN TALK TO ABOUT WHAT'S HAPPENING.
★ IF YOU'RE HURTING SOMEONE YOU LOVE, TAKE A BREAK FROM THEM. TRY AND FIND SOMEONE YOU CAN TALK TO ABOUT WHAT'S HAPPENING. LET THEM GET THE SPACE AND HELP THEY NEED.
★ IF THIS IS HAPPENING TO SOMEONE YOU KNOW, ASK THEM IF THEY WANT HELP.
REMEMBER: YOU ARE WORTHY OF LOVE. YOU DO NOT DESERVE TO BE HURT. IF YOU AREN'T SURE WHO YOU CAN TALK TO, THERE ARE SUPPORT LINES LISTED ON PAGE 428.

* IF YOU SKIPPED IT BEFORE, CHECK OUT THE BODY AUTONOMY CHAPTER, P. 71

SOMETIMES CRUSHES AND LOVE COME WITH FEELINGS IN OUR BODIES AND MINDS THAT ARE DIFFERENT FROM OTHER FEELINGS. IT'S A KIND OF EXCITEMENT AND ENERGY.

ADULTS USE WORDS LIKE DESIRE AND AROUSAL FOR THESE FEELINGS. IN THIS BOOK WE CALL THEM SEXY FEELINGS. SINCE EVERYBODY IS DIFFERENT, WE ALL EXPERIENCE SEXY FEELINGS DIFFERENTLY.

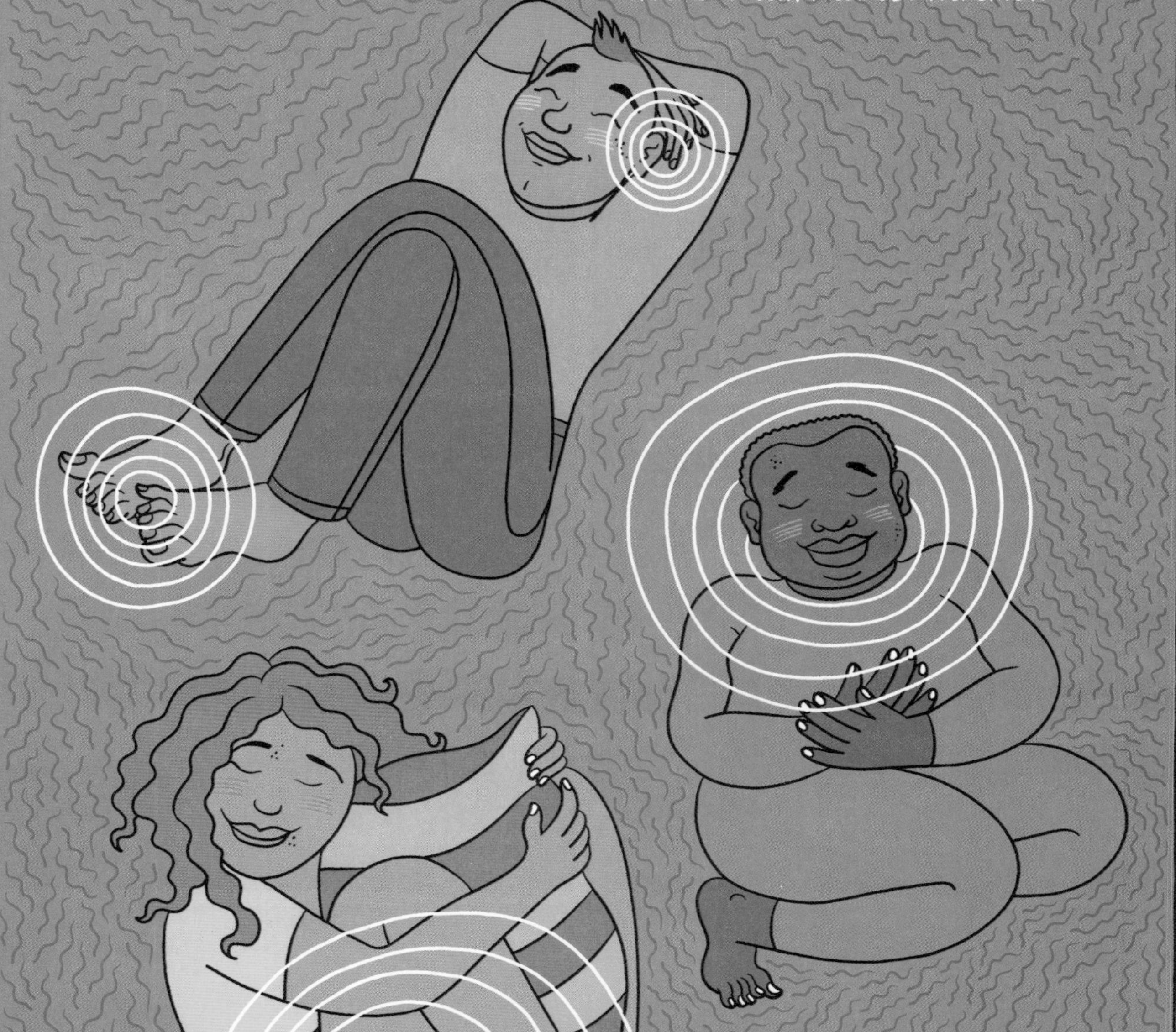

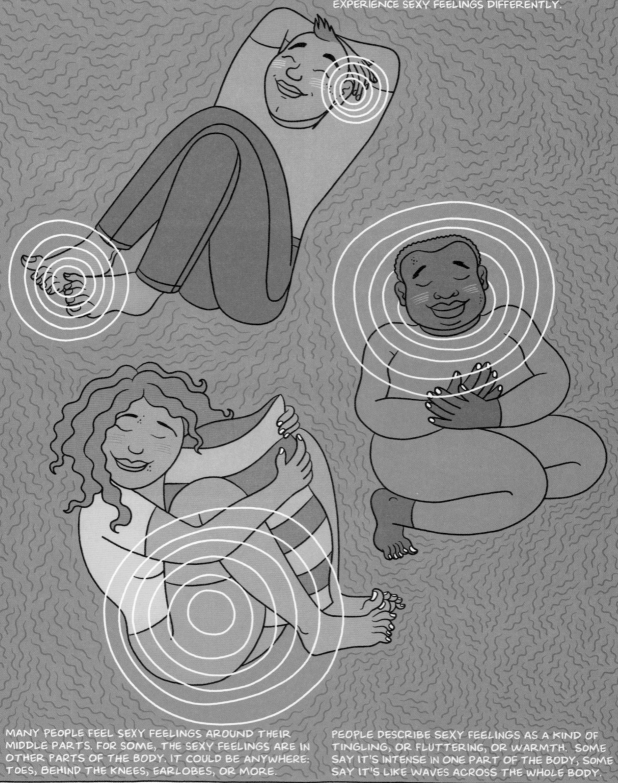

MANY PEOPLE FEEL SEXY FEELINGS AROUND THEIR MIDDLE PARTS. FOR SOME, THE SEXY FEELINGS ARE IN OTHER PARTS OF THE BODY. IT COULD BE ANYWHERE: TOES, BEHIND THE KNEES, EARLOBES, OR MORE.

PEOPLE DESCRIBE SEXY FEELINGS AS A KIND OF TINGLING, OR FLUTTERING, OR WARMTH. SOME SAY IT'S INTENSE IN ONE PART OF THE BODY, SOME SAY IT'S LIKE WAVES ACROSS THE WHOLE BODY.

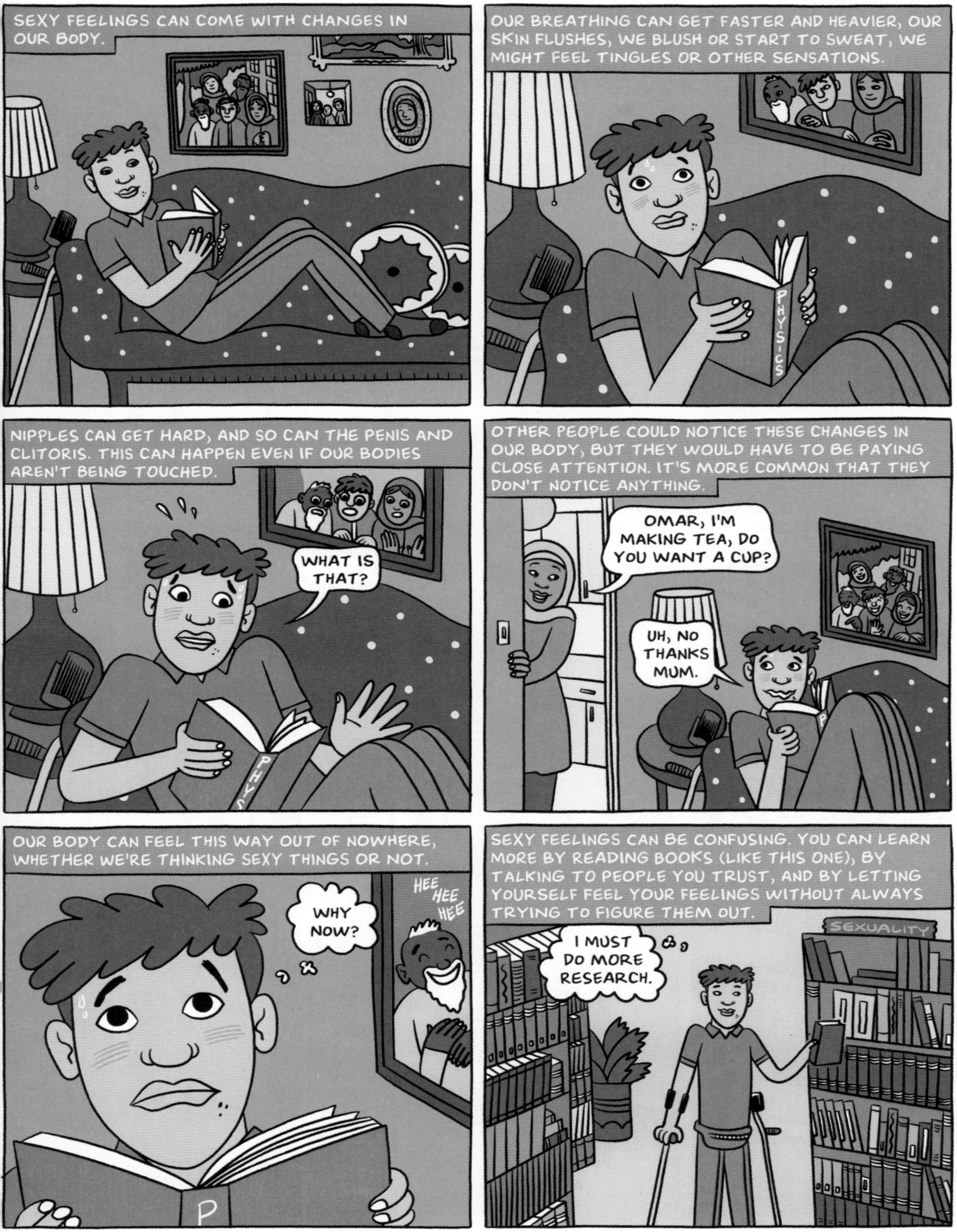
SEXY FEELINGS CAN COME WITH CHANGES IN OUR BODY.
OUR BREATHING CAN GET FASTER AND HEAVIER, OUR SKIN FLUSHES, WE BLUSH OR START TO SWEAT, WE MIGHT FEEL TINGLES OR OTHER SENSATIONS.
PHYSICS
NIPPLES CAN GET HARD, AND SO CAN THE PENIS AND CLITORIS. THIS CAN HAPPEN EVEN IF OUR BODIES AREN'T BEING TOUCHED.
WHAT IS THAT?
OTHER PEOPLE COULD NOTICE THESE CHANGES IN OUR BODY, BUT THEY WOULD HAVE TO BE PAYING CLOSE ATTENTION. IT'S MORE COMMON THAT THEY DON'T NOTICE ANYTHING.
OMAR, I'M MAKING TEA, DO YOU WANT A CUP?
UH, NO THANKS MUM.
OUR BODY CAN FEEL THIS WAY OUT OF NOWHERE, WHETHER WE'RE THINKING SEXY THINGS OR NOT.
WHY NOW?
HEE HEE HEE
SEXY FEELINGS CAN BE CONFUSING. YOU CAN LEARN MORE BY READING BOOKS (LIKE THIS ONE), BY TALKING TO PEOPLE YOU TRUST, AND BY LETTING YOURSELF FEEL YOUR FEELINGS WITHOUT ALWAYS TRYING TO FIGURE THEM OUT.
SEXUALITY
I MUST DO MORE RESEARCH.

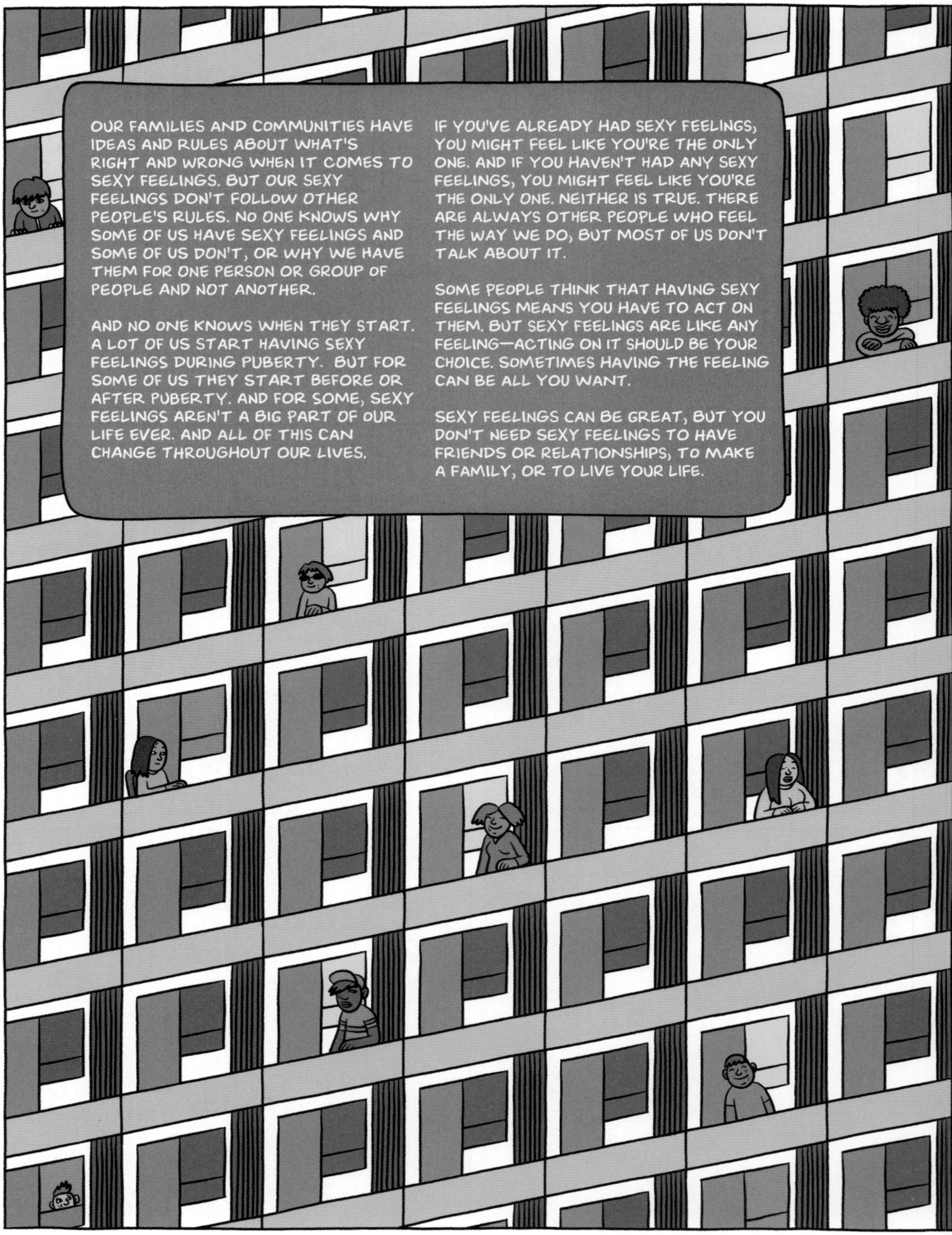
OUR FAMILIES AND COMMUNITIES HAVE IDEAS AND RULES ABOUT WHAT'S RIGHT AND WRONG WHEN IT COMES TO SEXY FEELINGS. BUT OUR SEXY FEELINGS DON'T FOLLOW OTHER PEOPLE'S RULES. NO ONE KNOWS WHY SOME OF US HAVE SEXY FEELINGS AND SOME OF US DON'T, OR WHY WE HAVE THEM FOR ONE PERSON OR GROUP OF PEOPLE AND NOT ANOTHER.
AND NO ONE KNOWS WHEN THEY START. A LOT OF US START HAVING SEXY FEELINGS DURING PUBERTY. BUT FOR SOME OF US THEY START BEFORE OR AFTER PUBERTY. AND FOR SOME, SEXY FEELINGS AREN'T A BIG PART OF OUR LIFE EVER. AND ALL OF THIS CAN CHANGE THROUGHOUT OUR LIVES.
IF YOU'VE ALREADY HAD SEXY FEELINGS, YOU MIGHT FEEL LIKE YOU'RE THE ONLY ONE. AND IF YOU HAVEN'T HAD ANY SEXY FEELINGS, YOU MIGHT FEEL LIKE YOU'RE THE ONLY ONE. NEITHER IS TRUE. THERE ARE ALWAYS OTHER PEOPLE WHO FEEL THE WAY WE DO, BUT MOST OF US DON'T TALK ABOUT IT.
SOME PEOPLE THINK THAT HAVING SEXY FEELINGS MEANS YOU HAVE TO ACT ON THEM. BUT SEXY FEELINGS ARE LIKE ANY FEELING—ACTING ON IT SHOULD BE YOUR CHOICE. SOMETIMES HAVING THE FEELING CAN BE ALL YOU WANT.
SEXY FEELINGS CAN BE GREAT, BUT YOU DON'T NEED SEXY FEELINGS TO HAVE FRIENDS OR RELATIONSHIPS, TO MAKE A FAMILY, OR TO LIVE YOUR LIFE.

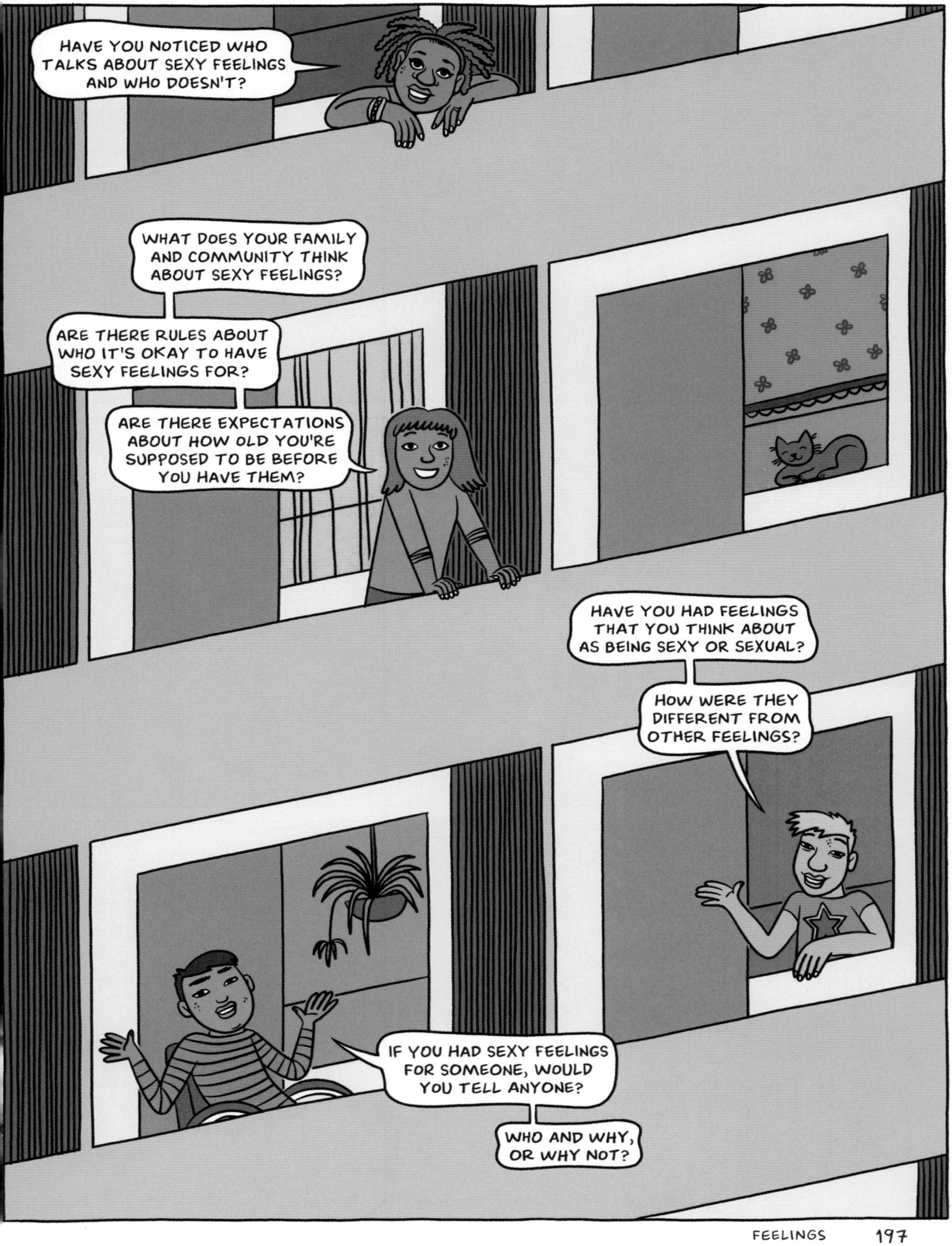
HAVE YOU NOTICED WHO TALKS ABOUT SEXY FEELINGS AND WHO DOESN'T?
WHAT DOES YOUR FAMILY AND COMMUNITY THINK ABOUT SEXY FEELINGS?
ARE THERE RULES ABOUT WHO IT'S OKAY TO HAVE SEXY FEELINGS FOR?
ARE THERE EXPECTATIONS ABOUT HOW OLD YOU'RE SUPPOSED TO BE BEFORE YOU HAVE THEM?
HAVE YOU HAD FEELINGS THAT YOU THINK ABOUT AS BEING SEXY OR SEXUAL?
HOW WERE THEY DIFFERENT FROM OTHER FEELINGS?
IF YOU HAD SEXY FEELINGS FOR SOMEONE, WOULD YOU TELL ANYONE?
WHO AND WHY, OR WHY NOT?

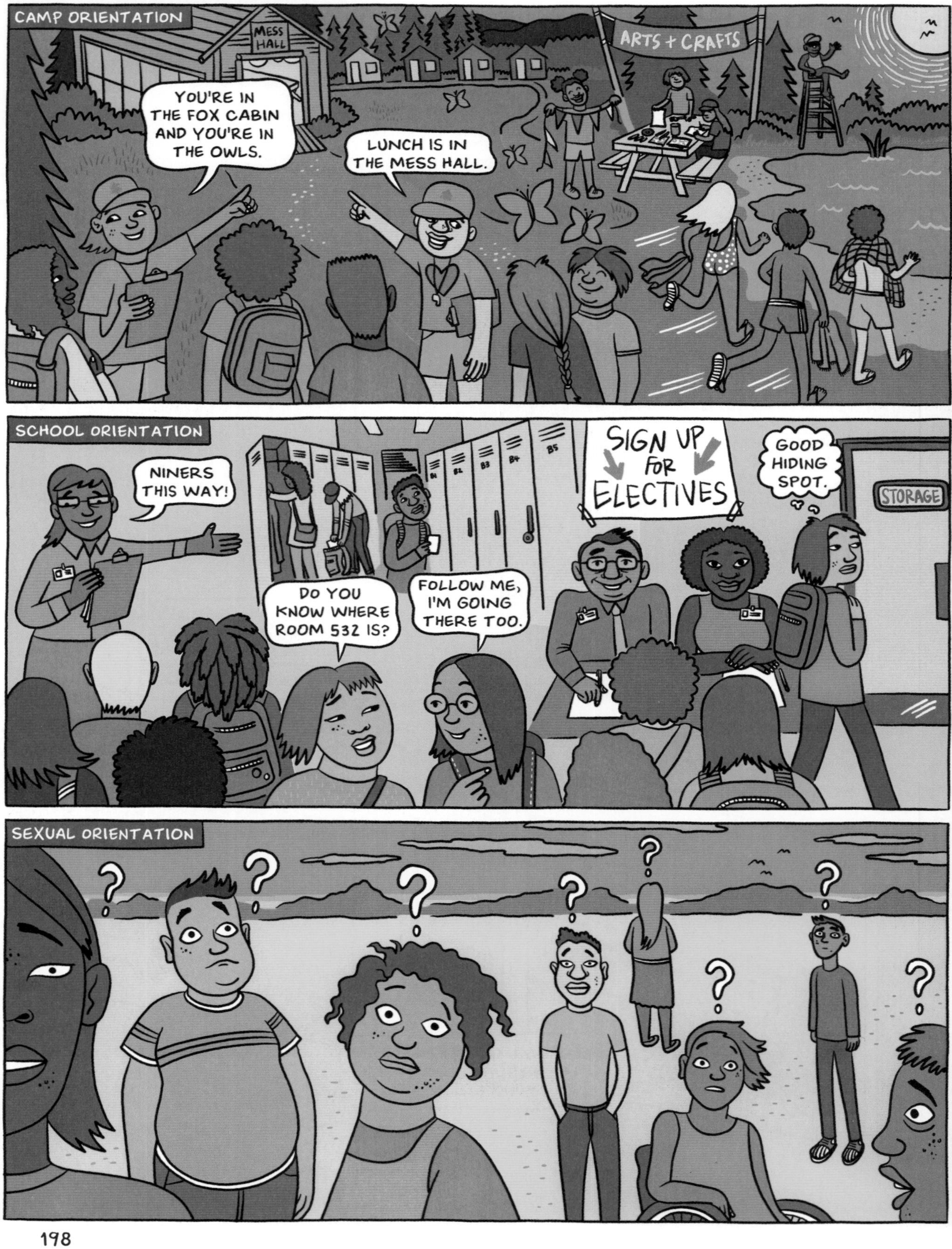
CAMP ORIENTATION
MESS HALL
ARTS + CRAFTS
YOU'RE IN THE FOX CABIN AND YOU'RE IN THE OWLS.
LUNCH IS IN THE MESS HALL.
SCHOOL ORIENTATION
NINERS THIS WAY!
SIGN UP FOR ELECTIVES
GOOD HIDING SPOT.
STORAGE
B1 B2 B3 B4 B5
DO YOU KNOW WHERE ROOM 532 IS?
FOLLOW ME, I'M GOING THERE TOO.
SEXUAL ORIENTATION

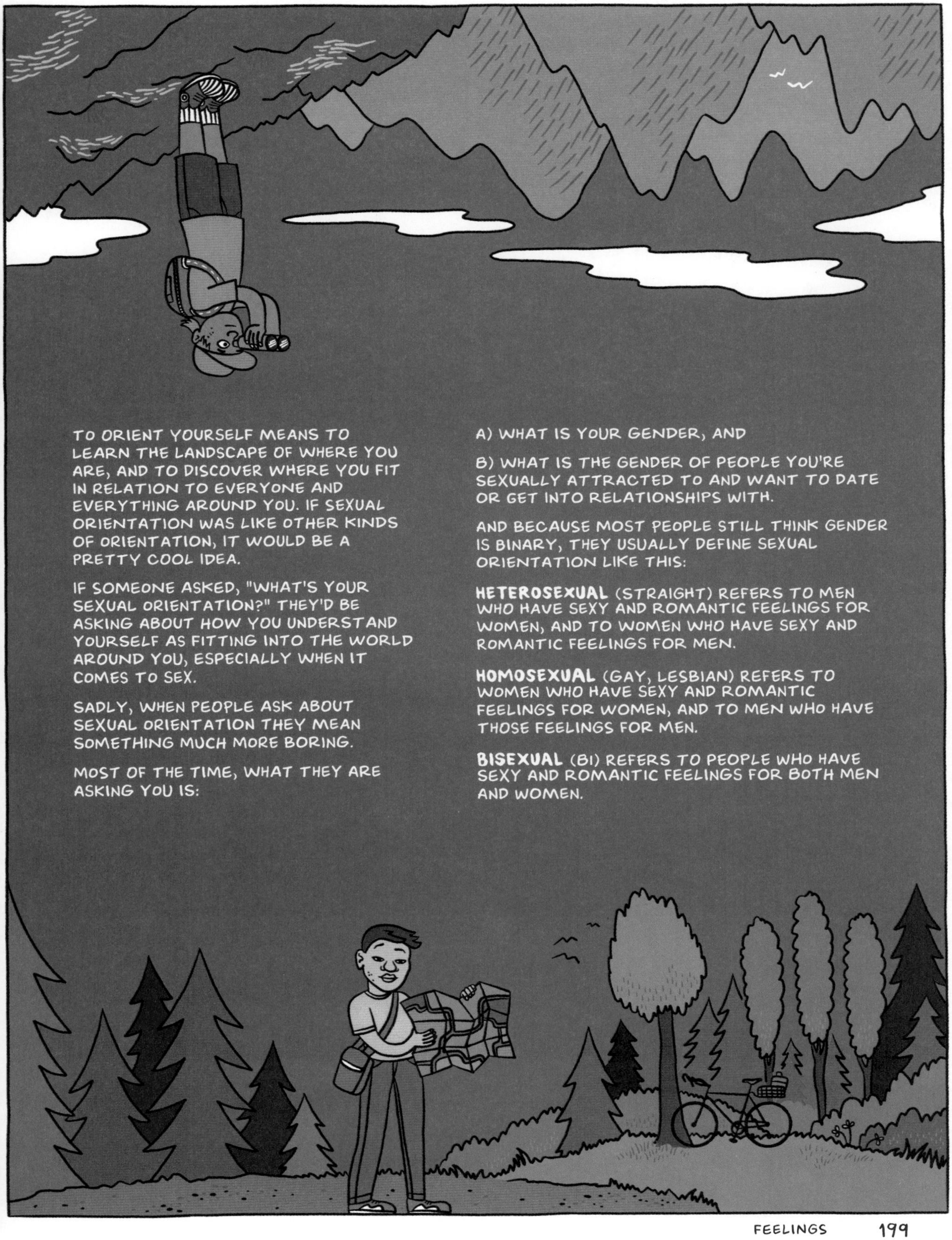
TO ORIENT YOURSELF MEANS TO LEARN THE LANDSCAPE OF WHERE YOU ARE, AND TO DISCOVER WHERE YOU FIT IN RELATION TO EVERYONE AND EVERYTHING AROUND YOU. IF SEXUAL ORIENTATION WAS LIKE OTHER KINDS OF ORIENTATION, IT WOULD BE A PRETTY COOL IDEA.
IF SOMEONE ASKED, "WHAT'S YOUR SEXUAL ORIENTATION?" THEY'D BE ASKING ABOUT HOW YOU UNDERSTAND YOURSELF AS FITTING INTO THE WORLD AROUND YOU, ESPECIALLY WHEN IT COMES TO SEX.
SADLY, WHEN PEOPLE ASK ABOUT SEXUAL ORIENTATION THEY MEAN SOMETHING MUCH MORE BORING.
MOST OF THE TIME, WHAT THEY ARE ASKING YOU IS:
A) WHAT IS YOUR GENDER, AND
B) WHAT IS THE GENDER OF PEOPLE YOU'RE SEXUALLY ATTRACTED TO AND WANT TO DATE OR GET INTO RELATIONSHIPS WITH.
AND BECAUSE MOST PEOPLE STILL THINK GENDER IS BINARY, THEY USUALLY DEFINE SEXUAL ORIENTATION LIKE THIS:
HETEROSEXUAL (STRAIGHT) REFERS TO MEN WHO HAVE SEXY AND ROMANTIC FEELINGS FOR WOMEN, AND TO WOMEN WHO HAVE SEXY AND ROMANTIC FEELINGS FOR MEN.
HOMOSEXUAL (GAY, LESBIAN) REFERS TO WOMEN WHO HAVE SEXY AND ROMANTIC FEELINGS FOR WOMEN, AND TO MEN WHO HAVE THOSE FEELINGS FOR MEN.
BISEXUAL (BI) REFERS TO PEOPLE WHO HAVE SEXY AND ROMANTIC FEELINGS FOR BOTH MEN AND WOMEN.

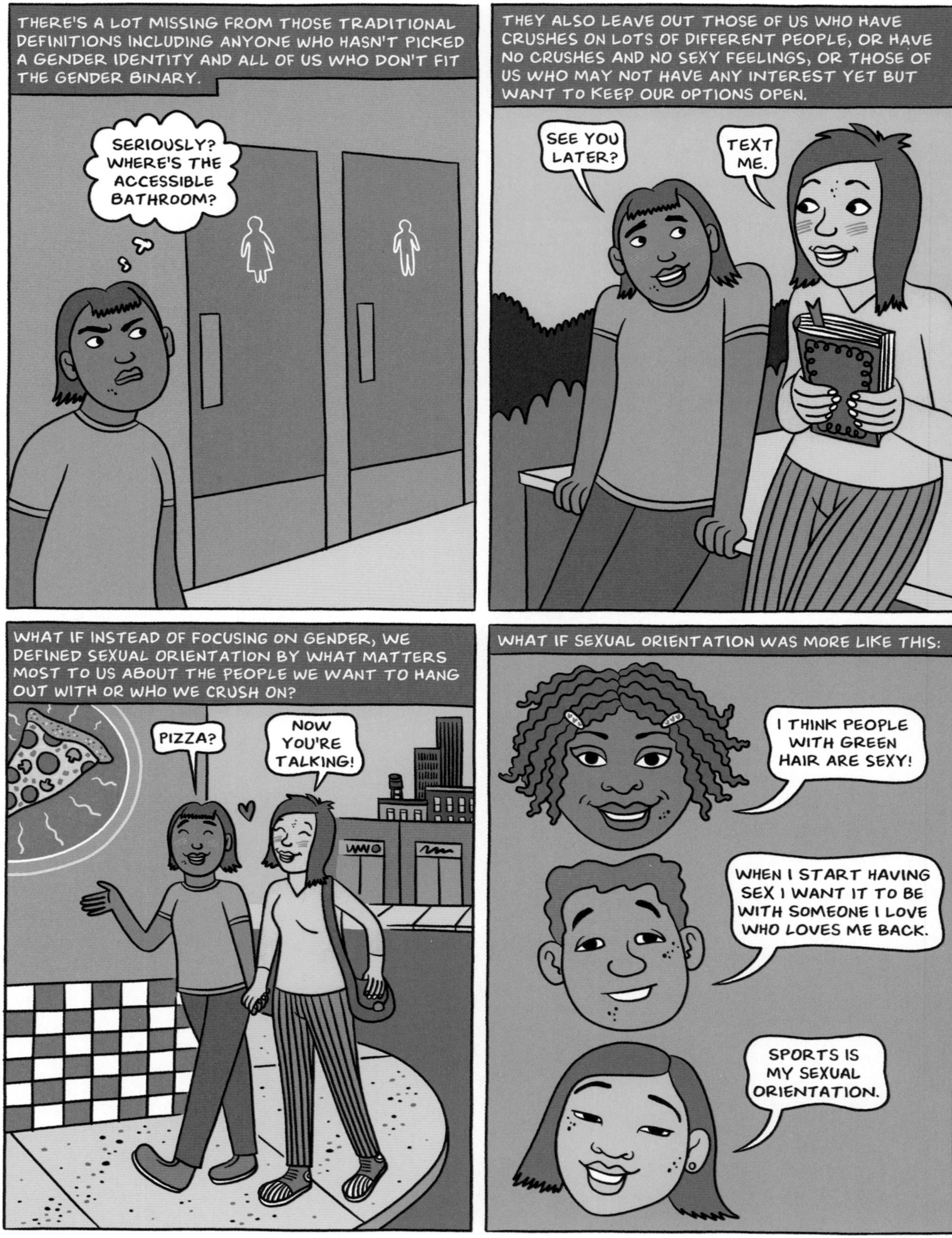
THERE'S A LOT MISSING FROM THOSE TRADITIONAL DEFINITIONS INCLUDING ANYONE WHO HASN'T PICKED A GENDER IDENTITY AND ALL OF US WHO DON'T FIT THE GENDER BINARY.
SERIOUSLY? WHERE'S THE ACCESSIBLE BATHROOM?
THEY ALSO LEAVE OUT THOSE OF US WHO HAVE CRUSHES ON LOTS OF DIFFERENT PEOPLE, OR HAVE NO CRUSHES AND NO SEXY FEELINGS, OR THOSE OF US WHO MAY NOT HAVE ANY INTEREST YET BUT WANT TO KEEP OUR OPTIONS OPEN.
SEE YOU LATER?
TEXT ME.
WHAT IF INSTEAD OF FOCUSING ON GENDER, WE DEFINED SEXUAL ORIENTATION BY WHAT MATTERS MOST TO US ABOUT THE PEOPLE WE WANT TO HANG OUT WITH OR WHO WE CRUSH ON?
PIZZA?
NOW YOU'RE TALKING!
WHAT IF SEXUAL ORIENTATION WAS MORE LIKE THIS:
I THINK PEOPLE WITH GREEN HAIR ARE SEXY!
WHEN I START HAVING SEX I WANT IT TO BE WITH SOMEONE I LOVE WHO LOVES ME BACK.
SPORTS IS MY SEXUAL ORIENTATION.

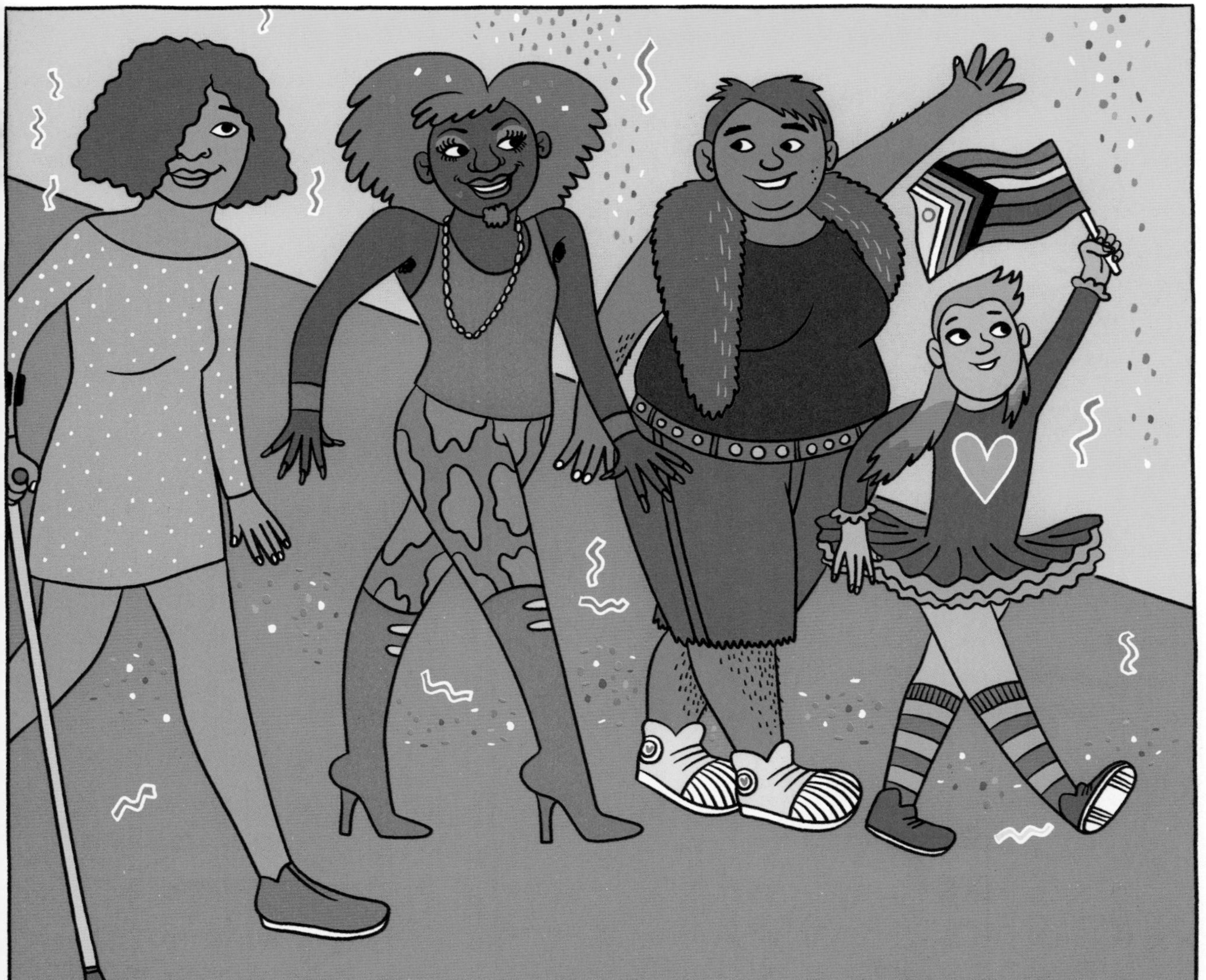

THE TRADITIONAL DEFINITIONS LIKE GAY, STRAIGHT, AND BISEXUAL WORK FOR SOME, BUT NOT ALL, OF US.

IF YOU DON'T ASK PEOPLE QUESTIONS ABOUT THEMSELVES, IT CAN SEEM LIKE EVERYONE AROUND YOU IS EITHER STRAIGHT OR GAY. BUT IF YOU TAKE THE TIME TO TALK TO PEOPLE ABOUT WHO THEY ARE, YOU FIND OUT THAT A LOT OF PEOPLE DON'T FIT INTO THOSE DEFINITIONS.

A LOT OF US COME UP WITH NEW WORDS TO DESCRIBE OURSELVES. PEOPLE—USUALLY YOUNG PEOPLE—ARE ALWAYS COMING UP WITH NEW WAYS TO IDENTIFY AND DESCRIBE WHO THEY ARE. HERE ARE THREE NEWER ORIENTATION WORDS:

ASEXUAL REFERS TO PEOPLE WHO DON'T EXPERIENCE SEXY FEELINGS TOWARD PEOPLE OF ANY GENDER.

PANSEXUAL (PAN) USUALLY REFERS TO SOMEONE OPEN TO CRUSHES, SEXY FEELINGS, DATING, AND RELATIONSHIPS WITH PEOPLE OF ANY AND ALL GENDERS. BY USING THE WORD PANSEXUAL THEY ARE REMINDING EVERYONE THAT THERE ARE MORE THAN TWO GENDERS AND MORE THAN ONE WAY TO LOVE OR HAVE SEXY FEELINGS.

QUEER IS AN OLD WORD THAT WAS USED FOR HURTING PEOPLE. IN SOME PLACES IT STILL IS. THE HURTING VERSION OF QUEER MEANT THAT SOMEONE SEEMED GAY OR THEIR GENDER EXPRESSION DIDN'T FIT WHAT WAS EXPECTED. EITHER WAY, PEOPLE USED IT AS A VIOLENT INSULT. YOU COULD GET CALLED QUEER WHETHER OR NOT YOU WERE GAY OR LESBIAN OR BI OR STRAIGHT.

BUT THEN SOME PEOPLE STARTED USING THE WORD QUEER WITH PRIDE, TO DESCRIBE NOT ONLY HOW THEY FEEL ABOUT SEX AND GENDER, BUT ALSO HOW THEY FEEL ABOUT THE RULES OF THE WORLD AND HOW THEY FEEL ABOUT THE PRESSURE TO BE NORMAL.

QUEER MIGHT MEAN YOU ARE ATTRACTED TO AND OPEN TO RELATIONSHIPS WITH PEOPLE OF ALL GENDERS AND ORIENTATIONS. IT IS ALSO A WAY OF SAYING THAT THE GENDER AND RELATIONSHIP RULES AND EXPECTATIONS OF THE WORLD DON'T WORK FOR YOU.

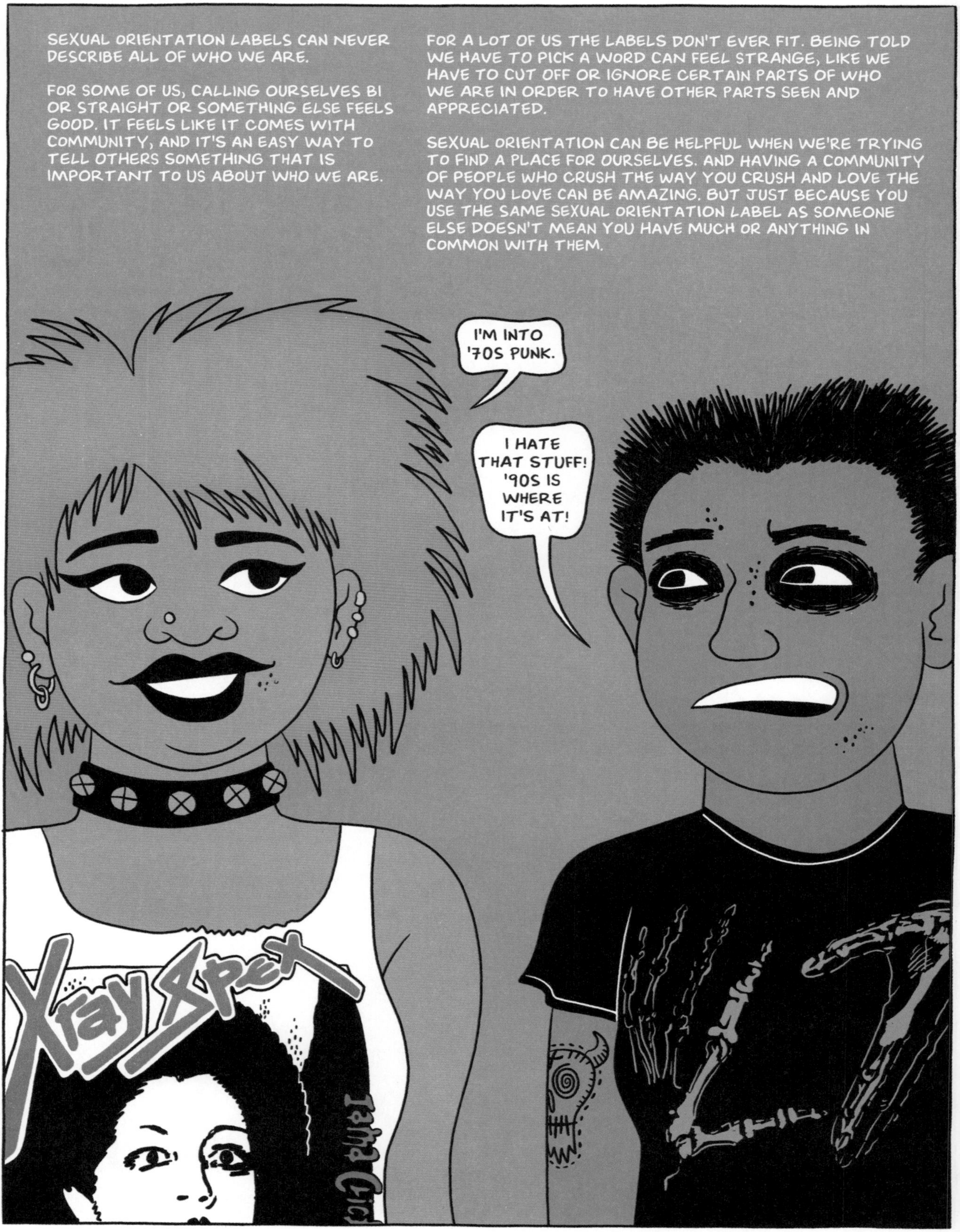
SEXUAL ORIENTATION LABELS CAN NEVER DESCRIBE ALL OF WHO WE ARE.
FOR SOME OF US, CALLING OURSELVES BI OR STRAIGHT OR SOMETHING ELSE FEELS GOOD. IT FEELS LIKE IT COMES WITH COMMUNITY, AND IT'S AN EASY WAY TO TELL OTHERS SOMETHING THAT IS IMPORTANT TO US ABOUT WHO WE ARE.
FOR A LOT OF US THE LABELS DON'T EVER FIT. BEING TOLD WE HAVE TO PICK A WORD CAN FEEL STRANGE, LIKE WE HAVE TO CUT OFF OR IGNORE CERTAIN PARTS OF WHO WE ARE IN ORDER TO HAVE OTHER PARTS SEEN AND APPRECIATED.
SEXUAL ORIENTATION CAN BE HELPFUL WHEN WE'RE TRYING TO FIND A PLACE FOR OURSELVES. AND HAVING A COMMUNITY OF PEOPLE WHO CRUSH THE WAY YOU CRUSH AND LOVE THE WAY YOU LOVE CAN BE AMAZING. BUT JUST BECAUSE YOU USE THE SAME SEXUAL ORIENTATION LABEL AS SOMEONE ELSE DOESN'T MEAN YOU HAVE MUCH OR ANYTHING IN COMMON WITH THEM.
I'M INTO '70S PUNK.
I HATE THAT STUFF! '90S IS WHERE IT'S AT!
Xray Spex

FIGURING OUT YOUR SEXUAL ORIENTATION ISN'T LIKE FIGURING OUT A MATH OR SCIENCE PROBLEM. THERE'S NO SECRET FORMULA, AND THERE'S NO ONLINE QUIZ YOU CAN TAKE THAT WILL TELL YOU YOUR ORIENTATION (EVEN THOUGH LOTS OF QUIZZES PROMISE TO DO JUST THAT). IF YOU WANT TO GO BEYOND THE LABELS AND THINK ABOUT WHERE YOU ARE AND WHERE YOU FIT IN, HERE ARE SOME QUESTIONS TO ASK YOURSELF.

IS SEX SOMETHING I CARE ABOUT?

DO I CARE ABOUT IT BECAUSE EVERYONE ELSE SEEMS TO, OR AM I INTERESTED IN IT FOR MYSELF?

DO I LIKE ANYONE IN A WAY THAT FEELS DIFFERENT FROM THE WAY I LIKE MY FRIENDS?

DO I THINK ABOUT PEOPLE IN WAYS THAT MAKE ME FEEL SEXY OR EXCITED?

DO I FIND MYSELF DRAWN TO CERTAIN GROUPS OF PEOPLE? ALWAYS ONE GROUP, OR DO I LIKE TO HAVE FRIENDS FROM LOTS OF DIFFERENT GROUPS?

WHAT KINDS OF PEOPLE AM I ATTRACTED TO/INTERESTED IN?

ARE THEY INTO CERTAIN THINGS? DO THEY THINK CERTAIN WAYS?

ARE THEY SHY OR OUTGOING? FUNNY OR SERIOUS? FRIENDLY OR MEAN?

IS THERE SOMETHING ABOUT THE WAY THEY DRESS, THEIR HAIR, HOW THEY MOVE, THAT MAKES ME WANT TO BE NEAR THEM?

ANSWERING THESE QUESTIONS WON'T MAGICALLY GIVE YOU A LABEL OR GROUP TO BELONG TO. SEX DOESN'T WORK THAT WAY. BUT STARTING TO ANSWER THESE QUESTIONS CAN HELP YOU FIGURE OUT MORE OF WHO YOU WANT IN YOUR LIFE AND WHAT YOU WANT TO DO WITH THEM. WHICH IS A GOOD PLACE TO START ANY JOURNEY, HOWEVER YOU ORIENT YOURSELF.

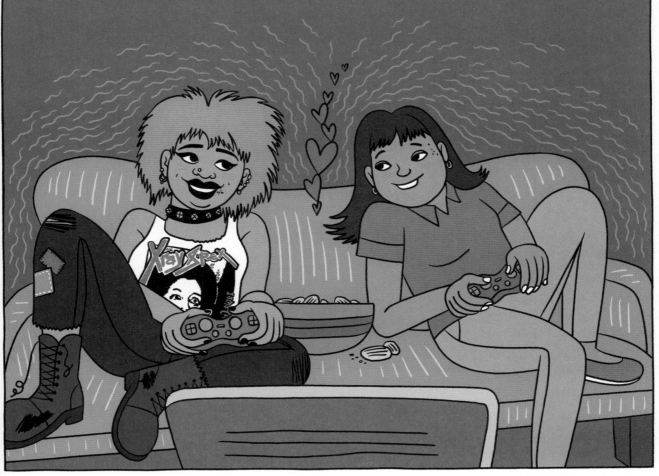

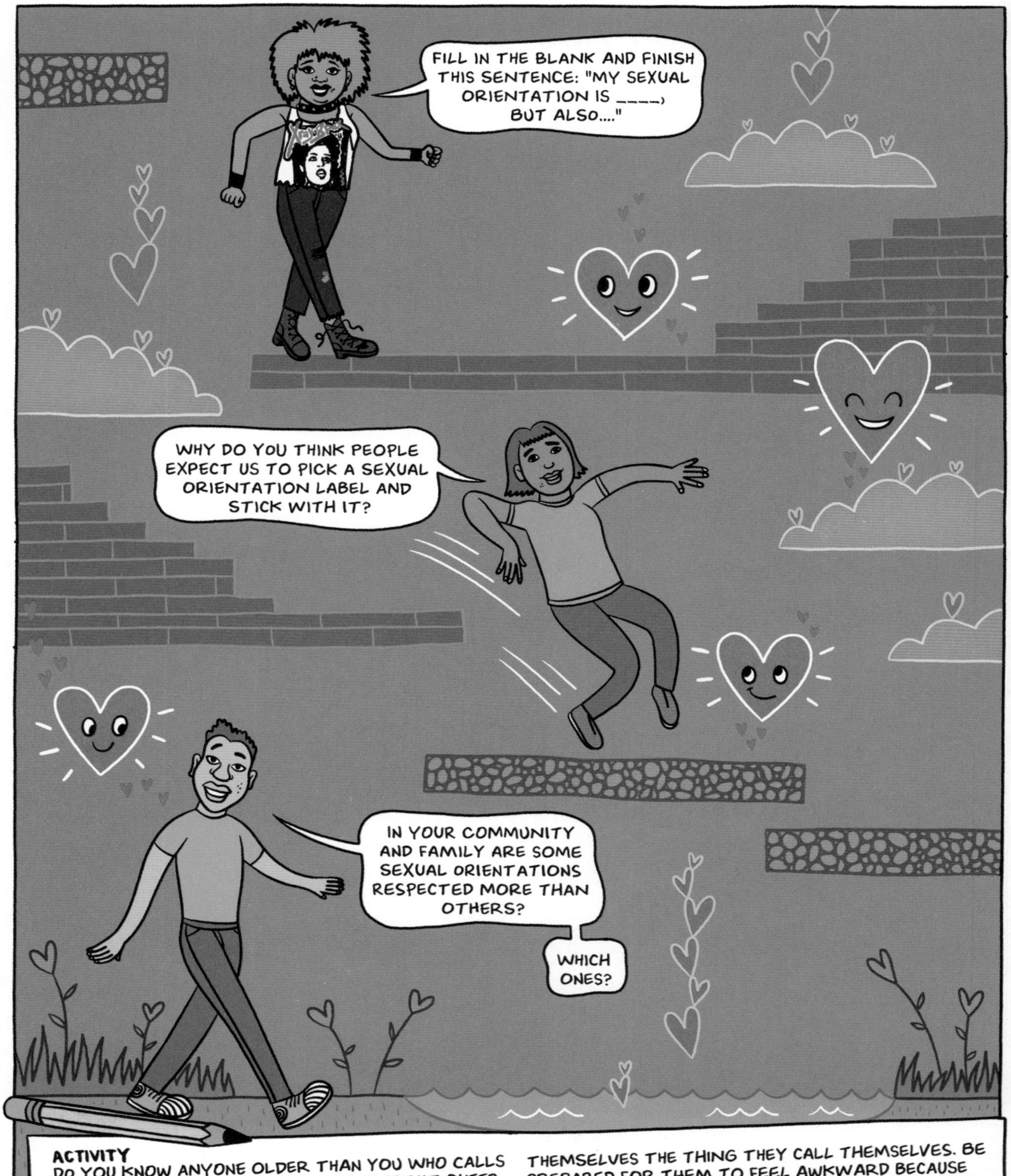

FILL IN THE BLANK AND FINISH THIS SENTENCE: "MY SEXUAL ORIENTATION IS ____, BUT ALSO...."
WHY DO YOU THINK PEOPLE EXPECT US TO PICK A SEXUAL ORIENTATION LABEL AND STICK WITH IT?
IN YOUR COMMUNITY AND FAMILY ARE SOME SEXUAL ORIENTATIONS RESPECTED MORE THAN OTHERS?
WHICH ONES?

ACTIVITY

DO YOU KNOW ANYONE OLDER THAN YOU WHO CALLS THEMSELVES GAY OR STRAIGHT? HOW ABOUT QUEER OR BISEXUAL? IF YOU DO, AND IF THEY ARE PEOPLE YOU CAN TALK TO, ASK THEM WHY THEY USE THOSE WORDS, AND WHAT THOSE WORDS MEAN TO THEM. ASK THEM WHAT IT WAS LIKE BEFORE THEY CALLED THEMSELVES THE THING THEY CALL THEMSELVES. BE PREPARED FOR THEM TO FEEL AWKWARD BECAUSE THEY MAY THINK YOU ARE ONLY ASKING ABOUT SEX. YOU CAN PUT THEM AT EASE BY SAYING YOU ARE ASKING ABOUT ALL THE FEELINGS, NOT JUST SEX. OR, YOU KNOW, YOU CAN WATCH THEM BE AWKWARD.

6

CONSENT

EVERYBODY READY?

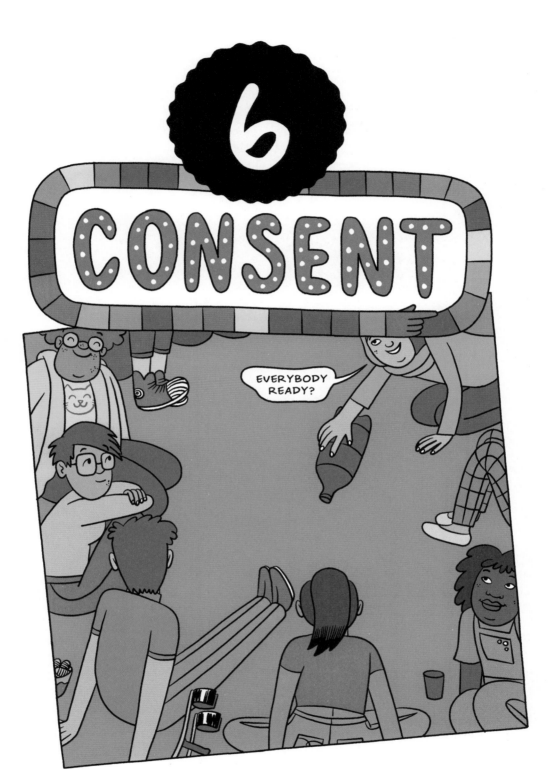

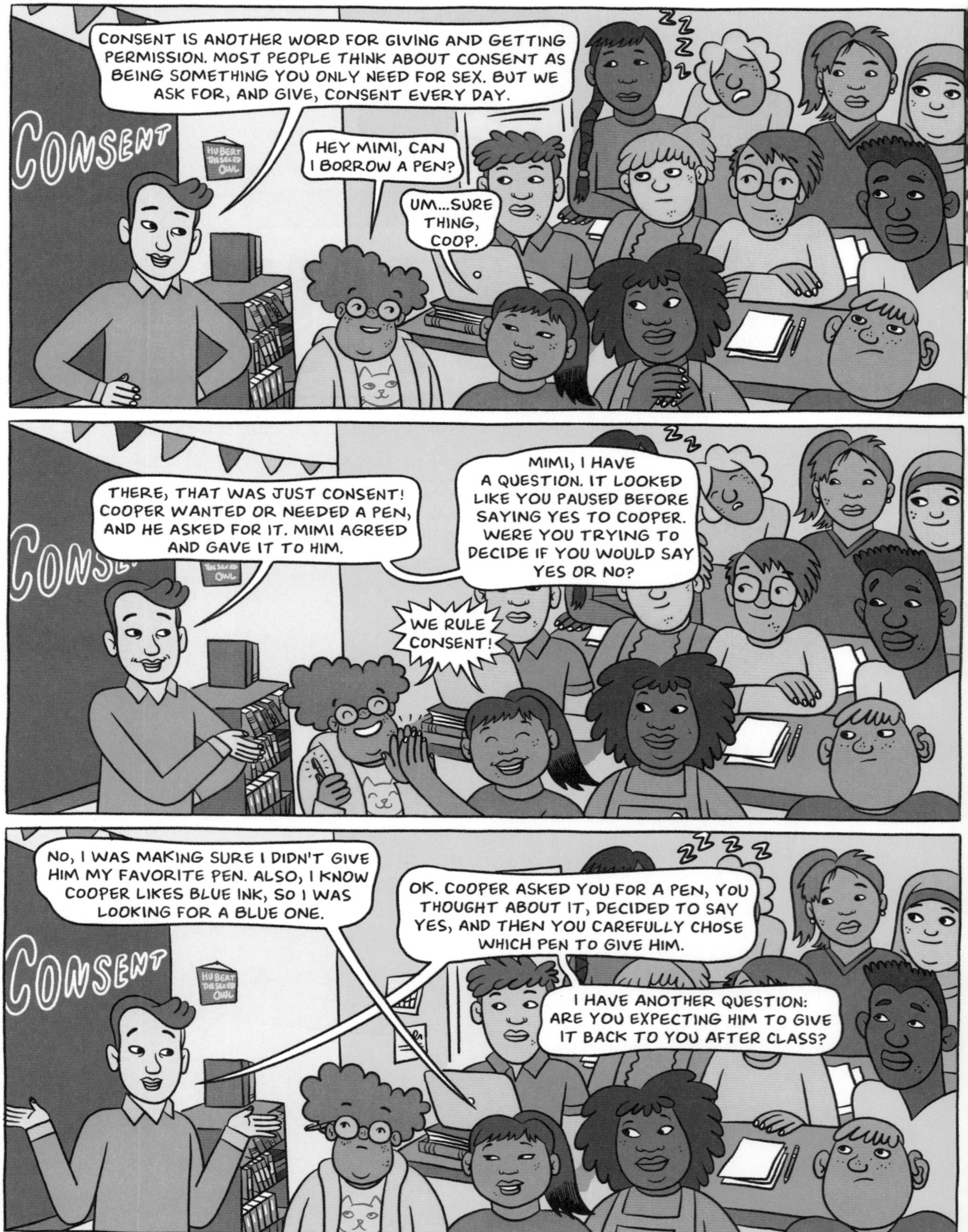
CONSENT IS ANOTHER WORD FOR GIVING AND GETTING PERMISSION. MOST PEOPLE THINK ABOUT CONSENT AS BEING SOMETHING YOU ONLY NEED FOR SEX. BUT WE ASK FOR, AND GIVE, CONSENT EVERY DAY.
CONSENT
HUBERT THE SEX ED OWL
HEY MIMI, CAN I BORROW A PEN?
UM...SURE THING, COOP.
Z Z Z
THERE, THAT WAS JUST CONSENT! COOPER WANTED OR NEEDED A PEN, AND HE ASKED FOR IT. MIMI AGREED AND GAVE IT TO HIM.
MIMI, I HAVE A QUESTION. IT LOOKED LIKE YOU PAUSED BEFORE SAYING YES TO COOPER. WERE YOU TRYING TO DECIDE IF YOU WOULD SAY YES OR NO?
WE RULE CONSENT!
NO, I WAS MAKING SURE I DIDN'T GIVE HIM MY FAVORITE PEN. ALSO, I KNOW COOPER LIKES BLUE INK, SO I WAS LOOKING FOR A BLUE ONE.
OK. COOPER ASKED YOU FOR A PEN, YOU THOUGHT ABOUT IT, DECIDED TO SAY YES, AND THEN YOU CAREFULLY CHOSE WHICH PEN TO GIVE HIM.
I HAVE ANOTHER QUESTION: ARE YOU EXPECTING HIM TO GIVE IT BACK TO YOU AFTER CLASS?
CONSENT
HUBERT THE SEX ED OWL

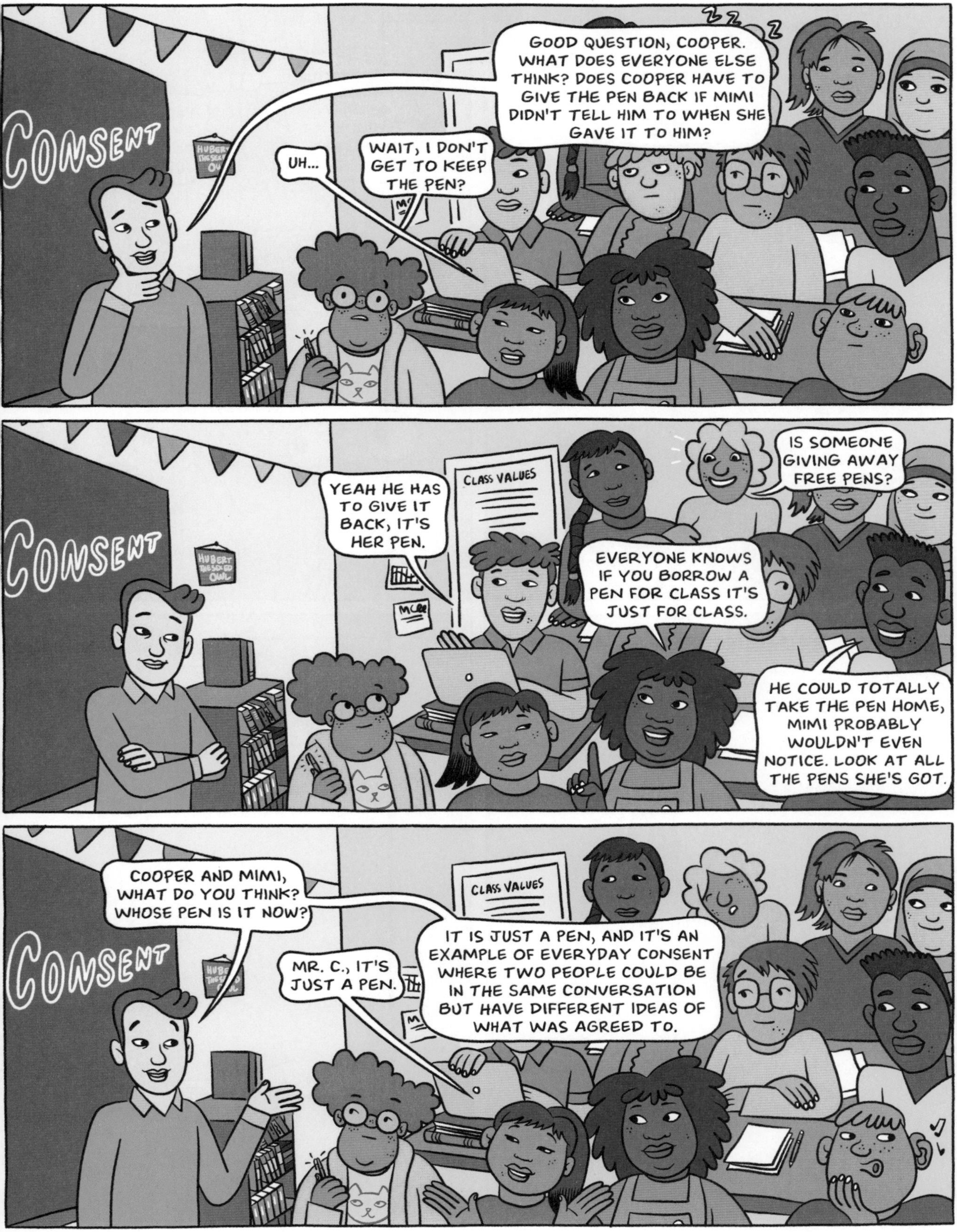
CONSENT
GOOD QUESTION, COOPER. WHAT DOES EVERYONE ELSE THINK? DOES COOPER HAVE TO GIVE THE PEN BACK IF MIMI DIDN'T TELL HIM TO WHEN SHE GAVE IT TO HIM?
UH...
WAIT, I DON'T GET TO KEEP THE PEN?
CONSENT
CLASS VALUES
YEAH HE HAS TO GIVE IT BACK, IT'S HER PEN.
IS SOMEONE GIVING AWAY FREE PENS?
EVERYONE KNOWS IF YOU BORROW A PEN FOR CLASS IT'S JUST FOR CLASS.
HE COULD TOTALLY TAKE THE PEN HOME, MIMI PROBABLY WOULDN'T EVEN NOTICE. LOOK AT ALL THE PENS SHE'S GOT.
CONSENT
CLASS VALUES
COOPER AND MIMI, WHAT DO YOU THINK? WHOSE PEN IS IT NOW?
MR. C., IT'S JUST A PEN.
IT IS JUST A PEN, AND IT'S AN EXAMPLE OF EVERYDAY CONSENT WHERE TWO PEOPLE COULD BE IN THE SAME CONVERSATION BUT HAVE DIFFERENT IDEAS OF WHAT WAS AGREED TO.

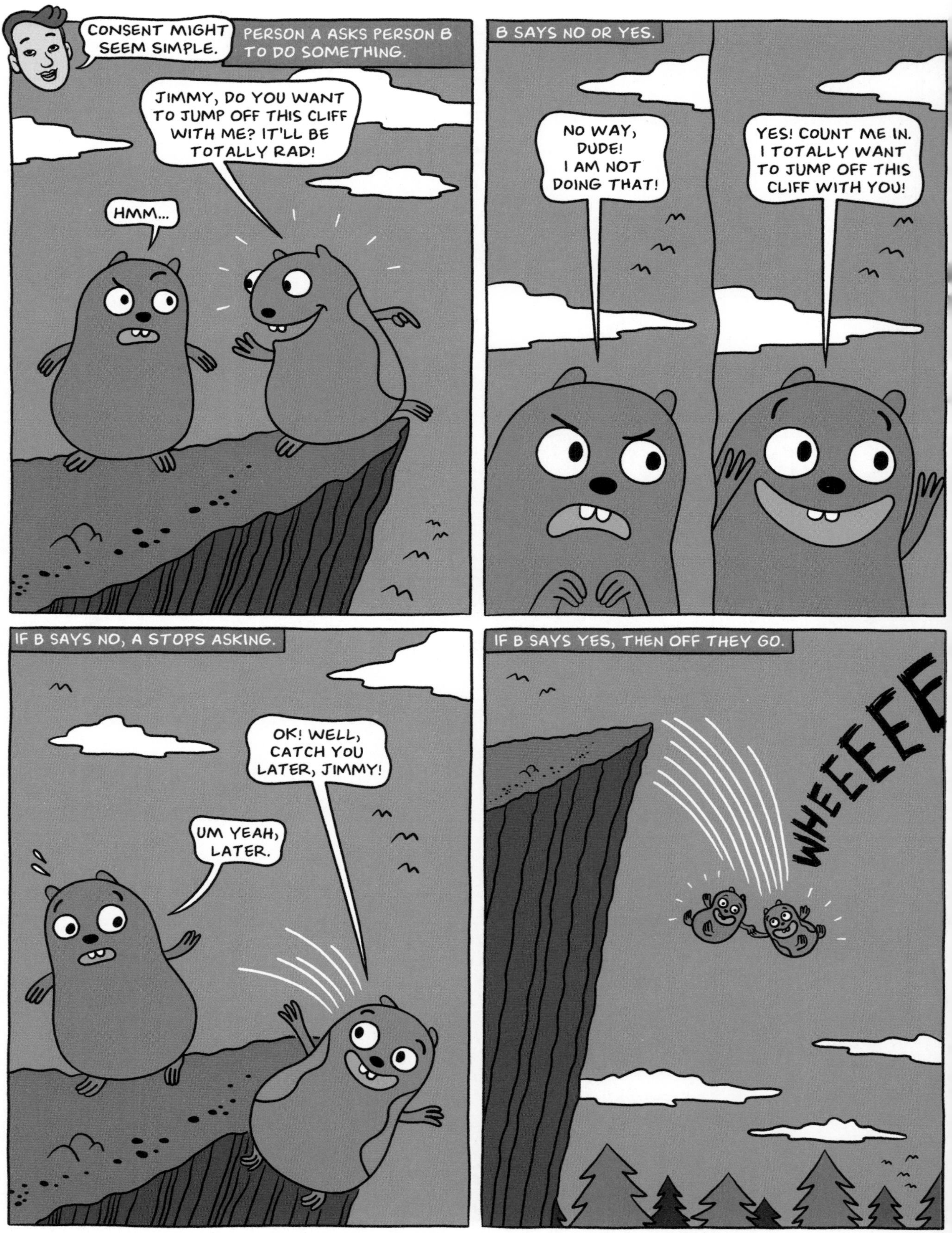
CONSENT MIGHT SEEM SIMPLE.
PERSON A ASKS PERSON B TO DO SOMETHING.
JIMMY, DO YOU WANT TO JUMP OFF THIS CLIFF WITH ME? IT'LL BE TOTALLY RAD!
HMM...
B SAYS NO OR YES.
NO WAY, DUDE! I AM NOT DOING THAT!
YES! COUNT ME IN. I TOTALLY WANT TO JUMP OFF THIS CLIFF WITH YOU!
IF B SAYS NO, A STOPS ASKING.
OK! WELL, CATCH YOU LATER, JIMMY!
UM YEAH, LATER.
IF B SAYS YES, THEN OFF THEY GO.
WHEEEEE

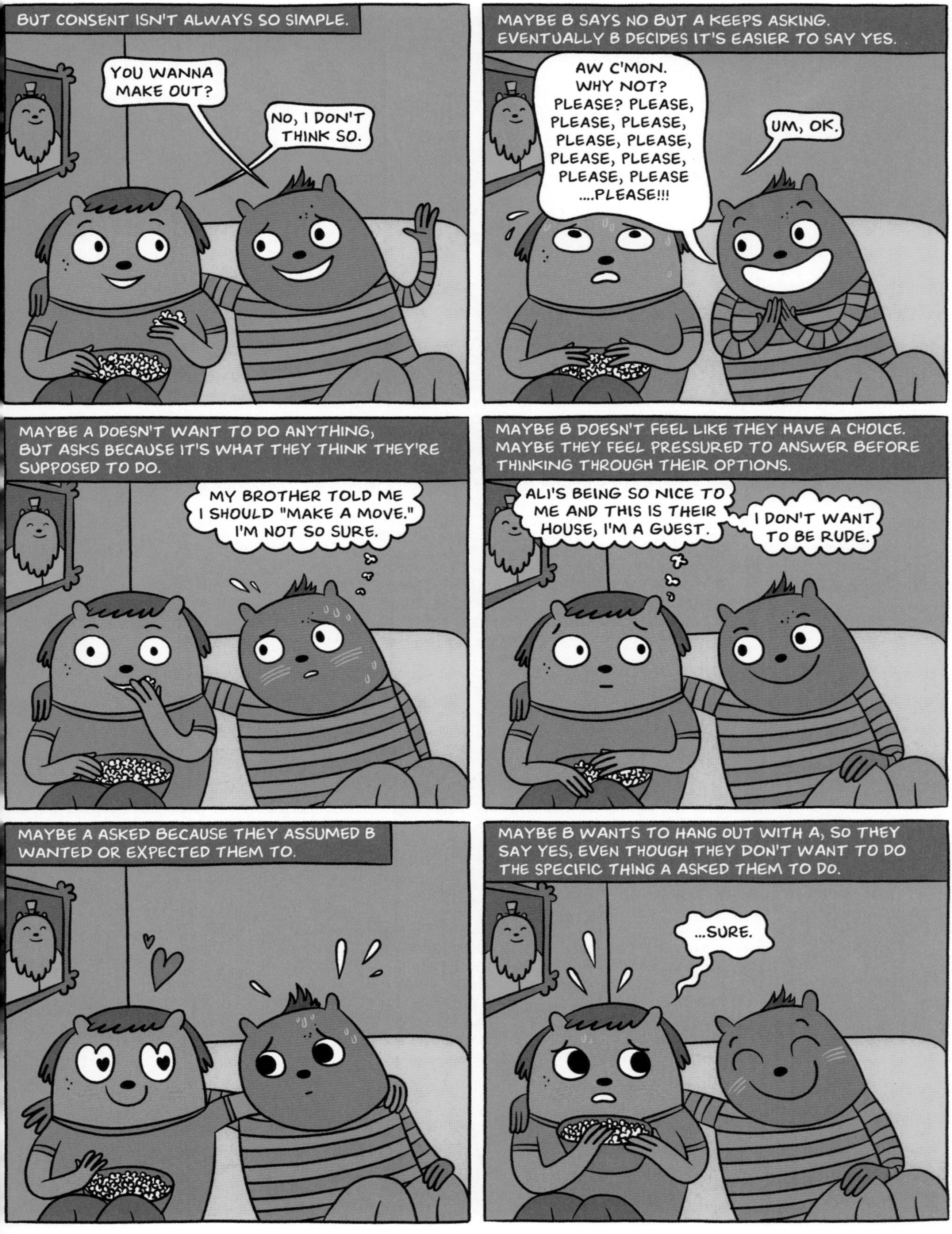
BUT CONSENT ISN'T ALWAYS SO SIMPLE.
YOU WANNA MAKE OUT?
NO, I DON'T THINK SO.
MAYBE B SAYS NO BUT A KEEPS ASKING. EVENTUALLY B DECIDES IT'S EASIER TO SAY YES.
AW C'MON. WHY NOT? PLEASE? PLEASE, PLEASE, PLEASE, PLEASE, PLEASE, PLEASE, PLEASE, PLEASE, PLEASE ....PLEASE!!!
UM, OK.
MAYBE A DOESN'T WANT TO DO ANYTHING, BUT ASKS BECAUSE IT'S WHAT THEY THINK THEY'RE SUPPOSED TO DO.
MY BROTHER TOLD ME I SHOULD "MAKE A MOVE." I'M NOT SO SURE.
MAYBE B DOESN'T FEEL LIKE THEY HAVE A CHOICE. MAYBE THEY FEEL PRESSURED TO ANSWER BEFORE THINKING THROUGH THEIR OPTIONS.
ALI'S BEING SO NICE TO ME AND THIS IS THEIR HOUSE, I'M A GUEST.
I DON'T WANT TO BE RUDE.
MAYBE A ASKED BECAUSE THEY ASSUMED B WANTED OR EXPECTED THEM TO.
MAYBE B WANTS TO HANG OUT WITH A, SO THEY SAY YES, EVEN THOUGH THEY DON'T WANT TO DO THE SPECIFIC THING A ASKED THEM TO DO.
...SURE.

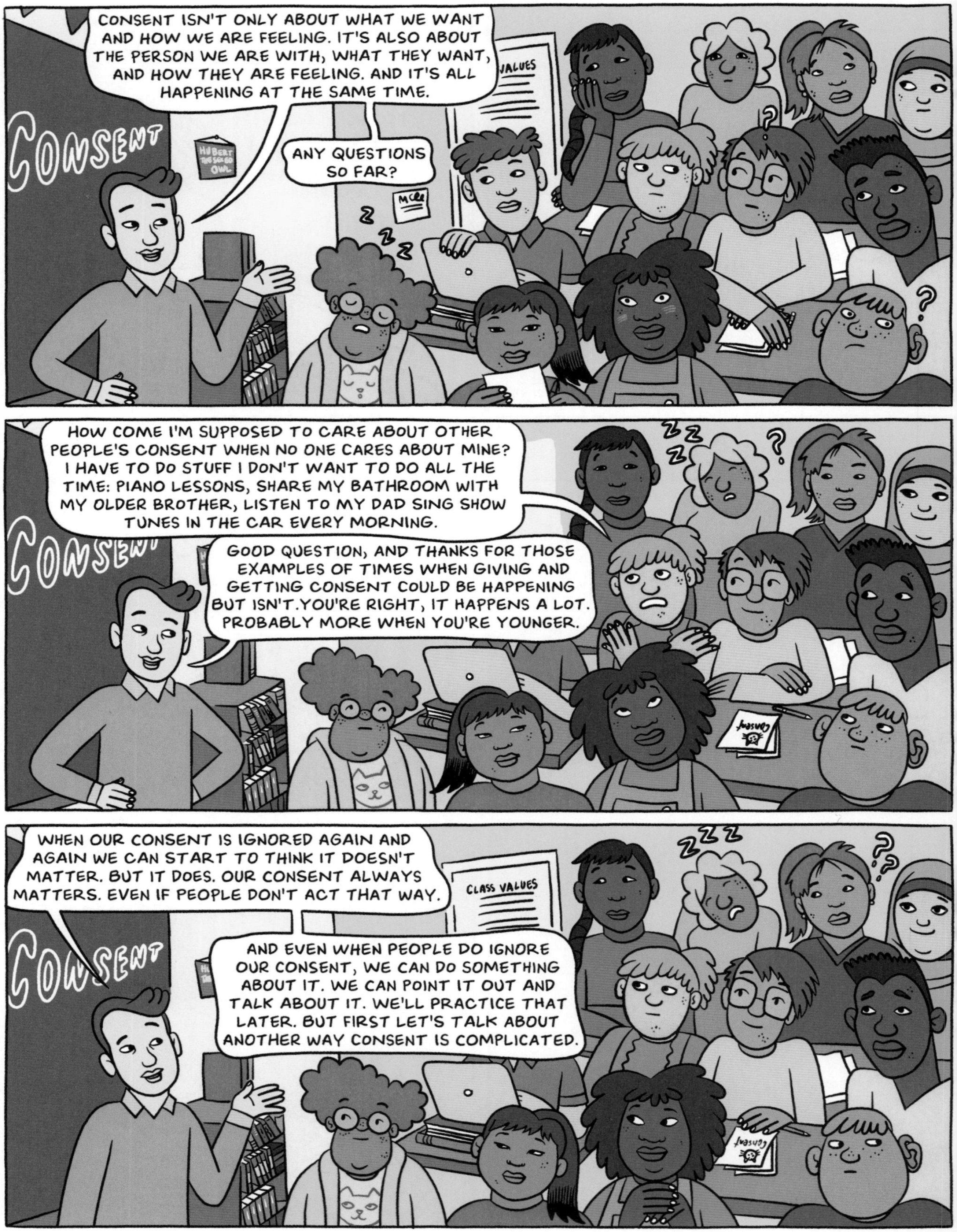
CONSENT ISN'T ONLY ABOUT WHAT WE WANT AND HOW WE ARE FEELING. IT'S ALSO ABOUT THE PERSON WE ARE WITH, WHAT THEY WANT, AND HOW THEY ARE FEELING. AND IT'S ALL HAPPENING AT THE SAME TIME.
ANY QUESTIONS SO FAR?
CONSENT
VALUES
HOW COME I'M SUPPOSED TO CARE ABOUT OTHER PEOPLE'S CONSENT WHEN NO ONE CARES ABOUT MINE? I HAVE TO DO STUFF I DON'T WANT TO DO ALL THE TIME: PIANO LESSONS, SHARE MY BATHROOM WITH MY OLDER BROTHER, LISTEN TO MY DAD SING SHOW TUNES IN THE CAR EVERY MORNING.
GOOD QUESTION, AND THANKS FOR THOSE EXAMPLES OF TIMES WHEN GIVING AND GETTING CONSENT COULD BE HAPPENING BUT ISN'T. YOU'RE RIGHT, IT HAPPENS A LOT. PROBABLY MORE WHEN YOU'RE YOUNGER.
WHEN OUR CONSENT IS IGNORED AGAIN AND AGAIN WE CAN START TO THINK IT DOESN'T MATTER. BUT IT DOES. OUR CONSENT ALWAYS MATTERS. EVEN IF PEOPLE DON'T ACT THAT WAY.
CLASS VALUES
AND EVEN WHEN PEOPLE DO IGNORE OUR CONSENT, WE CAN DO SOMETHING ABOUT IT. WE CAN POINT IT OUT AND TALK ABOUT IT. WE'LL PRACTICE THAT LATER. BUT FIRST LET'S TALK ABOUT ANOTHER WAY CONSENT IS COMPLICATED.

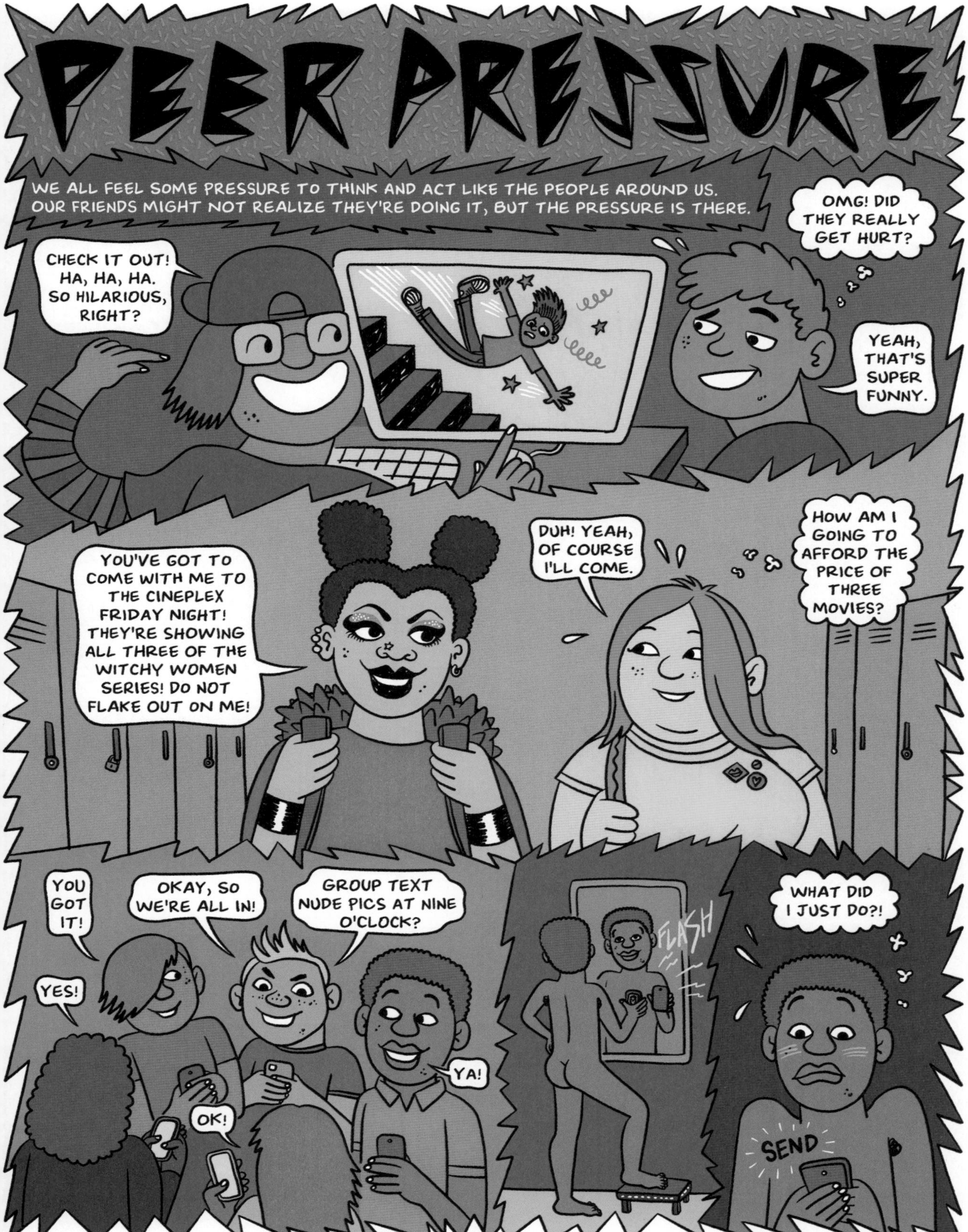
PEER PRESSURE
WE ALL FEEL SOME PRESSURE TO THINK AND ACT LIKE THE PEOPLE AROUND US. OUR FRIENDS MIGHT NOT REALIZE THEY'RE DOING IT, BUT THE PRESSURE IS THERE.
CHECK IT OUT! HA, HA, HA. SO HILARIOUS, RIGHT?
OMG! DID THEY REALLY GET HURT?
YEAH, THAT'S SUPER FUNNY.
YOU'VE GOT TO COME WITH ME TO THE CINEPLEX FRIDAY NIGHT! THEY'RE SHOWING ALL THREE OF THE WITCHY WOMEN SERIES! DO NOT FLAKE OUT ON ME!
DUH! YEAH, OF COURSE I'LL COME.
HOW AM I GOING TO AFFORD THE PRICE OF THREE MOVIES?
YOU GOT IT!
OKAY, SO WE'RE ALL IN!
GROUP TEXT NUDE PICS AT NINE O'CLOCK?
YES!
YA!
OK!
FLASH
WHAT DID I JUST DO?!
SEND

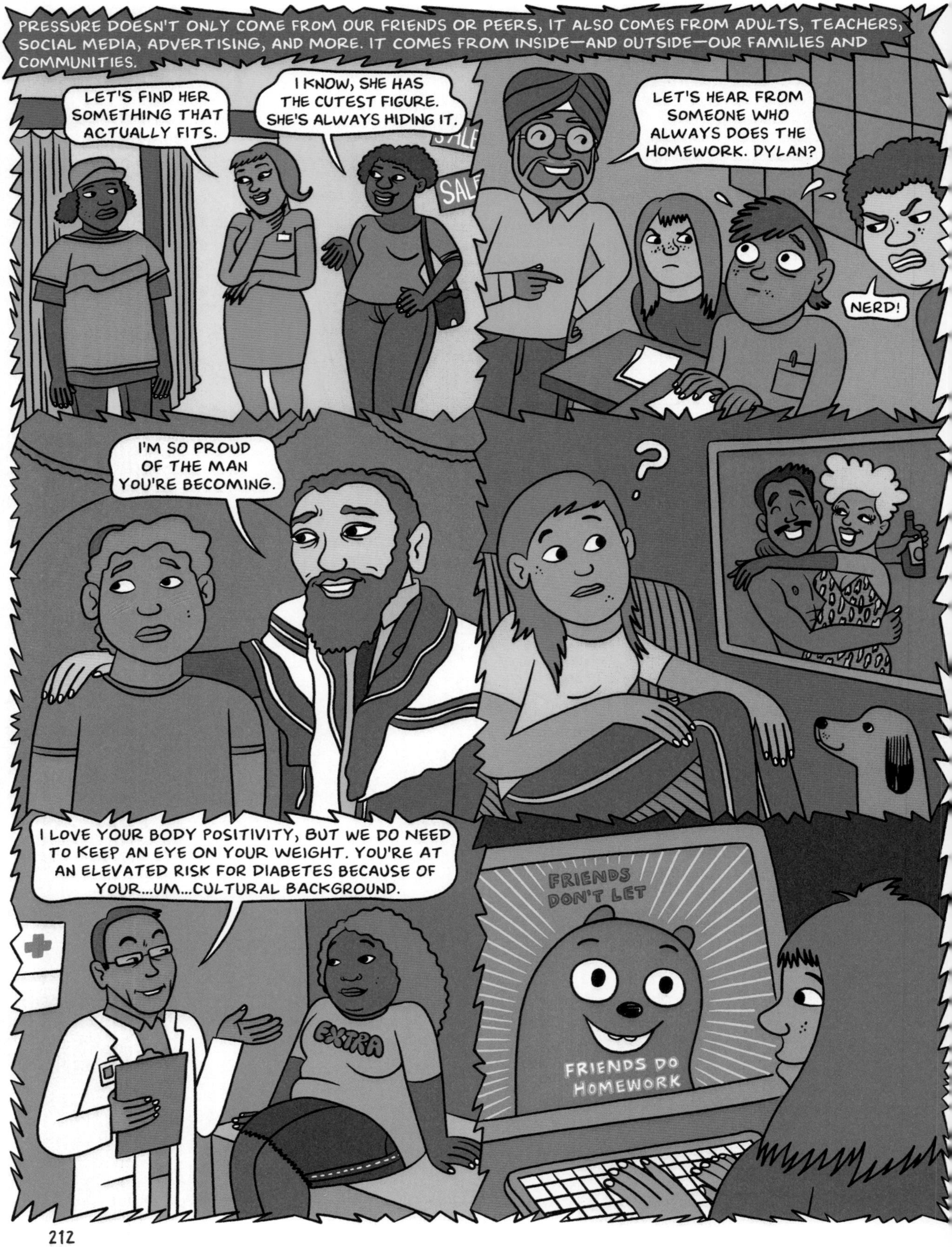
PRESSURE DOESN'T ONLY COME FROM OUR FRIENDS OR PEERS, IT ALSO COMES FROM ADULTS, TEACHERS, SOCIAL MEDIA, ADVERTISING, AND MORE. IT COMES FROM INSIDE—AND OUTSIDE—OUR FAMILIES AND COMMUNITIES.
LET'S FIND HER SOMETHING THAT ACTUALLY FITS.
I KNOW, SHE HAS THE CUTEST FIGURE. SHE'S ALWAYS HIDING IT.
SALE
SALE
LET'S HEAR FROM SOMEONE WHO ALWAYS DOES THE HOMEWORK. DYLAN?
NERD!
I'M SO PROUD OF THE MAN YOU'RE BECOMING.
?
I LOVE YOUR BODY POSITIVITY, BUT WE DO NEED TO KEEP AN EYE ON YOUR WEIGHT. YOU'RE AT AN ELEVATED RISK FOR DIABETES BECAUSE OF YOUR...UM...CULTURAL BACKGROUND.
EXTRA
FRIENDS DON'T LET
FRIENDS DO HOMEWORK

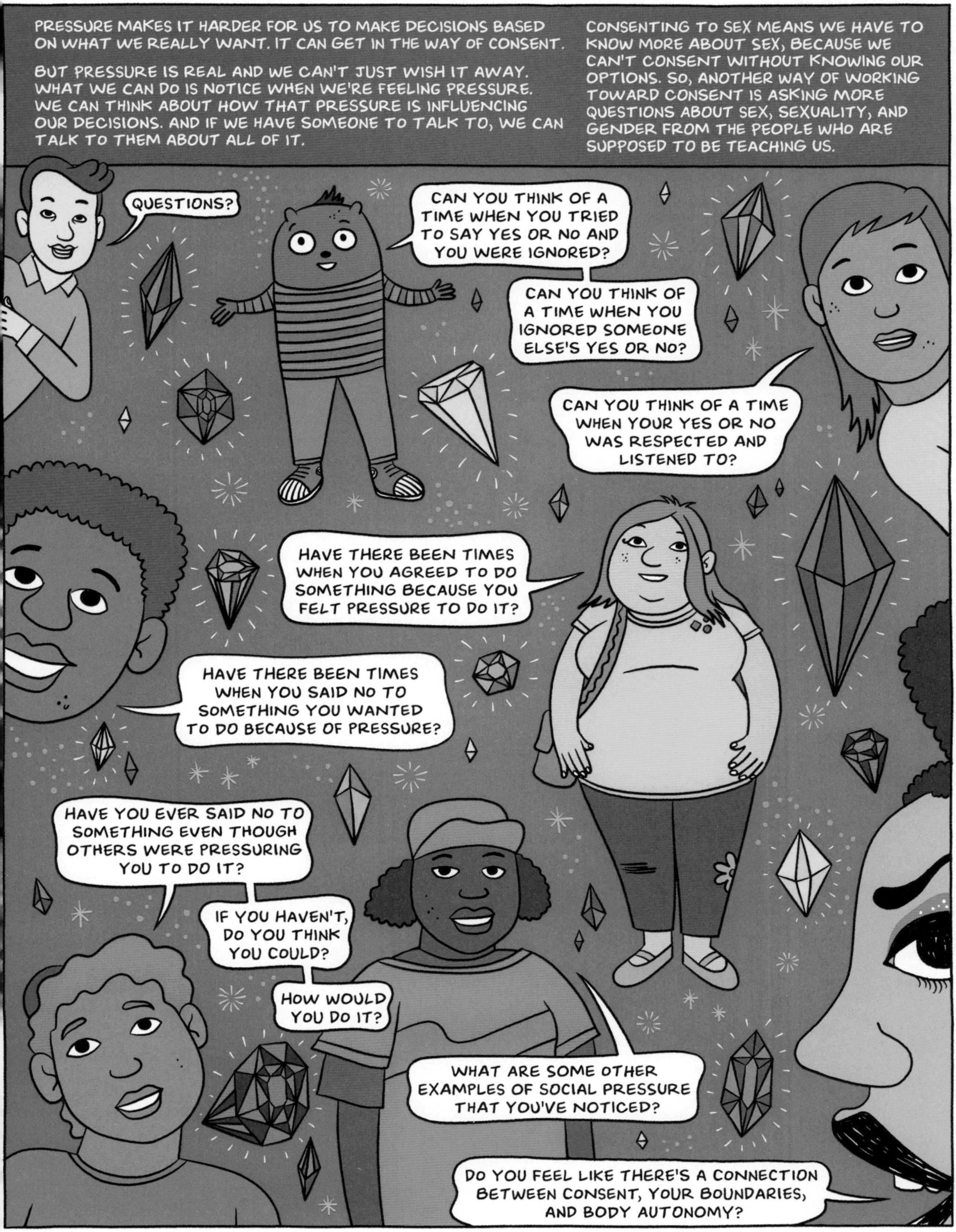
PRESSURE MAKES IT HARDER FOR US TO MAKE DECISIONS BASED ON WHAT WE REALLY WANT. IT CAN GET IN THE WAY OF CONSENT.
BUT PRESSURE IS REAL AND WE CAN'T JUST WISH IT AWAY. WHAT WE CAN DO IS NOTICE WHEN WE'RE FEELING PRESSURE. WE CAN THINK ABOUT HOW THAT PRESSURE IS INFLUENCING OUR DECISIONS. AND IF WE HAVE SOMEONE TO TALK TO, WE CAN TALK TO THEM ABOUT ALL OF IT.
CONSENTING TO SEX MEANS WE HAVE TO KNOW MORE ABOUT SEX, BECAUSE WE CAN'T CONSENT WITHOUT KNOWING OUR OPTIONS. SO, ANOTHER WAY OF WORKING TOWARD CONSENT IS ASKING MORE QUESTIONS ABOUT SEX, SEXUALITY, AND GENDER FROM THE PEOPLE WHO ARE SUPPOSED TO BE TEACHING US.
QUESTIONS?
CAN YOU THINK OF A TIME WHEN YOU TRIED TO SAY YES OR NO AND YOU WERE IGNORED?
CAN YOU THINK OF A TIME WHEN YOU IGNORED SOMEONE ELSE'S YES OR NO?
CAN YOU THINK OF A TIME WHEN YOUR YES OR NO WAS RESPECTED AND LISTENED TO?
HAVE THERE BEEN TIMES WHEN YOU AGREED TO DO SOMETHING BECAUSE YOU FELT PRESSURE TO DO IT?
HAVE THERE BEEN TIMES WHEN YOU SAID NO TO SOMETHING YOU WANTED TO DO BECAUSE OF PRESSURE?
HAVE YOU EVER SAID NO TO SOMETHING EVEN THOUGH OTHERS WERE PRESSURING YOU TO DO IT?
IF YOU HAVEN'T, DO YOU THINK YOU COULD?
HOW WOULD YOU DO IT?
WHAT ARE SOME OTHER EXAMPLES OF SOCIAL PRESSURE THAT YOU'VE NOTICED?
DO YOU FEEL LIKE THERE'S A CONNECTION BETWEEN CONSENT, YOUR BOUNDARIES, AND BODY AUTONOMY?

NERD ALERT BODY AUTONOMY AND CONSENT

SOME PEOPLE DON'T GET WHY CONSENT MATTERS. IF THEY WANT SOMETHING AND CAN GET IT, WHY SHOULD THEY CARE IF SOMEONE ELSE ISN'T HAVING A GOOD TIME? IF THE OTHER PERSON ISN'T PUTTING UP A FIGHT, ISN'T THAT ENOUGH?

THE ANSWER IS NO. CONSENT ISN'T ONLY ABOUT PAYING ATTENTION TO SOMEONE WHO IS FIGHTING YOU OFF. IT'S ABOUT RESPECTING BODY AUTONOMY.* BODY AUTONOMY ONLY WORKS IF WE ALL RESPECT EACH OTHER'S BODIES AND DECISIONS. PAYING ATTENTION TO HOW OTHER PEOPLE ARE FEELING AND WHAT THEY ARE SAYING—WITH THEIR WORDS AND WITH THEIR BODIES—IS A WAY OF SHOWING RESPECT AND PRACTICING BODY AUTONOMY.

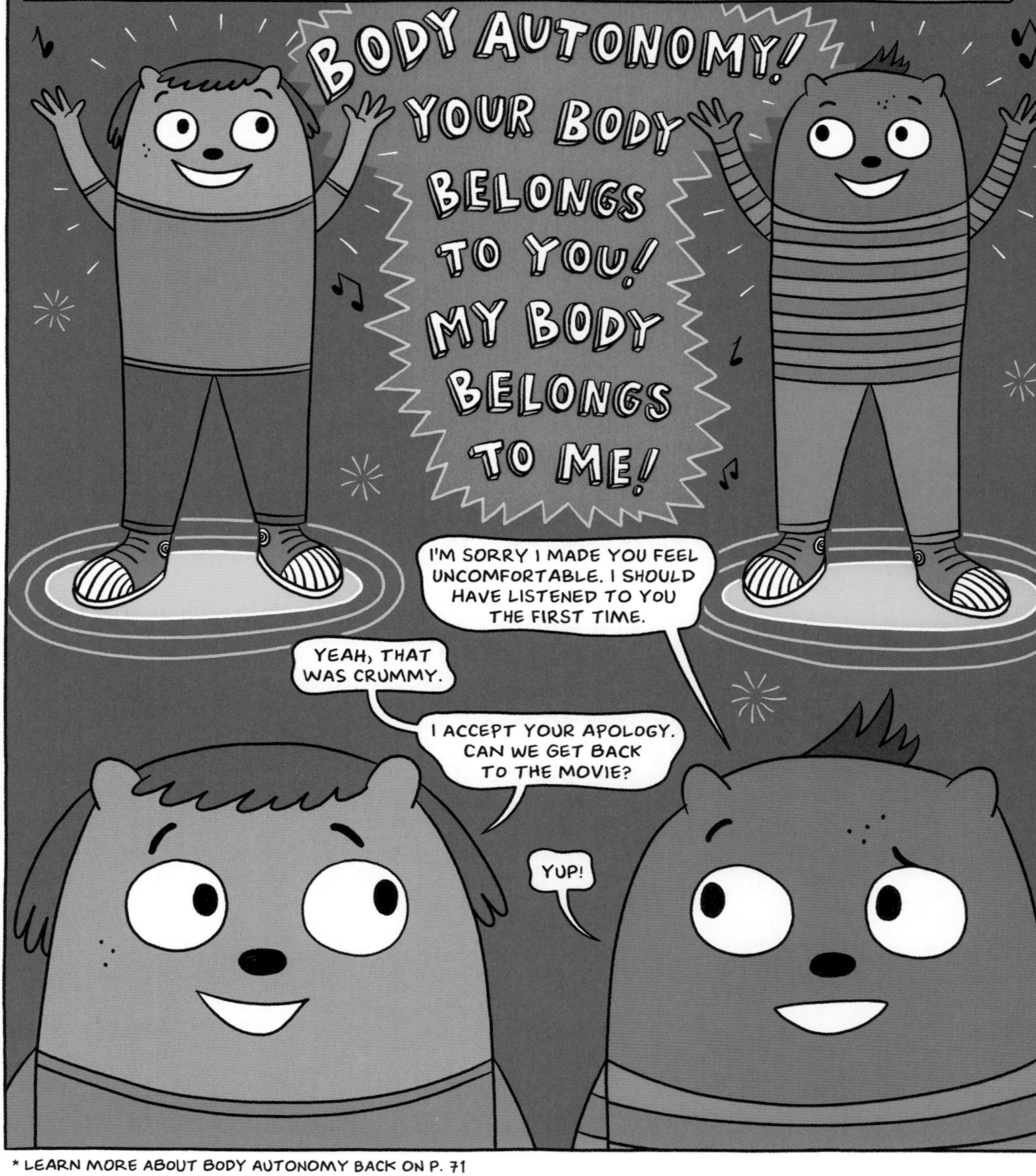
BODY AUTONOMY! YOUR BODY BELONGS TO YOU! MY BODY BELONGS TO ME!
I'M SORRY I MADE YOU FEEL UNCOMFORTABLE. I SHOULD HAVE LISTENED TO YOU THE FIRST TIME.
YEAH, THAT WAS CRUMMY.
I ACCEPT YOUR APOLOGY. CAN WE GET BACK TO THE MOVIE?
YUP!

* LEARN MORE ABOUT BODY AUTONOMY BACK ON P. 71

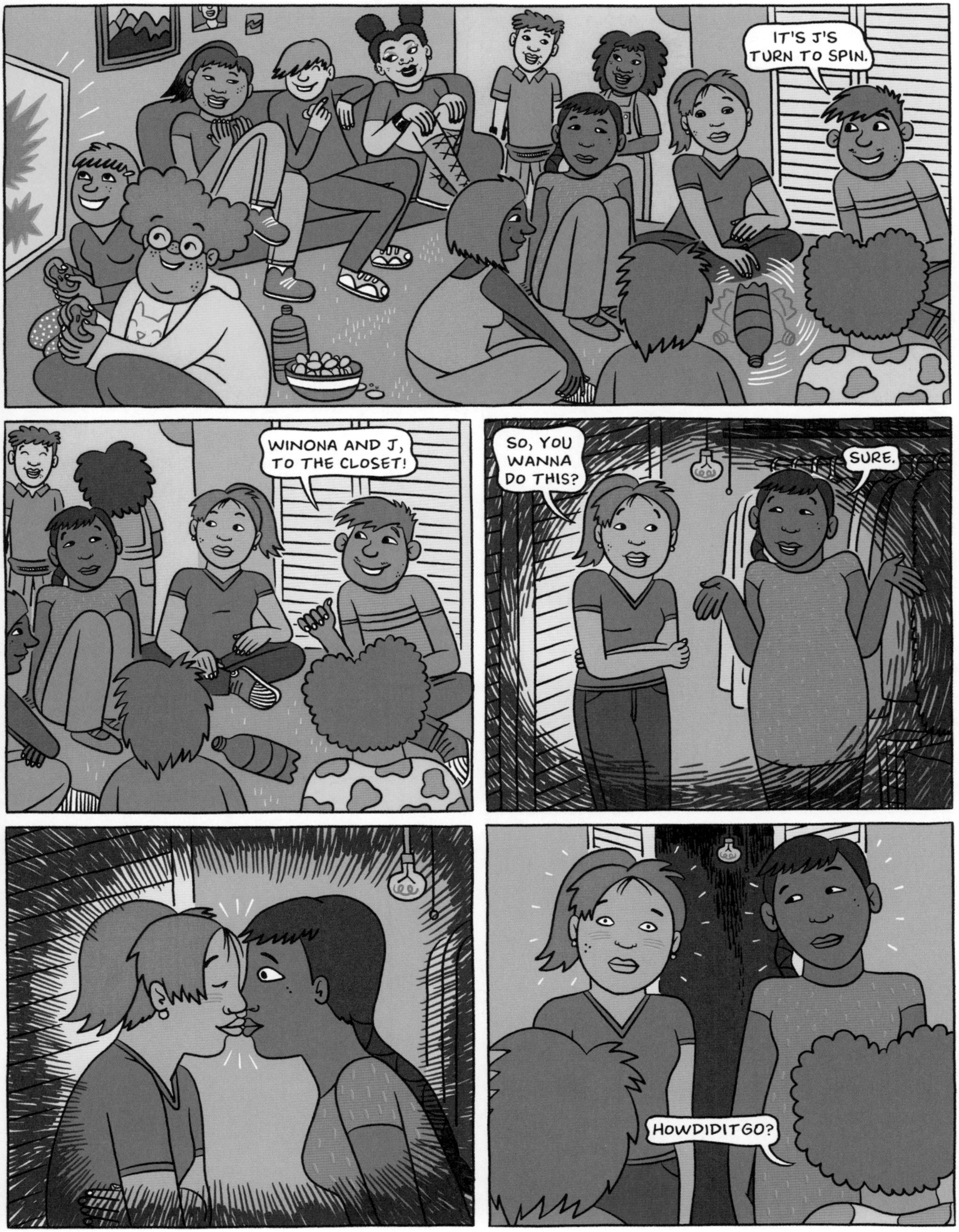
IT'S J'S TURN TO SPIN.
WINONA AND J, TO THE CLOSET!
SO, YOU WANNA DO THIS?
SURE.
HOWDIDITGO?

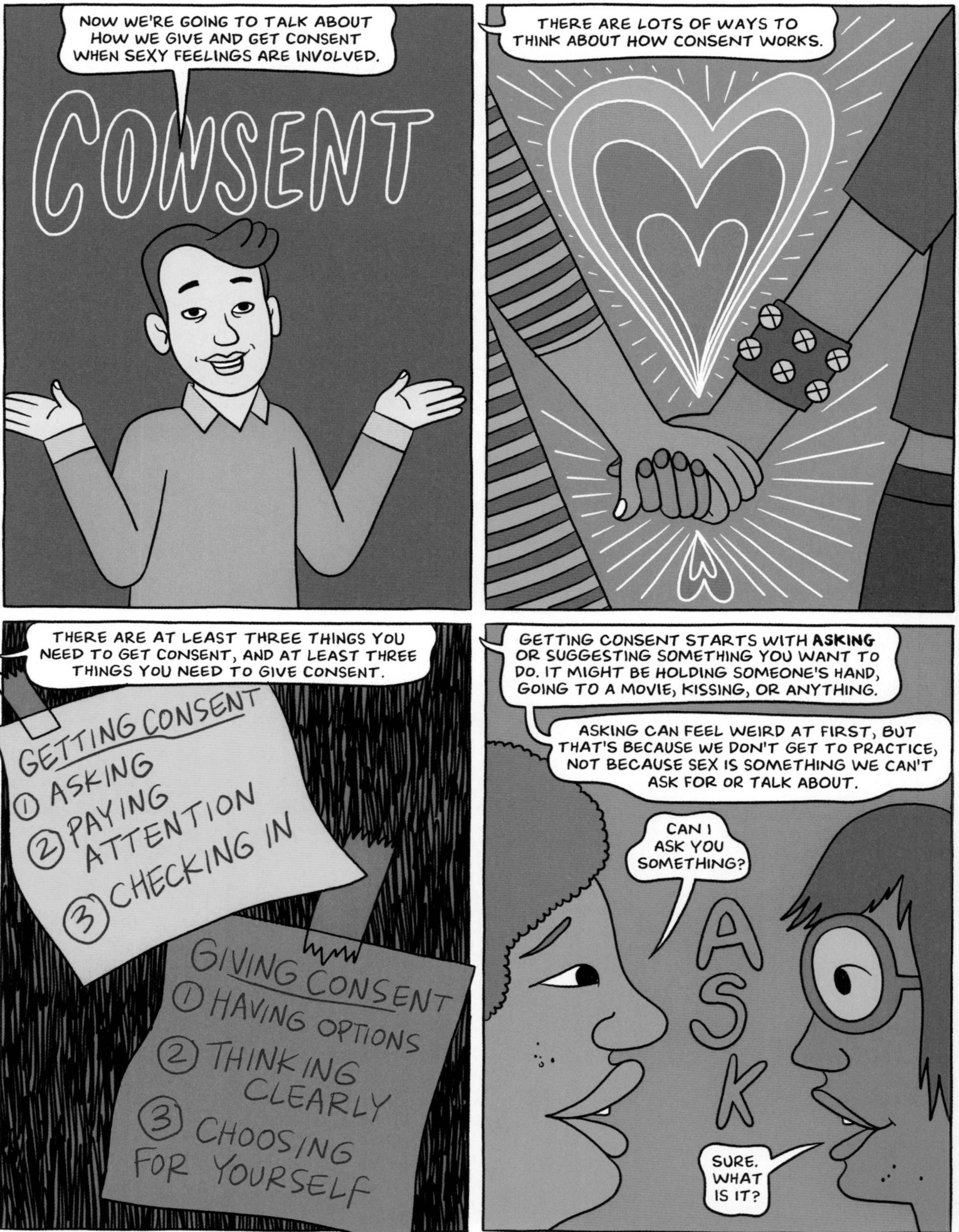
NOW WE'RE GOING TO TALK ABOUT HOW WE GIVE AND GET CONSENT WHEN SEXY FEELINGS ARE INVOLVED.
CONSENT
THERE ARE LOTS OF WAYS TO THINK ABOUT HOW CONSENT WORKS.
THERE ARE AT LEAST THREE THINGS YOU NEED TO GET CONSENT, AND AT LEAST THREE THINGS YOU NEED TO GIVE CONSENT.
GETTING CONSENT
① ASKING
② PAYING ATTENTION
③ CHECKING IN
GIVING CONSENT
① HAVING OPTIONS
② THINKING CLEARLY
③ CHOOSING FOR YOURSELF
GETTING CONSENT STARTS WITH **ASKING** OR SUGGESTING SOMETHING YOU WANT TO DO. IT MIGHT BE HOLDING SOMEONE'S HAND, GOING TO A MOVIE, KISSING, OR ANYTHING.
ASKING CAN FEEL WEIRD AT FIRST, BUT THAT'S BECAUSE WE DON'T GET TO PRACTICE, NOT BECAUSE SEX IS SOMETHING WE CAN'T ASK FOR OR TALK ABOUT.
CAN I ASK YOU SOMETHING?
ASK
SURE. WHAT IS IT?

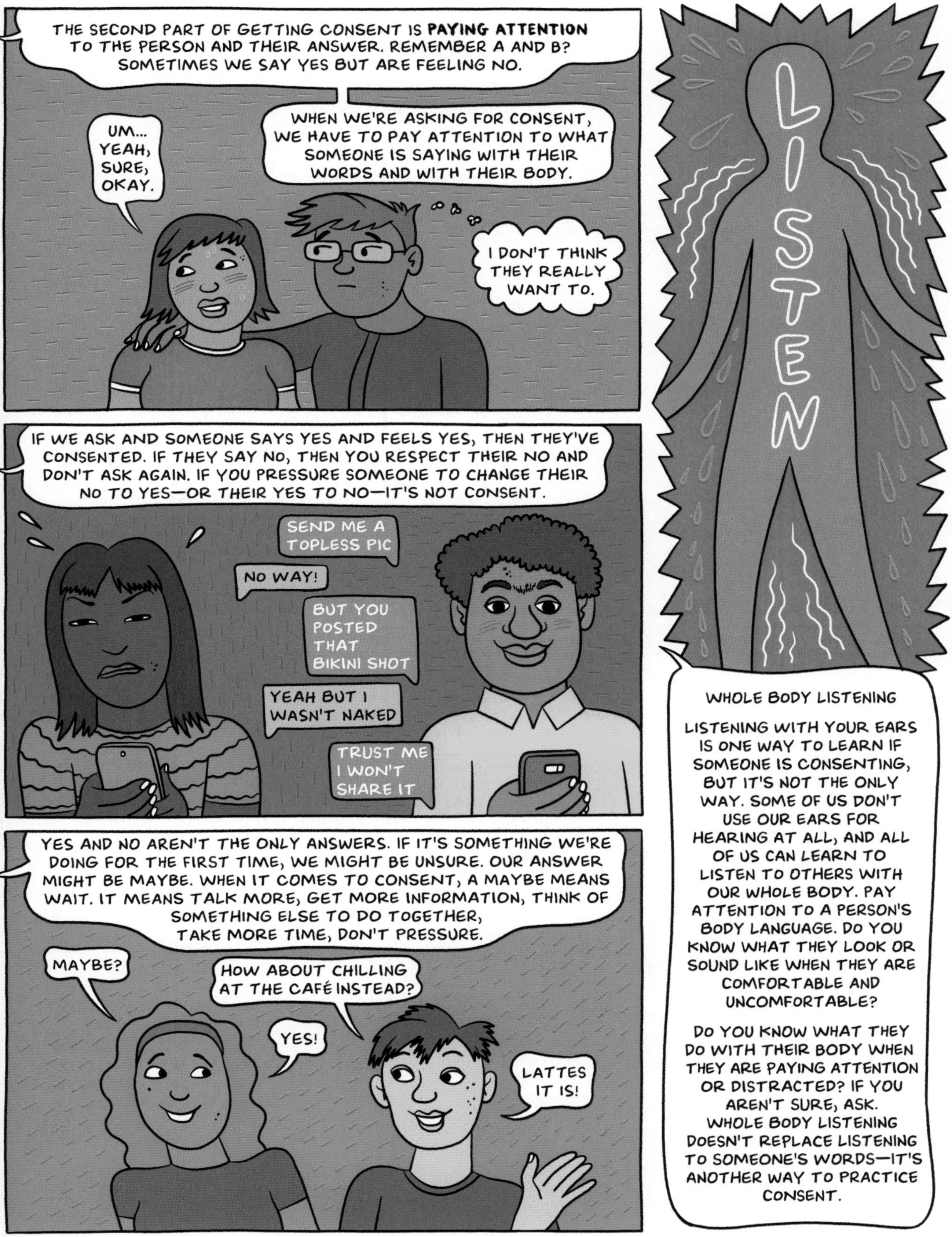
THE SECOND PART OF GETTING CONSENT IS **PAYING ATTENTION** TO THE PERSON AND THEIR ANSWER. REMEMBER A AND B? SOMETIMES WE SAY YES BUT ARE FEELING NO.
WHEN WE'RE ASKING FOR CONSENT, WE HAVE TO PAY ATTENTION TO WHAT SOMEONE IS SAYING WITH THEIR WORDS AND WITH THEIR BODY.
UM... YEAH, SURE, OKAY.
I DON'T THINK THEY REALLY WANT TO.
IF WE ASK AND SOMEONE SAYS YES AND FEELS YES, THEN THEY'VE CONSENTED. IF THEY SAY NO, THEN YOU RESPECT THEIR NO AND DON'T ASK AGAIN. IF YOU PRESSURE SOMEONE TO CHANGE THEIR NO TO YES—OR THEIR YES TO NO—IT'S NOT CONSENT.
SEND ME A TOPLESS PIC
NO WAY!
BUT YOU POSTED THAT BIKINI SHOT
YEAH BUT I WASN'T NAKED
TRUST ME I WON'T SHARE IT
YES AND NO AREN'T THE ONLY ANSWERS. IF IT'S SOMETHING WE'RE DOING FOR THE FIRST TIME, WE MIGHT BE UNSURE. OUR ANSWER MIGHT BE MAYBE. WHEN IT COMES TO CONSENT, A MAYBE MEANS WAIT. IT MEANS TALK MORE, GET MORE INFORMATION, THINK OF SOMETHING ELSE TO DO TOGETHER, TAKE MORE TIME, DON'T PRESSURE.
MAYBE?
HOW ABOUT CHILLING AT THE CAFÉ INSTEAD?
YES!
LATTES IT IS!
LISTEN
WHOLE BODY LISTENING
LISTENING WITH YOUR EARS IS ONE WAY TO LEARN IF SOMEONE IS CONSENTING, BUT IT'S NOT THE ONLY WAY. SOME OF US DON'T USE OUR EARS FOR HEARING AT ALL, AND ALL OF US CAN LEARN TO LISTEN TO OTHERS WITH OUR WHOLE BODY. PAY ATTENTION TO A PERSON'S BODY LANGUAGE. DO YOU KNOW WHAT THEY LOOK OR SOUND LIKE WHEN THEY ARE COMFORTABLE AND UNCOMFORTABLE?
DO YOU KNOW WHAT THEY DO WITH THEIR BODY WHEN THEY ARE PAYING ATTENTION OR DISTRACTED? IF YOU AREN'T SURE, ASK. WHOLE BODY LISTENING DOESN'T REPLACE LISTENING TO SOMEONE'S WORDS—IT'S ANOTHER WAY TO PRACTICE CONSENT.

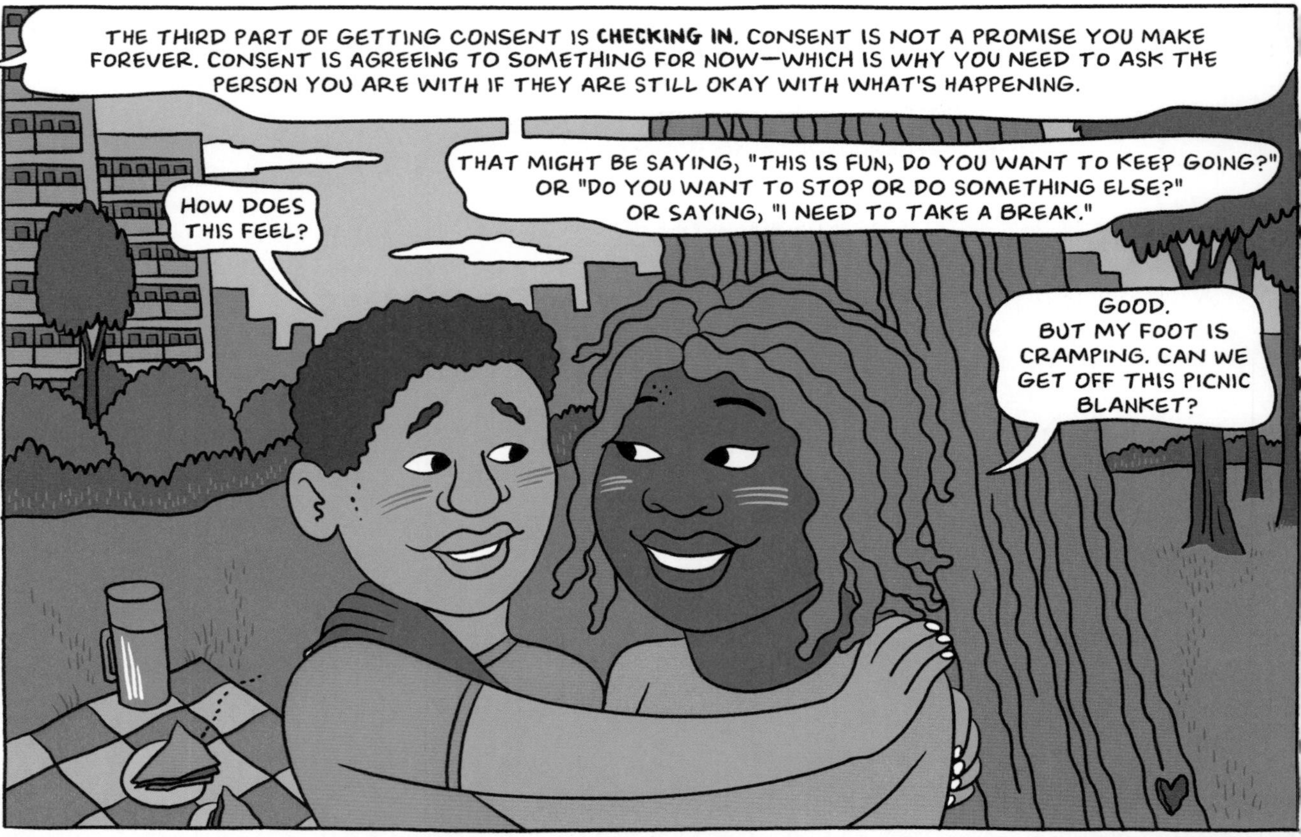
THE THIRD PART OF GETTING CONSENT IS **CHECKING IN**. CONSENT IS NOT A PROMISE YOU MAKE FOREVER. CONSENT IS AGREEING TO SOMETHING FOR NOW—WHICH IS WHY YOU NEED TO ASK THE PERSON YOU ARE WITH IF THEY ARE STILL OKAY WITH WHAT'S HAPPENING.
THAT MIGHT BE SAYING, "THIS IS FUN, DO YOU WANT TO KEEP GOING?" OR "DO YOU WANT TO STOP OR DO SOMETHING ELSE?" OR SAYING, "I NEED TO TAKE A BREAK."
HOW DOES THIS FEEL?
GOOD. BUT MY FOOT IS CRAMPING. CAN WE GET OFF THIS PICNIC BLANKET?

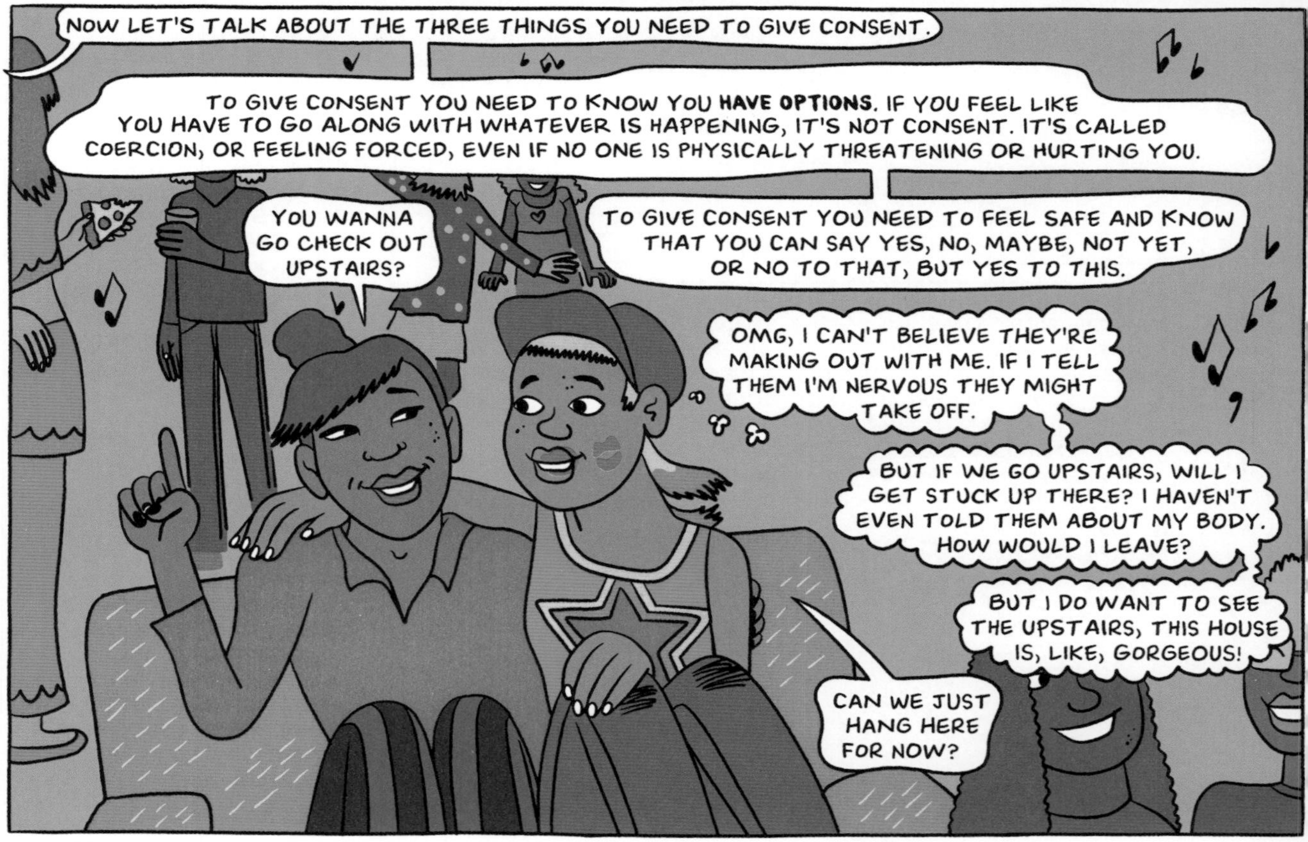
NOW LET'S TALK ABOUT THE THREE THINGS YOU NEED TO GIVE CONSENT.
TO GIVE CONSENT YOU NEED TO KNOW YOU **HAVE OPTIONS**. IF YOU FEEL LIKE YOU HAVE TO GO ALONG WITH WHATEVER IS HAPPENING, IT'S NOT CONSENT. IT'S CALLED COERCION, OR FEELING FORCED, EVEN IF NO ONE IS PHYSICALLY THREATENING OR HURTING YOU.
TO GIVE CONSENT YOU NEED TO FEEL SAFE AND KNOW THAT YOU CAN SAY YES, NO, MAYBE, NOT YET, OR NO TO THAT, BUT YES TO THIS.
YOU WANNA GO CHECK OUT UPSTAIRS?
OMG, I CAN'T BELIEVE THEY'RE MAKING OUT WITH ME. IF I TELL THEM I'M NERVOUS THEY MIGHT TAKE OFF.
BUT IF WE GO UPSTAIRS, WILL I GET STUCK UP THERE? I HAVEN'T EVEN TOLD THEM ABOUT MY BODY. HOW WOULD I LEAVE?
BUT I DO WANT TO SEE THE UPSTAIRS, THIS HOUSE IS, LIKE, GORGEOUS!
CAN WE JUST HANG HERE FOR NOW?

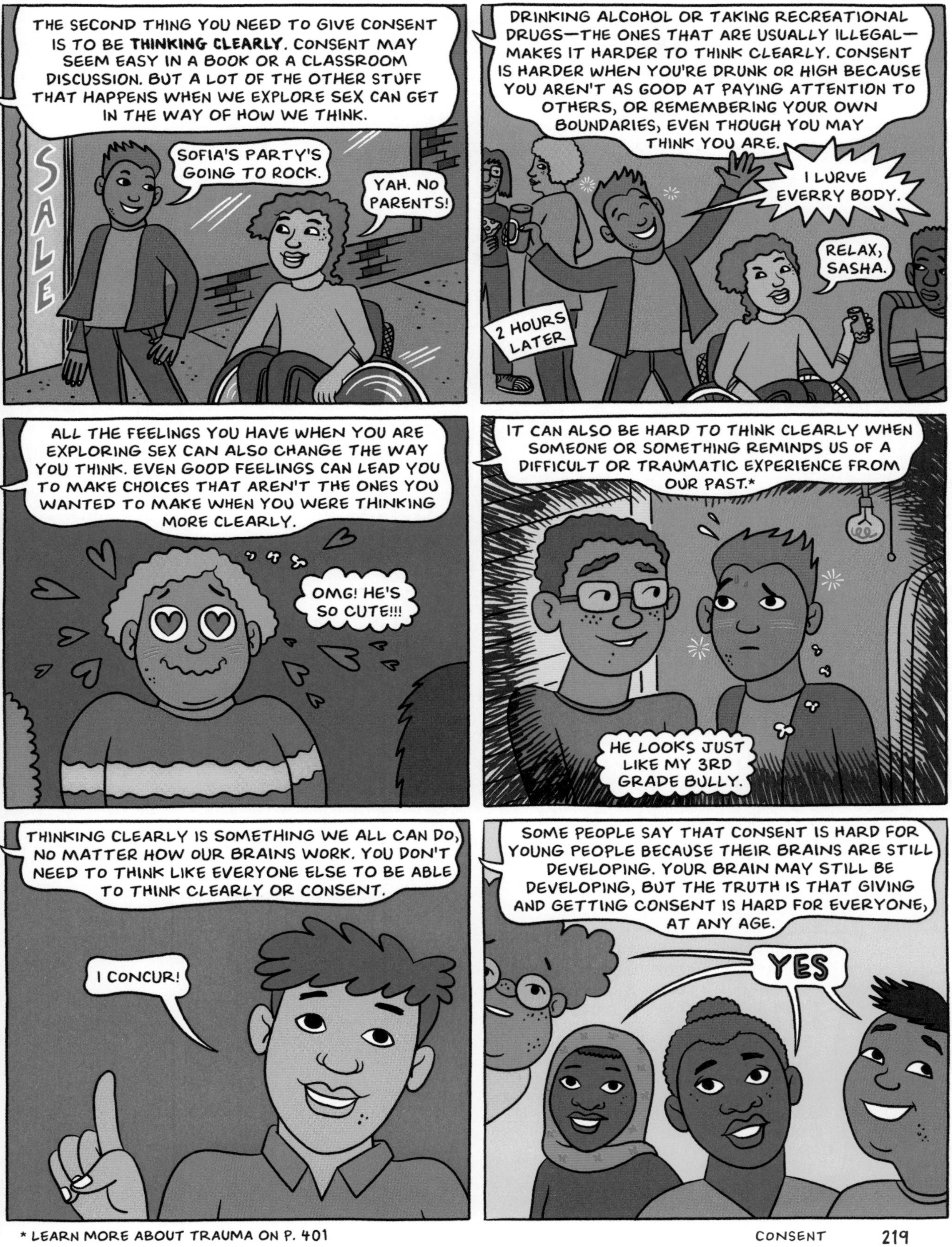
THE SECOND THING YOU NEED TO GIVE CONSENT IS TO BE **THINKING CLEARLY**. CONSENT MAY SEEM EASY IN A BOOK OR A CLASSROOM DISCUSSION. BUT A LOT OF THE OTHER STUFF THAT HAPPENS WHEN WE EXPLORE SEX CAN GET IN THE WAY OF HOW WE THINK.
SALE
SOFIA'S PARTY'S GOING TO ROCK.
YAH. NO PARENTS!
DRINKING ALCOHOL OR TAKING RECREATIONAL DRUGS—THE ONES THAT ARE USUALLY ILLEGAL—MAKES IT HARDER TO THINK CLEARLY. CONSENT IS HARDER WHEN YOU'RE DRUNK OR HIGH BECAUSE YOU AREN'T AS GOOD AT PAYING ATTENTION TO OTHERS, OR REMEMBERING YOUR OWN BOUNDARIES, EVEN THOUGH YOU MAY THINK YOU ARE.
2 HOURS LATER
I LURVE EVERRY BODY.
RELAX, SASHA.
ALL THE FEELINGS YOU HAVE WHEN YOU ARE EXPLORING SEX CAN ALSO CHANGE THE WAY YOU THINK. EVEN GOOD FEELINGS CAN LEAD YOU TO MAKE CHOICES THAT AREN'T THE ONES YOU WANTED TO MAKE WHEN YOU WERE THINKING MORE CLEARLY.
OMG! HE'S SO CUTE!!!
IT CAN ALSO BE HARD TO THINK CLEARLY WHEN SOMEONE OR SOMETHING REMINDS US OF A DIFFICULT OR TRAUMATIC EXPERIENCE FROM OUR PAST.*
HE LOOKS JUST LIKE MY 3RD GRADE BULLY.
THINKING CLEARLY IS SOMETHING WE ALL CAN DO, NO MATTER HOW OUR BRAINS WORK. YOU DON'T NEED TO THINK LIKE EVERYONE ELSE TO BE ABLE TO THINK CLEARLY OR CONSENT.
I CONCUR!
SOME PEOPLE SAY THAT CONSENT IS HARD FOR YOUNG PEOPLE BECAUSE THEIR BRAINS ARE STILL DEVELOPING. YOUR BRAIN MAY STILL BE DEVELOPING, BUT THE TRUTH IS THAT GIVING AND GETTING CONSENT IS HARD FOR EVERYONE, AT ANY AGE.
YES

* LEARN MORE ABOUT TRAUMA ON P. 401

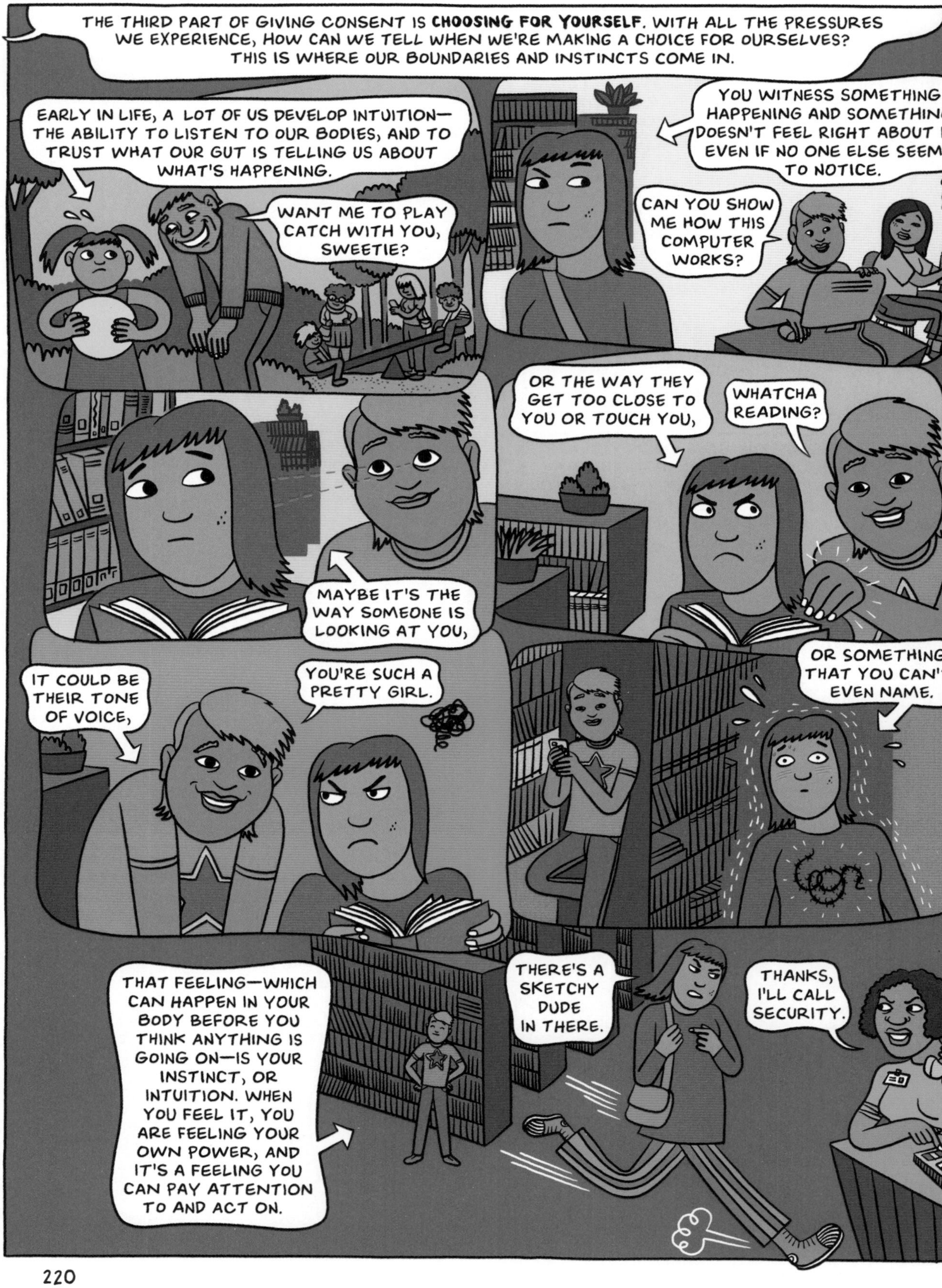
THE THIRD PART OF GIVING CONSENT IS **CHOOSING FOR YOURSELF**. WITH ALL THE PRESSURES WE EXPERIENCE, HOW CAN WE TELL WHEN WE'RE MAKING A CHOICE FOR OURSELVES? THIS IS WHERE OUR BOUNDARIES AND INSTINCTS COME IN.
EARLY IN LIFE, A LOT OF US DEVELOP INTUITION—THE ABILITY TO LISTEN TO OUR BODIES, AND TO TRUST WHAT OUR GUT IS TELLING US ABOUT WHAT'S HAPPENING.
WANT ME TO PLAY CATCH WITH YOU, SWEETIE?
YOU WITNESS SOMETHING HAPPENING AND SOMETHING DOESN'T FEEL RIGHT ABOUT IT, EVEN IF NO ONE ELSE SEEMS TO NOTICE.
CAN YOU SHOW ME HOW THIS COMPUTER WORKS?
?
MAYBE IT'S THE WAY SOMEONE IS LOOKING AT YOU,
OR THE WAY THEY GET TOO CLOSE TO YOU OR TOUCH YOU,
WHATCHA READING?
IT COULD BE THEIR TONE OF VOICE,
YOU'RE SUCH A PRETTY GIRL.
OR SOMETHING THAT YOU CAN'T EVEN NAME.
THAT FEELING—WHICH CAN HAPPEN IN YOUR BODY BEFORE YOU THINK ANYTHING IS GOING ON—IS YOUR INSTINCT, OR INTUITION. WHEN YOU FEEL IT, YOU ARE FEELING YOUR OWN POWER, AND IT'S A FEELING YOU CAN PAY ATTENTION TO AND ACT ON.
THERE'S A SKETCHY DUDE IN THERE.
THANKS, I'LL CALL SECURITY.

NERD ALERT INSTINCTS AND BIAS

LEARNING TO LISTEN TO YOUR INSTINCTS IS SOMETHING THAT YOU CAN DO TO KEEP YOURSELF, AND THE PEOPLE IN YOUR LIFE, SAFE. IT'S A SKILL TO BE PROUD OF. BUT NOT EVERY FEELING WE HAVE ABOUT OTHER PEOPLE COMES FROM INSIDE US. SOME OF THOSE FEELINGS ARE THINGS WE LEARNED.

THE WAY WE LOOK AT PEOPLE, AND JUDGE THEM TO BE SAFE OR DANGEROUS, HAS A LOT TO DO WITH THE DISCRIMINATION WE TALKED ABOUT IN THE BODY AUTONOMY CHAPTER (P. 71). SOME PEOPLE ARE TREATED AS SUSPICIOUS BECAUSE OF THEIR RACE, WHAT THEY LOOK LIKE, THEIR SIZE, HOW THEY TALK, HOW EASILY THEY FIT INTO THE GENDER BOXES OF MAN OR WOMAN, AND MORE. WHEN WE HOLD NEGATIVE BELIEFS ABOUT CERTAIN KINDS OF PEOPLE BECAUSE WE'VE BEEN RAISED TO BELIEVE THEM, IT'S CALLED BIAS. BEING SCARED OF SOMEONE BECAUSE WE'VE BEEN TAUGHT THEY LOOK DANGEROUS IS AN EXAMPLE OF BIAS.

SO IF WE GET A "BAD FEELING" ABOUT SOMEONE, HOW DO WE KNOW IF IT'S BECAUSE OF BIAS OR BECAUSE THEY WANT TO HARM US? THERE'S NO SIMPLE ANSWER.

WE NEED TO PAY ATTENTION AND LISTEN TO ALL OUR FEELINGS, AND WE ALSO NEED TO BE OPEN TO ASKING OURSELVES WHY WE FEEL THE WAY WE DO. OVER TIME, WE CAN LEARN THE DIFFERENCE BETWEEN WHAT TRUST AND BIAS FEELS LIKE IN OUR BODIES.

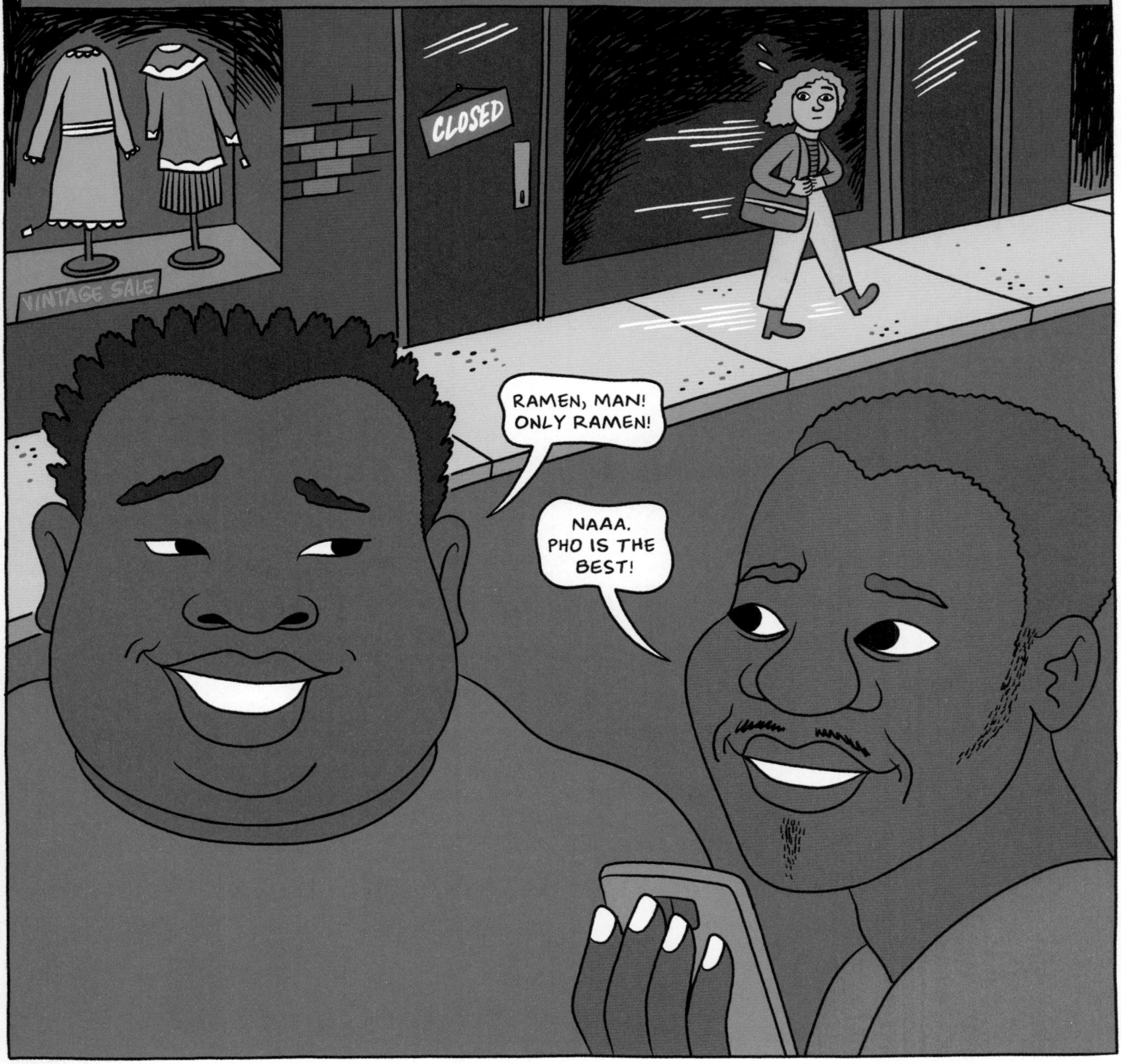
CLOSED
VINTAGE SALE
RAMEN, MAN! ONLY RAMEN!
NAAA. PHO IS THE BEST!

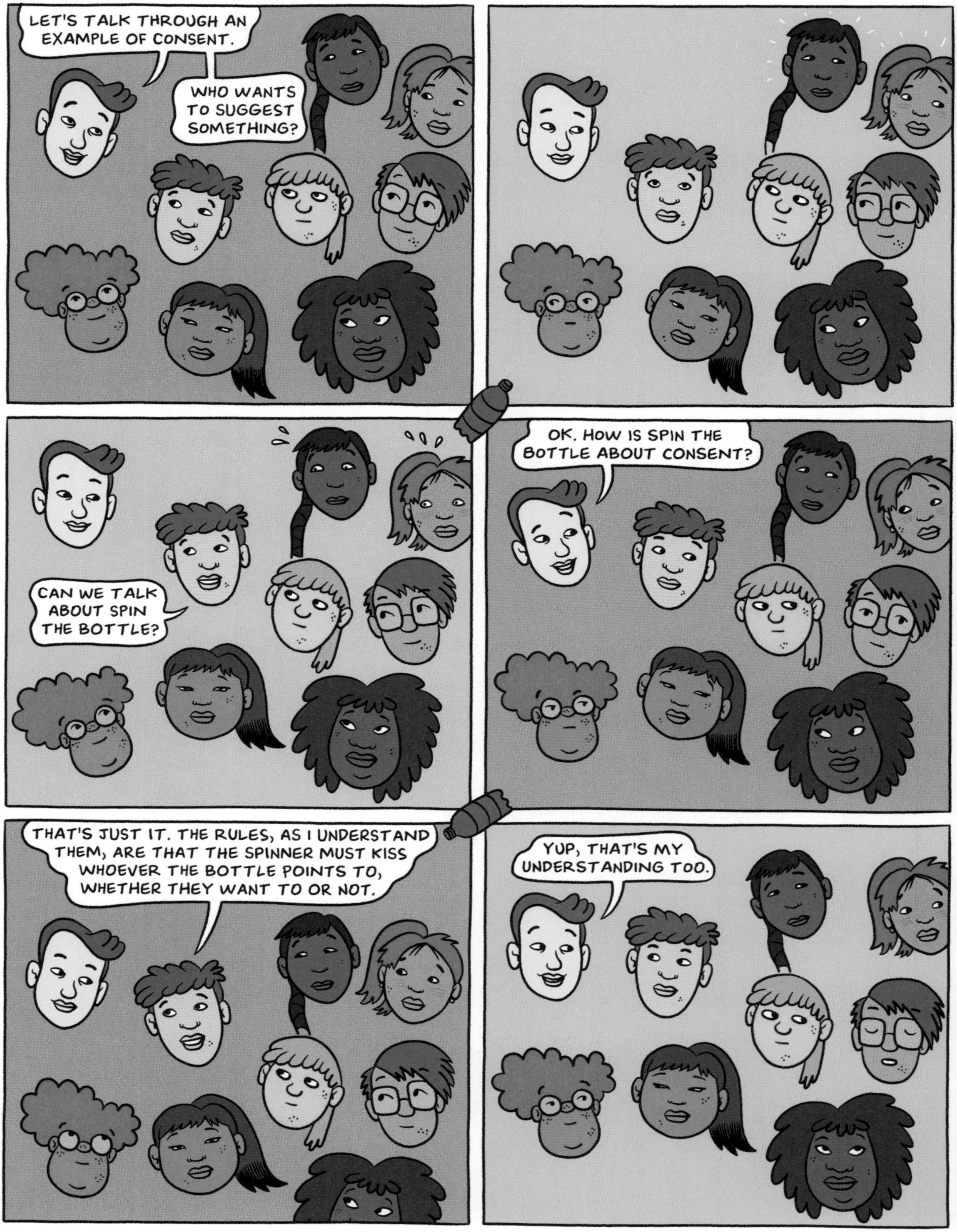
LET'S TALK THROUGH AN EXAMPLE OF CONSENT.
WHO WANTS TO SUGGEST SOMETHING?
CAN WE TALK ABOUT SPIN THE BOTTLE?
OK. HOW IS SPIN THE BOTTLE ABOUT CONSENT?
THAT'S JUST IT. THE RULES, AS I UNDERSTAND THEM, ARE THAT THE SPINNER MUST KISS WHOEVER THE BOTTLE POINTS TO, WHETHER THEY WANT TO OR NOT.
YUP, THAT'S MY UNDERSTANDING TOO.

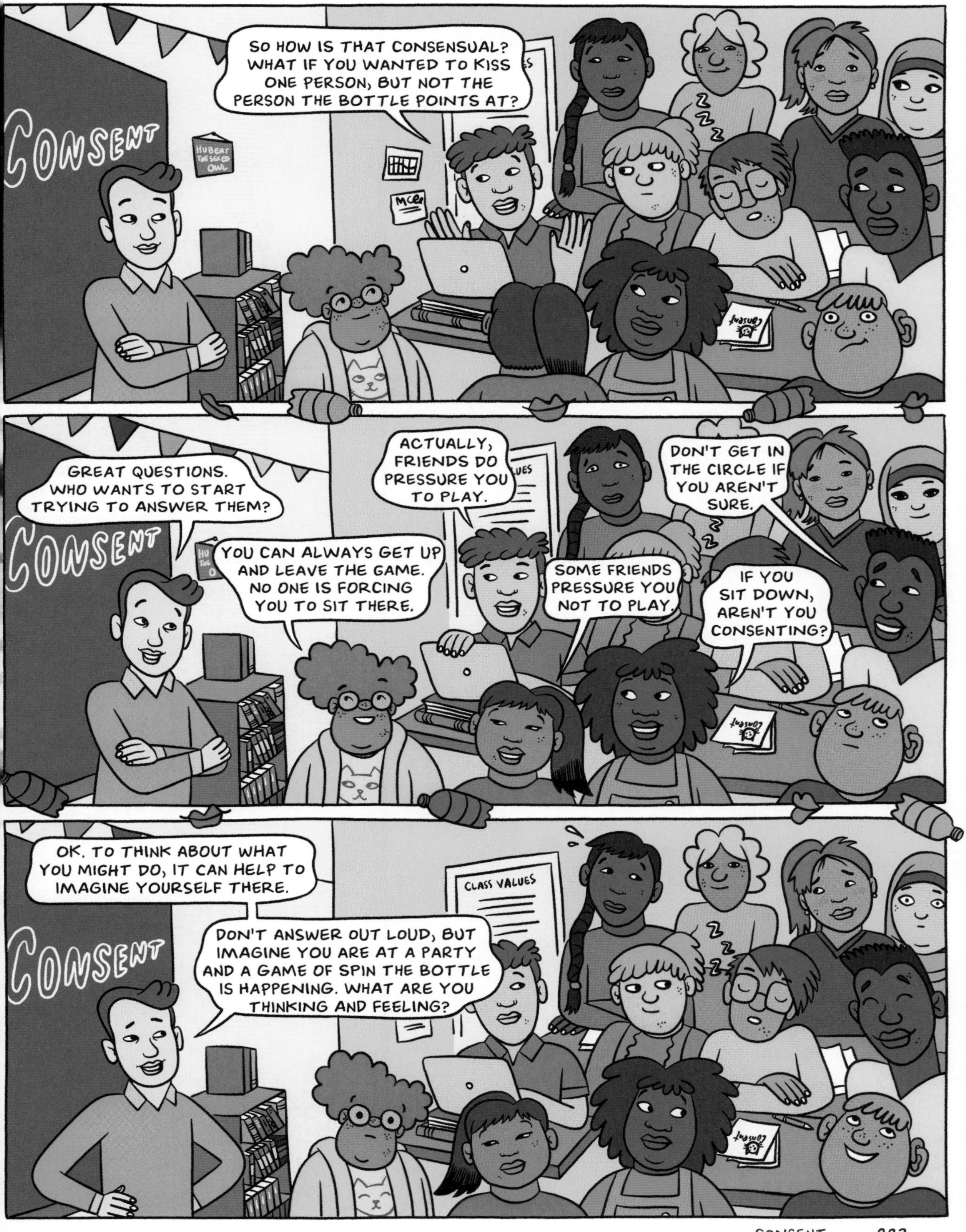
CONSENT
HUBERT THE SEXED OWL
SO HOW IS THAT CONSENSUAL? WHAT IF YOU WANTED TO KISS ONE PERSON, BUT NOT THE PERSON THE BOTTLE POINTS AT?
GREAT QUESTIONS. WHO WANTS TO START TRYING TO ANSWER THEM?
ACTUALLY, FRIENDS DO PRESSURE YOU TO PLAY.
DON'T GET IN THE CIRCLE IF YOU AREN'T SURE.
YOU CAN ALWAYS GET UP AND LEAVE THE GAME. NO ONE IS FORCING YOU TO SIT THERE.
SOME FRIENDS PRESSURE YOU NOT TO PLAY.
IF YOU SIT DOWN, AREN'T YOU CONSENTING?
OK. TO THINK ABOUT WHAT YOU MIGHT DO, IT CAN HELP TO IMAGINE YOURSELF THERE.
CLASS VALUES
DON'T ANSWER OUT LOUD, BUT IMAGINE YOU ARE AT A PARTY AND A GAME OF SPIN THE BOTTLE IS HAPPENING. WHAT ARE YOU THINKING AND FEELING?

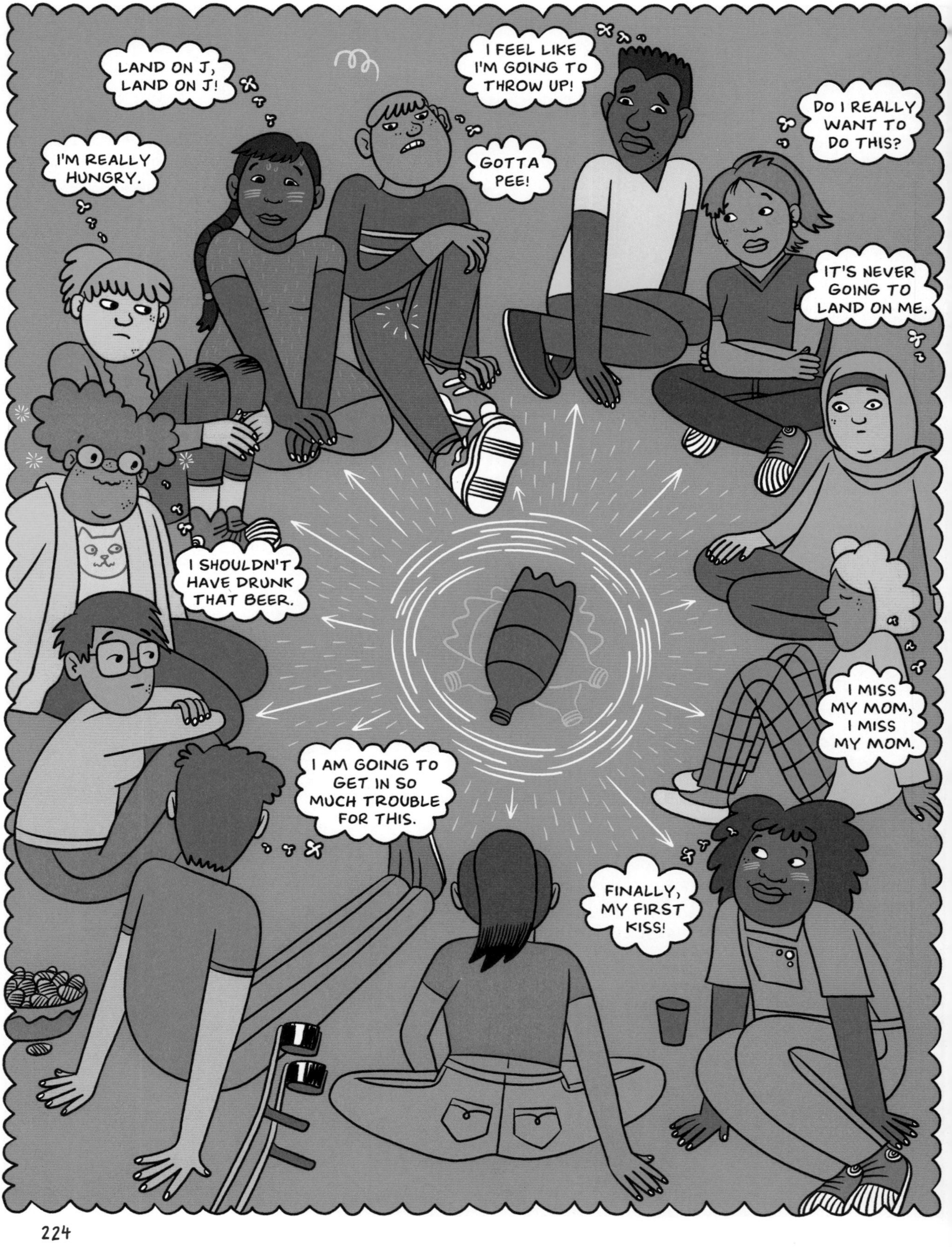
LAND ON J, LAND ON J!
I FEEL LIKE I'M GOING TO THROW UP!
DO I REALLY WANT TO DO THIS?
I'M REALLY HUNGRY.
GOTTA PEE!
IT'S NEVER GOING TO LAND ON ME.
I SHOULDN'T HAVE DRUNK THAT BEER.
I MISS MY MOM, I MISS MY MOM.
I AM GOING TO GET IN SO MUCH TROUBLE FOR THIS.
FINALLY, MY FIRST KISS!

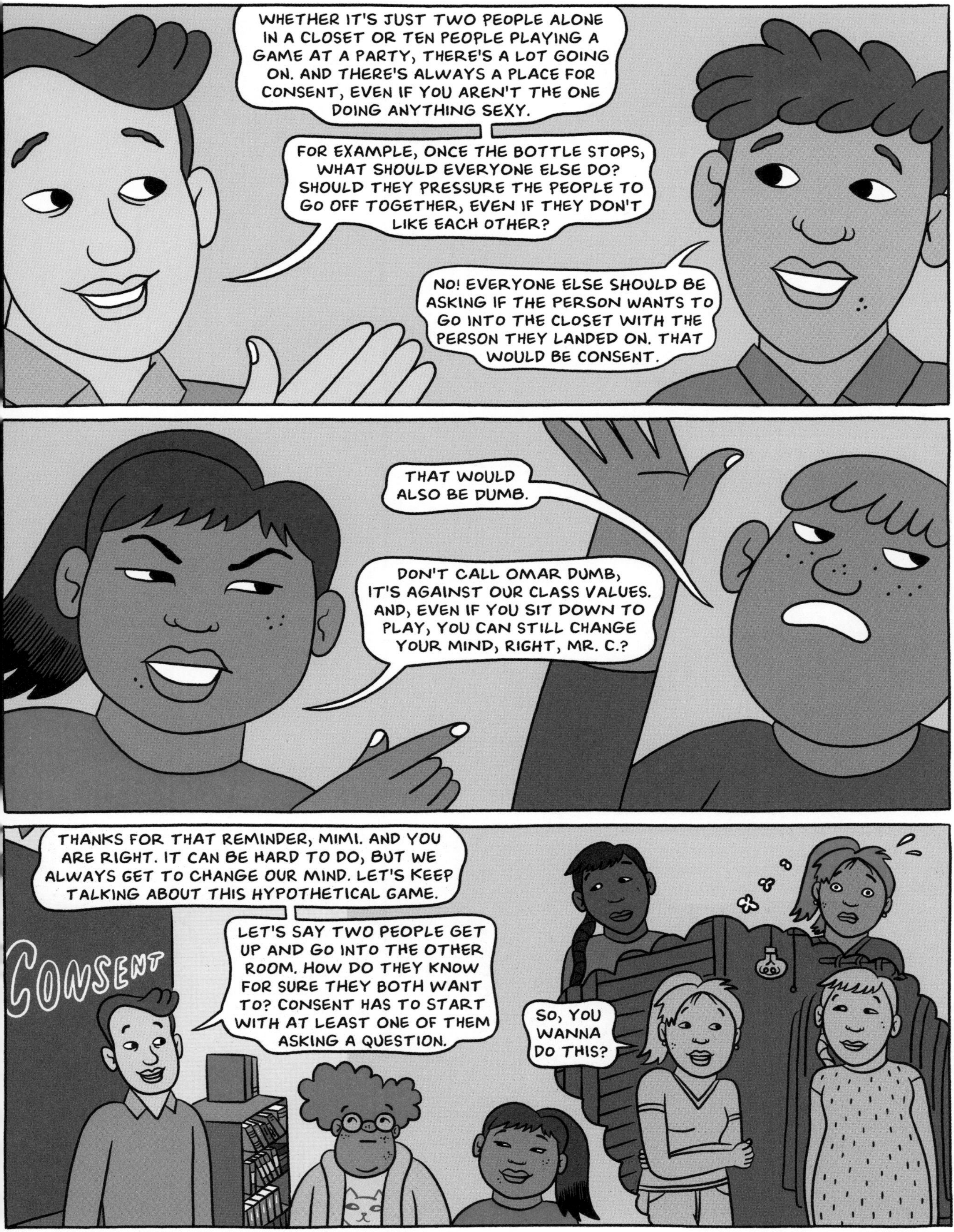
WHETHER IT'S JUST TWO PEOPLE ALONE IN A CLOSET OR TEN PEOPLE PLAYING A GAME AT A PARTY, THERE'S A LOT GOING ON. AND THERE'S ALWAYS A PLACE FOR CONSENT, EVEN IF YOU AREN'T THE ONE DOING ANYTHING SEXY.
FOR EXAMPLE, ONCE THE BOTTLE STOPS, WHAT SHOULD EVERYONE ELSE DO? SHOULD THEY PRESSURE THE PEOPLE TO GO OFF TOGETHER, EVEN IF THEY DON'T LIKE EACH OTHER?
NO! EVERYONE ELSE SHOULD BE ASKING IF THE PERSON WANTS TO GO INTO THE CLOSET WITH THE PERSON THEY LANDED ON. THAT WOULD BE CONSENT.
THAT WOULD ALSO BE DUMB.
DON'T CALL OMAR DUMB, IT'S AGAINST OUR CLASS VALUES. AND, EVEN IF YOU SIT DOWN TO PLAY, YOU CAN STILL CHANGE YOUR MIND, RIGHT, MR. C.?
THANKS FOR THAT REMINDER, MIMI. AND YOU ARE RIGHT. IT CAN BE HARD TO DO, BUT WE ALWAYS GET TO CHANGE OUR MIND. LET'S KEEP TALKING ABOUT THIS HYPOTHETICAL GAME.
LET'S SAY TWO PEOPLE GET UP AND GO INTO THE OTHER ROOM. HOW DO THEY KNOW FOR SURE THEY BOTH WANT TO? CONSENT HAS TO START WITH AT LEAST ONE OF THEM ASKING A QUESTION.
CONSENT
SO, YOU WANNA DO THIS?

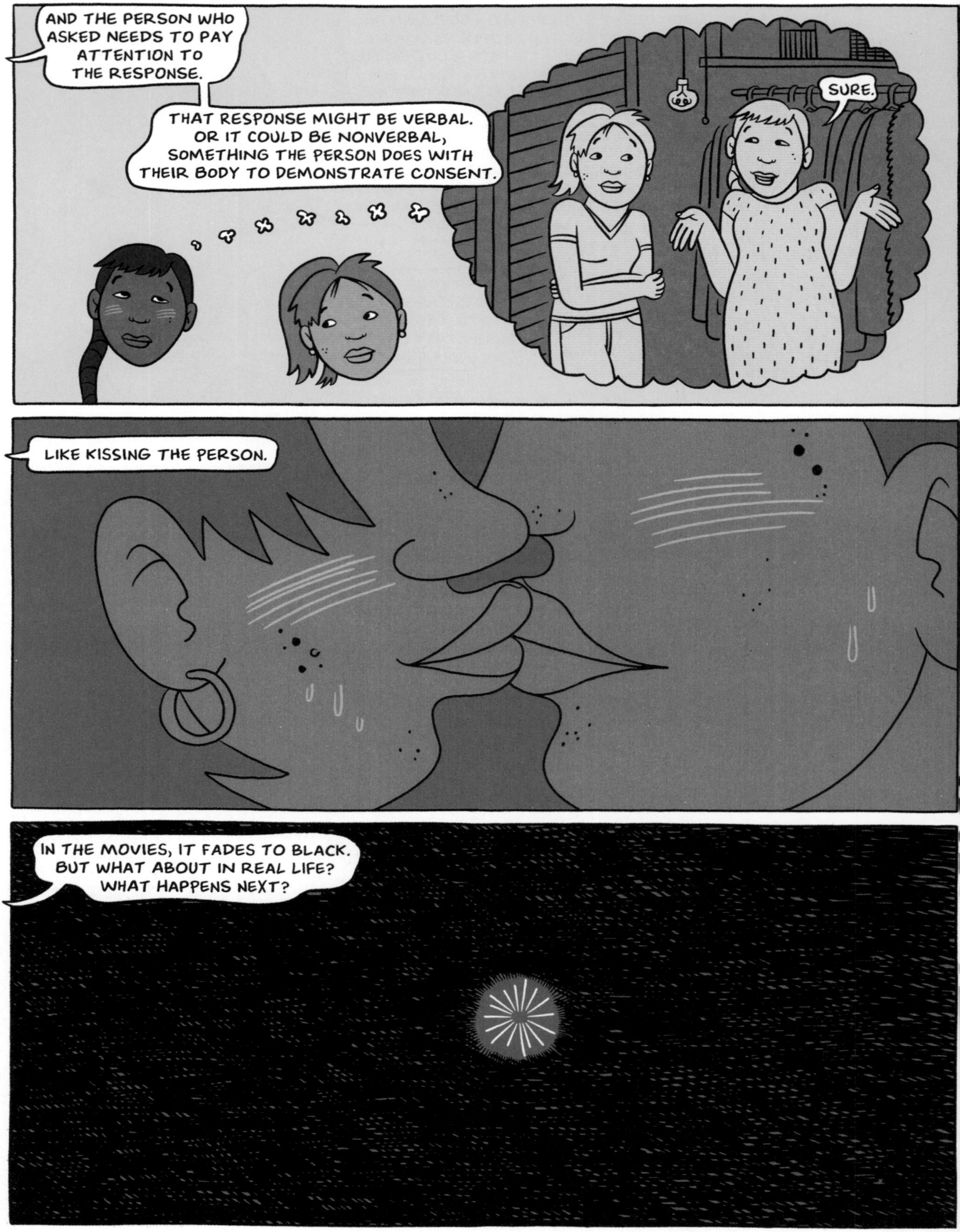
AND THE PERSON WHO ASKED NEEDS TO PAY ATTENTION TO THE RESPONSE.
THAT RESPONSE MIGHT BE VERBAL. OR IT COULD BE NONVERBAL, SOMETHING THE PERSON DOES WITH THEIR BODY TO DEMONSTRATE CONSENT.
SURE.
LIKE KISSING THE PERSON.
IN THE MOVIES, IT FADES TO BLACK. BUT WHAT ABOUT IN REAL LIFE? WHAT HAPPENS NEXT?

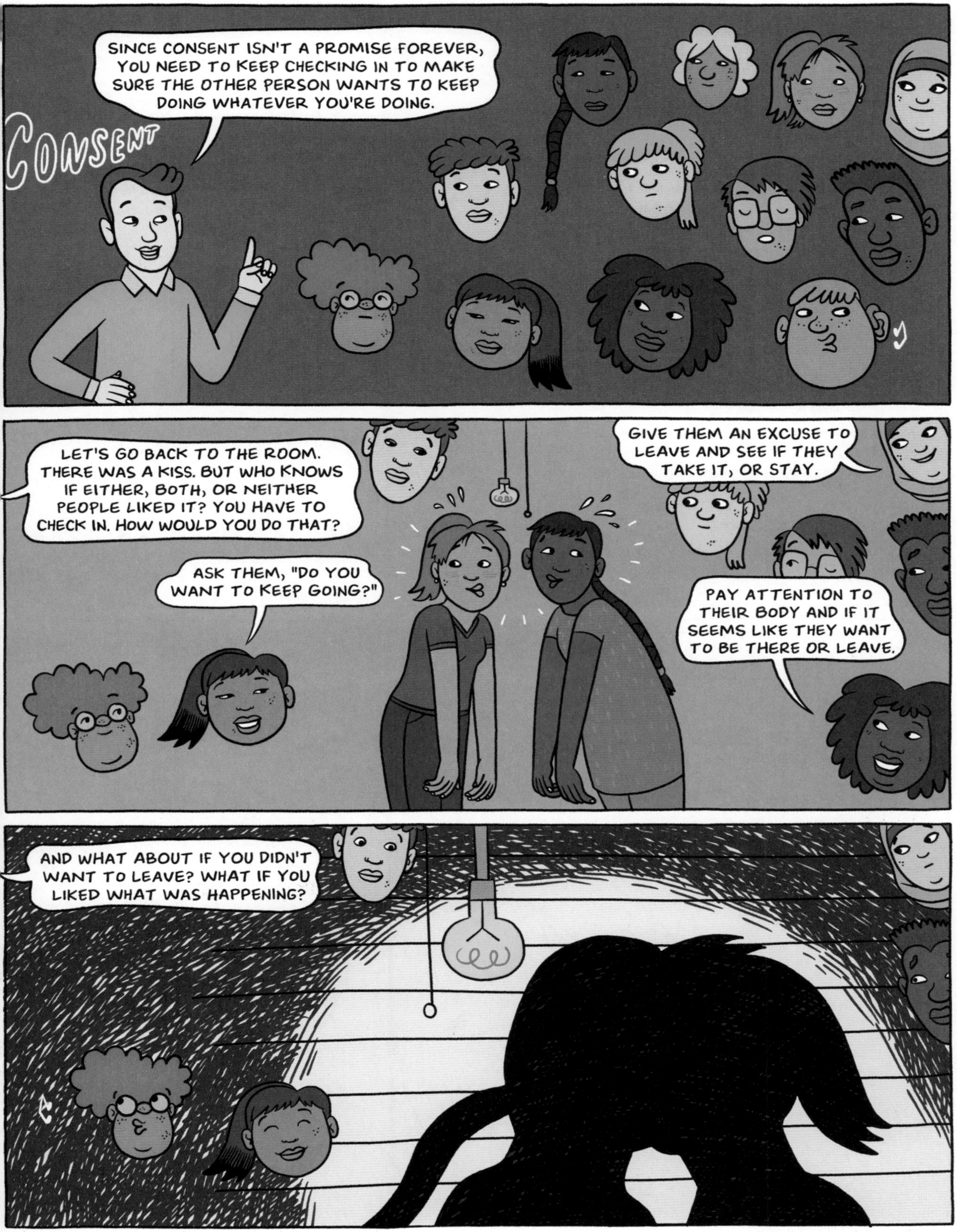
SINCE CONSENT ISN'T A PROMISE FOREVER, YOU NEED TO KEEP CHECKING IN TO MAKE SURE THE OTHER PERSON WANTS TO KEEP DOING WHATEVER YOU'RE DOING.
CONSENT
LET'S GO BACK TO THE ROOM. THERE WAS A KISS. BUT WHO KNOWS IF EITHER, BOTH, OR NEITHER PEOPLE LIKED IT? YOU HAVE TO CHECK IN. HOW WOULD YOU DO THAT?
ASK THEM, "DO YOU WANT TO KEEP GOING?"
GIVE THEM AN EXCUSE TO LEAVE AND SEE IF THEY TAKE IT, OR STAY.
PAY ATTENTION TO THEIR BODY AND IF IT SEEMS LIKE THEY WANT TO BE THERE OR LEAVE.
AND WHAT ABOUT IF YOU DIDN'T WANT TO LEAVE? WHAT IF YOU LIKED WHAT WAS HAPPENING?

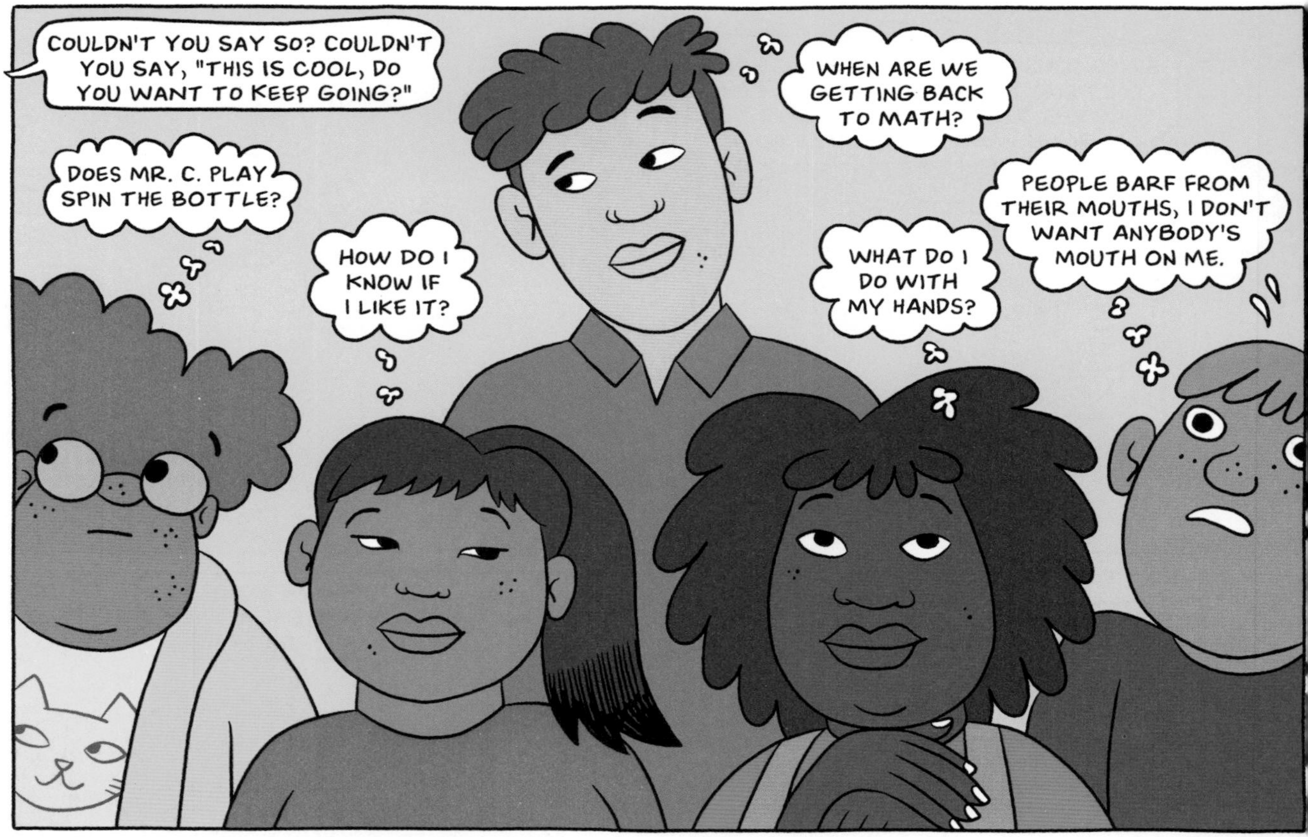
COULDN'T YOU SAY SO? COULDN'T YOU SAY, "THIS IS COOL, DO YOU WANT TO KEEP GOING?"
WHEN ARE WE GETTING BACK TO MATH?
DOES MR. C. PLAY SPIN THE BOTTLE?
HOW DO I KNOW IF I LIKE IT?
WHAT DO I DO WITH MY HANDS?
PEOPLE BARF FROM THEIR MOUTHS, I DON'T WANT ANYBODY'S MOUTH ON ME.

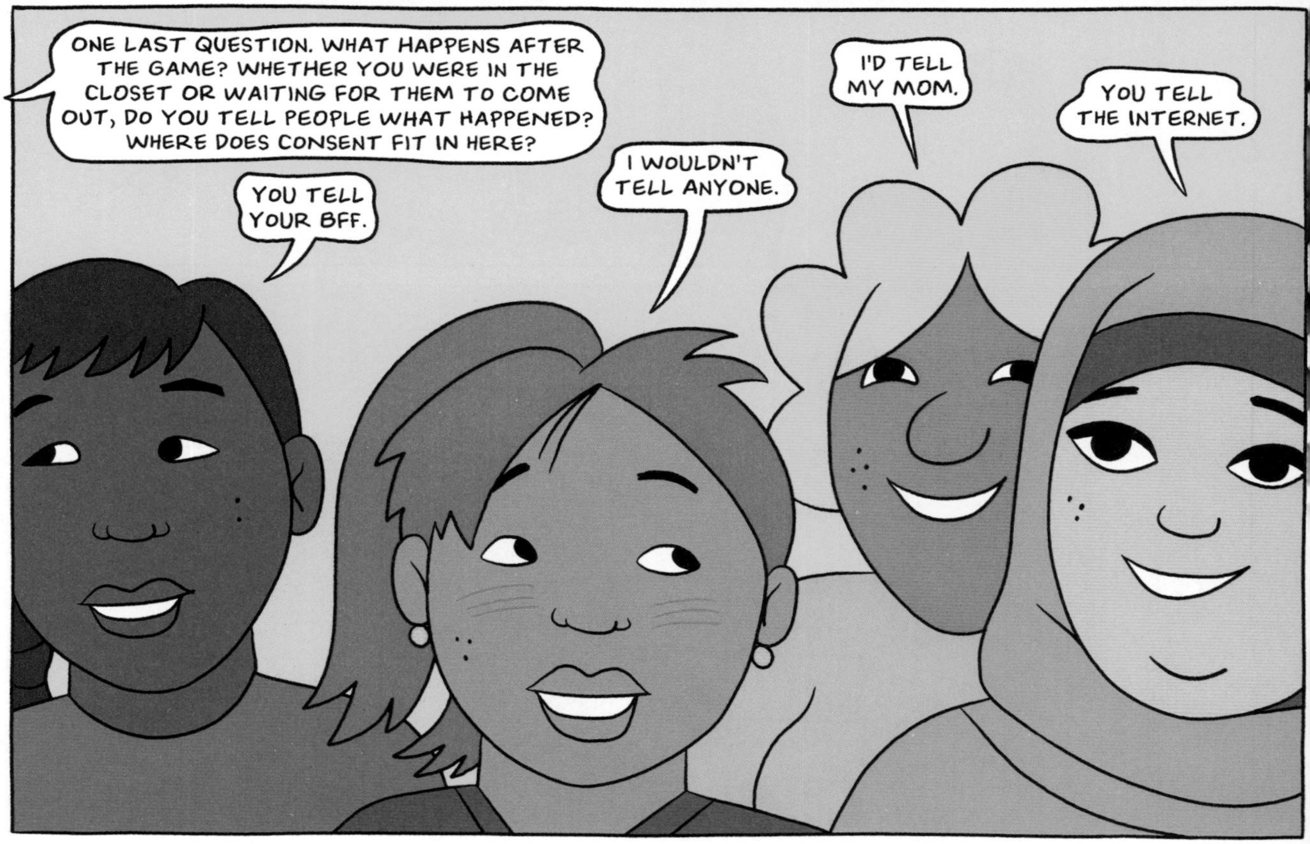
ONE LAST QUESTION. WHAT HAPPENS AFTER THE GAME? WHETHER YOU WERE IN THE CLOSET OR WAITING FOR THEM TO COME OUT, DO YOU TELL PEOPLE WHAT HAPPENED? WHERE DOES CONSENT FIT IN HERE?
YOU TELL YOUR BFF.
I WOULDN'T TELL ANYONE.
I'D TELL MY MOM.
YOU TELL THE INTERNET.

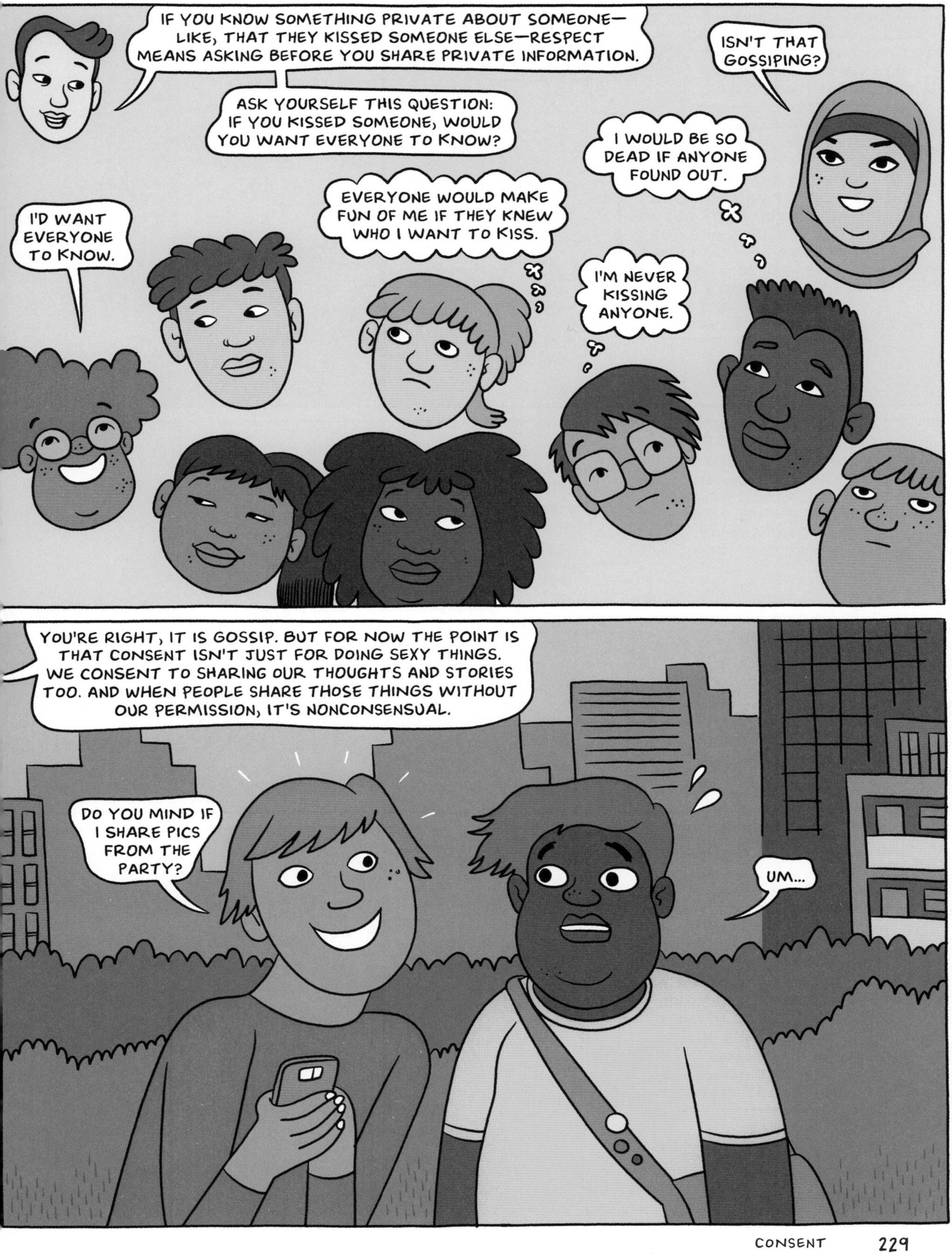
IF YOU KNOW SOMETHING PRIVATE ABOUT SOMEONE—LIKE, THAT THEY KISSED SOMEONE ELSE—RESPECT MEANS ASKING BEFORE YOU SHARE PRIVATE INFORMATION.
ASK YOURSELF THIS QUESTION: IF YOU KISSED SOMEONE, WOULD YOU WANT EVERYONE TO KNOW?
ISN'T THAT GOSSIPING?
I WOULD BE SO DEAD IF ANYONE FOUND OUT.
EVERYONE WOULD MAKE FUN OF ME IF THEY KNEW WHO I WANT TO KISS.
I'D WANT EVERYONE TO KNOW.
I'M NEVER KISSING ANYONE.
YOU'RE RIGHT, IT IS GOSSIP. BUT FOR NOW THE POINT IS THAT CONSENT ISN'T JUST FOR DOING SEXY THINGS. WE CONSENT TO SHARING OUR THOUGHTS AND STORIES TOO. AND WHEN PEOPLE SHARE THOSE THINGS WITHOUT OUR PERMISSION, IT'S NONCONSENSUAL.
DO YOU MIND IF I SHARE PICS FROM THE PARTY?
UM...

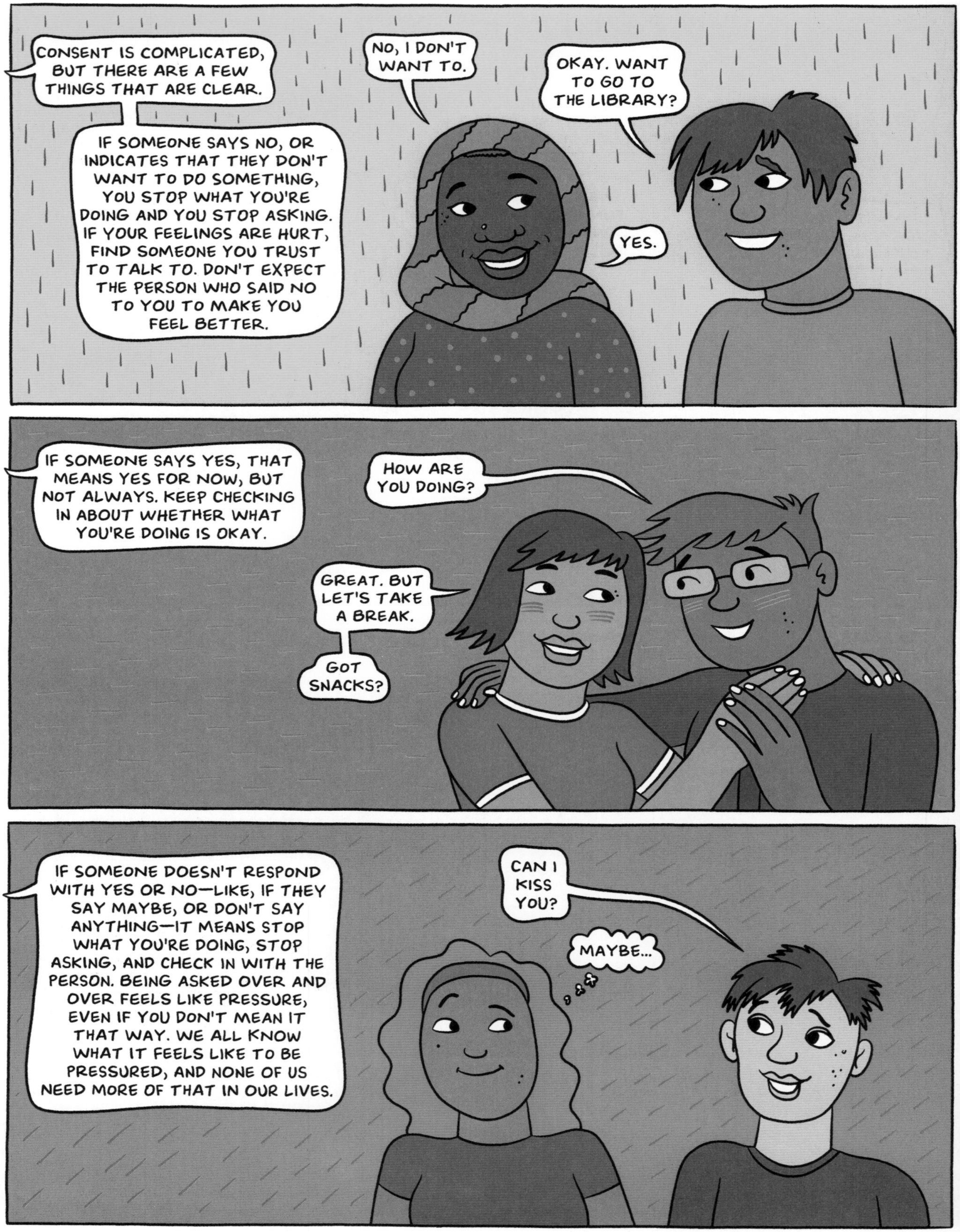
CONSENT IS COMPLICATED, BUT THERE ARE A FEW THINGS THAT ARE CLEAR.
IF SOMEONE SAYS NO, OR INDICATES THAT THEY DON'T WANT TO DO SOMETHING, YOU STOP WHAT YOU'RE DOING AND YOU STOP ASKING. IF YOUR FEELINGS ARE HURT, FIND SOMEONE YOU TRUST TO TALK TO. DON'T EXPECT THE PERSON WHO SAID NO TO YOU TO MAKE YOU FEEL BETTER.
NO, I DON'T WANT TO.
OKAY. WANT TO GO TO THE LIBRARY?
YES.
IF SOMEONE SAYS YES, THAT MEANS YES FOR NOW, BUT NOT ALWAYS. KEEP CHECKING IN ABOUT WHETHER WHAT YOU'RE DOING IS OKAY.
HOW ARE YOU DOING?
GREAT. BUT LET'S TAKE A BREAK.
GOT SNACKS?
IF SOMEONE DOESN'T RESPOND WITH YES OR NO—LIKE, IF THEY SAY MAYBE, OR DON'T SAY ANYTHING—IT MEANS STOP WHAT YOU'RE DOING, STOP ASKING, AND CHECK IN WITH THE PERSON. BEING ASKED OVER AND OVER FEELS LIKE PRESSURE, EVEN IF YOU DON'T MEAN IT THAT WAY. WE ALL KNOW WHAT IT FEELS LIKE TO BE PRESSURED, AND NONE OF US NEED MORE OF THAT IN OUR LIVES.
CAN I KISS YOU?
MAYBE...

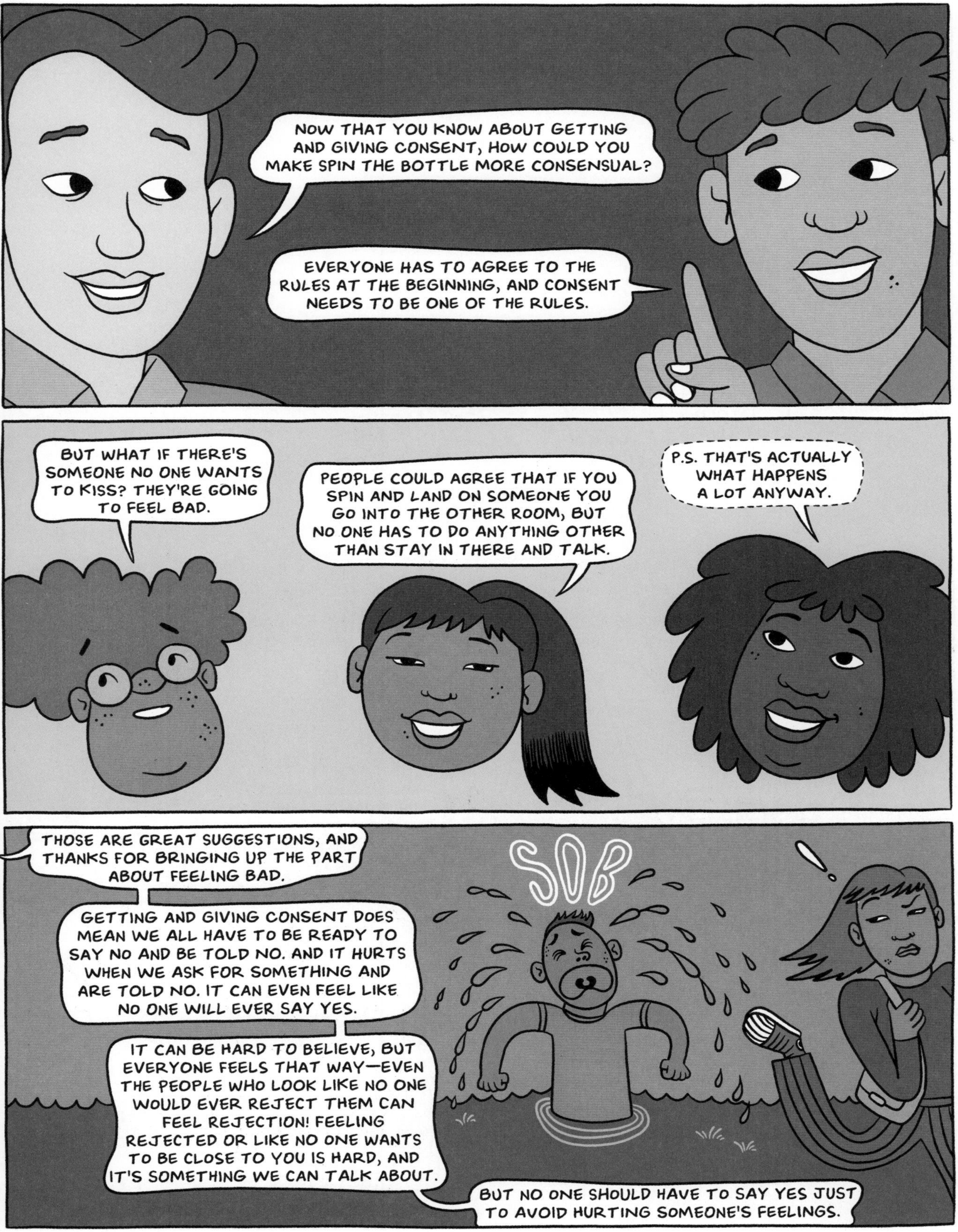
NOW THAT YOU KNOW ABOUT GETTING AND GIVING CONSENT, HOW COULD YOU MAKE SPIN THE BOTTLE MORE CONSENSUAL?
EVERYONE HAS TO AGREE TO THE RULES AT THE BEGINNING, AND CONSENT NEEDS TO BE ONE OF THE RULES.
BUT WHAT IF THERE'S SOMEONE NO ONE WANTS TO KISS? THEY'RE GOING TO FEEL BAD.
PEOPLE COULD AGREE THAT IF YOU SPIN AND LAND ON SOMEONE YOU GO INTO THE OTHER ROOM, BUT NO ONE HAS TO DO ANYTHING OTHER THAN STAY IN THERE AND TALK.
P.S. THAT'S ACTUALLY WHAT HAPPENS A LOT ANYWAY.
THOSE ARE GREAT SUGGESTIONS, AND THANKS FOR BRINGING UP THE PART ABOUT FEELING BAD.
GETTING AND GIVING CONSENT DOES MEAN WE ALL HAVE TO BE READY TO SAY NO AND BE TOLD NO. AND IT HURTS WHEN WE ASK FOR SOMETHING AND ARE TOLD NO. IT CAN EVEN FEEL LIKE NO ONE WILL EVER SAY YES.
SOB
!
IT CAN BE HARD TO BELIEVE, BUT EVERYONE FEELS THAT WAY—EVEN THE PEOPLE WHO LOOK LIKE NO ONE WOULD EVER REJECT THEM CAN FEEL REJECTION! FEELING REJECTED OR LIKE NO ONE WANTS TO BE CLOSE TO YOU IS HARD, AND IT'S SOMETHING WE CAN TALK ABOUT.
BUT NO ONE SHOULD HAVE TO SAY YES JUST TO AVOID HURTING SOMEONE'S FEELINGS.

WHEN THEY DON'T EVEN ASK

IN REAL LIFE, PEOPLE DON'T ALWAYS ASK BEFORE HOLDING HANDS, KISSING, OR TRYING OTHER SEXY THINGS. THEY MIGHT BE SHY, OR NO ONE HAS TAUGHT THEM ABOUT CONSENT, OR THEY KNOW ABOUT IT BUT DON'T KNOW HOW TO DO IT.

WHEN SOMEONE SAYS OR DOES SOMETHING TO US WITHOUT OUR CONSENT IT MIGHT BE HARASSMENT, ASSAULT, OR RAPE. YOU CAN FIND OUT MORE ABOUT THOSE WORDS IN THE SAFETY SECTION ON P. 371.

IT WOULD BE BETTER IF EVERYONE KNEW ABOUT AND PRACTICED CONSENT. BUT BECAUSE THEY DON'T, WE ALL NEED TO THINK ABOUT WHAT WE'LL DO IF SOMEONE TOUCHES US WITHOUT ASKING.

WHEN SOMEONE TOUCHES US WITHOUT ASKING, LEARNING TO SAY YES, NO, AND MAYBE TAKES PRACTICE AND POWER. IT'S POWER WE ALL HAVE, BUT WITHOUT PRACTICE, WE CAN FORGET WE HAVE IT.

ANYTIME YOU EXPERIENCE SOMETHING THAT DOESN'T FEEL LIKE A CHOICE YOU CAN ALWAYS:

- ★ TRY TO STOP WHAT'S HAPPENING.
- ★ FIND ANOTHER PLACE TO GO/LEAVE THE SPACE IF YOU CAN.
- ★ TALK TO SOMEONE YOU TRUST.
- ★ GET HELP TO FIGURE OUT HOW THINGS CAN CHANGE.

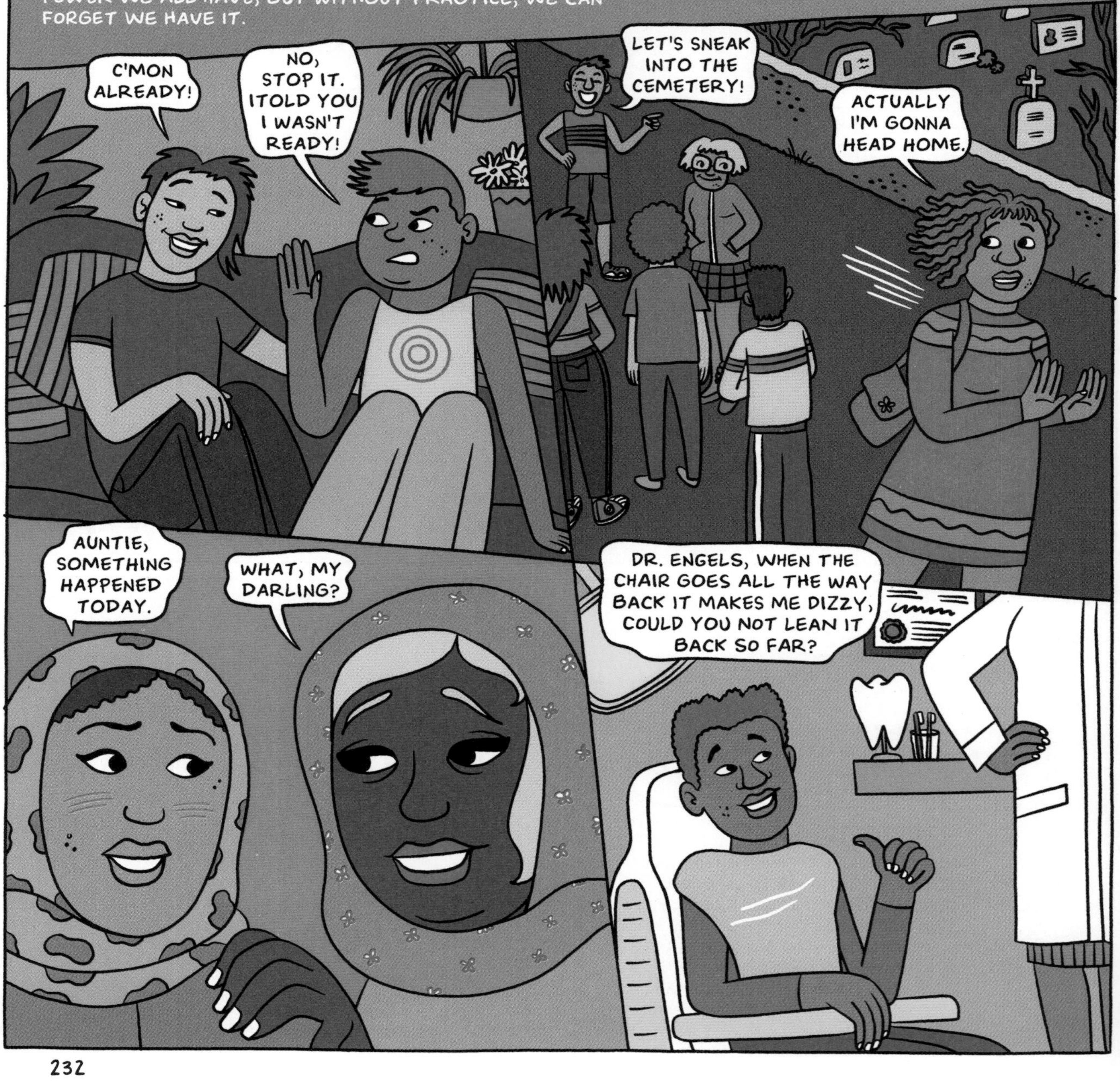
C'MON ALREADY!
NO, STOP IT. I TOLD YOU I WASN'T READY!
LET'S SNEAK INTO THE CEMETERY!
ACTUALLY I'M GONNA HEAD HOME.
AUNTIE, SOMETHING HAPPENED TODAY.
WHAT, MY DARLING?
DR. ENGELS, WHEN THE CHAIR GOES ALL THE WAY BACK IT MAKES ME DIZZY, COULD YOU NOT LEAN IT BACK SO FAR?

NERD ALERT CONSENT AND JUSTICE

SOME OF US ARE TAUGHT EARLY IN OUR LIVES THAT OUR VOICE, OUR CONSENT, DOESN'T MATTER. WE SAY NO A HUNDRED TIMES AND NO ONE LISTENS. WE DON'T SEE PEOPLE WHO LOOK LIKE US GETTING RESPECT. THAT'S NOT JUSTICE, BUT IT IS THE WORLD TODAY.

THE MORE POWER YOU HAVE ACCESS TO, THE MORE LIKELY OTHER PEOPLE WILL PAY ATTENTION TO YOUR CONSENT. HAVING ACCESS TO POWER ISN'T JUST ABOUT US. IT'S ABOUT OUR RACE, HOW MUCH MONEY OUR FAMILY HAS, WHETHER OR NOT WE WERE BORN IN THE COUNTRY WE LIVE IN, HOW MUCH OUR BODY FITS IN OR STICKS OUT, AND OUR MANY IDENTITIES, INCLUDING GENDER AND SEXUAL ORIENTATION.

WE ALL HAVE EXPERIENCES WHERE WE DO AND DON'T HAVE POWER. BUT COMPARED TO ADULTS, ALL YOUNG PEOPLE HAVE LESS ACCESS TO POWER AND FEWER CHANCES TO CONSENT. MANY OF US GO THROUGH LIFE GETTING THE MESSAGE THAT WE ARE LESS DESERVING THAN OTHERS WHEN IT COMES TO CHOICES—THAT WE SHOULD FEEL LUCKY IF ANYONE IS PAYING ATTENTION TO US, AND SHOULD SAY YES TO WHATEVER IS OFFERED. WE MAY NOT EVEN REALIZE SAYING NO OR MAYBE IS AN OPTION. JUSTICE MEANS EVERY PERSON FEELS LIKE THEY CAN SPEAK THEIR MIND AND FOLLOW THEIR HEART.

WHEN THERE IS JUSTICE, EVERYONE KNOWS THAT THEY ARE WORTHY OF CONSENT, RESPECT, AND BODY AUTONOMY. WHEN THERE IS JUSTICE, EVERYONE GETS TO SAY YES, NO, AND MAYBE WITHOUT FEAR.

CAN YOU BELIEVE IT? THE COP TOTALLY LET ME GO WITH A WARNING. HE WAS SO NICE!
YEAH, I CAN BELIEVE IT.
BLM
BLACK TRANS LIVES MATTER
YES.
NO.
WHAT ARE YOU SEARCHING NOW?
AGE OF CONSENT IN NEW YORK STATE.
MAYBE.
...

NERD ALERT CONSENT AND THE LAW

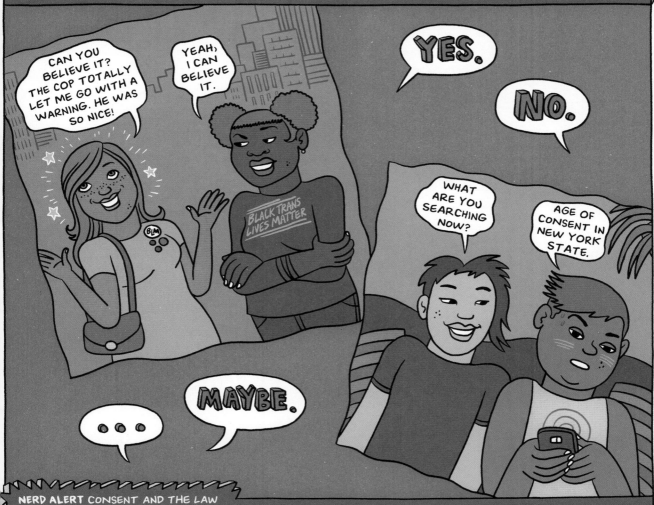

MOST COUNTRIES HAVE LAWS ABOUT HOW OLD YOU HAVE TO BE IN ORDER TO BE ABLE TO CONSENT TO SEX. IF YOU ARE UNDER THE AGE OF CONSENT THAT MEANS THAT EVEN IF YOU CHOOSE TO DO SEXY THINGS WITH SOMEONE, THEY COULD BE ARRESTED FOR IT, AND THE LAW WOULDN'T CONSIDER IT SEX—IT WOULD BE ASSAULT OR RAPE.

THE LAWS ARE DIFFERENT FROM PLACE TO PLACE. IN SOME PLACES, IF YOU ARE DOING SEXY THINGS WITH SOMEONE CLOSE TO YOUR AGE, THEN THE LAW ALLOWS IT. DIFFERENT PLACES DEFINE "SEXY THINGS" DIFFERENTLY. IF YOU WANT TO KNOW MORE ABOUT THE LAW WHERE YOU LIVE, YOU CAN SEARCH FOR "AGE OF CONSENT LAWS" AND YOUR COUNTRY OR STATE.

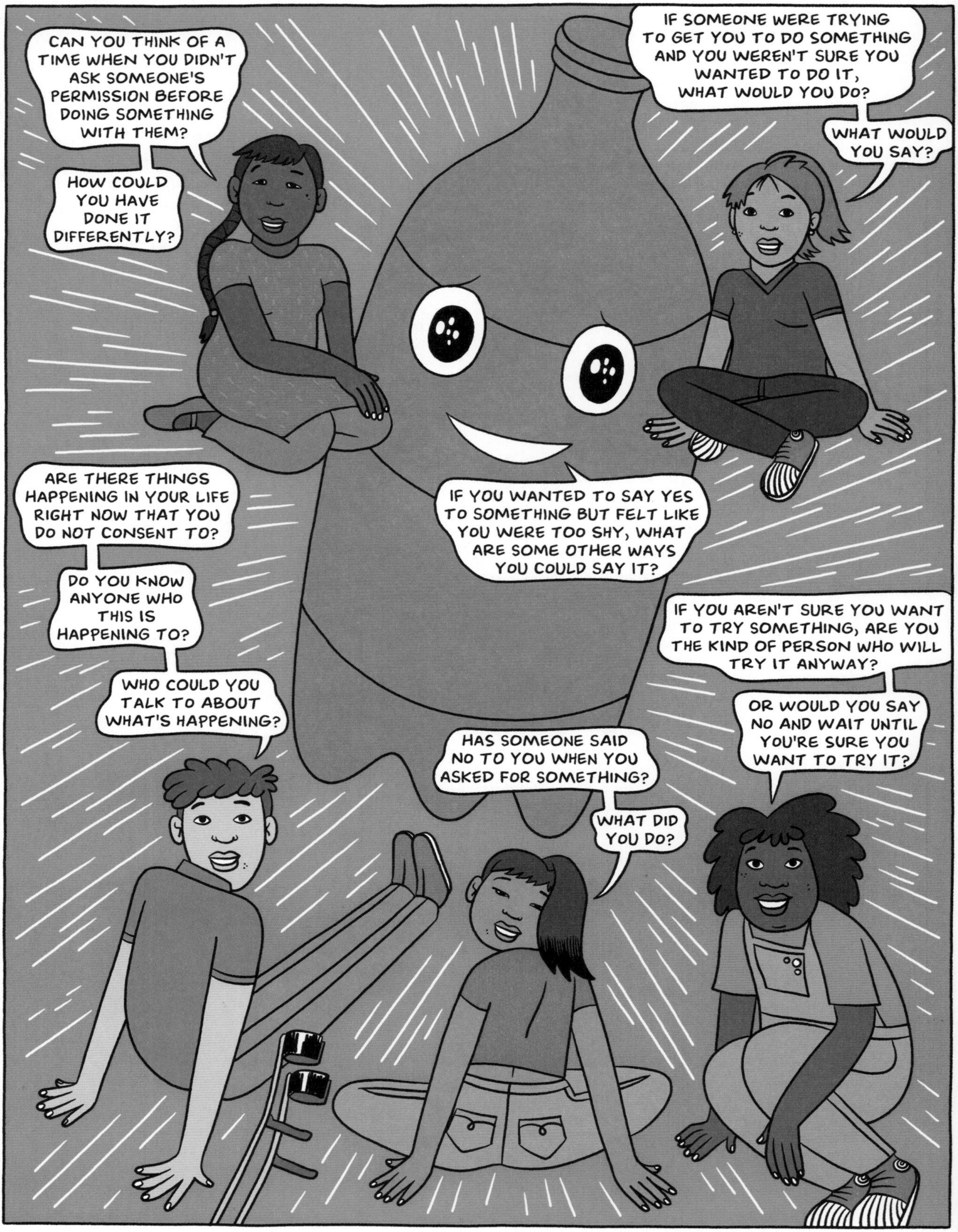
CAN YOU THINK OF A TIME WHEN YOU DIDN'T ASK SOMEONE'S PERMISSION BEFORE DOING SOMETHING WITH THEM?
HOW COULD YOU HAVE DONE IT DIFFERENTLY?
IF SOMEONE WERE TRYING TO GET YOU TO DO SOMETHING AND YOU WEREN'T SURE YOU WANTED TO DO IT, WHAT WOULD YOU DO?
WHAT WOULD YOU SAY?
IF YOU WANTED TO SAY YES TO SOMETHING BUT FELT LIKE YOU WERE TOO SHY, WHAT ARE SOME OTHER WAYS YOU COULD SAY IT?
ARE THERE THINGS HAPPENING IN YOUR LIFE RIGHT NOW THAT YOU DO NOT CONSENT TO?
DO YOU KNOW ANYONE WHO THIS IS HAPPENING TO?
WHO COULD YOU TALK TO ABOUT WHAT'S HAPPENING?
IF YOU AREN'T SURE YOU WANT TO TRY SOMETHING, ARE YOU THE KIND OF PERSON WHO WILL TRY IT ANYWAY?
OR WOULD YOU SAY NO AND WAIT UNTIL YOU'RE SURE YOU WANT TO TRY IT?
HAS SOMEONE SAID NO TO YOU WHEN YOU ASKED FOR SOMETHING?
WHAT DID YOU DO?

ACTIVITY
CHECK OUT THESE CLASSIC EXAMPLES OF PEOPLE NOT ASKING FOR CONSENT. HOW COULD YOU CHANGE THE DIALOGUE TO MAKE IT MORE CONSENSUAL?

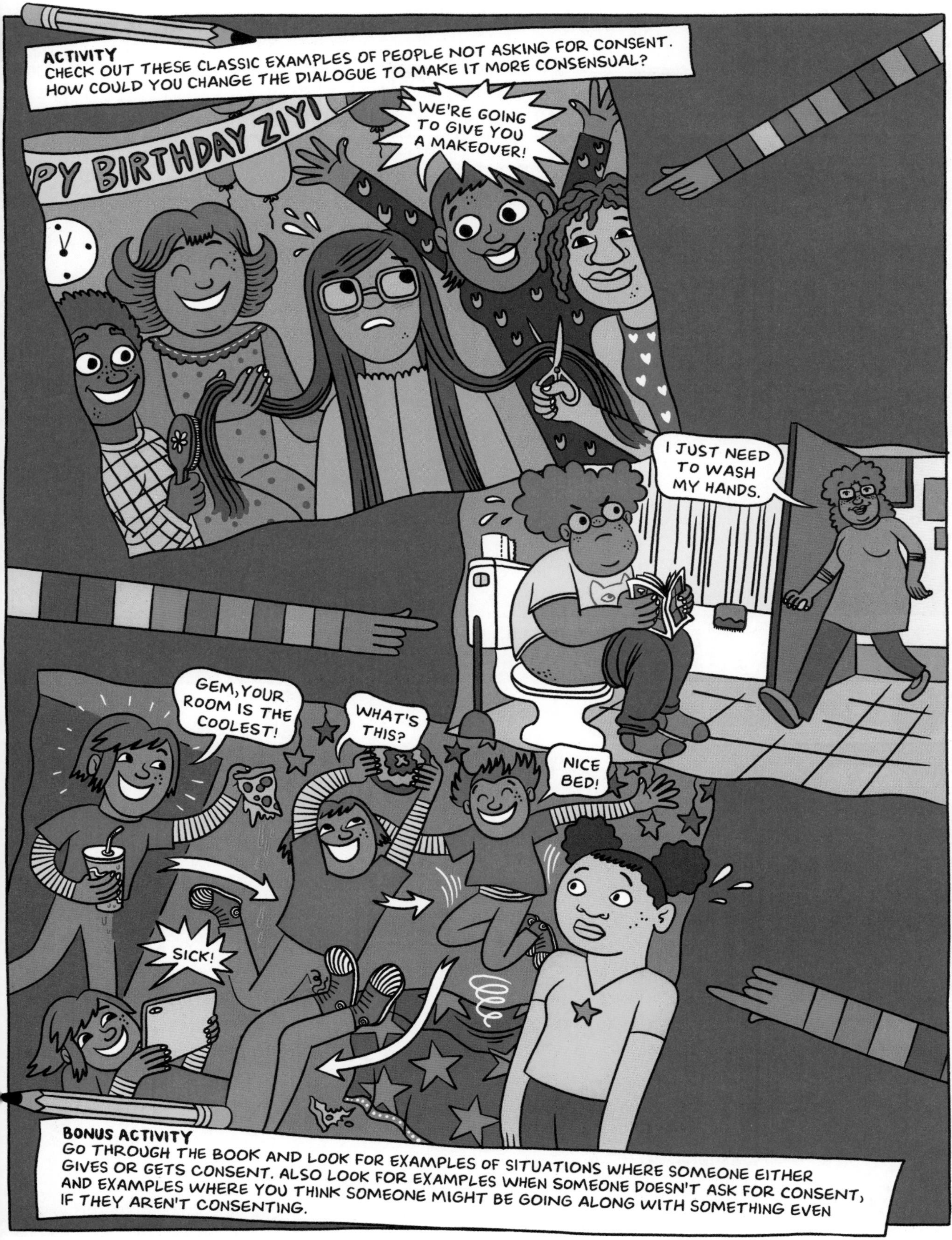
PY BIRTHDAY ZIYI
WE'RE GOING TO GIVE YOU A MAKEOVER!
I JUST NEED TO WASH MY HANDS.
GEM, YOUR ROOM IS THE COOLEST!
WHAT'S THIS?
NICE BED!
SICK!

BONUS ACTIVITY
GO THROUGH THE BOOK AND LOOK FOR EXAMPLES OF SITUATIONS WHERE SOMEONE EITHER GIVES OR GETS CONSENT. ALSO LOOK FOR EXAMPLES WHEN SOMEONE DOESN'T ASK FOR CONSENT, AND EXAMPLES WHERE YOU THINK SOMEONE MIGHT BE GOING ALONG WITH SOMETHING EVEN IF THEY AREN'T CONSENTING.

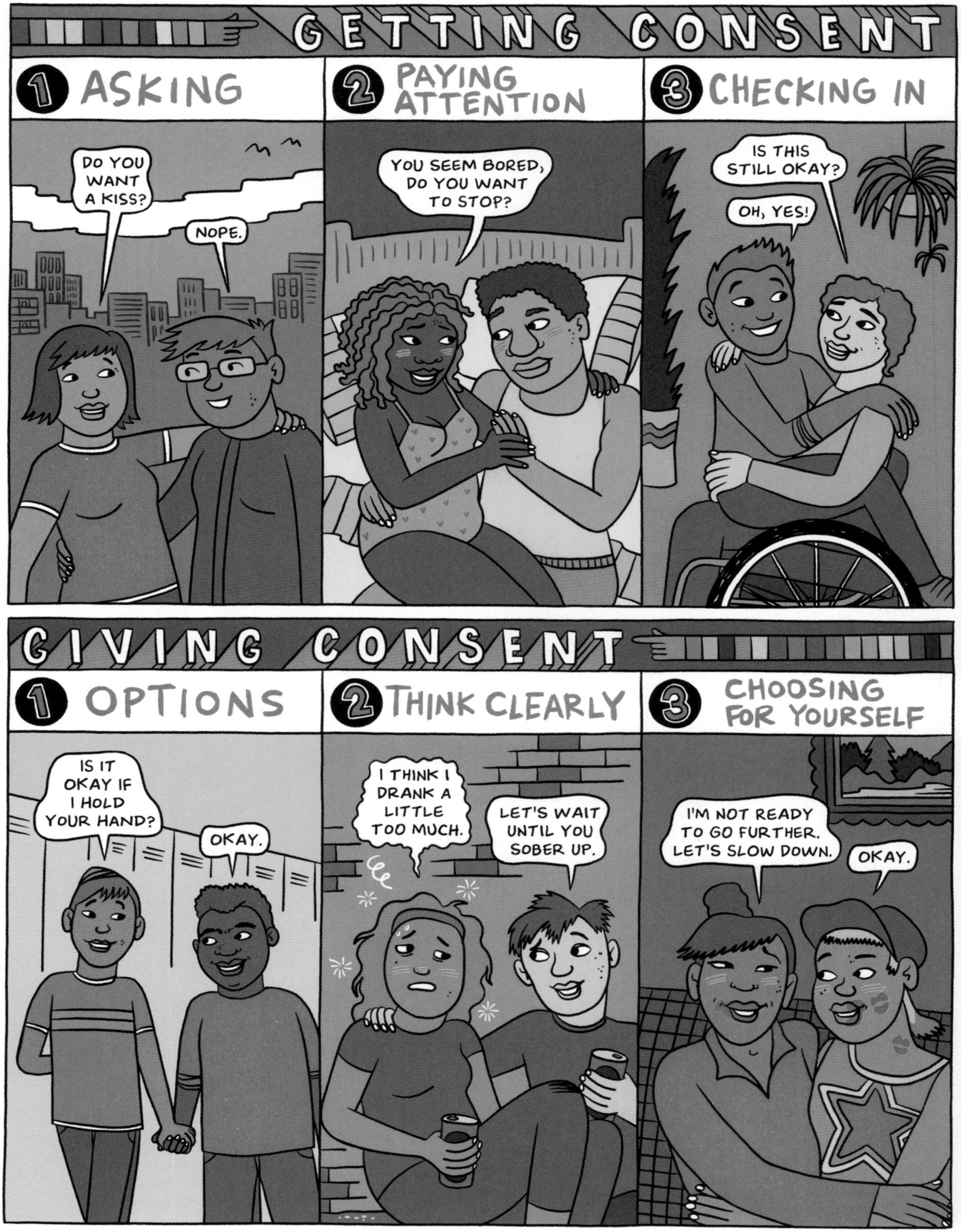
GETTING CONSENT
1 ASKING
DO YOU WANT A KISS?
NOPE.
2 PAYING ATTENTION
YOU SEEM BORED, DO YOU WANT TO STOP?
3 CHECKING IN
IS THIS STILL OKAY?
OH, YES!
GIVING CONSENT
1 OPTIONS
IS IT OKAY IF I HOLD YOUR HAND?
OKAY.
2 THINK CLEARLY
I THINK I DRANK A LITTLE TOO MUCH.
LET'S WAIT UNTIL YOU SOBER UP.
3 CHOOSING FOR YOURSELF
I'M NOT READY TO GO FURTHER. LET'S SLOW DOWN.
OKAY.

7

TALKING

WHAT'S THE WORD FOR WHEN YOU LIKE SOMEONE BUT YOU DON'T LIKE THEIR TASTE IN MUSIC?

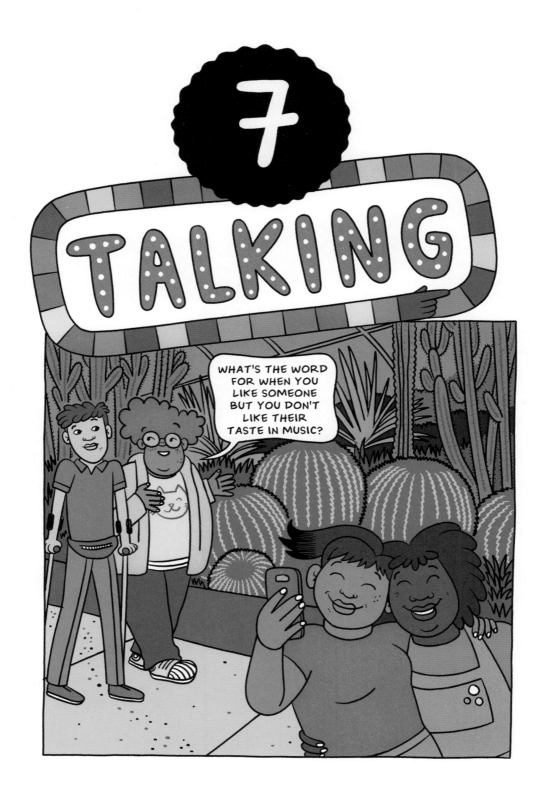

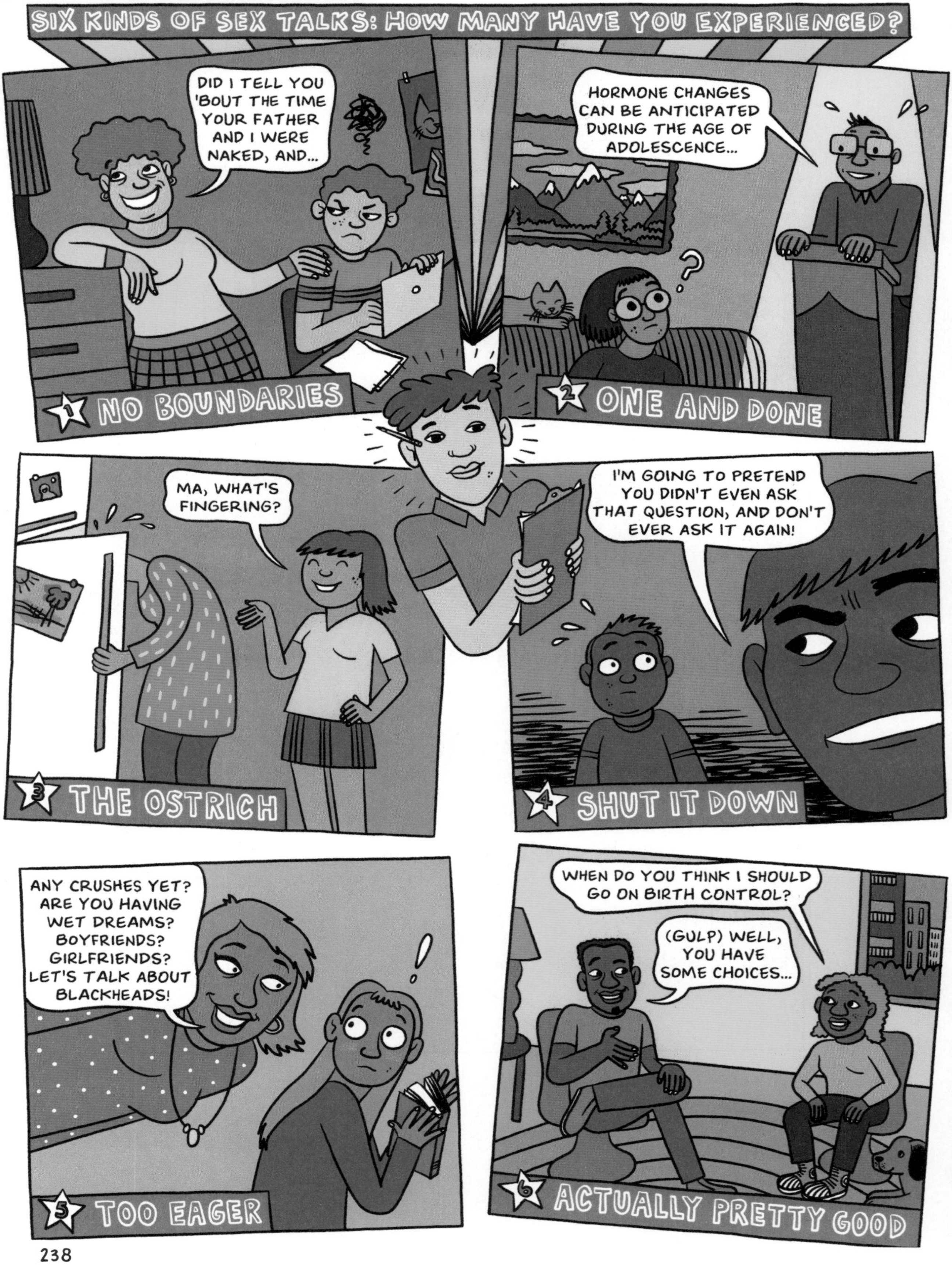
SIX KINDS OF SEX TALKS: HOW MANY HAVE YOU EXPERIENCED?
DID I TELL YOU 'BOUT THE TIME YOUR FATHER AND I WERE NAKED, AND...
1 NO BOUNDARIES
HORMONE CHANGES CAN BE ANTICIPATED DURING THE AGE OF ADOLESCENCE...
?
2 ONE AND DONE
MA, WHAT'S FINGERING?
3 THE OSTRICH
I'M GOING TO PRETEND YOU DIDN'T EVEN ASK THAT QUESTION, AND DON'T EVER ASK IT AGAIN!
4 SHUT IT DOWN
ANY CRUSHES YET? ARE YOU HAVING WET DREAMS? BOYFRIENDS? GIRLFRIENDS? LET'S TALK ABOUT BLACKHEADS!
!
5 TOO EAGER
WHEN DO YOU THINK I SHOULD GO ON BIRTH CONTROL?
(GULP) WELL, YOU HAVE SOME CHOICES...
6 ACTUALLY PRETTY GOOD

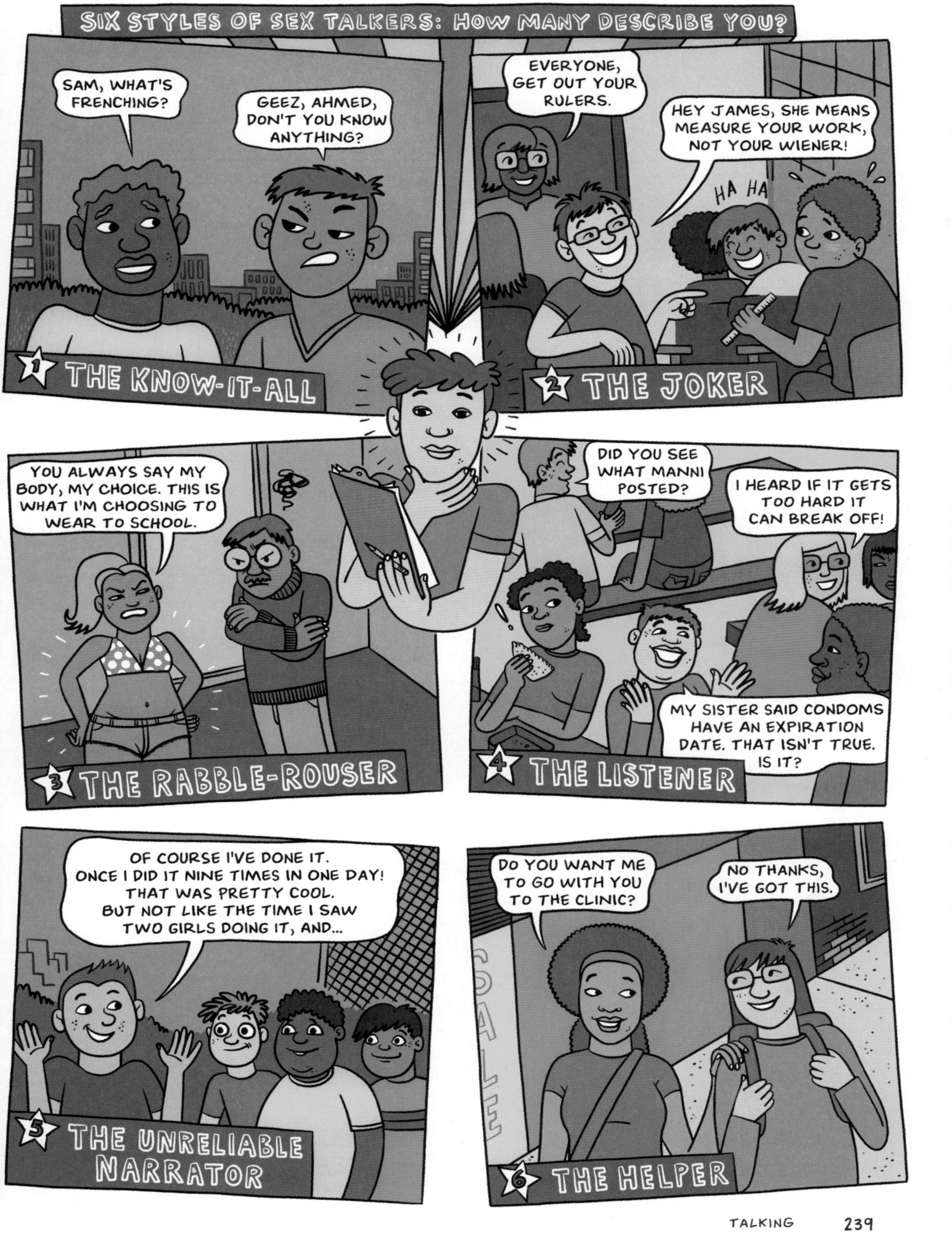
SIX STYLES OF SEX TALKERS: HOW MANY DESCRIBE YOU?
SAM, WHAT'S FRENCHING?
GEEZ, AHMED, DON'T YOU KNOW ANYTHING?
1 THE KNOW-IT-ALL
EVERYONE, GET OUT YOUR RULERS.
HEY JAMES, SHE MEANS MEASURE YOUR WORK, NOT YOUR WIENER!
HA HA
2 THE JOKER
YOU ALWAYS SAY MY BODY, MY CHOICE. THIS IS WHAT I'M CHOOSING TO WEAR TO SCHOOL.
3 THE RABBLE-ROUSER
DID YOU SEE WHAT MANNI POSTED?
I HEARD IF IT GETS TOO HARD IT CAN BREAK OFF!
MY SISTER SAID CONDOMS HAVE AN EXPIRATION DATE. THAT ISN'T TRUE. IS IT?
4 THE LISTENER
OF COURSE I'VE DONE IT. ONCE I DID IT NINE TIMES IN ONE DAY! THAT WAS PRETTY COOL. BUT NOT LIKE THE TIME I SAW TWO GIRLS DOING IT, AND...
5 THE UNRELIABLE NARRATOR
DO YOU WANT ME TO GO WITH YOU TO THE CLINIC?
NO THANKS, I'VE GOT THIS.
SALE
6 THE HELPER

THERE ARE LOTS OF REASONS IT'S DIFFICULT TO TALK ABOUT SEX.

- PEOPLE SAY SEX IS PRIVATE, BUT IT'S OBVIOUSLY ALSO PUBLIC, BECAUSE IT'S IN MOVIES, ON TV, AND ONLINE. THIS IS CONFUSING AND LEAVES MOST OF US UNSURE ABOUT HOW MUCH WE'RE ALLOWED TO TALK ABOUT IT, WITH WHOM, AND WHEN.
- PEOPLE TREAT SEX LIKE IT'S OKAY TO JOKE ABOUT, BUT THEN CALL YOU A PERVERT IF YOU'RE CURIOUS OR ASK HONEST QUESTIONS.
- BECAUSE SO MANY PEOPLE THINK YOUNG PEOPLE SHOULDN'T TALK ABOUT SEX, WE DON'T GET TO HAVE ENOUGH CHANCES TO PRACTICE AND LEARN WHAT WORKS.

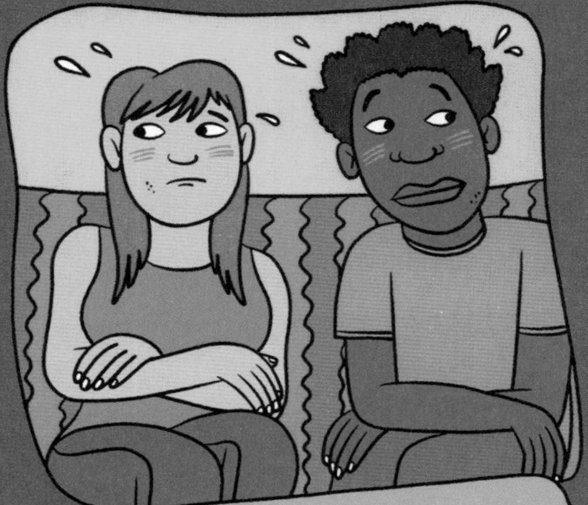

TALKING ABOUT SEX IS ONE OF THOSE THINGS YOU GET BETTER AT BY DOING IT. YOUR FIRST TIMES TALKING ABOUT SEX DON'T HAVE TO BE WITH SOMEONE YOU HAVE SEXY FEELINGS FOR. YOU CAN PRACTICE WITH FRIENDS OR FAMILY MEMBERS YOU TRUST.

IF YOU'RE CURIOUS ABOUT SEX AND WISH YOU COULD FIND PEOPLE TO TALK TO, REMEMBER THAT CONSENT ISN'T JUST FOR HAVING SEX, IT'S FOR TALKING ABOUT IT TOO. ASK BEFORE YOU START TALKING ABOUT IT, AND CHECK IN WHILE YOU'RE TALKING ABOUT IT TO MAKE SURE YOU AND THE PEOPLE YOU'RE TALKING TO ARE STILL FEELING OKAY WITH THE CONVERSATION.

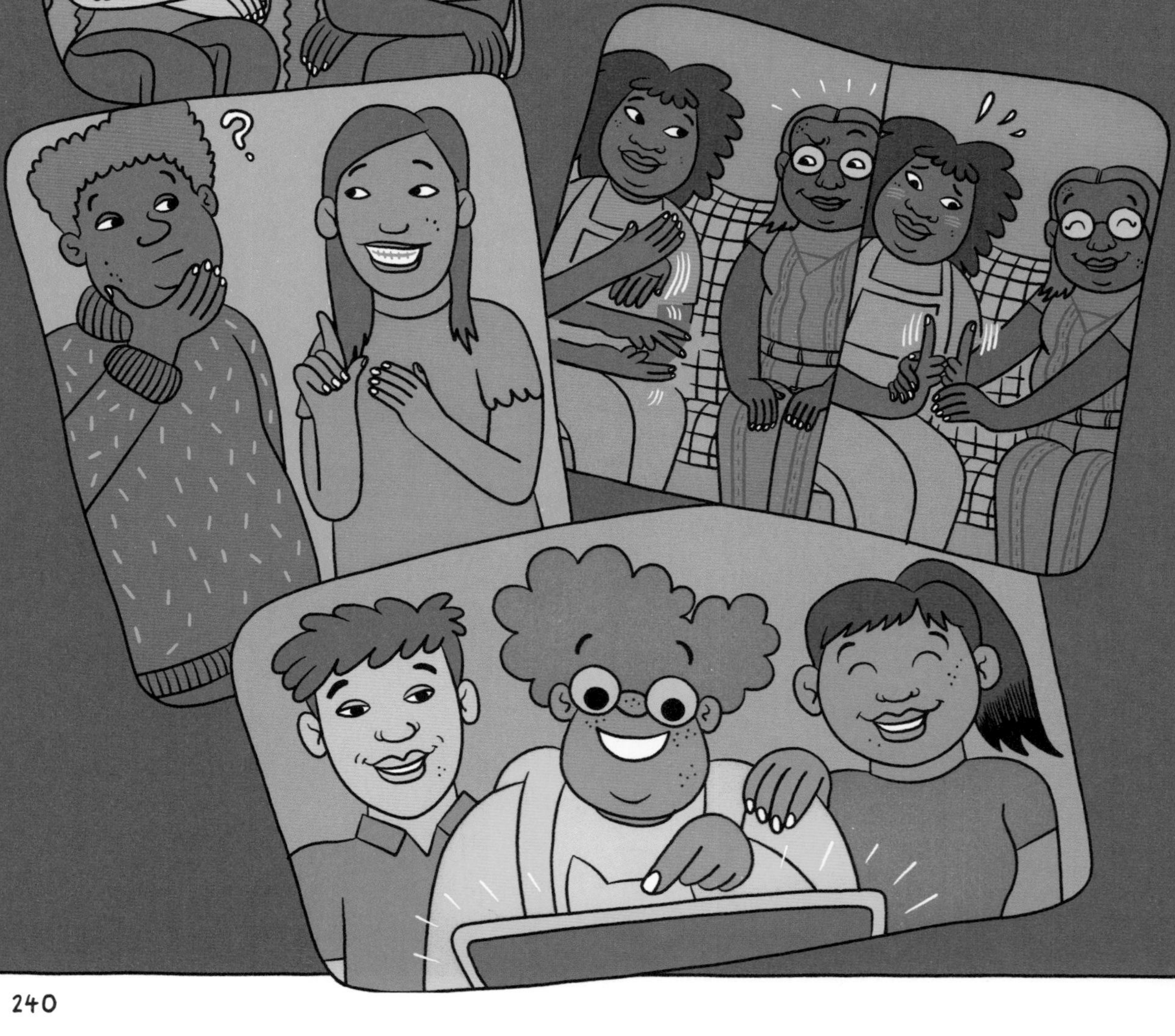

WE PROBABLY TALK ABOUT SEX MORE ONLINE THAN
ANYWHERE ELSE. THE INTERNET IS FULL OF INFORMATION
ABOUT SEX, AS WELL AS OPPORTUNITIES TO ASK QUESTIONS,
SHARE STORIES, AND FIND OTHER PEOPLE WHO ARE
FIGURING STUFF OUT ABOUT SEX AND GENDER.

IT'S ALSO A PLACE FULL OF MISINFORMATION, SCAMS, AND
PEOPLE BEING THEIR WORST SELVES.
SO HOW DO YOU KNOW WHAT TO TRUST?

WHO WROTE IT?

IS THERE AN AUTHOR WHOSE NAME IS ATTACHED TO WHAT
YOU'RE READING? WHEN YOU SEARCH FOR THEM, WHAT ELSE
DO YOU FIND? HAVE THEY WRITTEN OTHER THINGS, OR DONE
WORK IN THE AREA THAT THEY'RE WRITING ABOUT? WHAT DO
PEOPLE YOU KNOW AND TRUST THINK OF THE AUTHOR OR
SITE? WHO LIKES OR FOLLOWS THEM, AND WHO DO THEY LIKE
OR FOLLOW? IF IT'S A WEBSITE, IS THERE AN "ABOUT" PAGE
WITH A DETAILED BIO?

HOW IS IT WRITTEN?

DOES IT SEEM LIKE THE AUTHOR IS TRYING TO CONVINCE YOU
OF SOMETHING, OR ARE THEY SHARING INFORMATION AND
ENCOURAGING YOU TO MAKE UP YOUR OWN MIND?

THE LANGUAGE PEOPLE USE CAN ALSO TELL YOU SOMETHING
ABOUT THEIR TRUSTWORTHINESS. ARE THEY TALKING DOWN
TO YOU, OR TO ANY GROUP? ARE THEY USING LANGUAGE
THAT SEEMS INTENDED TO SHOCK OR HURT, OR ARE THEY
USING LANGUAGE IN A WAY THAT INVITES PEOPLE TO
ENGAGE WITH THEM?

DO THE AUTHORS LINK TO OTHER PEOPLE'S WORK ONLINE?
DO THEY LINK TO PAGES YOU ALREADY KNOW?
DO THE PAGES THEY LINK TO SEEM TRUSTWORTHY?

WHAT ELSE IS ON THE PAGE?

IF THERE ARE IMAGES OF PEOPLE, DO THEY LOOK LIKE YOU OR
PEOPLE WHO ARE IN YOUR COMMUNITIES? DOES EVERYONE
LOOK THE SAME?

IS THERE ADVERTISING ON THE PAGE? DO ALL THE ADS
SEEM THE SAME?

DOES THE PAGE INCLUDE A DATE IT WAS MOST
RECENTLY UPDATED?

THE INTERNET IS PUBLIC

BEING ONLINE CAN FEEL PRIVATE AND INTIMATE, ESPECIALLY
IF YOU'RE SHARING WITH ONE PERSON AT A TIME. BUT THE
INTERNET IS A PUBLIC SPACE, AND YOU SHOULD TREAT IT THAT
WAY WHEN YOU DECIDE WHAT KINDS OF SEX TALK YOU'RE
GOING TO HAVE THERE. WHAT YOU DO ONLINE DOESN'T EVER
DISAPPEAR, EVEN IF YOU DELETE SOMETHING. AND UNLESS
YOU KNOW HOW TO AVOID THEM, THERE ARE ALWAYS
COMPANIES TRACKING YOUR EVERY CLICK AND RECORDING
WHAT YOU READ, WATCH, AND LISTEN TO. THIS GOES FOR
TEXTING TOO.

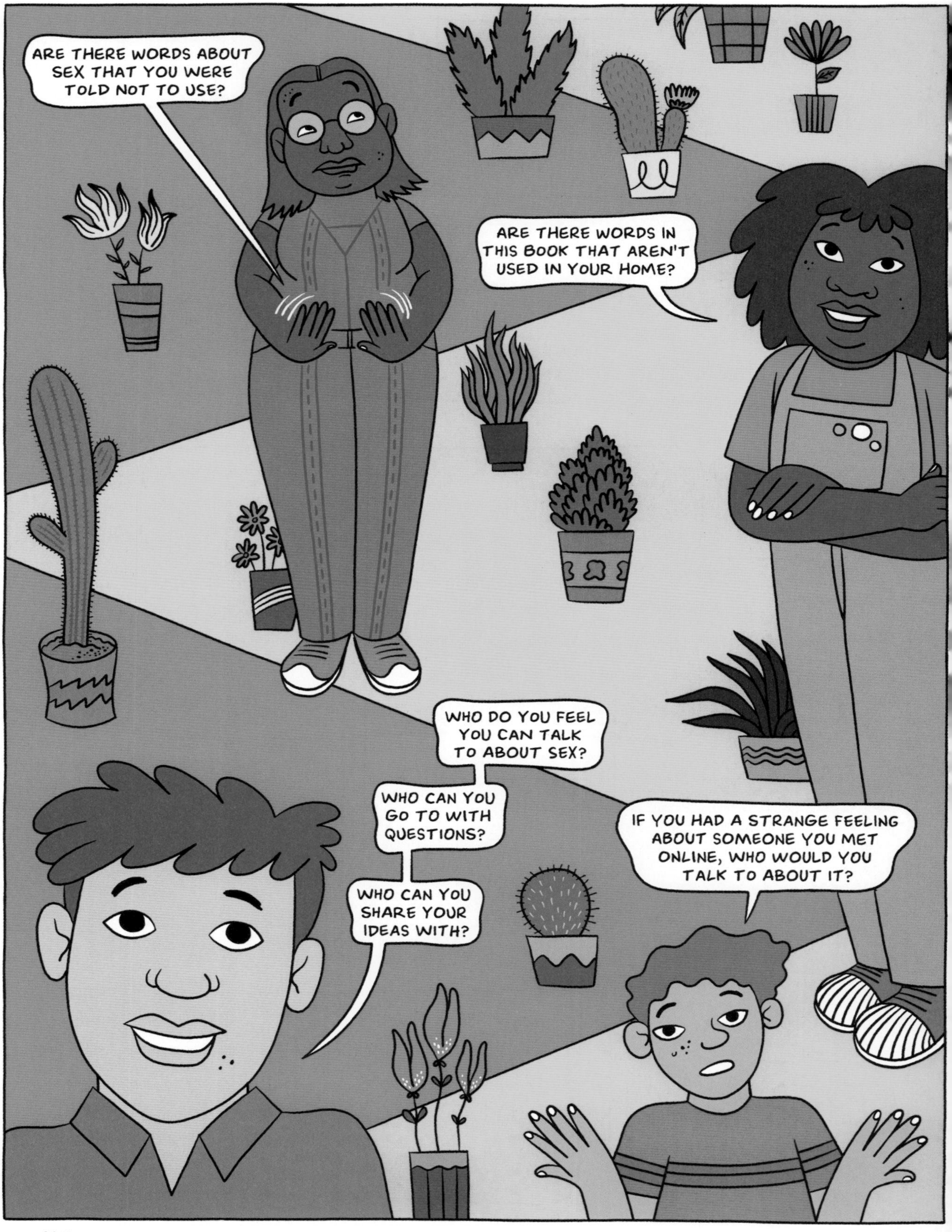
ARE THERE WORDS ABOUT SEX THAT YOU WERE TOLD NOT TO USE?
ARE THERE WORDS IN THIS BOOK THAT AREN'T USED IN YOUR HOME?
WHO DO YOU FEEL YOU CAN TALK TO ABOUT SEX?
WHO CAN YOU GO TO WITH QUESTIONS?
WHO CAN YOU SHARE YOUR IDEAS WITH?
IF YOU HAD A STRANGE FEELING ABOUT SOMEONE YOU MET ONLINE, WHO WOULD YOU TALK TO ABOUT IT?

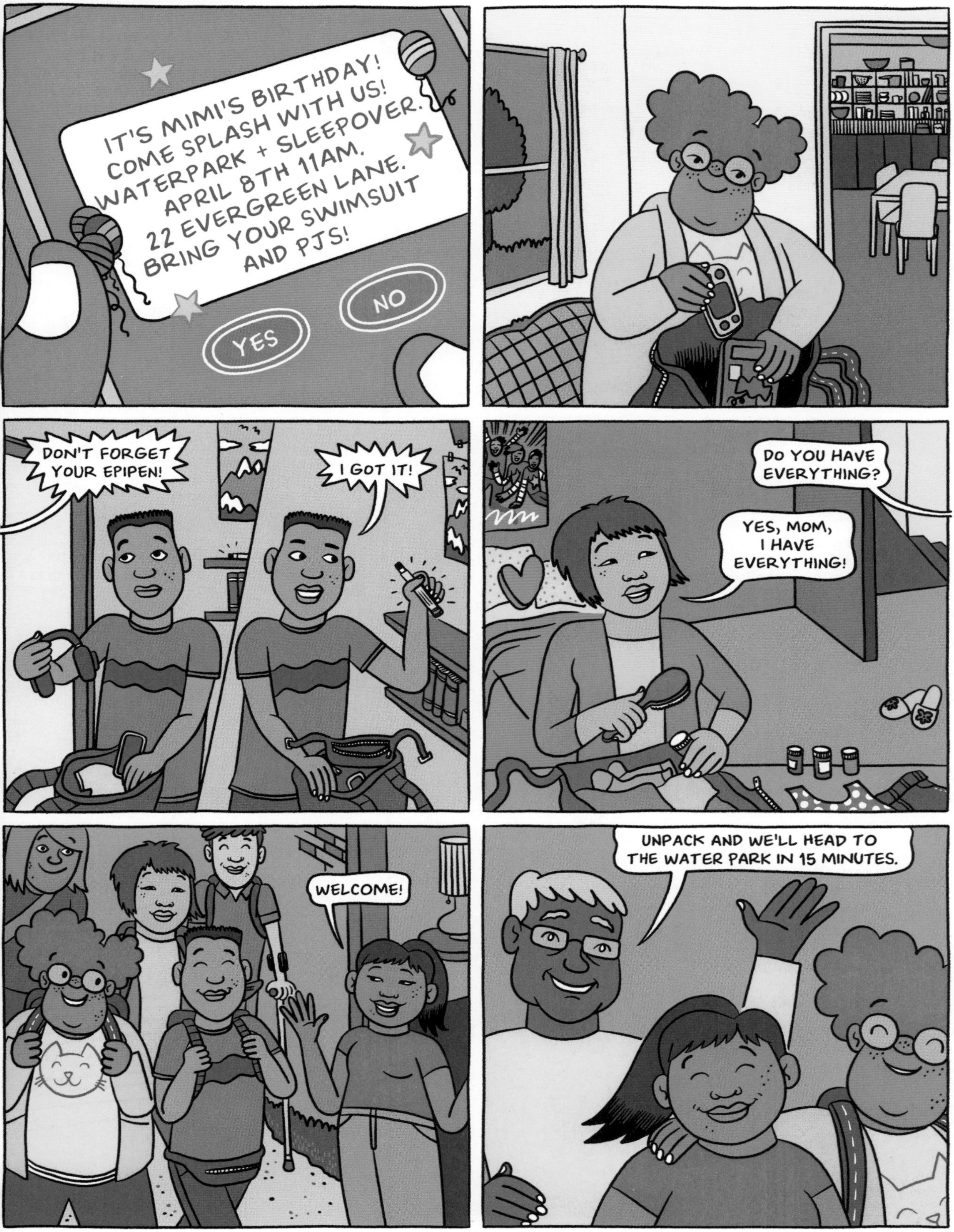
IT'S MIMI'S BIRTHDAY!
COME SPLASH WITH US!
WATERPARK + SLEEPOVER.
APRIL 8TH 11AM.
22 EVERGREEN LANE.
BRING YOUR SWIMSUIT
AND PJS!
YES
NO
DON'T FORGET YOUR EPIPEN!
I GOT IT!
DO YOU HAVE EVERYTHING?
YES, MOM, I HAVE EVERYTHING!
WELCOME!
UNPACK AND WE'LL HEAD TO THE WATER PARK IN 15 MINUTES.

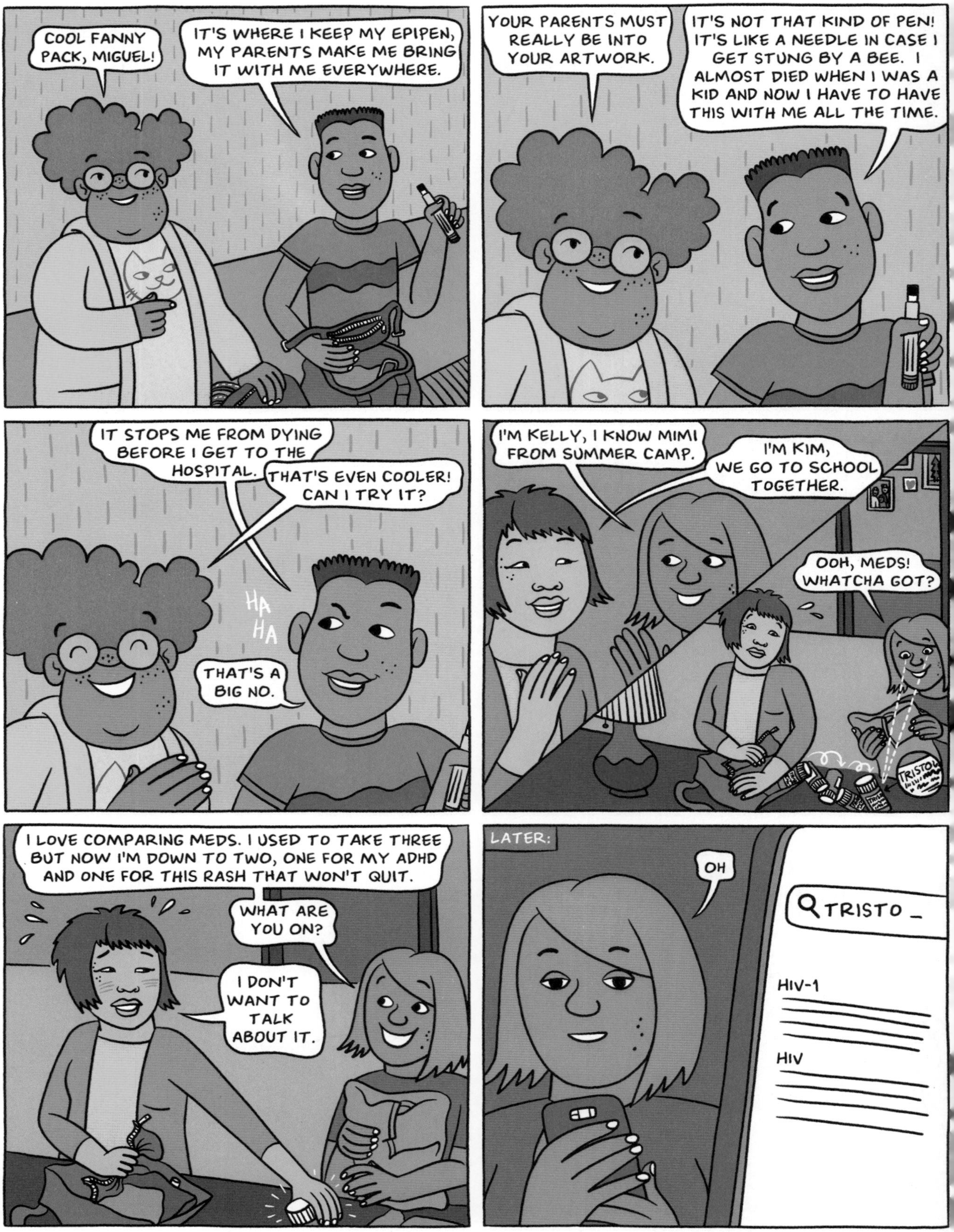
COOL FANNY PACK, MIGUEL!
IT'S WHERE I KEEP MY EPIPEN, MY PARENTS MAKE ME BRING IT WITH ME EVERYWHERE.
YOUR PARENTS MUST REALLY BE INTO YOUR ARTWORK.
IT'S NOT THAT KIND OF PEN! IT'S LIKE A NEEDLE IN CASE I GET STUNG BY A BEE. I ALMOST DIED WHEN I WAS A KID AND NOW I HAVE TO HAVE THIS WITH ME ALL THE TIME.
IT STOPS ME FROM DYING BEFORE I GET TO THE HOSPITAL.
THAT'S EVEN COOLER! CAN I TRY IT?
HA HA
THAT'S A BIG NO.
I'M KELLY, I KNOW MIMI FROM SUMMER CAMP.
I'M KIM, WE GO TO SCHOOL TOGETHER.
OOH, MEDS! WHATCHA GOT?
I LOVE COMPARING MEDS. I USED TO TAKE THREE BUT NOW I'M DOWN TO TWO, ONE FOR MY ADHD AND ONE FOR THIS RASH THAT WON'T QUIT.
WHAT ARE YOU ON?
I DON'T WANT TO TALK ABOUT IT.
LATER:
OH
TRISTO _
HIV-1
HIV

WHEN WE FEEL EMBARRASSED OF OUR BODIES AND MINDS, MOST OF US THINK THAT THE PROBLEM IS US. WE THINK THAT WE SHOULD FEEL ASHAMED BECAUSE WE'RE DIFFERENT AND WE'RE NOT WHAT OTHER PEOPLE THINK OF AS NORMAL.

BUT NO BODY IS WRONG. SHAME IS SOMETHING WE LEARN, AND ONE WAY WE'RE TAUGHT TO FEEL SHAME IS THROUGH STIGMA.

THE WORD STIGMA COMES FROM AN OLD GREEK WORD FOR A MARK OR WOUND. STIGMA REFERS TO THE WAY SOME PEOPLE ARE "MARKED" AND TREATED BADLY BECAUSE THEY ARE DIFFERENT.

WE MIGHT BE MARKED BY THE COLOR OF OUR SKIN, WHERE WE GREW UP, HOW MUCH MONEY OUR FAMILIES HAVE, OR WHO WE LOVE. WE MIGHT BE MARKED BY THE SIZE AND SHAPE OF OUR BODIES, OR THE WAYS WE MOVE AROUND OR COMMUNICATE OR THINK.

WHATEVER MAKES US STAND OUT AS DIFFERENT CAN MARK US AND MAKE US A TARGET OF STIGMA.

SSSSTIGMA!
SSSSTIGMA!
SSSSTIGMA!

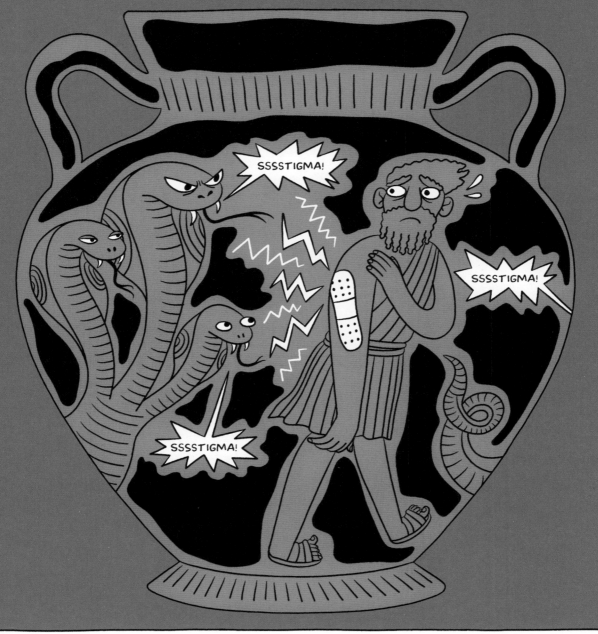

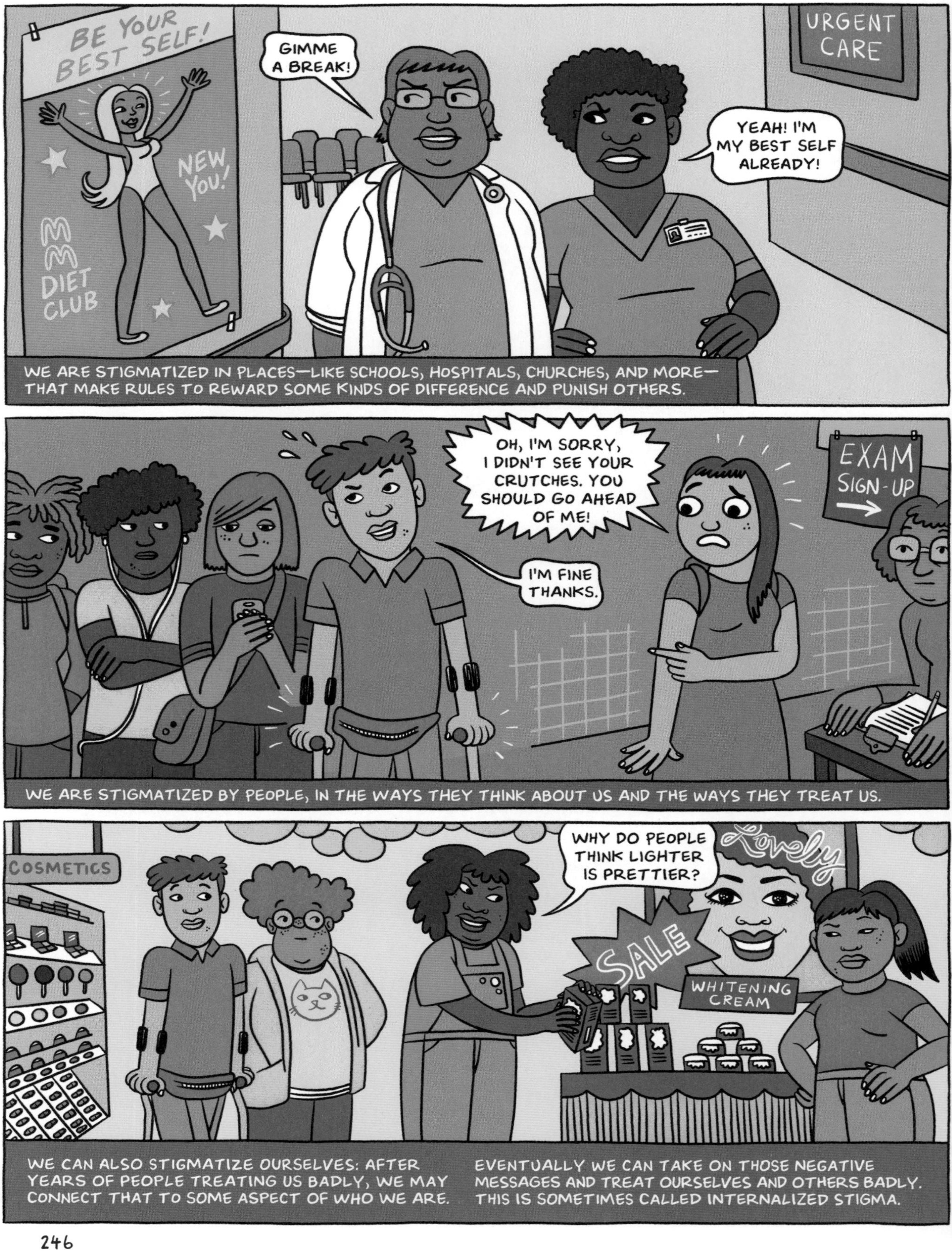

BE YOUR BEST SELF!
NEW YOU!
DIET CLUB
GIMME A BREAK!
URGENT CARE
YEAH! I'M MY BEST SELF ALREADY!
WE ARE STIGMATIZED IN PLACES—LIKE SCHOOLS, HOSPITALS, CHURCHES, AND MORE—THAT MAKE RULES TO REWARD SOME KINDS OF DIFFERENCE AND PUNISH OTHERS.
OH, I'M SORRY, I DIDN'T SEE YOUR CRUTCHES. YOU SHOULD GO AHEAD OF ME!
I'M FINE THANKS.
EXAM SIGN-UP →
WE ARE STIGMATIZED BY PEOPLE, IN THE WAYS THEY THINK ABOUT US AND THE WAYS THEY TREAT US.
COSMETICS
WHY DO PEOPLE THINK LIGHTER IS PRETTIER?
Lovely
SALE
WHITENING CREAM
WE CAN ALSO STIGMATIZE OURSELVES: AFTER YEARS OF PEOPLE TREATING US BADLY, WE MAY CONNECT THAT TO SOME ASPECT OF WHO WE ARE.
EVENTUALLY WE CAN TAKE ON THOSE NEGATIVE MESSAGES AND TREAT OURSELVES AND OTHERS BADLY. THIS IS SOMETIMES CALLED INTERNALIZED STIGMA.

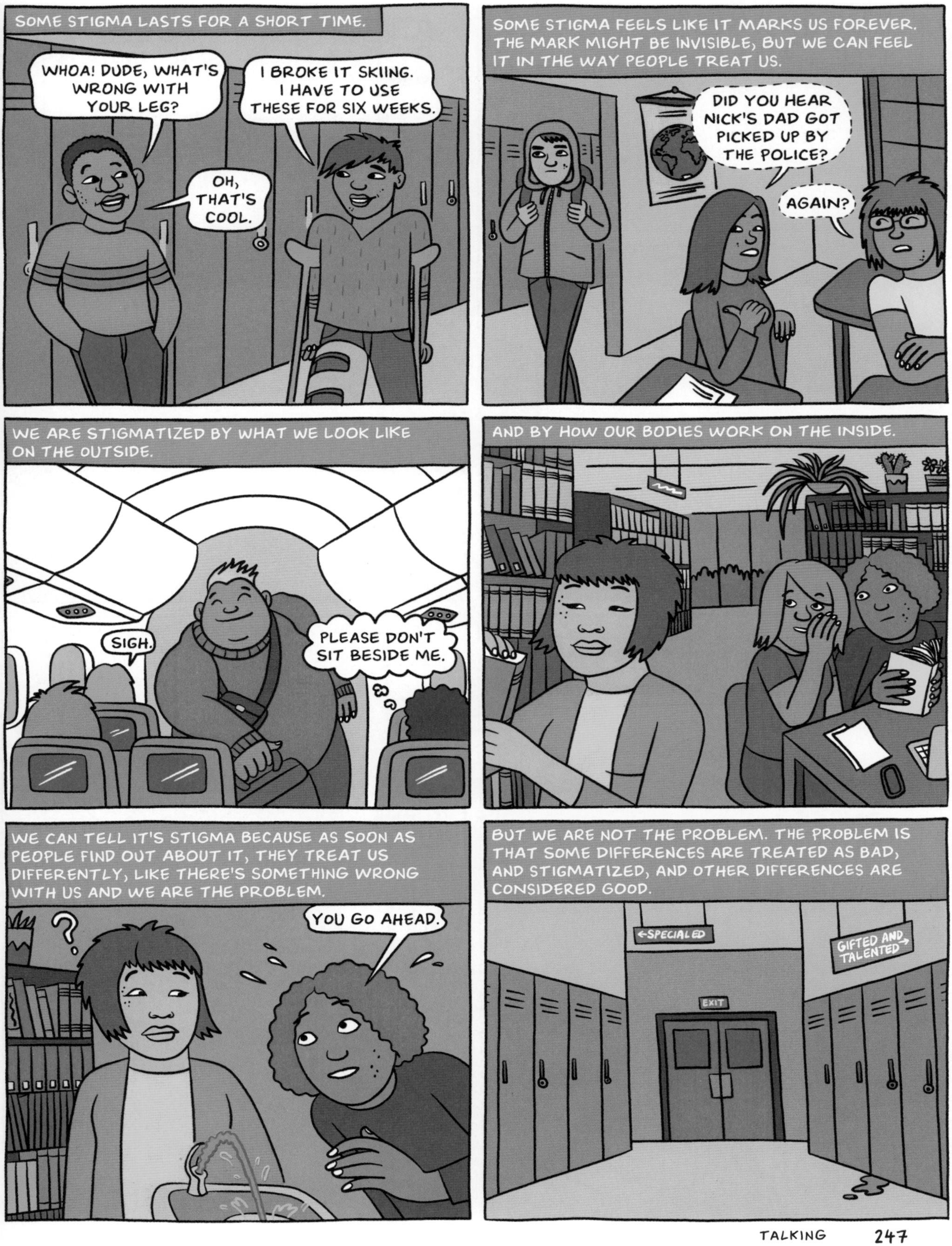
SOME STIGMA LASTS FOR A SHORT TIME.
WHOA! DUDE, WHAT'S WRONG WITH YOUR LEG?
I BROKE IT SKIING. I HAVE TO USE THESE FOR SIX WEEKS.
OH, THAT'S COOL.
SOME STIGMA FEELS LIKE IT MARKS US FOREVER. THE MARK MIGHT BE INVISIBLE, BUT WE CAN FEEL IT IN THE WAY PEOPLE TREAT US.
DID YOU HEAR NICK'S DAD GOT PICKED UP BY THE POLICE?
AGAIN?
WE ARE STIGMATIZED BY WHAT WE LOOK LIKE ON THE OUTSIDE.
SIGH.
PLEASE DON'T SIT BESIDE ME.
AND BY HOW OUR BODIES WORK ON THE INSIDE.
WE CAN TELL IT'S STIGMA BECAUSE AS SOON AS PEOPLE FIND OUT ABOUT IT, THEY TREAT US DIFFERENTLY, LIKE THERE'S SOMETHING WRONG WITH US AND WE ARE THE PROBLEM.
?
YOU GO AHEAD.
BUT WE ARE NOT THE PROBLEM. THE PROBLEM IS THAT SOME DIFFERENCES ARE TREATED AS BAD, AND STIGMATIZED, AND OTHER DIFFERENCES ARE CONSIDERED GOOD.
←SPECIAL ED
GIFTED AND TALENTED→
EXIT

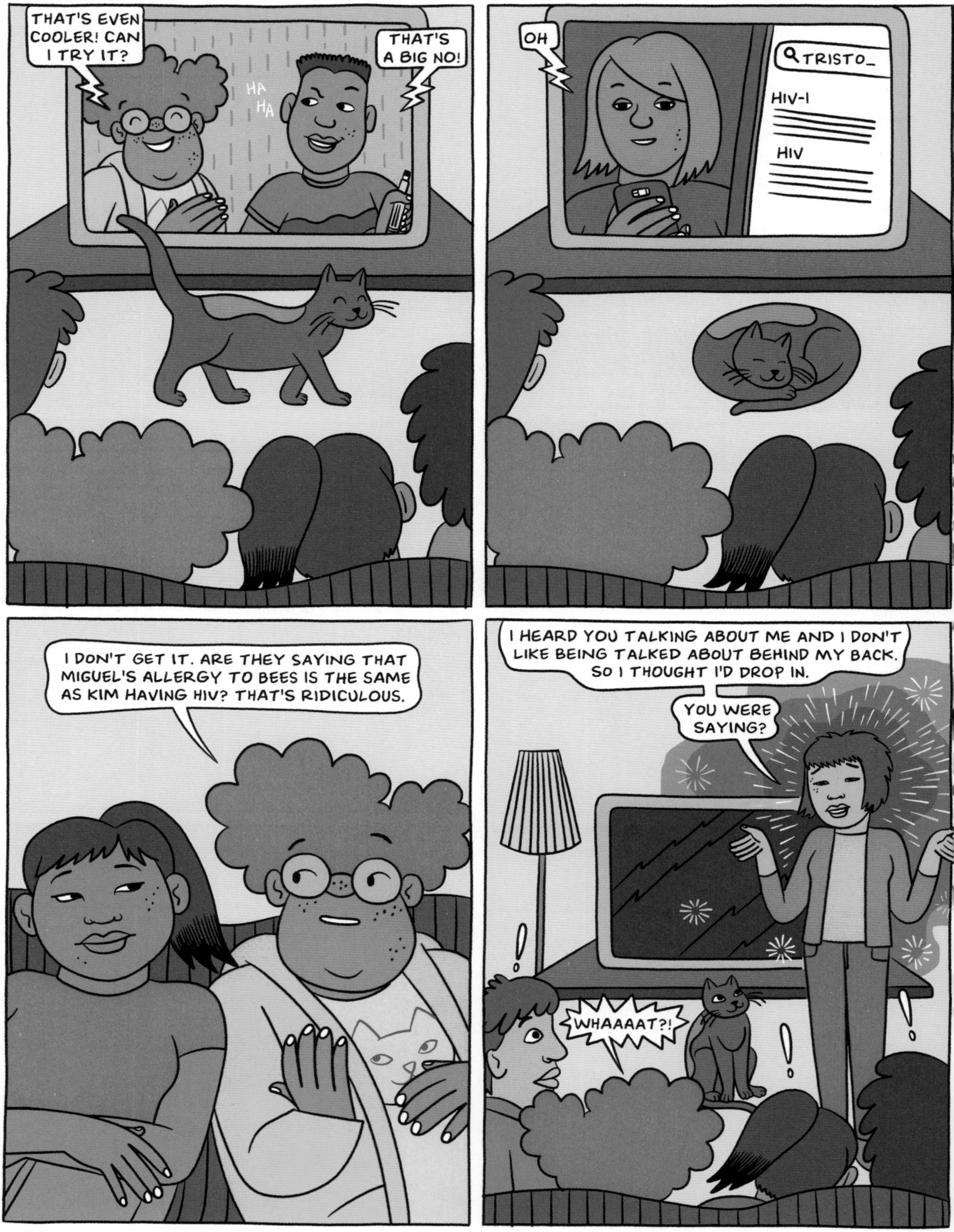
THAT'S EVEN COOLER! CAN I TRY IT?
THAT'S A BIG NO!
HA HA
OH
TRISTO_
HIV-1
HIV
I DON'T GET IT. ARE THEY SAYING THAT MIGUEL'S ALLERGY TO BEES IS THE SAME AS KIM HAVING HIV? THAT'S RIDICULOUS.
I HEARD YOU TALKING ABOUT ME AND I DON'T LIKE BEING TALKED ABOUT BEHIND MY BACK. SO I THOUGHT I'D DROP IN.
YOU WERE SAYING?
WHAAAAT?!

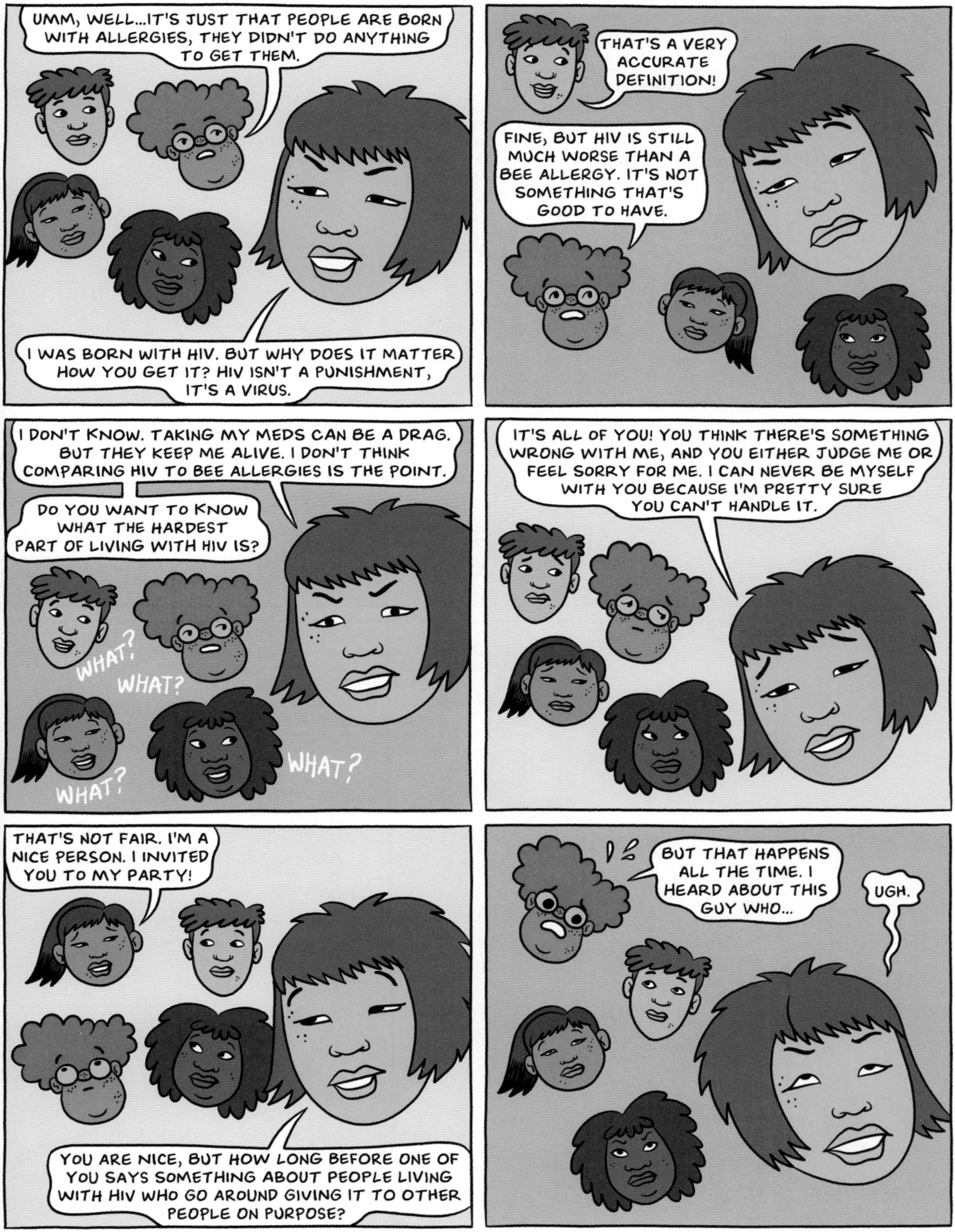
UMM, WELL...IT'S JUST THAT PEOPLE ARE BORN WITH ALLERGIES, THEY DIDN'T DO ANYTHING TO GET THEM.
I WAS BORN WITH HIV. BUT WHY DOES IT MATTER HOW YOU GET IT? HIV ISN'T A PUNISHMENT, IT'S A VIRUS.
THAT'S A VERY ACCURATE DEFINITION!
FINE, BUT HIV IS STILL MUCH WORSE THAN A BEE ALLERGY. IT'S NOT SOMETHING THAT'S GOOD TO HAVE.
I DON'T KNOW. TAKING MY MEDS CAN BE A DRAG. BUT THEY KEEP ME ALIVE. I DON'T THINK COMPARING HIV TO BEE ALLERGIES IS THE POINT.
DO YOU WANT TO KNOW WHAT THE HARDEST PART OF LIVING WITH HIV IS?
WHAT?
WHAT?
WHAT?
WHAT?
IT'S ALL OF YOU! YOU THINK THERE'S SOMETHING WRONG WITH ME, AND YOU EITHER JUDGE ME OR FEEL SORRY FOR ME. I CAN NEVER BE MYSELF WITH YOU BECAUSE I'M PRETTY SURE YOU CAN'T HANDLE IT.
THAT'S NOT FAIR. I'M A NICE PERSON. I INVITED YOU TO MY PARTY!
YOU ARE NICE, BUT HOW LONG BEFORE ONE OF YOU SAYS SOMETHING ABOUT PEOPLE LIVING WITH HIV WHO GO AROUND GIVING IT TO OTHER PEOPLE ON PURPOSE?
BUT THAT HAPPENS ALL THE TIME. I HEARD ABOUT THIS GUY WHO...
UGH.

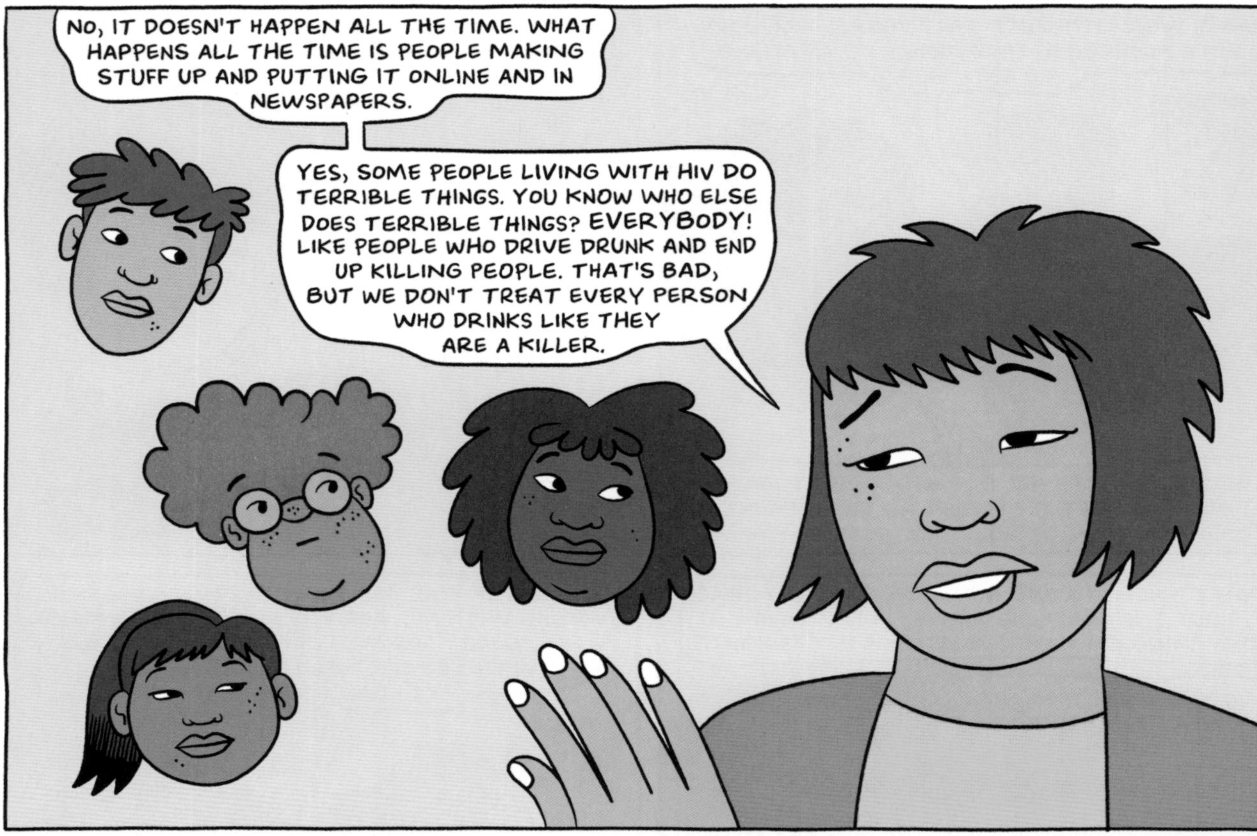
NO, IT DOESN'T HAPPEN ALL THE TIME. WHAT HAPPENS ALL THE TIME IS PEOPLE MAKING STUFF UP AND PUTTING IT ONLINE AND IN NEWSPAPERS.
YES, SOME PEOPLE LIVING WITH HIV DO TERRIBLE THINGS. YOU KNOW WHO ELSE DOES TERRIBLE THINGS? EVERYBODY! LIKE PEOPLE WHO DRIVE DRUNK AND END UP KILLING PEOPLE. THAT'S BAD, BUT WE DON'T TREAT EVERY PERSON WHO DRINKS LIKE THEY ARE A KILLER.

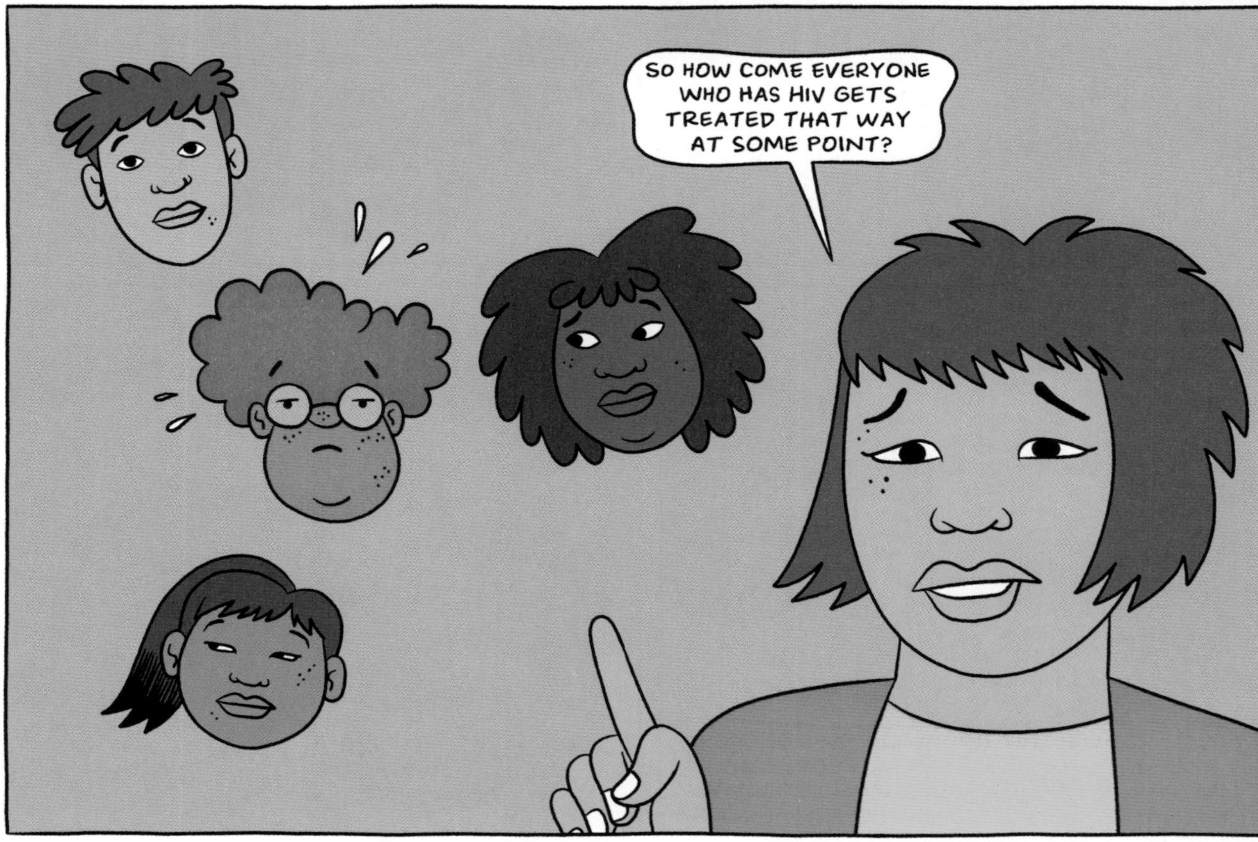
SO HOW COME EVERYONE WHO HAS HIV GETS TREATED THAT WAY AT SOME POINT?

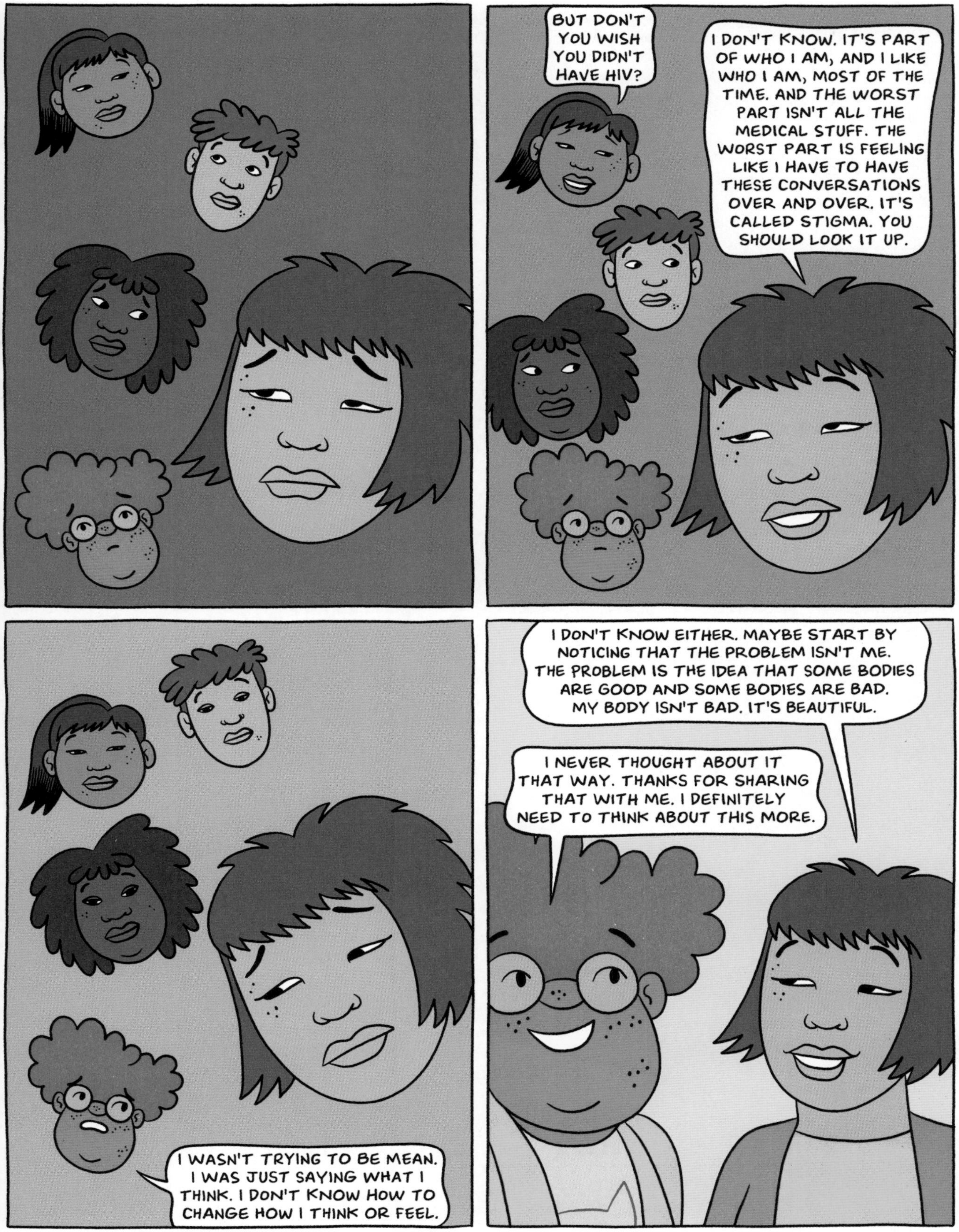
BUT DON'T YOU WISH YOU DIDN'T HAVE HIV?
I DON'T KNOW. IT'S PART OF WHO I AM, AND I LIKE WHO I AM, MOST OF THE TIME. AND THE WORST PART ISN'T ALL THE MEDICAL STUFF. THE WORST PART IS FEELING LIKE I HAVE TO HAVE THESE CONVERSATIONS OVER AND OVER. IT'S CALLED STIGMA. YOU SHOULD LOOK IT UP.
I WASN'T TRYING TO BE MEAN. I WAS JUST SAYING WHAT I THINK. I DON'T KNOW HOW TO CHANGE HOW I THINK OR FEEL.
I DON'T KNOW EITHER. MAYBE START BY NOTICING THAT THE PROBLEM ISN'T ME. THE PROBLEM IS THE IDEA THAT SOME BODIES ARE GOOD AND SOME BODIES ARE BAD. MY BODY ISN'T BAD. IT'S BEAUTIFUL.
I NEVER THOUGHT ABOUT IT THAT WAY. THANKS FOR SHARING THAT WITH ME. I DEFINITELY NEED TO THINK ABOUT THIS MORE.

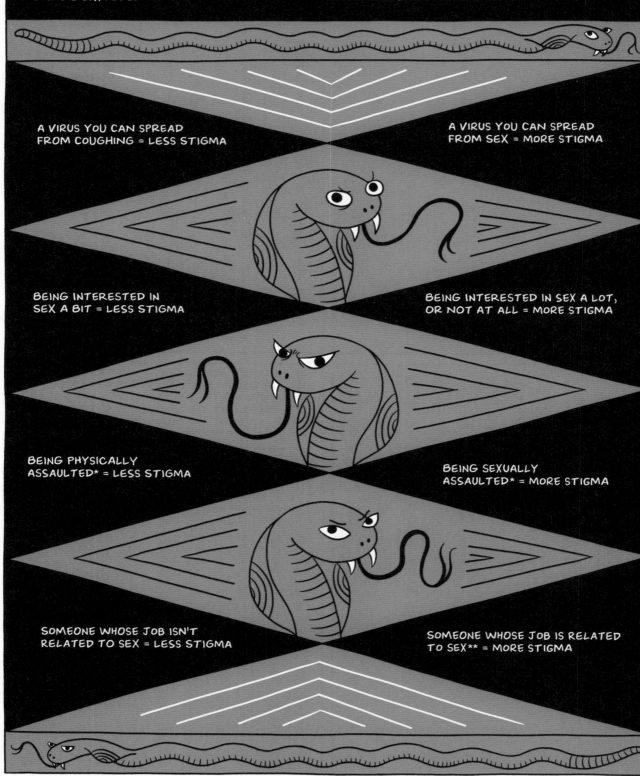

STIGMA IS TRICKY—ESPECIALLY IN A WORLD THAT SAYS THERE'S SOMETHING WRONG WITH US BECAUSE WE DON'T FIT THE NORM OR WHAT'S EXPECTED.

PEOPLE ARE STIGMATIZED FOR ALL SORTS OF DIFFERENCE, BUT WHEN THAT DIFFERENCE HAS SOMETHING TO DO WITH SEX OR GENDER, THERE'S USUALLY MORE STIGMA.

A VIRUS YOU CAN SPREAD FROM COUGHING = LESS STIGMA

A VIRUS YOU CAN SPREAD FROM SEX = MORE STIGMA

BEING INTERESTED IN SEX A BIT = LESS STIGMA

BEING INTERESTED IN SEX A LOT, OR NOT AT ALL = MORE STIGMA

BEING PHYSICALLY ASSAULTED* = LESS STIGMA

BEING SEXUALLY ASSAULTED* = MORE STIGMA

SOMEONE WHOSE JOB ISN'T RELATED TO SEX = LESS STIGMA

SOMEONE WHOSE JOB IS RELATED TO SEX** = MORE STIGMA

* MORE ABOUT ASSAULT ON P. 384   ** MORE ABOUT SEX WORK ON P. 424

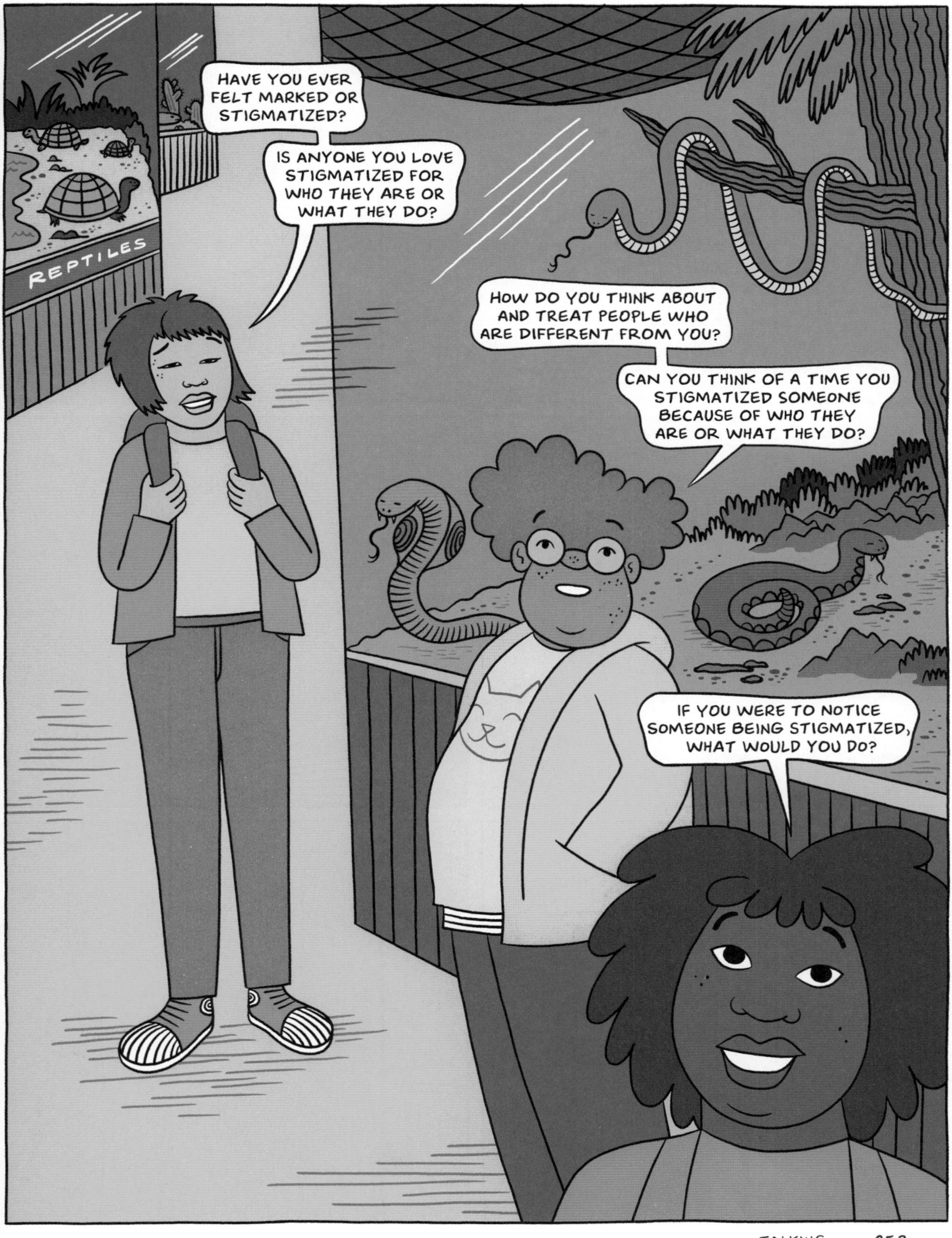
REPTILES
HAVE YOU EVER FELT MARKED OR STIGMATIZED?
IS ANYONE YOU LOVE STIGMATIZED FOR WHO THEY ARE OR WHAT THEY DO?
HOW DO YOU THINK ABOUT AND TREAT PEOPLE WHO ARE DIFFERENT FROM YOU?
CAN YOU THINK OF A TIME YOU STIGMATIZED SOMEONE BECAUSE OF WHO THEY ARE OR WHAT THEY DO?
IF YOU WERE TO NOTICE SOMEONE BEING STIGMATIZED, WHAT WOULD YOU DO?

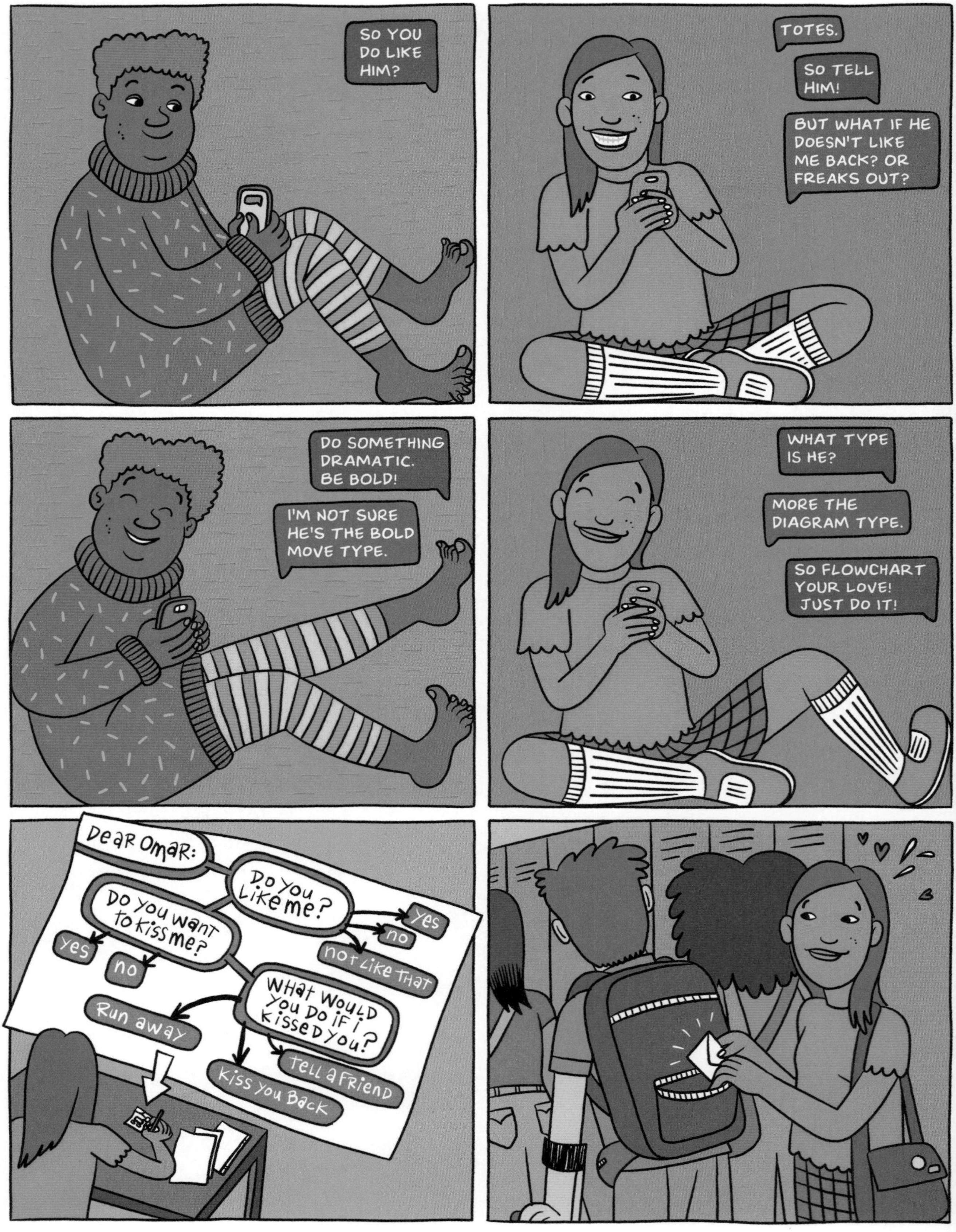
SO YOU DO LIKE HIM?
TOTES.
SO TELL HIM!
BUT WHAT IF HE DOESN'T LIKE ME BACK? OR FREAKS OUT?
DO SOMETHING DRAMATIC. BE BOLD!
I'M NOT SURE HE'S THE BOLD MOVE TYPE.
WHAT TYPE IS HE?
MORE THE DIAGRAM TYPE.
SO FLOWCHART YOUR LOVE! JUST DO IT!
Dear Omar:
Do you Like me?
yes
no
not Like That
Do you want to kiss me?
yes
no
What would you Do if i kissed you?
Run away
tell a Friend
Kiss you Back

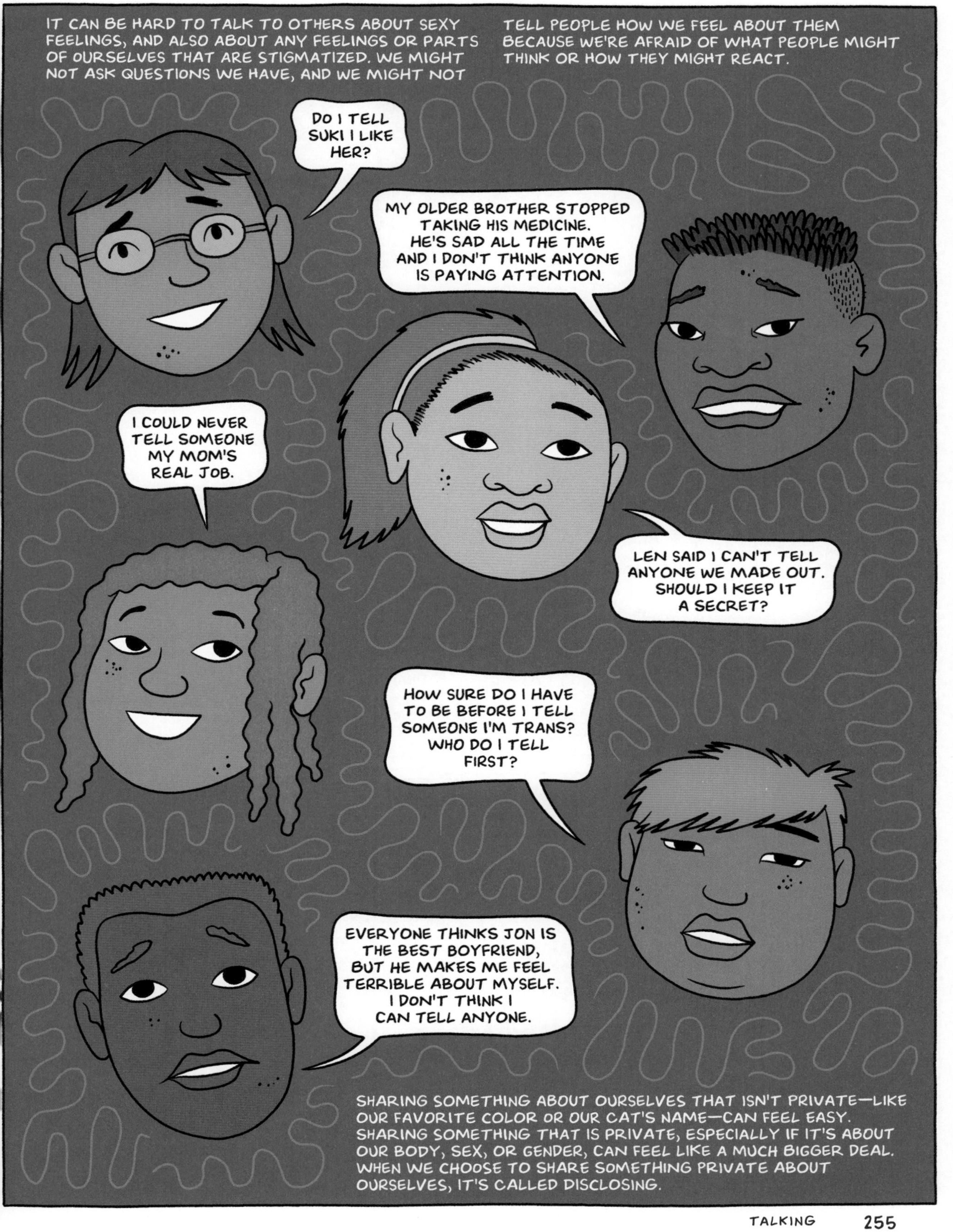
IT CAN BE HARD TO TALK TO OTHERS ABOUT SEXY FEELINGS, AND ALSO ABOUT ANY FEELINGS OR PARTS OF OURSELVES THAT ARE STIGMATIZED. WE MIGHT NOT ASK QUESTIONS WE HAVE, AND WE MIGHT NOT TELL PEOPLE HOW WE FEEL ABOUT THEM BECAUSE WE'RE AFRAID OF WHAT PEOPLE MIGHT THINK OR HOW THEY MIGHT REACT.
DO I TELL SUKI I LIKE HER?
MY OLDER BROTHER STOPPED TAKING HIS MEDICINE. HE'S SAD ALL THE TIME AND I DON'T THINK ANYONE IS PAYING ATTENTION.
I COULD NEVER TELL SOMEONE MY MOM'S REAL JOB.
LEN SAID I CAN'T TELL ANYONE WE MADE OUT. SHOULD I KEEP IT A SECRET?
HOW SURE DO I HAVE TO BE BEFORE I TELL SOMEONE I'M TRANS? WHO DO I TELL FIRST?
EVERYONE THINKS JON IS THE BEST BOYFRIEND, BUT HE MAKES ME FEEL TERRIBLE ABOUT MYSELF. I DON'T THINK I CAN TELL ANYONE.
SHARING SOMETHING ABOUT OURSELVES THAT ISN'T PRIVATE—LIKE OUR FAVORITE COLOR OR OUR CAT'S NAME—CAN FEEL EASY. SHARING SOMETHING THAT IS PRIVATE, ESPECIALLY IF IT'S ABOUT OUR BODY, SEX, OR GENDER, CAN FEEL LIKE A MUCH BIGGER DEAL. WHEN WE CHOOSE TO SHARE SOMETHING PRIVATE ABOUT OURSELVES, IT'S CALLED DISCLOSING.

MOST PEOPLE WONDER WHEN IS THE RIGHT TIME TO DISCLOSE OR SHARE SOMETHING PRIVATE. THE SHORT ANSWER IS THAT THERE ISN'T ONE RIGHT TIME.

IT DEPENDS ON YOU, ON THE PERSON YOU WANT TO DISCLOSE TO, ON THE COMMUNITY YOU'RE IN, AND ON WHAT YOU'RE DISCLOSING.

THE MOST IMPORTANT PART OF MAKING THE DECISION IS THAT IT'S YOUR CHOICE AND YOU'VE THOUGHT IT THROUGH.

YOU CAN'T KNOW HOW A PERSON WILL REACT, BUT YOU CAN PLAN FOR A RESPONSE THAT'S POSITIVE, NEGATIVE, OR NEUTRAL AND THINK ABOUT HOW IT WILL FEEL. IT CAN ALSO HELP TO TALK THROUGH SCENARIOS AND POSSIBILITIES WITH SOMEONE YOU TRUST.

ONE WAY TO BREAK IT DOWN IS TO THINK ABOUT:
★ WHY ARE YOU DISCLOSING?
★ WHAT ARE YOU HOPING WILL HAPPEN?
★ HOW CAN YOU PREPARE FOR REACTIONS THAT YOU MIGHT NOT EXPECT?

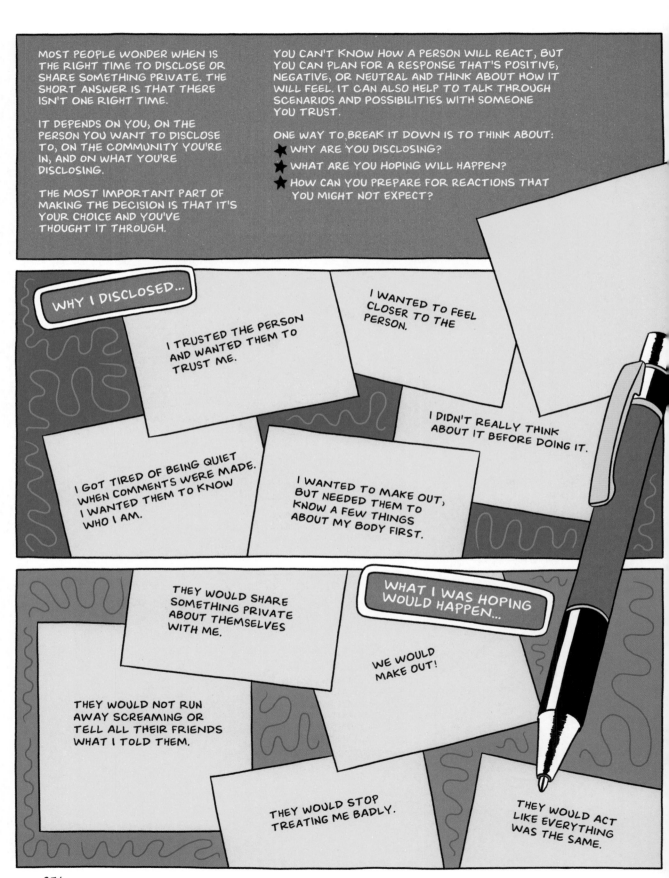

WHY I DISCLOSED...

I TRUSTED THE PERSON AND WANTED THEM TO TRUST ME.

I WANTED TO FEEL CLOSER TO THE PERSON.

I DIDN'T REALLY THINK ABOUT IT BEFORE DOING IT.

I GOT TIRED OF BEING QUIET WHEN COMMENTS WERE MADE. I WANTED THEM TO KNOW WHO I AM.

I WANTED TO MAKE OUT, BUT NEEDED THEM TO KNOW A FEW THINGS ABOUT MY BODY FIRST.

THEY WOULD SHARE SOMETHING PRIVATE ABOUT THEMSELVES WITH ME.

WHAT I WAS HOPING WOULD HAPPEN...

WE WOULD MAKE OUT!

THEY WOULD NOT RUN AWAY SCREAMING OR TELL ALL THEIR FRIENDS WHAT I TOLD THEM.

THEY WOULD STOP TREATING ME BADLY.

THEY WOULD ACT LIKE EVERYTHING WAS THE SAME.

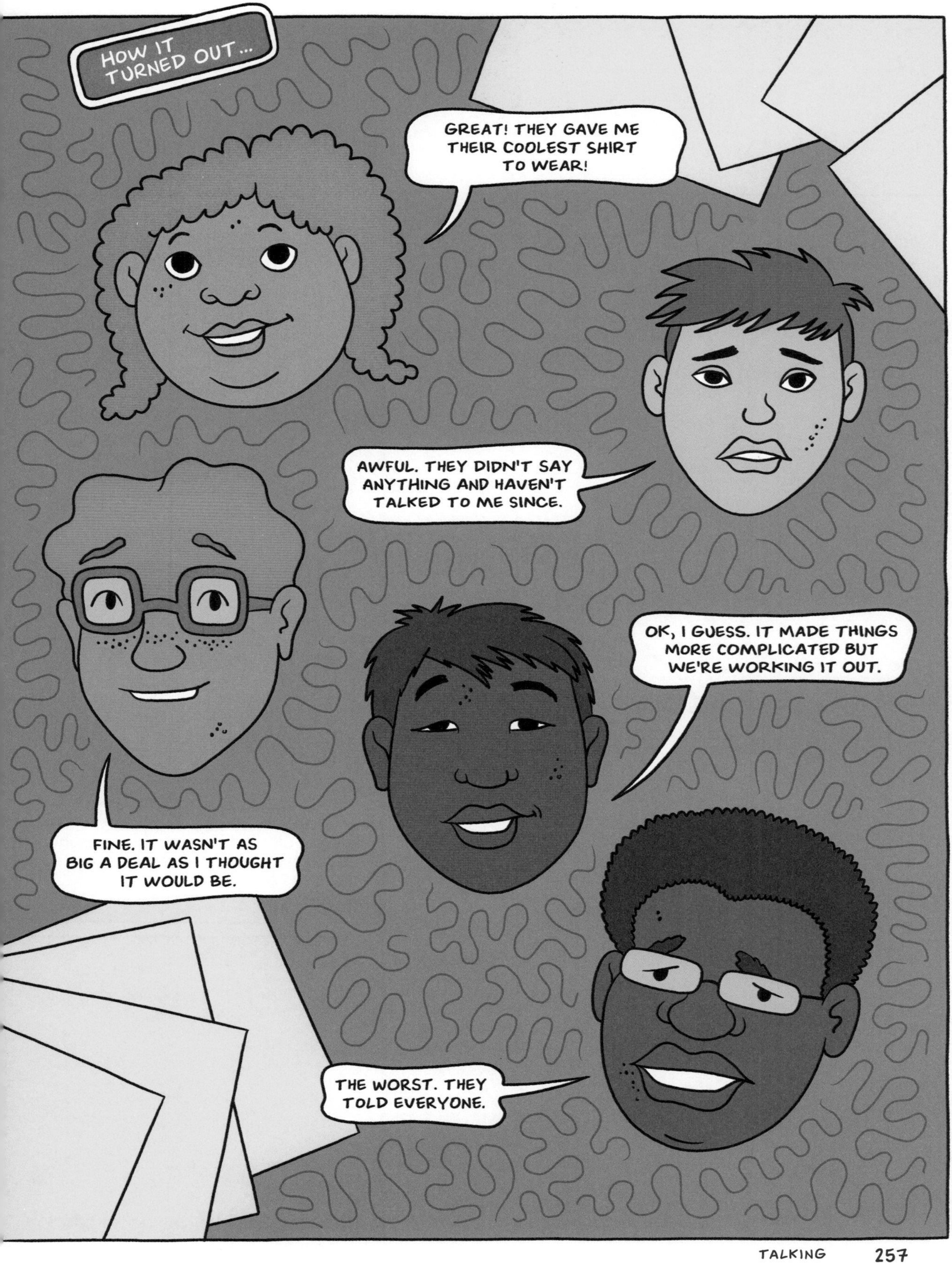
HOW IT TURNED OUT...
GREAT! THEY GAVE ME THEIR COOLEST SHIRT TO WEAR!
AWFUL. THEY DIDN'T SAY ANYTHING AND HAVEN'T TALKED TO ME SINCE.
OK, I GUESS. IT MADE THINGS MORE COMPLICATED BUT WE'RE WORKING IT OUT.
FINE. IT WASN'T AS BIG A DEAL AS I THOUGHT IT WOULD BE.
THE WORST. THEY TOLD EVERYONE.

DISCLOSING FEELS SCARY AND RISKY BECAUSE IT IS. TAKING RISKS IS PART OF LIFE, AND WE ALL DESERVE TO BE ABLE TO CHOOSE TO TAKE RISKS.

BUT SOME OF US DON'T GET TO TAKE AS MANY RISKS AS OTHERS. JUSTICE WOULD MEAN EVERYONE HAVING THE FREEDOM TO TAKE RISKS—AND TO DECIDE WHAT LEVEL OF RISK TO TAKE.

PEOPLE IN OUR LIVES WHO CARE ABOUT US MIGHT DISCOURAGE US FROM DISCLOSING THINGS THEY THINK WILL END BADLY FOR US. IT'S UNDERSTANDABLE. BUT RESPECT MEANS LETTING US MAKE OUR OWN CHOICES, NOT ONLY THE CHOICES OTHERS WANT US TO MAKE.

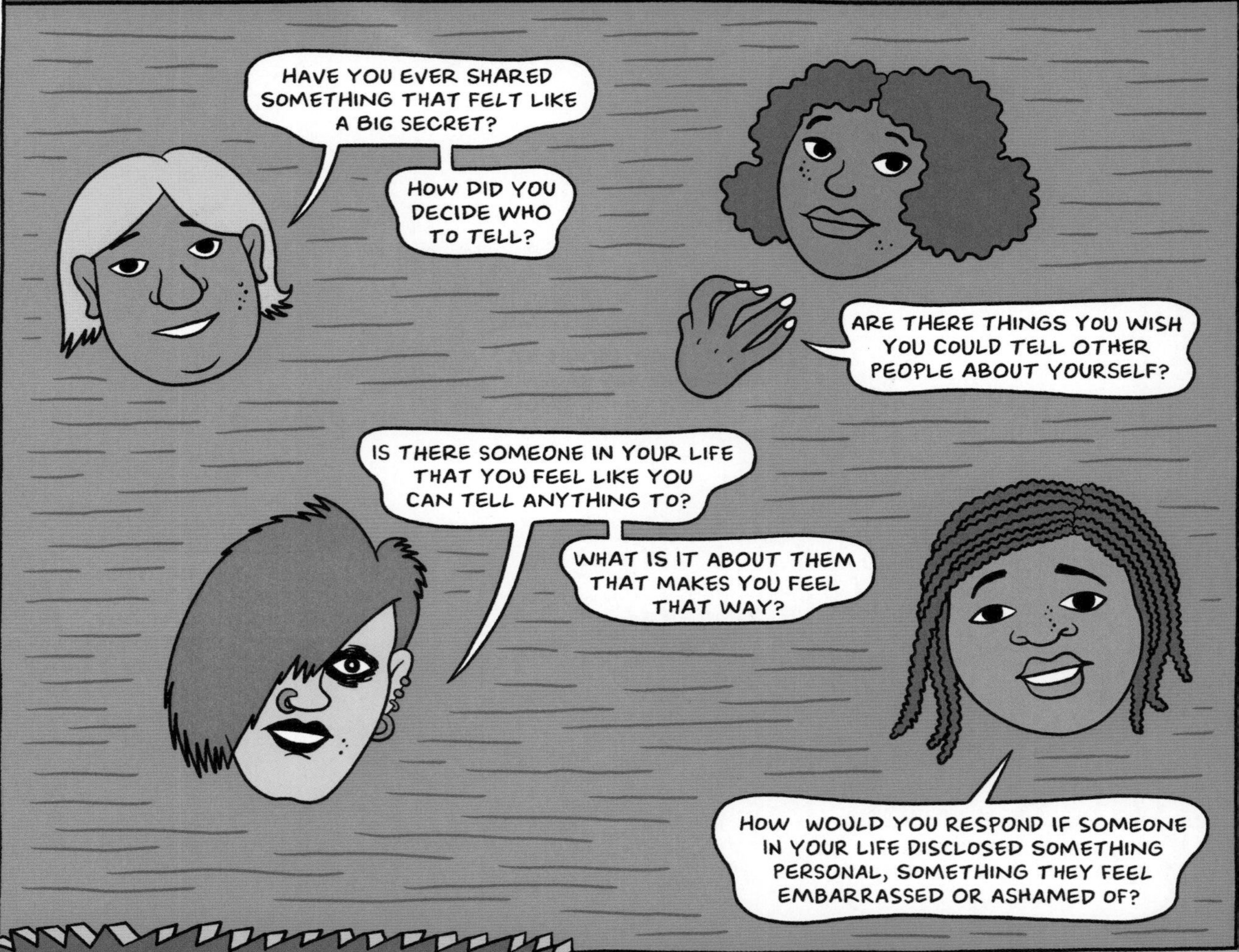
HAVE YOU EVER SHARED SOMETHING THAT FELT LIKE A BIG SECRET?
HOW DID YOU DECIDE WHO TO TELL?
ARE THERE THINGS YOU WISH YOU COULD TELL OTHER PEOPLE ABOUT YOURSELF?
IS THERE SOMEONE IN YOUR LIFE THAT YOU FEEL LIKE YOU CAN TELL ANYTHING TO?
WHAT IS IT ABOUT THEM THAT MAKES YOU FEEL THAT WAY?
HOW WOULD YOU RESPOND IF SOMEONE IN YOUR LIFE DISCLOSED SOMETHING PERSONAL, SOMETHING THEY FEEL EMBARRASSED OR ASHAMED OF?

NERD ALERT HOW TO RECEIVE A DISCLOSURE

WE CAN ALL MAKE DISCLOSING A BIT EASIER BY BEING THE KIND OF PERSON WHO RECEIVES A DISCLOSURE WITH RESPECT AND KINDNESS. EVEN IF WE DON'T GIVE THE PERSON SHARING WHAT THEY WANT, THE WAY WE REACT CAN MAKE THE EXPERIENCE LESS PAINFUL. HERE ARE FOUR WAYS TO MAKE DISCLOSING LESS PAINFUL FOR OTHERS:

1. THANK THEM FOR SHARING WITH YOU.
2. ACKNOWLEDGE THAT THE PERSON TOOK A RISK IN SHARING SOMETHING PRIVATE WITH YOU. YOU COULD POINT OUT IT'S A BRAVE THING TO DO.
3. IF YOU AREN'T SURE HOW TO RESPOND, SAY SO. LET THEM KNOW YOU NEED TIME BUT THAT YOU WILL RESPOND IN A BIT. AND THEN FOLLOW THROUGH AND RESPOND.
4. DON'T SHARE WHAT THEY TOLD YOU WITH FRIENDS. YOU MAY NEED AND WANT TO TALK TO SOMEONE ABOUT IT, BUT PICK EITHER AN ADULT OR AT LEAST SOMEONE IN YOUR LIFE WHO DOESN'T KNOW THIS PERSON THAT WELL. RESPECT THEIR PRIVACY BY NOT GOSSIPING.

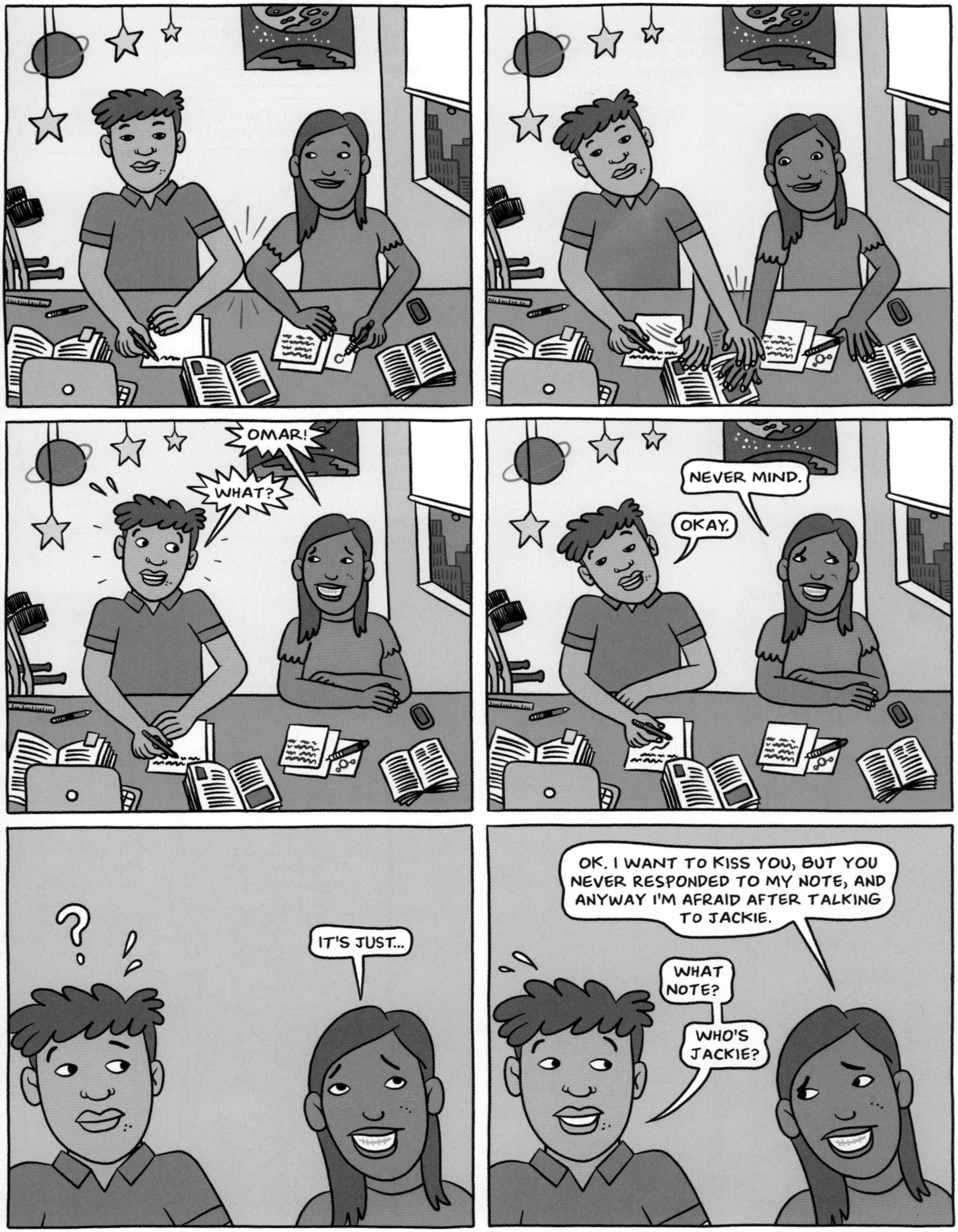
OMAR!
WHAT?
NEVER MIND.
OKAY.
IT'S JUST...
OK. I WANT TO KISS YOU, BUT YOU NEVER RESPONDED TO MY NOTE, AND ANYWAY I'M AFRAID AFTER TALKING TO JACKIE.
WHAT NOTE?
WHO'S JACKIE?

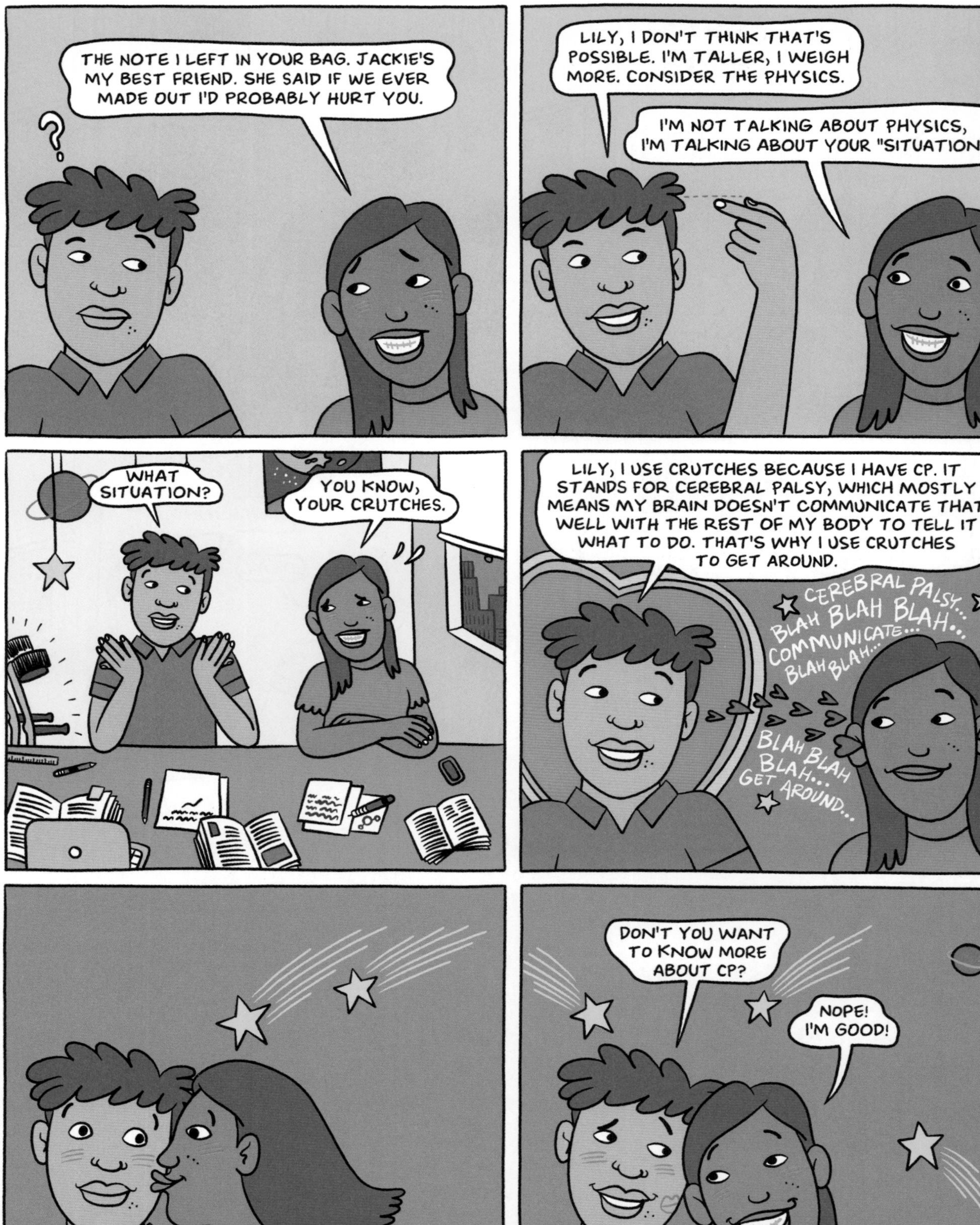

THE NOTE I LEFT IN YOUR BAG. JACKIE'S MY BEST FRIEND. SHE SAID IF WE EVER MADE OUT I'D PROBABLY HURT YOU.
?
LILY, I DON'T THINK THAT'S POSSIBLE. I'M TALLER, I WEIGH MORE. CONSIDER THE PHYSICS.
I'M NOT TALKING ABOUT PHYSICS, I'M TALKING ABOUT YOUR "SITUATION."
WHAT SITUATION?
YOU KNOW, YOUR CRUTCHES.
LILY, I USE CRUTCHES BECAUSE I HAVE CP. IT STANDS FOR CEREBRAL PALSY, WHICH MOSTLY MEANS MY BRAIN DOESN'T COMMUNICATE THAT WELL WITH THE REST OF MY BODY TO TELL IT WHAT TO DO. THAT'S WHY I USE CRUTCHES TO GET AROUND.
CEREBRAL PALSY... BLAH BLAH BLAH... COMMUNICATE... BLAH BLAH...
BLAH BLAH BLAH... GET AROUND...
DON'T YOU WANT TO KNOW MORE ABOUT CP?
NOPE! I'M GOOD!

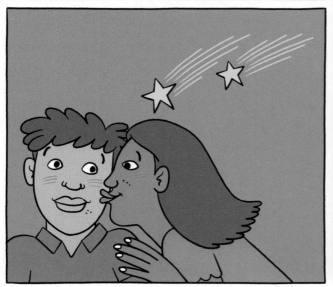

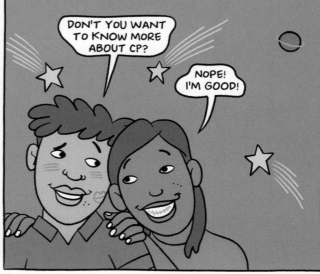

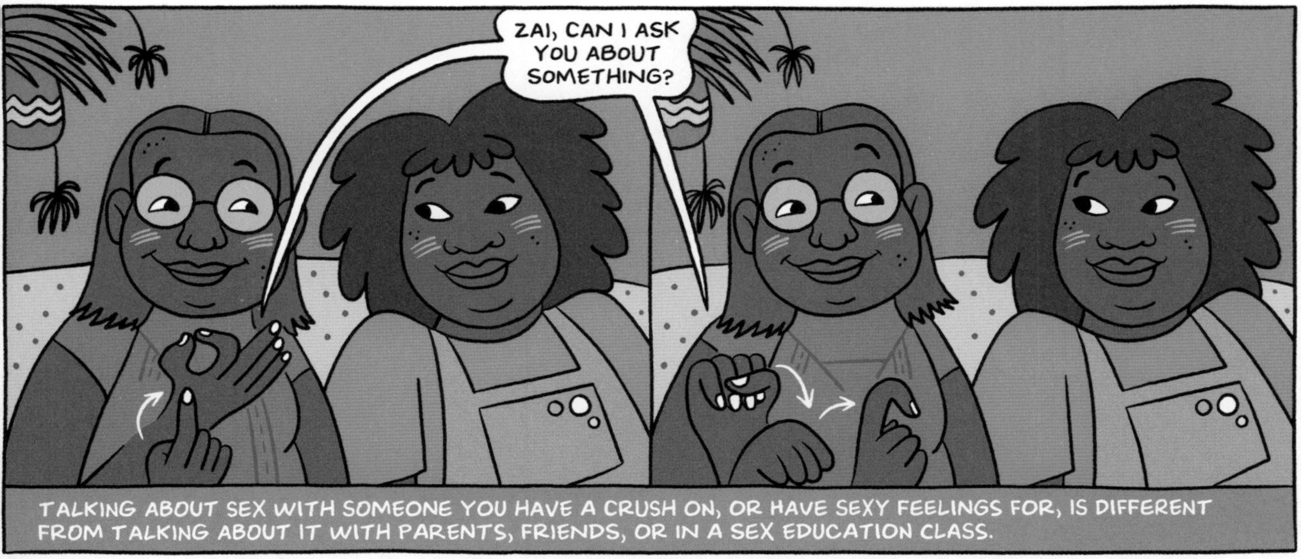
ZAI, CAN I ASK YOU ABOUT SOMETHING?
TALKING ABOUT SEX WITH SOMEONE YOU HAVE A CRUSH ON, OR HAVE SEXY FEELINGS FOR, IS DIFFERENT FROM TALKING ABOUT IT WITH PARENTS, FRIENDS, OR IN A SEX EDUCATION CLASS.

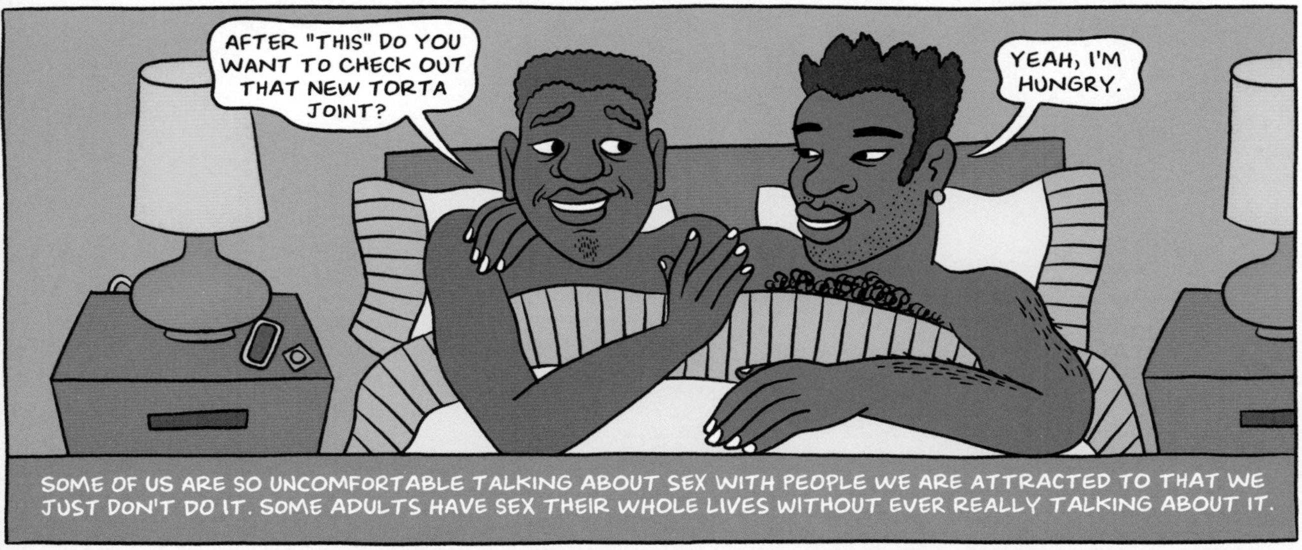
AFTER "THIS" DO YOU WANT TO CHECK OUT THAT NEW TORTA JOINT?
YEAH, I'M HUNGRY.
SOME OF US ARE SO UNCOMFORTABLE TALKING ABOUT SEX WITH PEOPLE WE ARE ATTRACTED TO THAT WE JUST DON'T DO IT. SOME ADULTS HAVE SEX THEIR WHOLE LIVES WITHOUT EVER REALLY TALKING ABOUT IT.

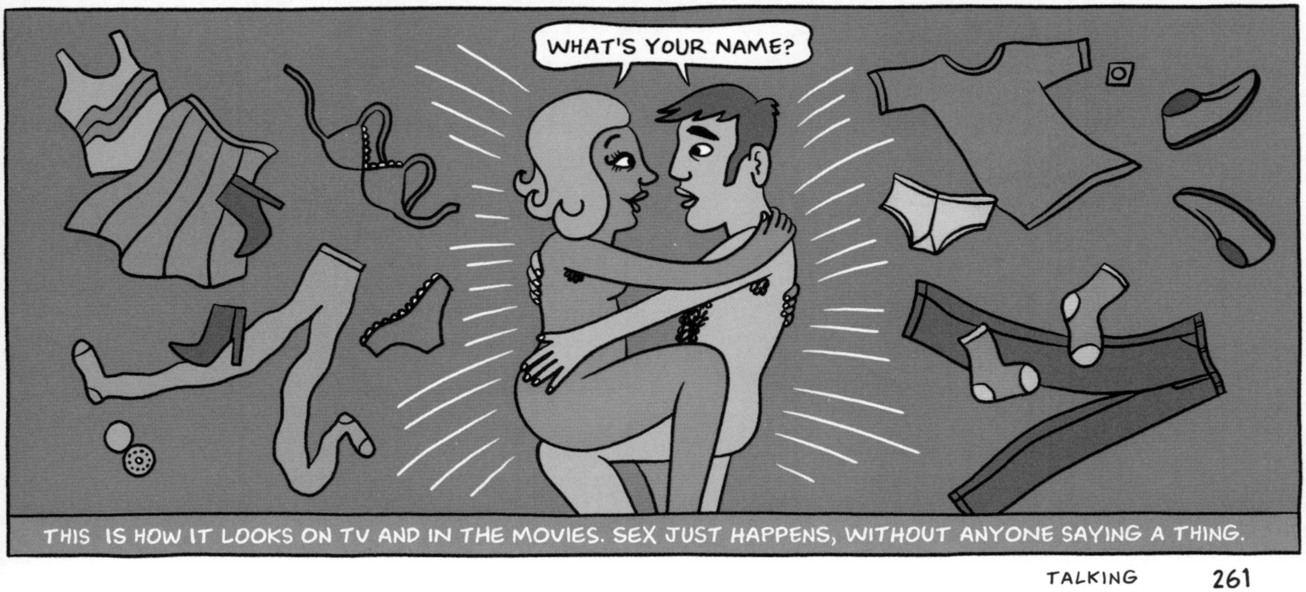
WHAT'S YOUR NAME?
THIS IS HOW IT LOOKS ON TV AND IN THE MOVIES. SEX JUST HAPPENS, WITHOUT ANYONE SAYING A THING.

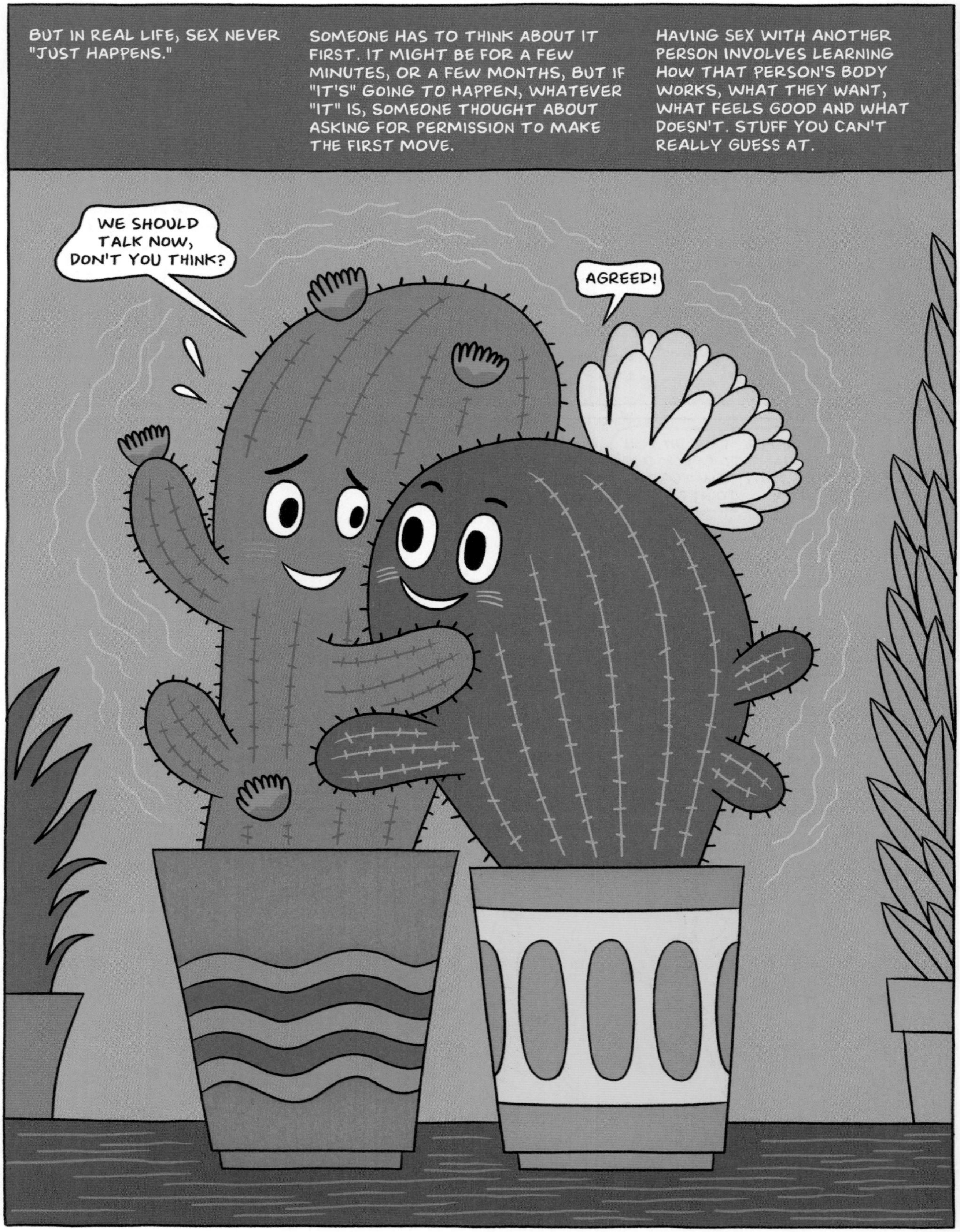
BUT IN REAL LIFE, SEX NEVER "JUST HAPPENS."
SOMEONE HAS TO THINK ABOUT IT FIRST. IT MIGHT BE FOR A FEW MINUTES, OR A FEW MONTHS, BUT IF "IT'S" GOING TO HAPPEN, WHATEVER "IT" IS, SOMEONE THOUGHT ABOUT ASKING FOR PERMISSION TO MAKE THE FIRST MOVE.
HAVING SEX WITH ANOTHER PERSON INVOLVES LEARNING HOW THAT PERSON'S BODY WORKS, WHAT THEY WANT, WHAT FEELS GOOD AND WHAT DOESN'T. STUFF YOU CAN'T REALLY GUESS AT.
WE SHOULD TALK NOW, DON'T YOU THINK?
AGREED!

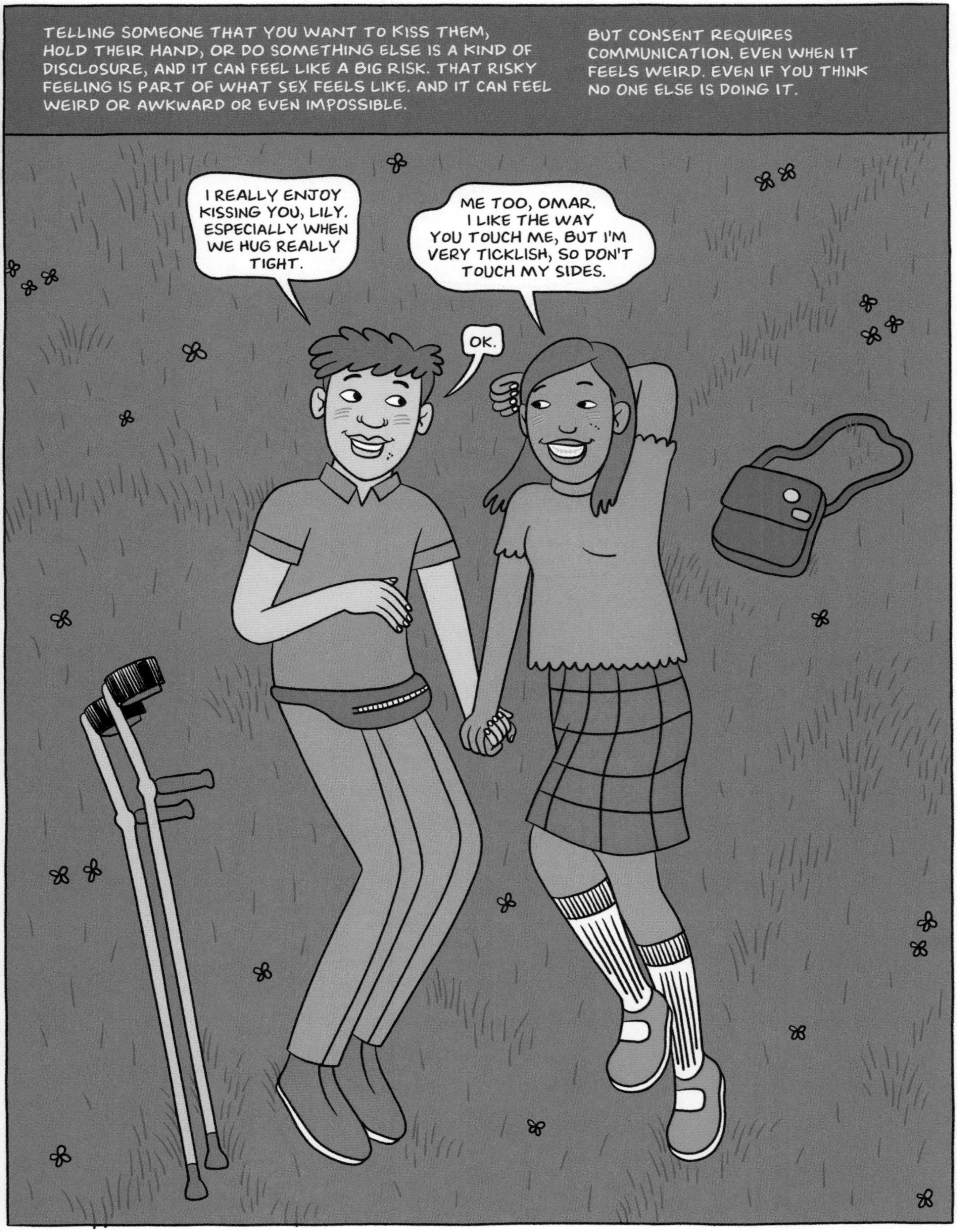
TELLING SOMEONE THAT YOU WANT TO KISS THEM, HOLD THEIR HAND, OR DO SOMETHING ELSE IS A KIND OF DISCLOSURE, AND IT CAN FEEL LIKE A BIG RISK. THAT RISKY FEELING IS PART OF WHAT SEX FEELS LIKE. AND IT CAN FEEL WEIRD OR AWKWARD OR EVEN IMPOSSIBLE.
BUT CONSENT REQUIRES COMMUNICATION. EVEN WHEN IT FEELS WEIRD. EVEN IF YOU THINK NO ONE ELSE IS DOING IT.
I REALLY ENJOY KISSING YOU, LILY. ESPECIALLY WHEN WE HUG REALLY TIGHT.
ME TOO, OMAR. I LIKE THE WAY YOU TOUCH ME, BUT I'M VERY TICKLISH, SO DON'T TOUCH MY SIDES.
OK.

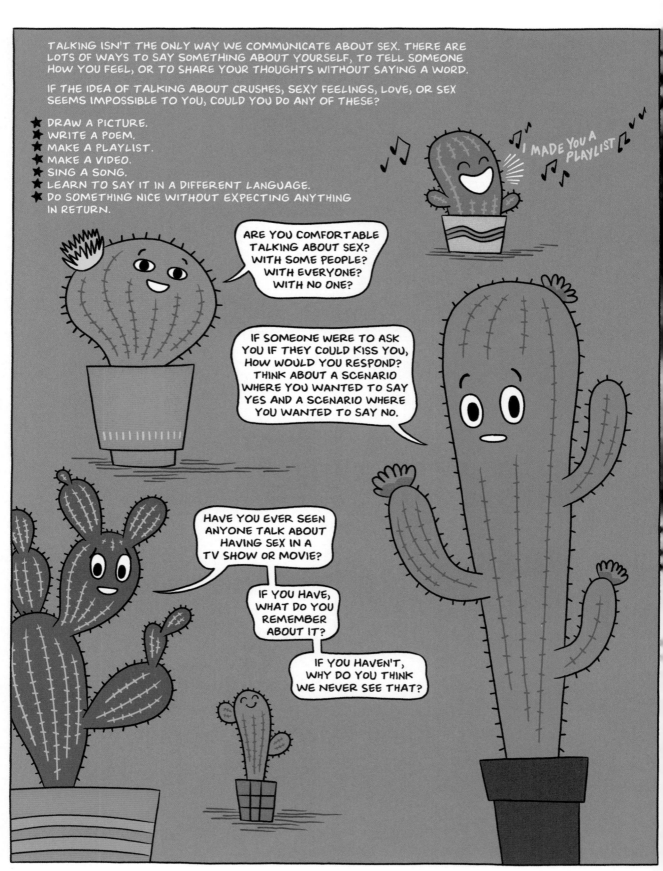

TALKING ISN'T THE ONLY WAY WE COMMUNICATE ABOUT SEX. THERE ARE LOTS OF WAYS TO SAY SOMETHING ABOUT YOURSELF, TO TELL SOMEONE HOW YOU FEEL, OR TO SHARE YOUR THOUGHTS WITHOUT SAYING A WORD.

IF THE IDEA OF TALKING ABOUT CRUSHES, SEXY FEELINGS, LOVE, OR SEX SEEMS IMPOSSIBLE TO YOU, COULD YOU DO ANY OF THESE?

★ DRAW A PICTURE.
★ WRITE A POEM.
★ MAKE A PLAYLIST.
★ MAKE A VIDEO.
★ SING A SONG.
★ LEARN TO SAY IT IN A DIFFERENT LANGUAGE.
★ DO SOMETHING NICE WITHOUT EXPECTING ANYTHING IN RETURN.

I MADE YOU A PLAYLIST

ARE YOU COMFORTABLE TALKING ABOUT SEX? WITH SOME PEOPLE? WITH EVERYONE? WITH NO ONE?

IF SOMEONE WERE TO ASK YOU IF THEY COULD KISS YOU, HOW WOULD YOU RESPOND? THINK ABOUT A SCENARIO WHERE YOU WANTED TO SAY YES AND A SCENARIO WHERE YOU WANTED TO SAY NO.

HAVE YOU EVER SEEN ANYONE TALK ABOUT HAVING SEX IN A TV SHOW OR MOVIE?

IF YOU HAVE, WHAT DO YOU REMEMBER ABOUT IT?

IF YOU HAVEN'T, WHY DO YOU THINK WE NEVER SEE THAT?

8 RELATIONSHIPS

HI KIDS, NEED ANYTHING?
HI MRS. S.
NO THANKS, MOM, WE'RE GOOD.
HI MRS. S.
HI MRS. S!

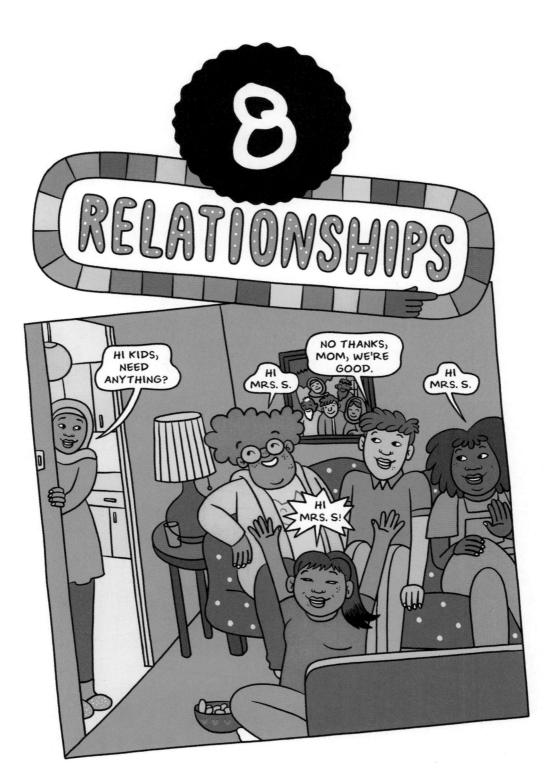

HAVING A "RELATIONSHIP" SOUNDS LIKE A SERIOUS THING—SOMETHING THAT INVOLVES LOVE, COMMITMENT, AND THE GIVING OF GIFTS. BUT SAYING YOU HAVE A RELATIONSHIP, OR ARE IN A RELATIONSHIP, IS JUST ANOTHER WAY OF SAYING YOU ARE CONNECTED TO SOMEONE.

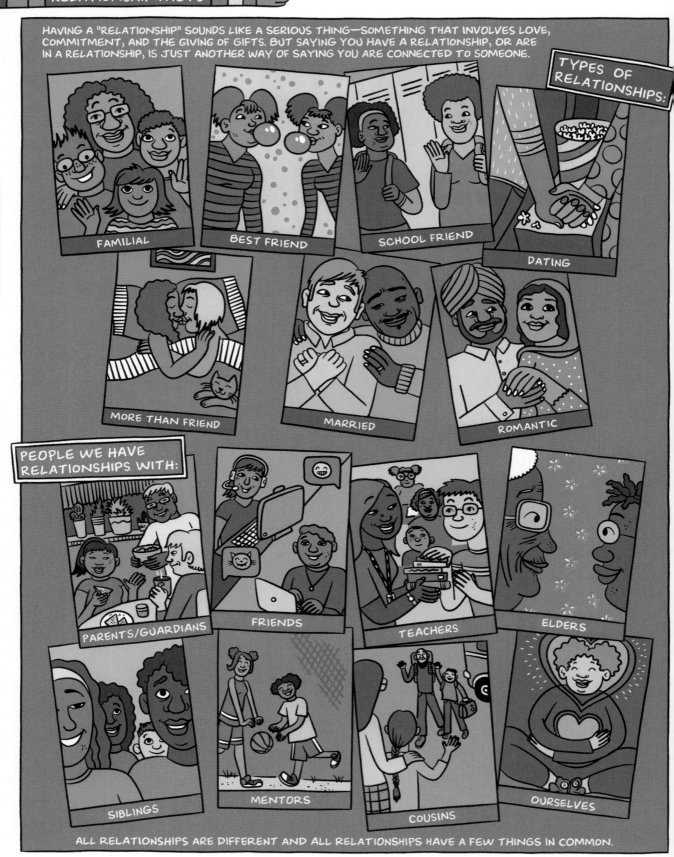

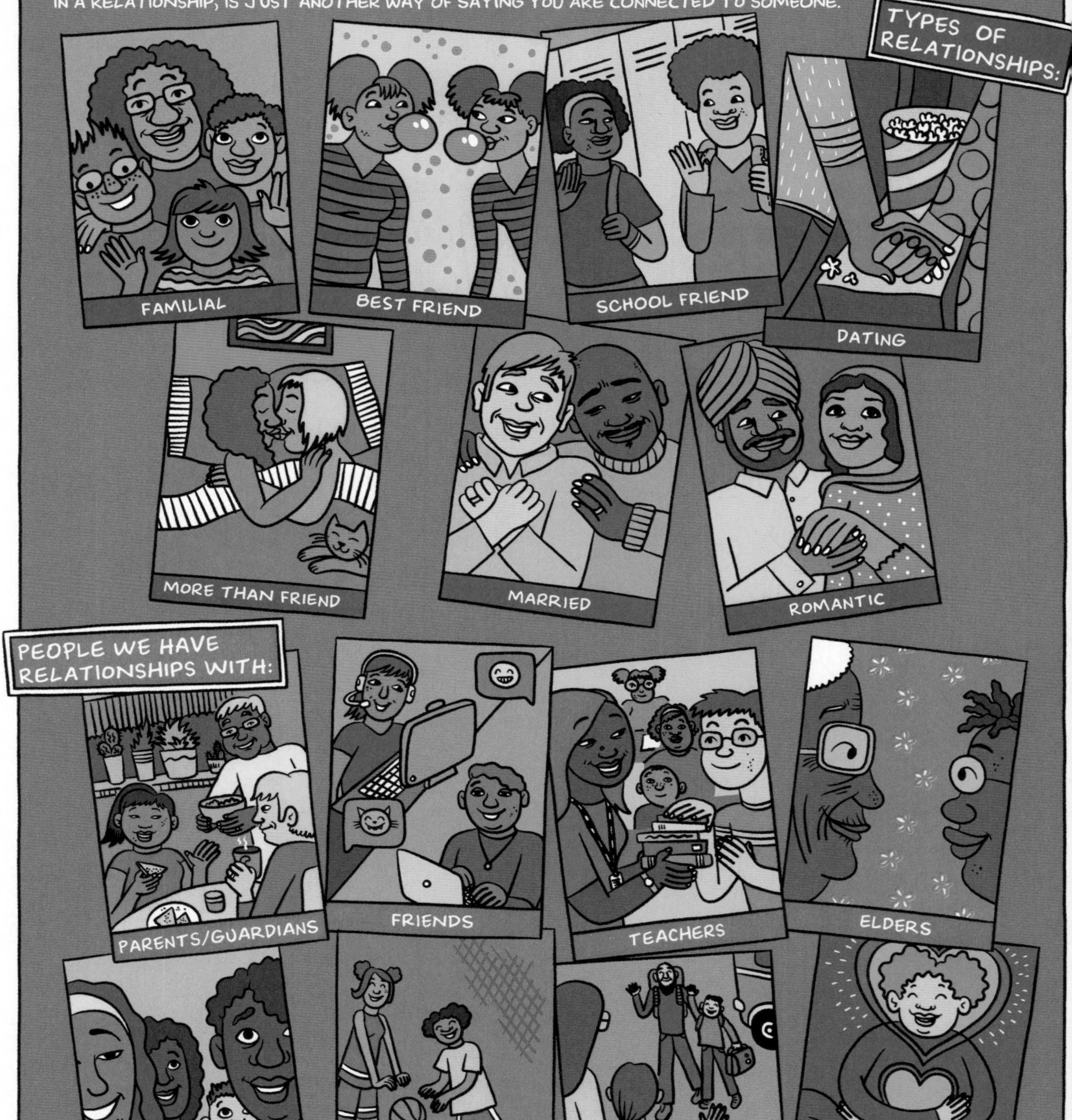
TYPES OF RELATIONSHIPS:
FAMILIAL
BEST FRIEND
SCHOOL FRIEND
DATING
MORE THAN FRIEND
MARRIED
ROMANTIC
PEOPLE WE HAVE RELATIONSHIPS WITH:
PARENTS/GUARDIANS
FRIENDS
TEACHERS
ELDERS
SIBLINGS
MENTORS
COUSINS
OURSELVES

ALL RELATIONSHIPS ARE DIFFERENT AND ALL RELATIONSHIPS HAVE A FEW THINGS IN COMMON.

EVERY RELATIONSHIP HAS PROS AND CONS.

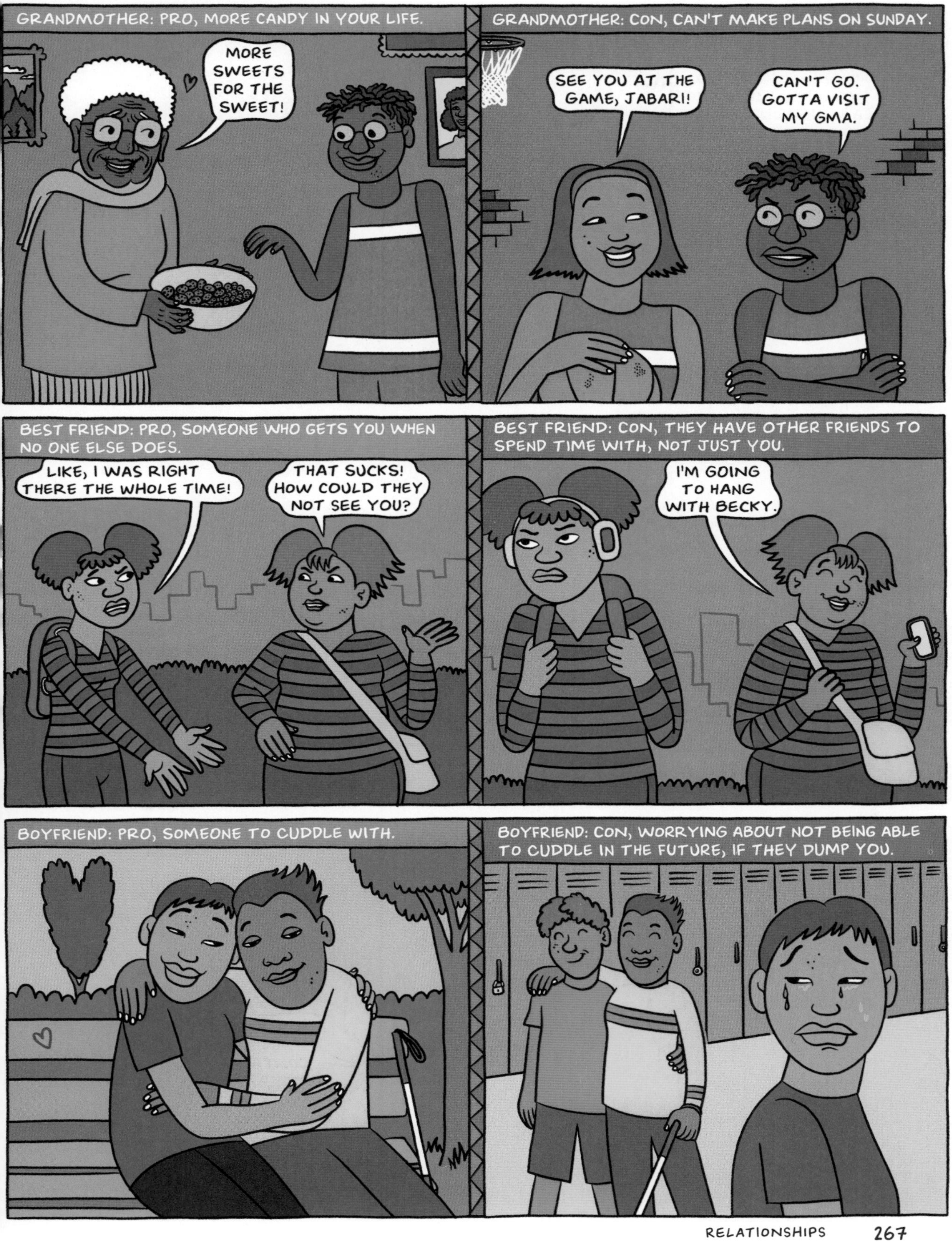
GRANDMOTHER: PRO, MORE CANDY IN YOUR LIFE.
MORE SWEETS FOR THE SWEET!
GRANDMOTHER: CON, CAN'T MAKE PLANS ON SUNDAY.
SEE YOU AT THE GAME, JABARI!
CAN'T GO. GOTTA VISIT MY GMA.
BEST FRIEND: PRO, SOMEONE WHO GETS YOU WHEN NO ONE ELSE DOES.
LIKE, I WAS RIGHT THERE THE WHOLE TIME!
THAT SUCKS! HOW COULD THEY NOT SEE YOU?
BEST FRIEND: CON, THEY HAVE OTHER FRIENDS TO SPEND TIME WITH, NOT JUST YOU.
I'M GOING TO HANG WITH BECKY.
BOYFRIEND: PRO, SOMEONE TO CUDDLE WITH.
BOYFRIEND: CON, WORRYING ABOUT NOT BEING ABLE TO CUDDLE IN THE FUTURE, IF THEY DUMP YOU.

EVERY RELATIONSHIP HAS EXPECTATIONS.

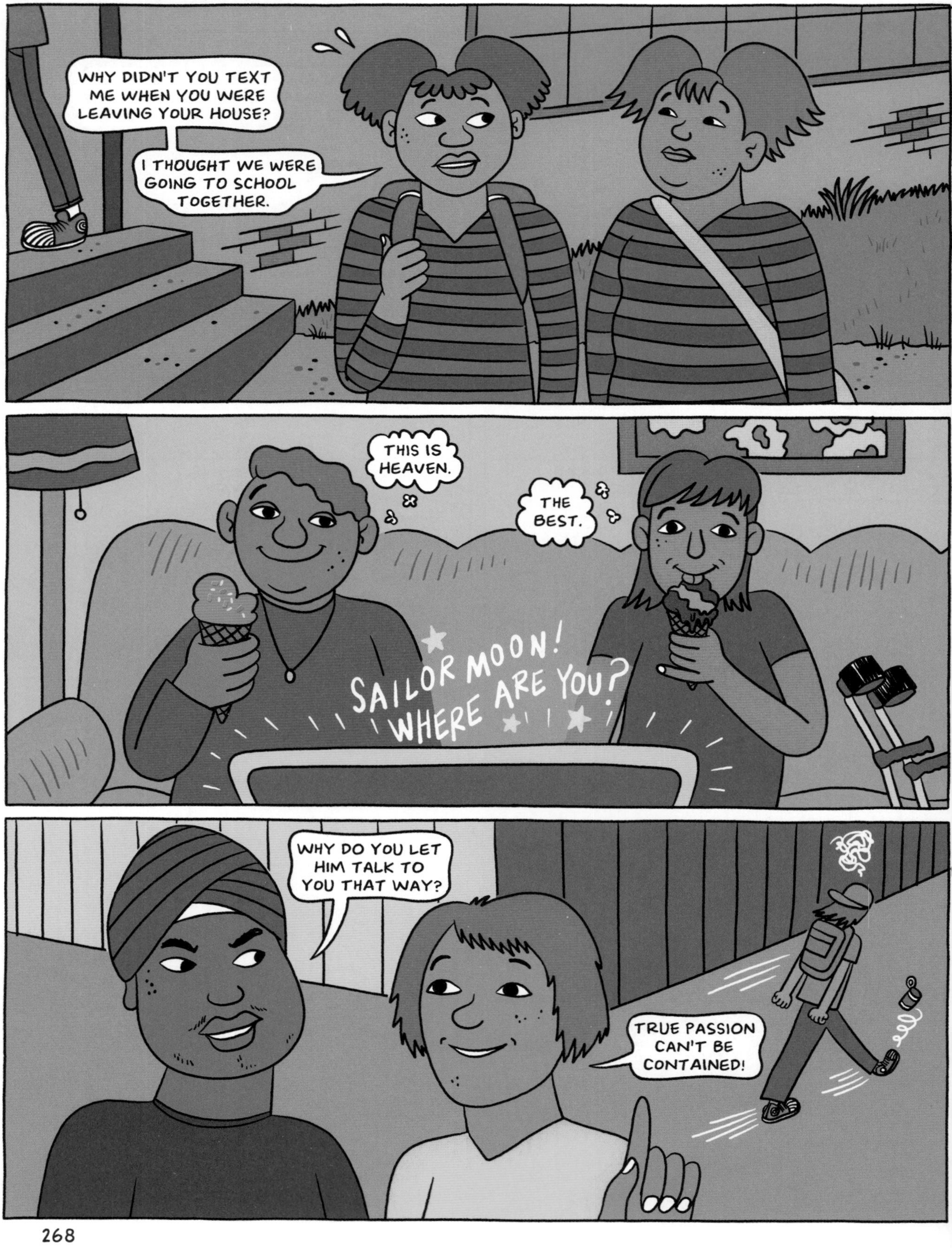
WHY DIDN'T YOU TEXT ME WHEN YOU WERE LEAVING YOUR HOUSE?
I THOUGHT WE WERE GOING TO SCHOOL TOGETHER.
THIS IS HEAVEN.
THE BEST.
SAILOR MOON! WHERE ARE YOU?
WHY DO YOU LET HIM TALK TO YOU THAT WAY?
TRUE PASSION CAN'T BE CONTAINED!

EVERY RELATIONSHIP CAN HOLD EVERY KIND OF FEELING.

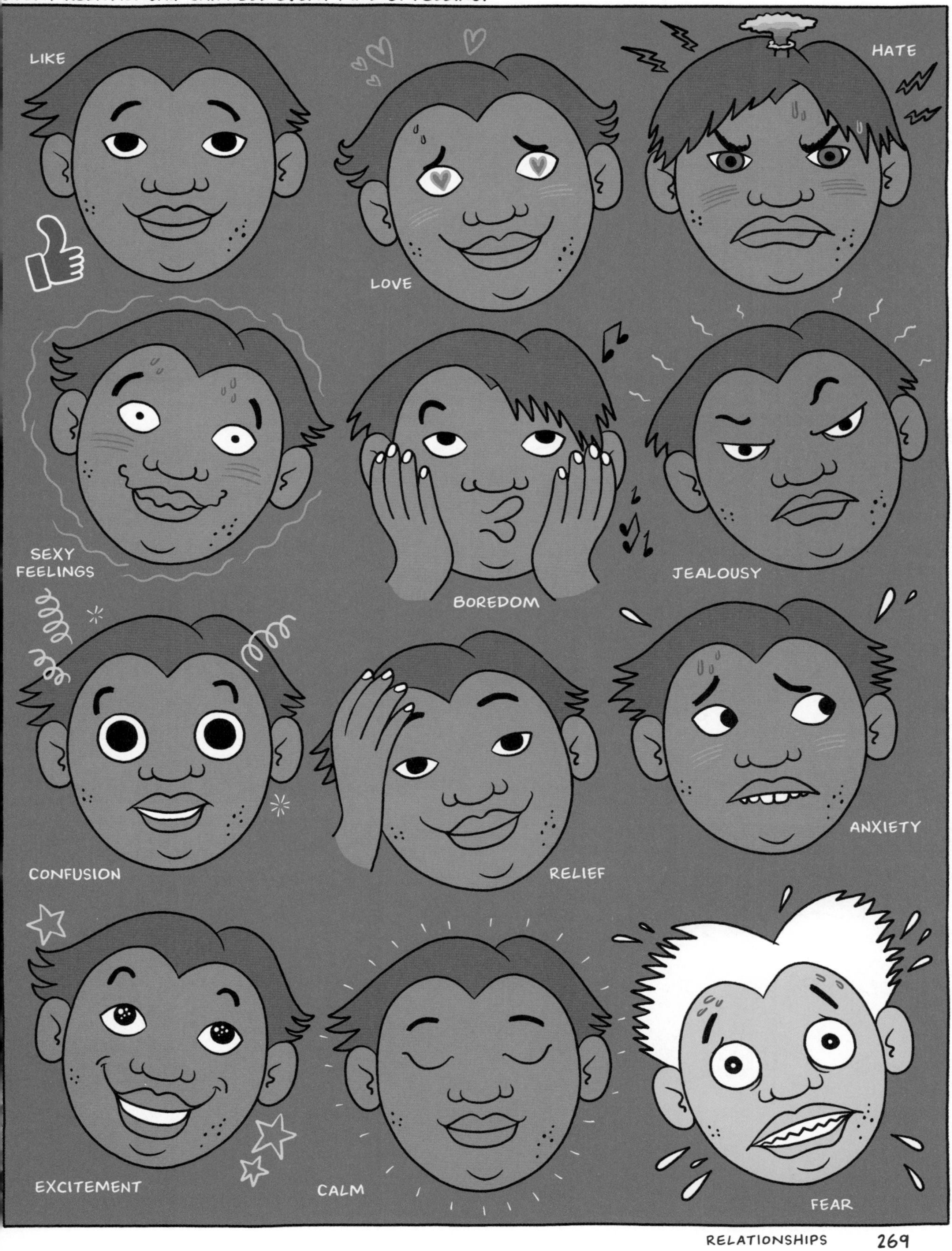
LIKE
LOVE
HATE
SEXY FEELINGS
BOREDOM
JEALOUSY
CONFUSION
RELIEF
ANXIETY
EXCITEMENT
CALM
FEAR

AND EVERY RELATIONSHIP CHANGES.

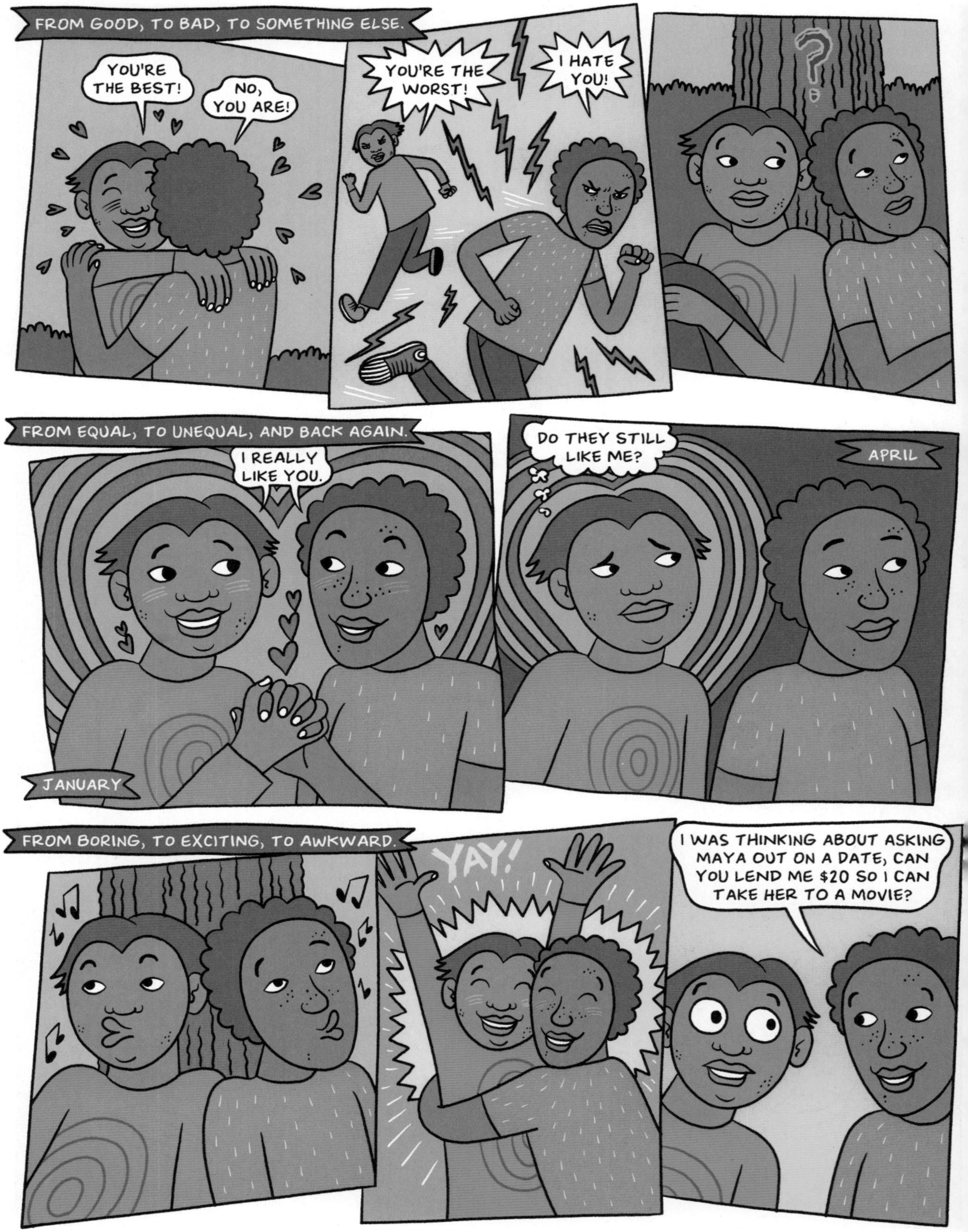
FROM GOOD, TO BAD, TO SOMETHING ELSE.
YOU'RE THE BEST!
NO, YOU ARE!
YOU'RE THE WORST!
I HATE YOU!
?
FROM EQUAL, TO UNEQUAL, AND BACK AGAIN.
I REALLY LIKE YOU.
JANUARY
DO THEY STILL LIKE ME?
APRIL
FROM BORING, TO EXCITING, TO AWKWARD.
YAY!
I WAS THINKING ABOUT ASKING MAYA OUT ON A DATE, CAN YOU LEND ME $20 SO I CAN TAKE HER TO A MOVIE?

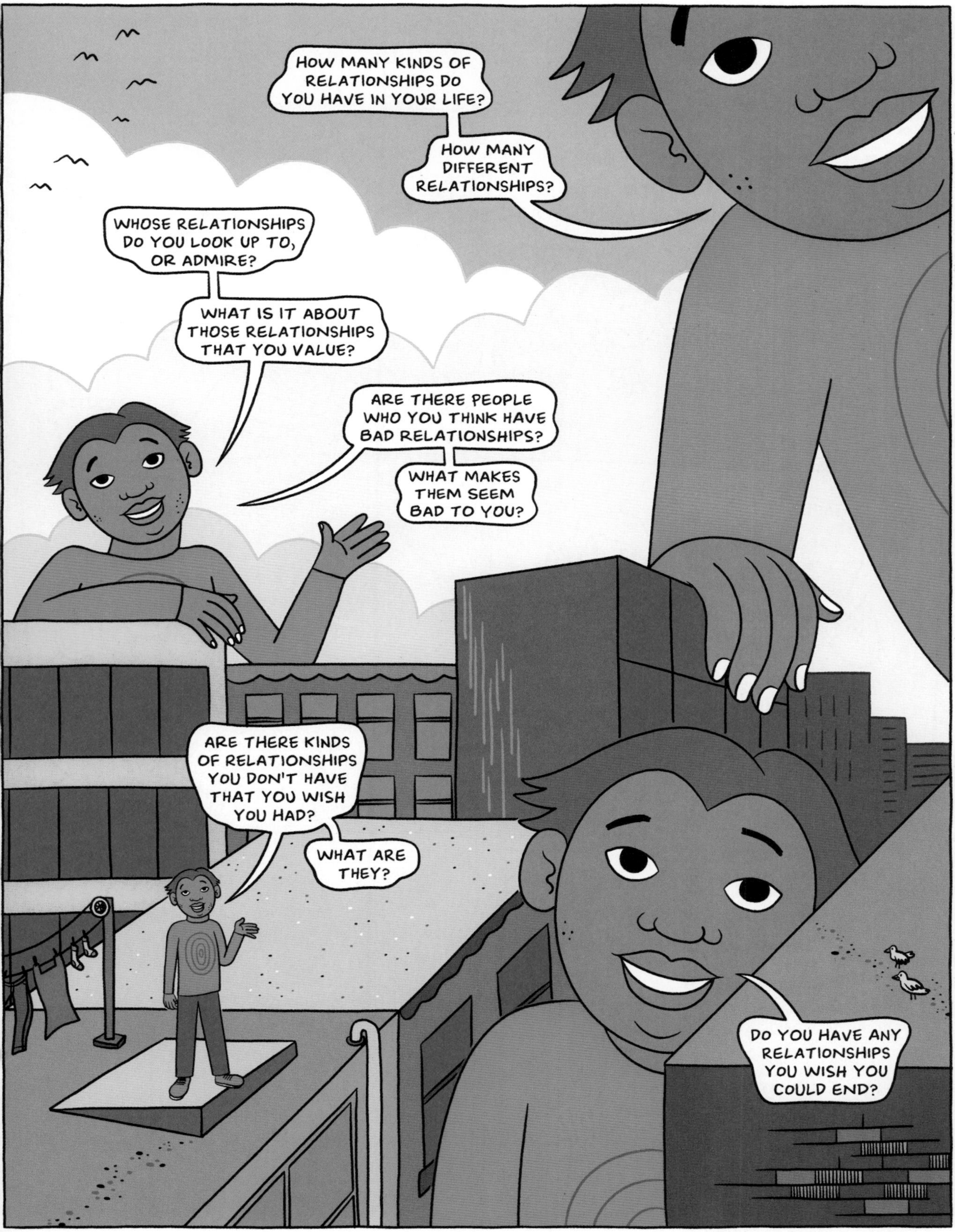
HOW MANY KINDS OF RELATIONSHIPS DO YOU HAVE IN YOUR LIFE?
HOW MANY DIFFERENT RELATIONSHIPS?
WHOSE RELATIONSHIPS DO YOU LOOK UP TO, OR ADMIRE?
WHAT IS IT ABOUT THOSE RELATIONSHIPS THAT YOU VALUE?
ARE THERE PEOPLE WHO YOU THINK HAVE BAD RELATIONSHIPS?
WHAT MAKES THEM SEEM BAD TO YOU?
ARE THERE KINDS OF RELATIONSHIPS YOU DON'T HAVE THAT YOU WISH YOU HAD?
WHAT ARE THEY?
DO YOU HAVE ANY RELATIONSHIPS YOU WISH YOU COULD END?

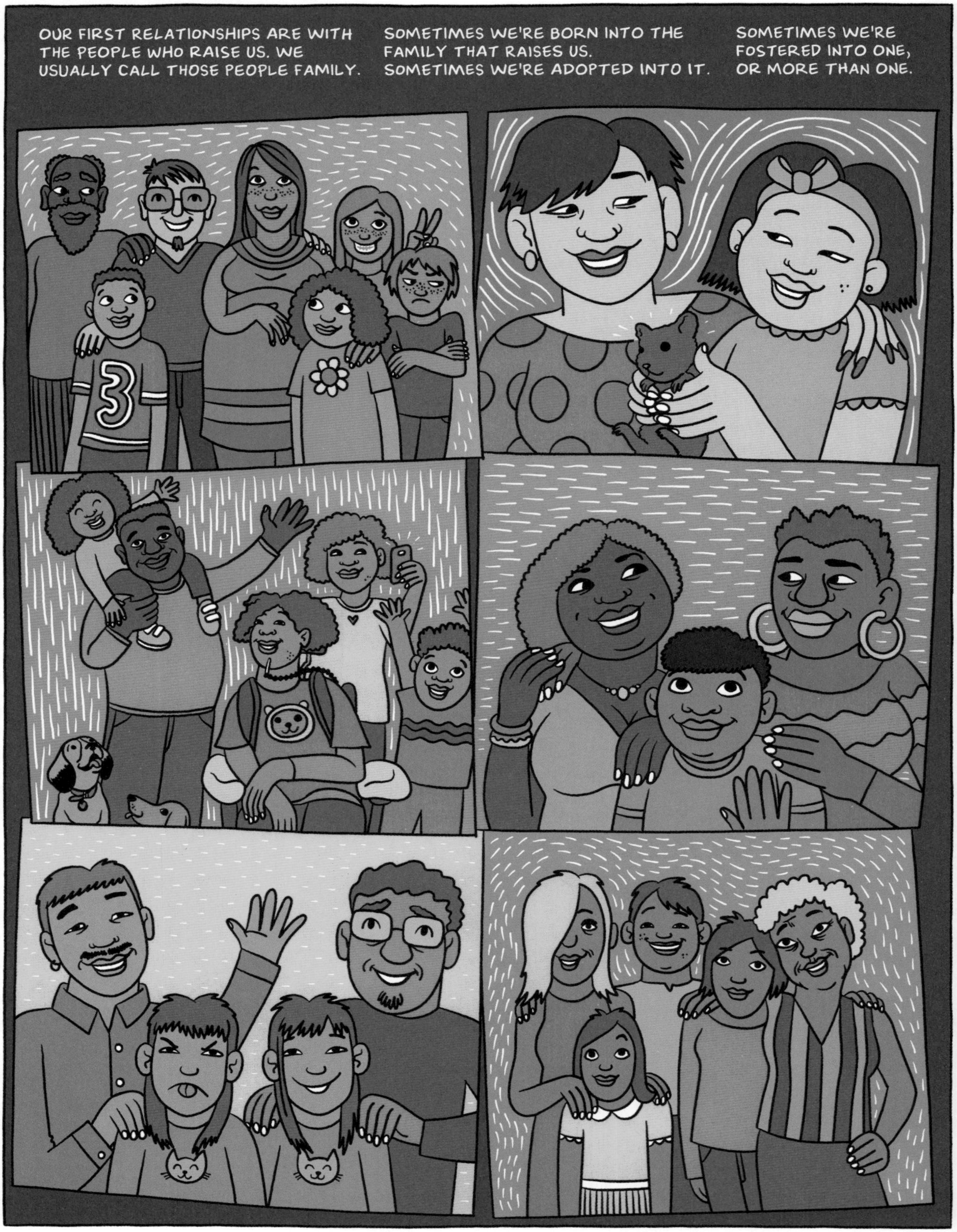
OUR FIRST RELATIONSHIPS ARE WITH THE PEOPLE WHO RAISE US. WE USUALLY CALL THOSE PEOPLE FAMILY.
SOMETIMES WE'RE BORN INTO THE FAMILY THAT RAISES US. SOMETIMES WE'RE ADOPTED INTO IT.
SOMETIMES WE'RE FOSTERED INTO ONE, OR MORE THAN ONE.

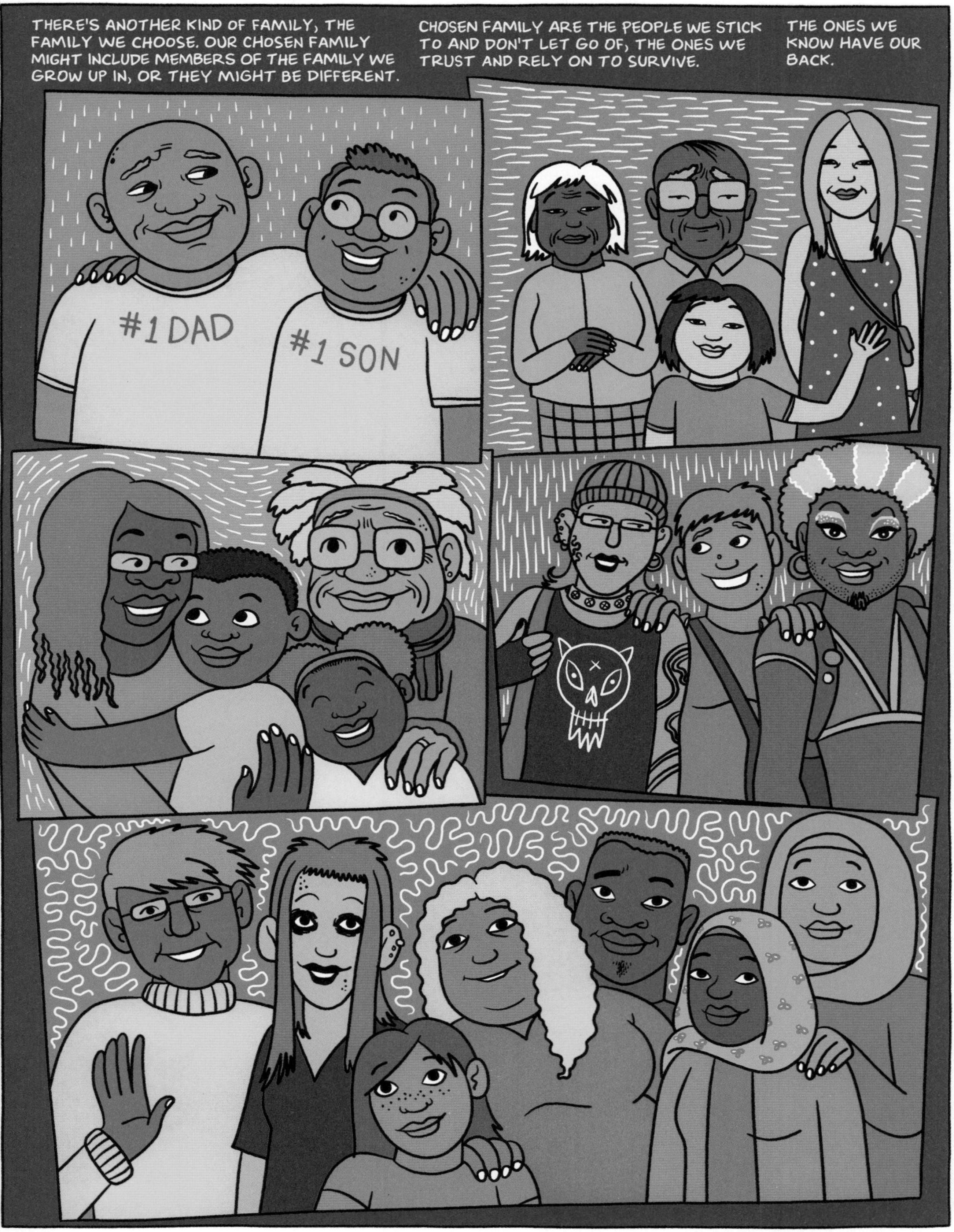
THERE'S ANOTHER KIND OF FAMILY, THE FAMILY WE CHOOSE. OUR CHOSEN FAMILY MIGHT INCLUDE MEMBERS OF THE FAMILY WE GROW UP IN, OR THEY MIGHT BE DIFFERENT.
CHOSEN FAMILY ARE THE PEOPLE WE STICK TO AND DON'T LET GO OF, THE ONES WE TRUST AND RELY ON TO SURVIVE.
THE ONES WE KNOW HAVE OUR BACK.
#1 DAD
#1 SON

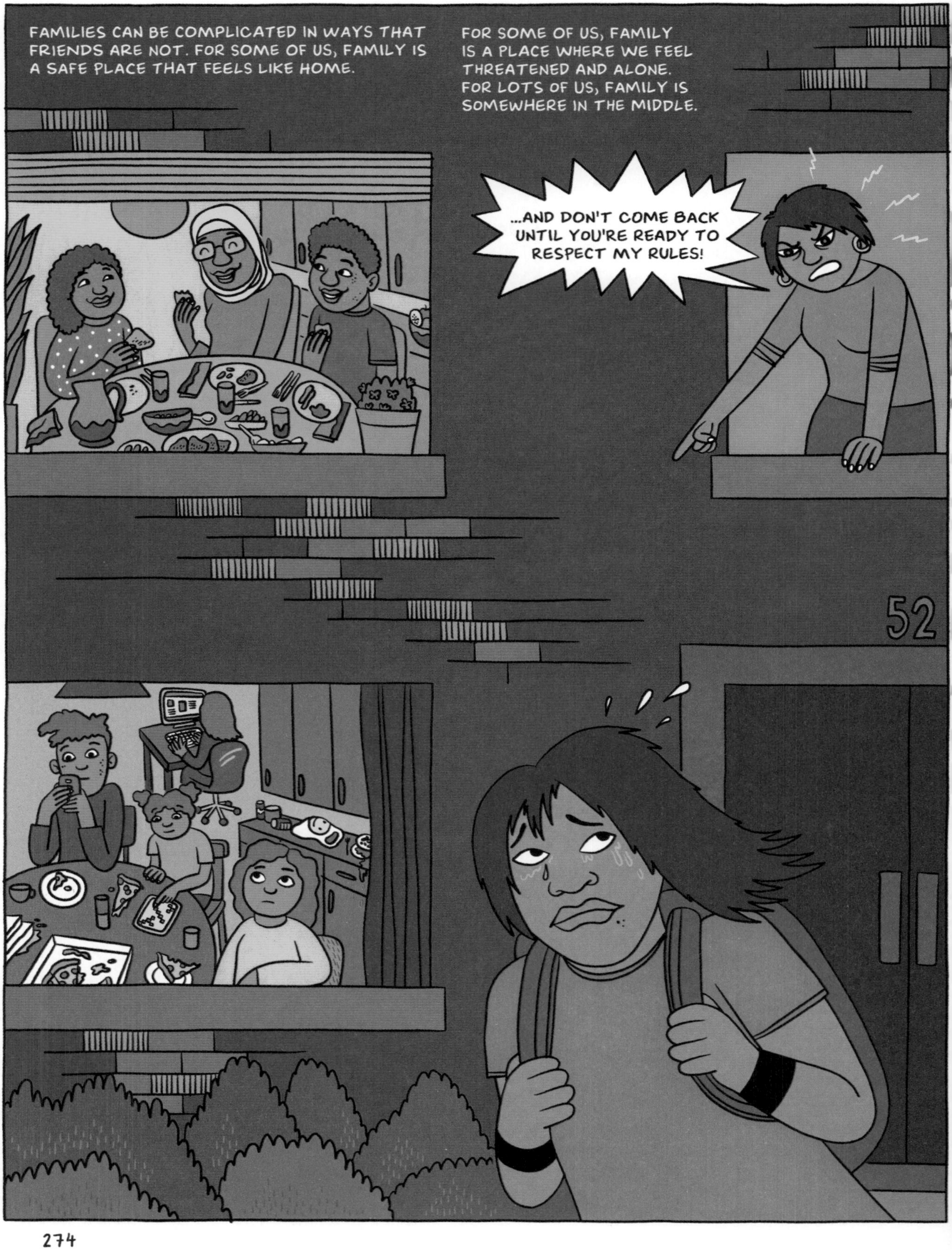
FAMILIES CAN BE COMPLICATED IN WAYS THAT FRIENDS ARE NOT. FOR SOME OF US, FAMILY IS A SAFE PLACE THAT FEELS LIKE HOME.
FOR SOME OF US, FAMILY IS A PLACE WHERE WE FEEL THREATENED AND ALONE. FOR LOTS OF US, FAMILY IS SOMEWHERE IN THE MIDDLE.
...AND DON'T COME BACK UNTIL YOU'RE READY TO RESPECT MY RULES!
52

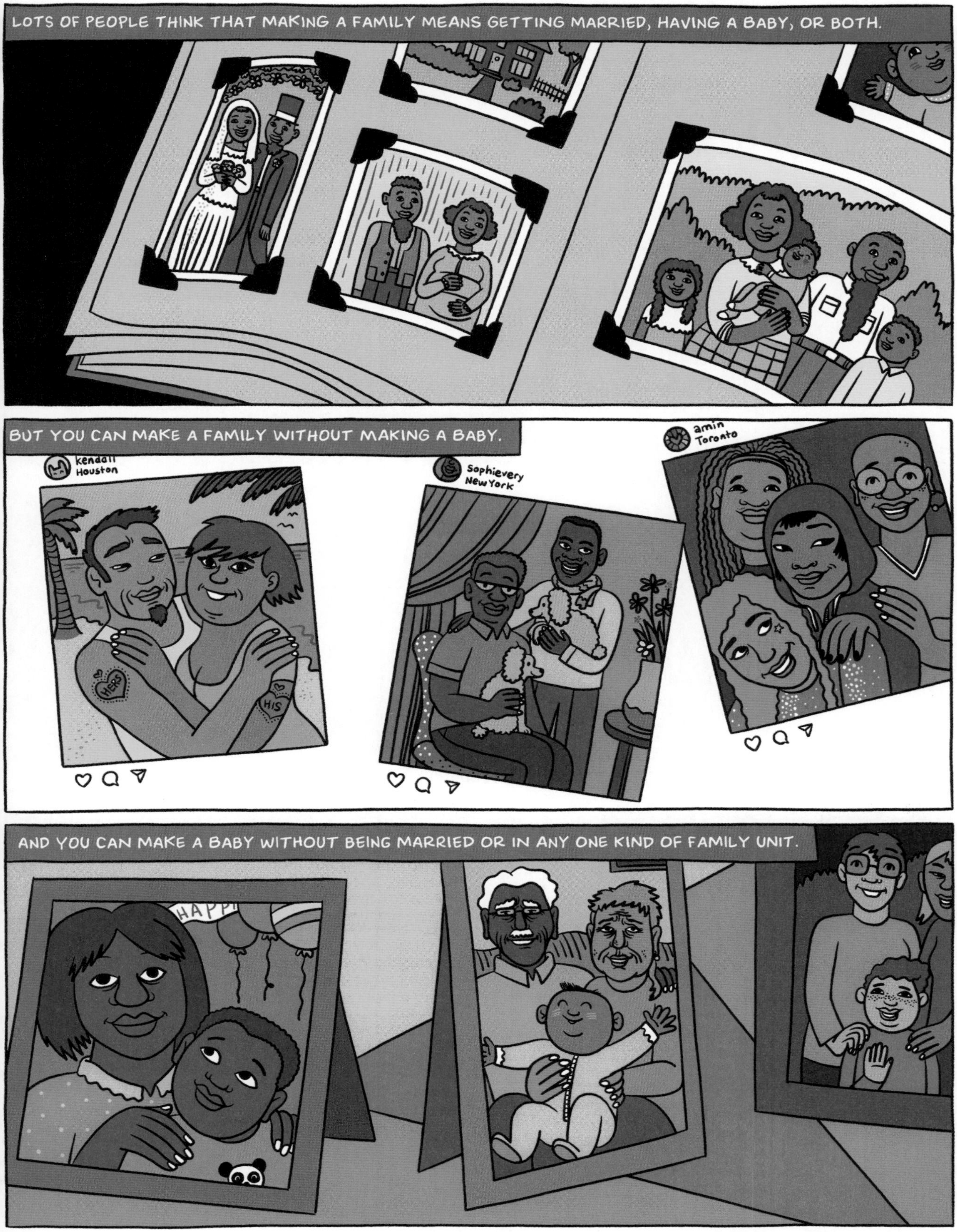
LOTS OF PEOPLE THINK THAT MAKING A FAMILY MEANS GETTING MARRIED, HAVING A BABY, OR BOTH.
BUT YOU CAN MAKE A FAMILY WITHOUT MAKING A BABY.
kendall
Houston
HERS
HIS
Sophievery
New York
amin
Toronto
AND YOU CAN MAKE A BABY WITHOUT BEING MARRIED OR IN ANY ONE KIND OF FAMILY UNIT.

NERD ALERT WHERE DID CHOSEN FAMILY COME FROM?

CHOSEN FAMILY IS FOR EVERYONE, BUT IT PROBABLY STARTED WITH PEOPLE WHO MADE CHOSEN FAMILY TO SURVIVE. YOUNG PEOPLE WHO ARE KICKED OUT OF THEIR HOMES, OR HAD TO LEAVE TO ESCAPE VIOLENCE, MAKE CHOSEN FAMILY FOR A PLACE OF SAFETY AND CELEBRATION.

DISABLED PEOPLE OF ALL AGES HAVE ALSO CREATED CHOSEN FAMILY AND NETWORKS OF SUPPORT WHEN THE GOVERNMENT MAKES IT HARD FOR THEM TO LIVE WITH OR MARRY THE PEOPLE THEY LOVE WITHOUT LOSING HEALTH CARE.

THERE HAVE ALWAYS BEEN THOSE OF US WHO FEEL LIKE WE DON'T HAVE A PLACE IN THE WORLD. SOMETIMES IT'S HARD TO FIND IT, BUT IT'S GOOD TO REMEMBER THAT OUR ELDERS WHO FELT THE SAME WAY MANAGED, AND WE CAN TOO. CHOSEN FAMILY IS PART OF THIS TRADITION OF SURVIVAL AND RESISTANCE.

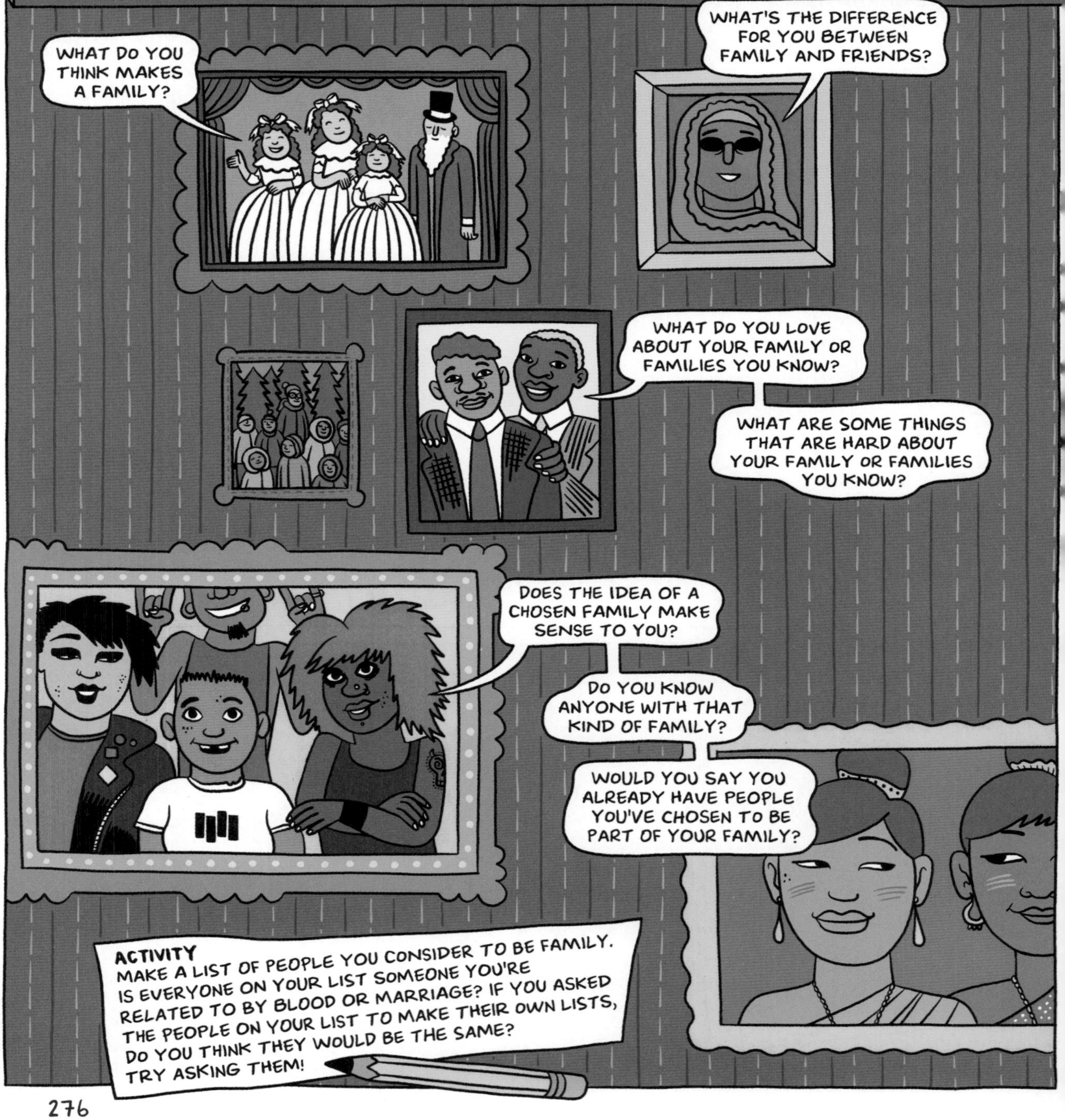
WHAT DO YOU THINK MAKES A FAMILY?
WHAT'S THE DIFFERENCE FOR YOU BETWEEN FAMILY AND FRIENDS?
WHAT DO YOU LOVE ABOUT YOUR FAMILY OR FAMILIES YOU KNOW?
WHAT ARE SOME THINGS THAT ARE HARD ABOUT YOUR FAMILY OR FAMILIES YOU KNOW?
DOES THE IDEA OF A CHOSEN FAMILY MAKE SENSE TO YOU?
DO YOU KNOW ANYONE WITH THAT KIND OF FAMILY?
WOULD YOU SAY YOU ALREADY HAVE PEOPLE YOU'VE CHOSEN TO BE PART OF YOUR FAMILY?

ACTIVITY
MAKE A LIST OF PEOPLE YOU CONSIDER TO BE FAMILY. IS EVERYONE ON YOUR LIST SOMEONE YOU'RE RELATED TO BY BLOOD OR MARRIAGE? IF YOU ASKED THE PEOPLE ON YOUR LIST TO MAKE THEIR OWN LISTS, DO YOU THINK THEY WOULD BE THE SAME? TRY ASKING THEM!

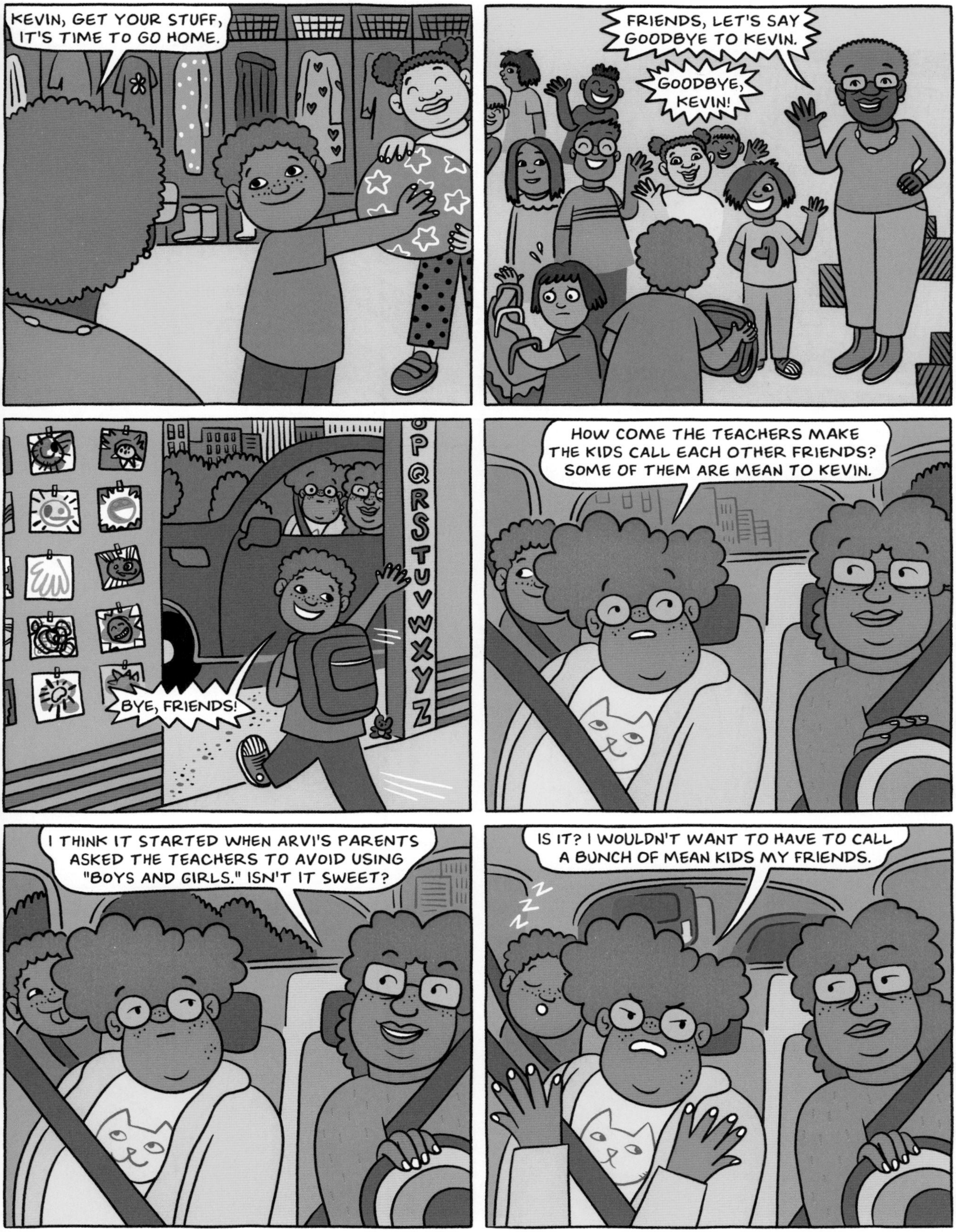
KEVIN, GET YOUR STUFF, IT'S TIME TO GO HOME.
FRIENDS, LET'S SAY GOODBYE TO KEVIN.
GOODBYE, KEVIN!
O P Q R S T U V W X Y Z
BYE, FRIENDS!
HOW COME THE TEACHERS MAKE THE KIDS CALL EACH OTHER FRIENDS? SOME OF THEM ARE MEAN TO KEVIN.
I THINK IT STARTED WHEN ARVI'S PARENTS ASKED THE TEACHERS TO AVOID USING "BOYS AND GIRLS." ISN'T IT SWEET?
Z Z Z
IS IT? I WOULDN'T WANT TO HAVE TO CALL A BUNCH OF MEAN KIDS MY FRIENDS.

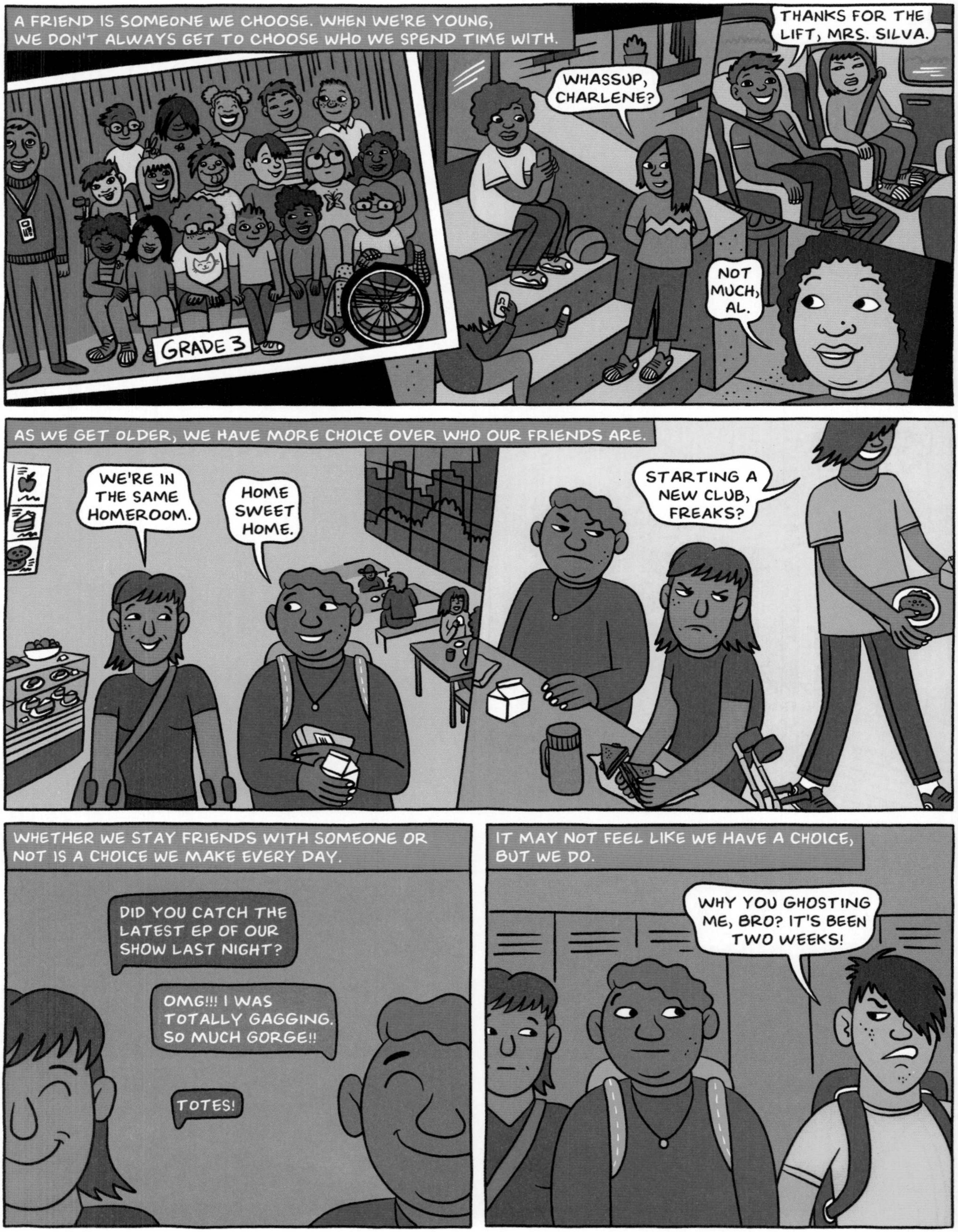
A FRIEND IS SOMEONE WE CHOOSE. WHEN WE'RE YOUNG, WE DON'T ALWAYS GET TO CHOOSE WHO WE SPEND TIME WITH.
GRADE 3
WHASSUP, CHARLENE?
NOT MUCH, AL.
THANKS FOR THE LIFT, MRS. SILVA.
AS WE GET OLDER, WE HAVE MORE CHOICE OVER WHO OUR FRIENDS ARE.
WE'RE IN THE SAME HOMEROOM.
HOME SWEET HOME.
STARTING A NEW CLUB, FREAKS?
WHETHER WE STAY FRIENDS WITH SOMEONE OR NOT IS A CHOICE WE MAKE EVERY DAY.
DID YOU CATCH THE LATEST EP OF OUR SHOW LAST NIGHT?
OMG!!! I WAS TOTALLY GAGGING. SO MUCH GORGE!!
TOTES!
IT MAY NOT FEEL LIKE WE HAVE A CHOICE, BUT WE DO.
WHY YOU GHOSTING ME, BRO? IT'S BEEN TWO WEEKS!

HOW MANY? WHAT KIND?

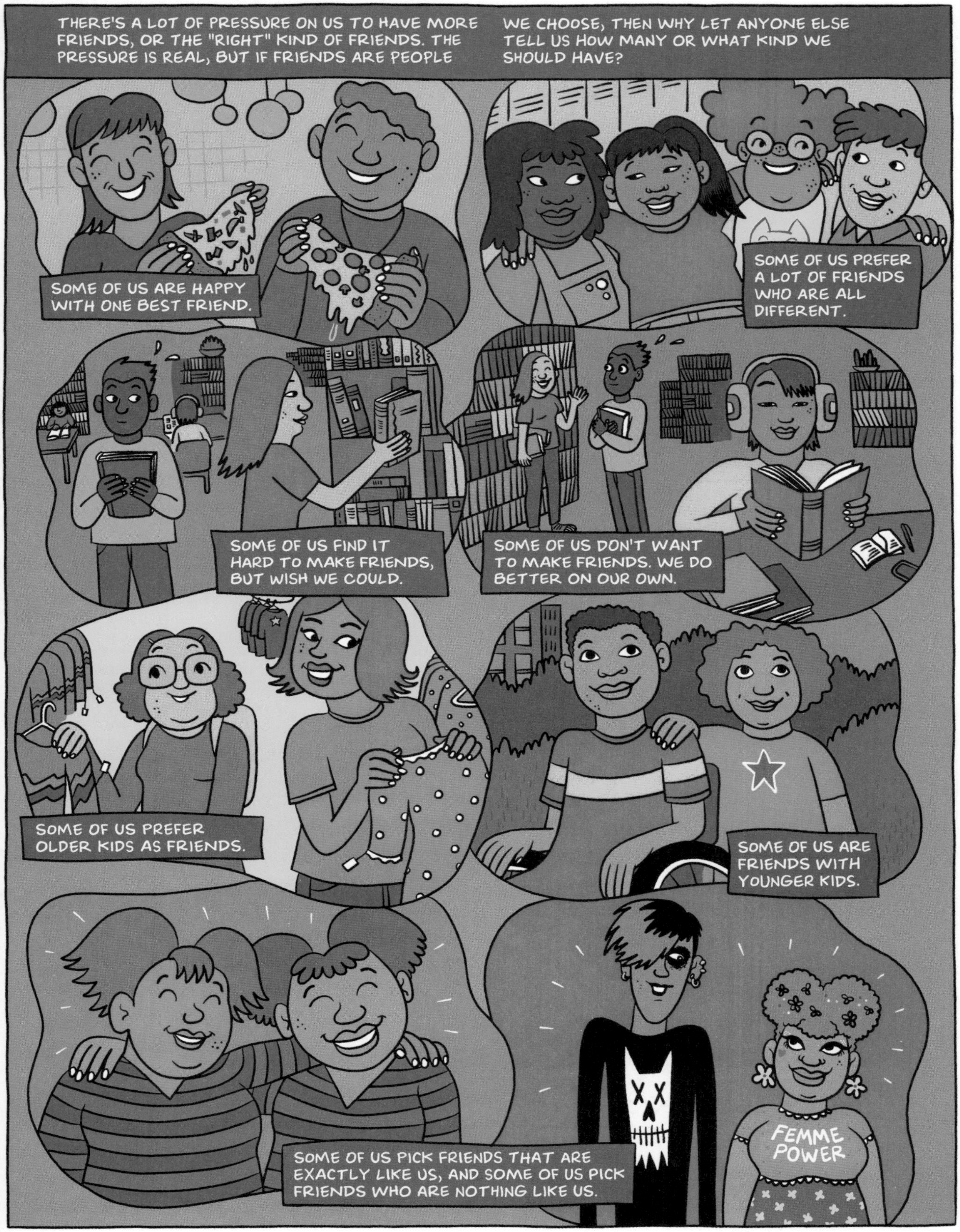
THERE'S A LOT OF PRESSURE ON US TO HAVE MORE FRIENDS, OR THE "RIGHT" KIND OF FRIENDS. THE PRESSURE IS REAL, BUT IF FRIENDS ARE PEOPLE WE CHOOSE, THEN WHY LET ANYONE ELSE TELL US HOW MANY OR WHAT KIND WE SHOULD HAVE?
SOME OF US ARE HAPPY WITH ONE BEST FRIEND.
SOME OF US PREFER A LOT OF FRIENDS WHO ARE ALL DIFFERENT.
SOME OF US FIND IT HARD TO MAKE FRIENDS, BUT WISH WE COULD.
SOME OF US DON'T WANT TO MAKE FRIENDS. WE DO BETTER ON OUR OWN.
SOME OF US PREFER OLDER KIDS AS FRIENDS.
SOME OF US ARE FRIENDS WITH YOUNGER KIDS.
FEMME POWER
SOME OF US PICK FRIENDS THAT ARE EXACTLY LIKE US, AND SOME OF US PICK FRIENDS WHO ARE NOTHING LIKE US.

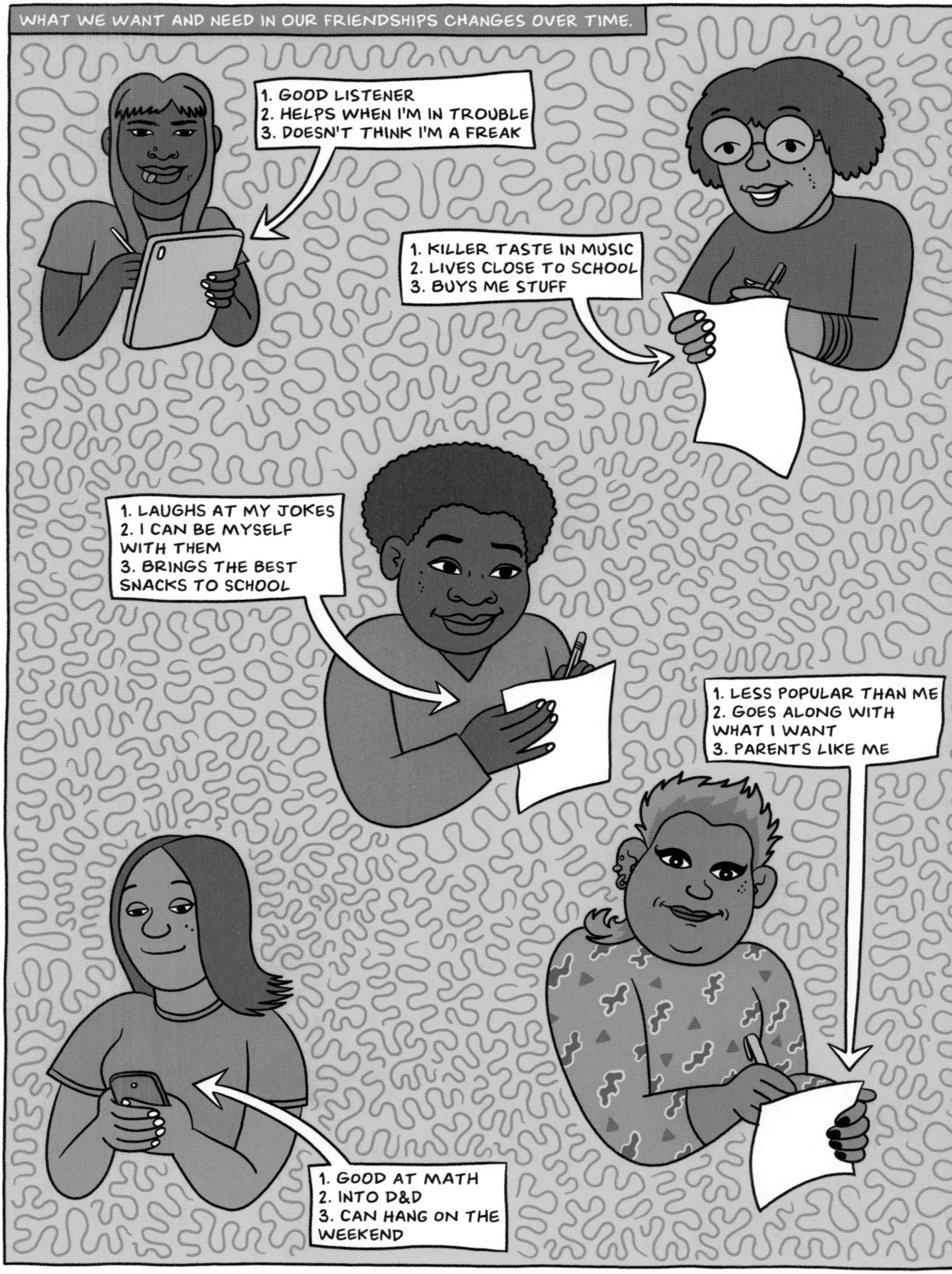
WHAT WE WANT AND NEED IN OUR FRIENDSHIPS CHANGES OVER TIME.
1. GOOD LISTENER 2. HELPS WHEN I'M IN TROUBLE 3. DOESN'T THINK I'M A FREAK
1. KILLER TASTE IN MUSIC 2. LIVES CLOSE TO SCHOOL 3. BUYS ME STUFF
1. LAUGHS AT MY JOKES 2. I CAN BE MYSELF WITH THEM 3. BRINGS THE BEST SNACKS TO SCHOOL
1. LESS POPULAR THAN ME 2. GOES ALONG WITH WHAT I WANT 3. PARENTS LIKE ME
1. GOOD AT MATH 2. INTO D&D 3. CAN HANG ON THE WEEKEND

SOME OF US ACT LIKE WE HAVE NO CHOICE WHEN IT COMES TO FRIENDS. WE BECOME FRIENDS WITH WHOEVER IS AROUND OR WHOEVER WANTS TO BE OUR FRIEND. CHOOSING A FRIEND MEANS THINKING ABOUT WHAT YOU WANT AND WHAT YOU ARE WILLING TO OFFER IN A FRIENDSHIP.

IT CAN BE HARD TO TELL IF SOMEONE IS GOING TO BE A GOOD FRIEND UNTIL WE GET TO KNOW THEM. AND WHEN WE FIND OURSELVES STUCK WITH A BAD FRIEND—IT HAPPENS TO ALL OF US AT SOME POINT—IT CAN BE HARD TO KNOW WHAT TO DO. DO YOU DROP THEM? DO YOU HOPE THEY CHANGE? DO YOU ASK THEM TO CHANGE?

THERE ARE LOTS OF WAYS TO BE A FRIEND, BUT MOST OF US WANT A FRIEND WHO MAKES US FEEL GOOD MORE OFTEN THAN BAD, A FRIEND WHO LISTENS, AND A FRIEND WE CAN TRUST. TRUST LOOKS DIFFERENT WITH DIFFERENT PEOPLE, BUT THERE ARE A FEW THINGS WE CAN LOOK FOR.

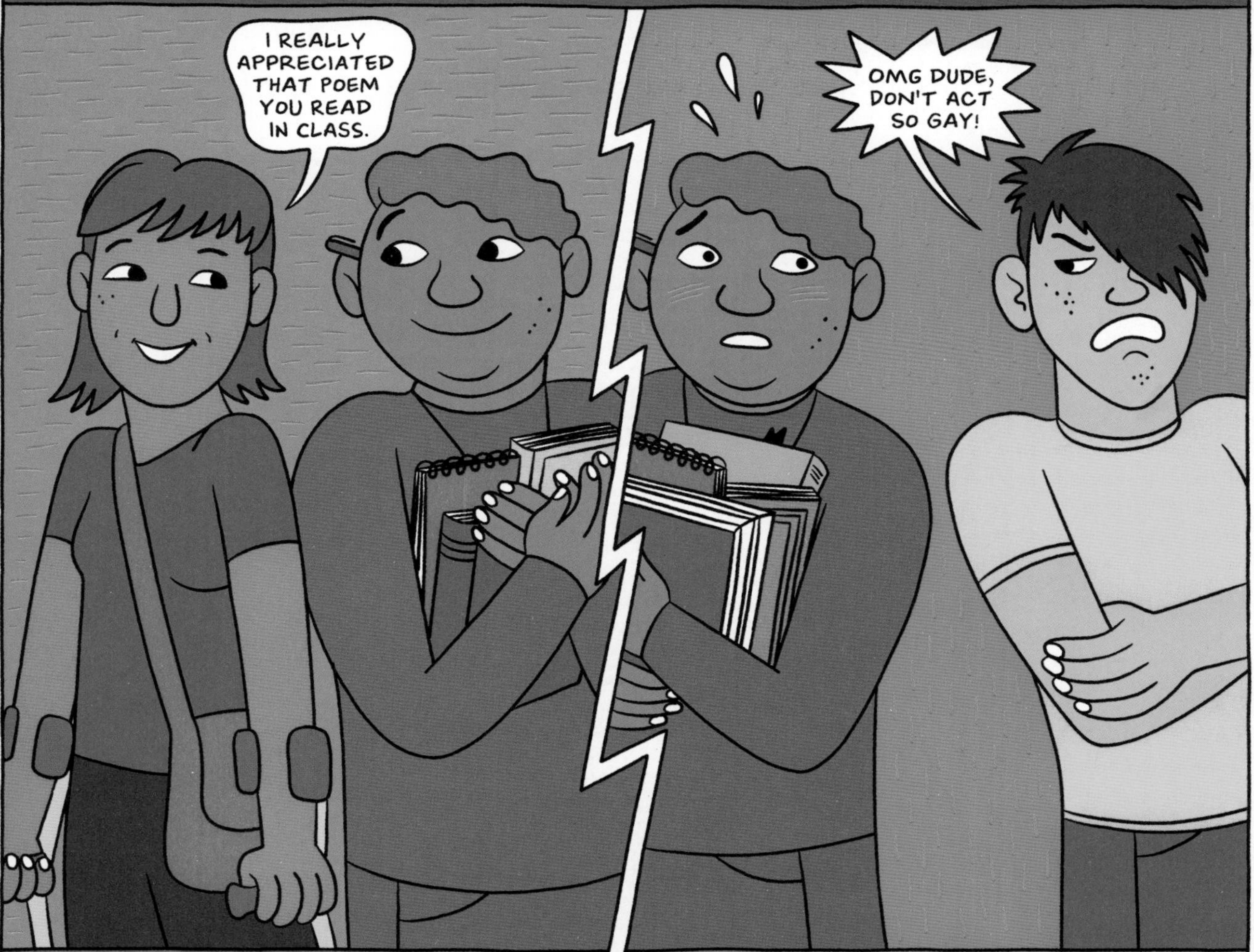
I REALLY APPRECIATED THAT POEM YOU READ IN CLASS.
OMG DUDE, DON'T ACT SO GAY!

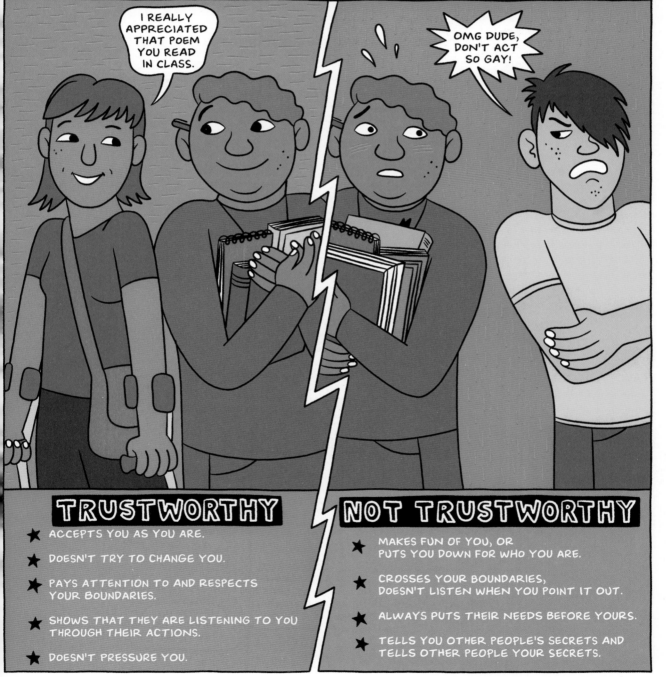

TRUSTWORTHY

- ★ ACCEPTS YOU AS YOU ARE.
- ★ DOESN'T TRY TO CHANGE YOU.
- ★ PAYS ATTENTION TO AND RESPECTS YOUR BOUNDARIES.
- ★ SHOWS THAT THEY ARE LISTENING TO YOU THROUGH THEIR ACTIONS.
- ★ DOESN'T PRESSURE YOU.

NOT TRUSTWORTHY

- ★ MAKES FUN OF YOU, OR PUTS YOU DOWN FOR WHO YOU ARE.
- ★ CROSSES YOUR BOUNDARIES, DOESN'T LISTEN WHEN YOU POINT IT OUT.
- ★ ALWAYS PUTS THEIR NEEDS BEFORE YOURS.
- ★ TELLS YOU OTHER PEOPLE'S SECRETS AND TELLS OTHER PEOPLE YOUR SECRETS.

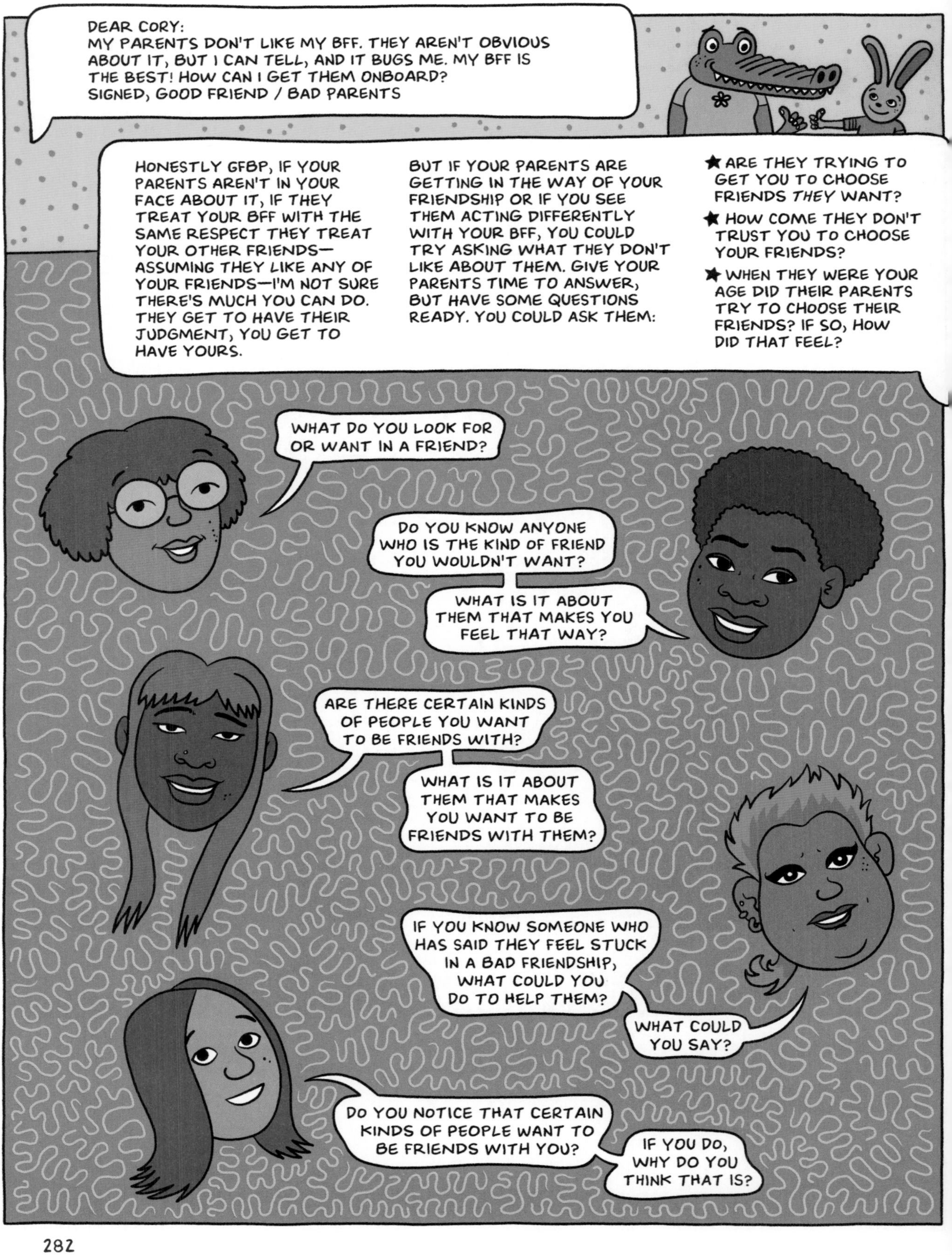
DEAR CORY:
MY PARENTS DON'T LIKE MY BFF. THEY AREN'T OBVIOUS ABOUT IT, BUT I CAN TELL, AND IT BUGS ME. MY BFF IS THE BEST! HOW CAN I GET THEM ONBOARD?
SIGNED, GOOD FRIEND / BAD PARENTS
HONESTLY GFBP, IF YOUR PARENTS AREN'T IN YOUR FACE ABOUT IT, IF THEY TREAT YOUR BFF WITH THE SAME RESPECT THEY TREAT YOUR OTHER FRIENDS—ASSUMING THEY LIKE ANY OF YOUR FRIENDS—I'M NOT SURE THERE'S MUCH YOU CAN DO. THEY GET TO HAVE THEIR JUDGMENT, YOU GET TO HAVE YOURS.
BUT IF YOUR PARENTS ARE GETTING IN THE WAY OF YOUR FRIENDSHIP OR IF YOU SEE THEM ACTING DIFFERENTLY WITH YOUR BFF, YOU COULD TRY ASKING WHAT THEY DON'T LIKE ABOUT THEM. GIVE YOUR PARENTS TIME TO ANSWER, BUT HAVE SOME QUESTIONS READY. YOU COULD ASK THEM:
★ ARE THEY TRYING TO GET YOU TO CHOOSE FRIENDS *THEY* WANT?
★ HOW COME THEY DON'T TRUST YOU TO CHOOSE YOUR FRIENDS?
★ WHEN THEY WERE YOUR AGE DID THEIR PARENTS TRY TO CHOOSE THEIR FRIENDS? IF SO, HOW DID THAT FEEL?
WHAT DO YOU LOOK FOR OR WANT IN A FRIEND?
DO YOU KNOW ANYONE WHO IS THE KIND OF FRIEND YOU WOULDN'T WANT?
WHAT IS IT ABOUT THEM THAT MAKES YOU FEEL THAT WAY?
ARE THERE CERTAIN KINDS OF PEOPLE YOU WANT TO BE FRIENDS WITH?
WHAT IS IT ABOUT THEM THAT MAKES YOU WANT TO BE FRIENDS WITH THEM?
IF YOU KNOW SOMEONE WHO HAS SAID THEY FEEL STUCK IN A BAD FRIENDSHIP, WHAT COULD YOU DO TO HELP THEM?
WHAT COULD YOU SAY?
DO YOU NOTICE THAT CERTAIN KINDS OF PEOPLE WANT TO BE FRIENDS WITH YOU?
IF YOU DO, WHY DO YOU THINK THAT IS?

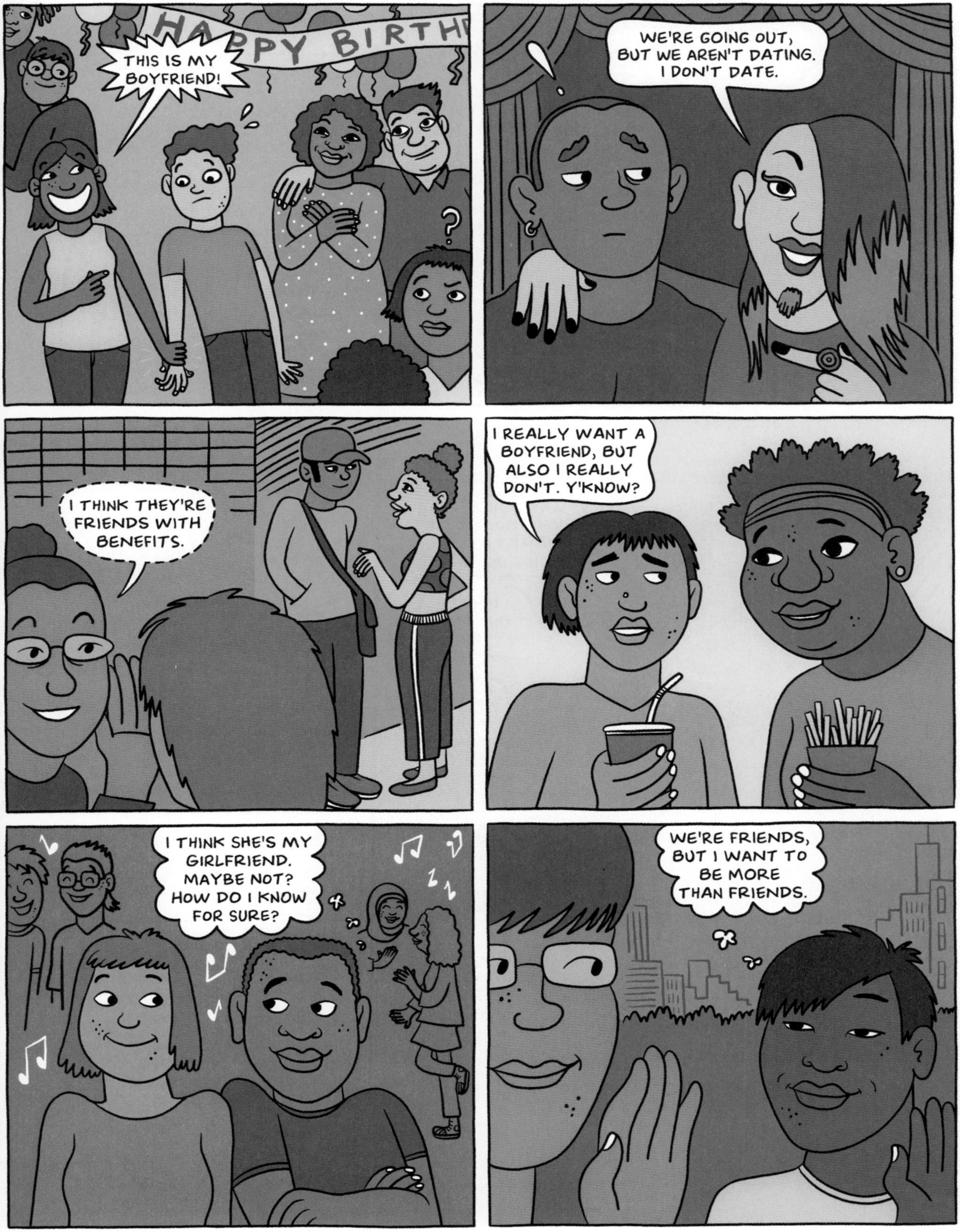
HAPPY BIRTH
THIS IS MY BOYFRIEND!
WE'RE GOING OUT, BUT WE AREN'T DATING. I DON'T DATE.
I THINK THEY'RE FRIENDS WITH BENEFITS.
I REALLY WANT A BOYFRIEND, BUT ALSO I REALLY DON'T. Y'KNOW?
I THINK SHE'S MY GIRLFRIEND. MAYBE NOT? HOW DO I KNOW FOR SURE?
WE'RE FRIENDS, BUT I WANT TO BE MORE THAN FRIENDS.

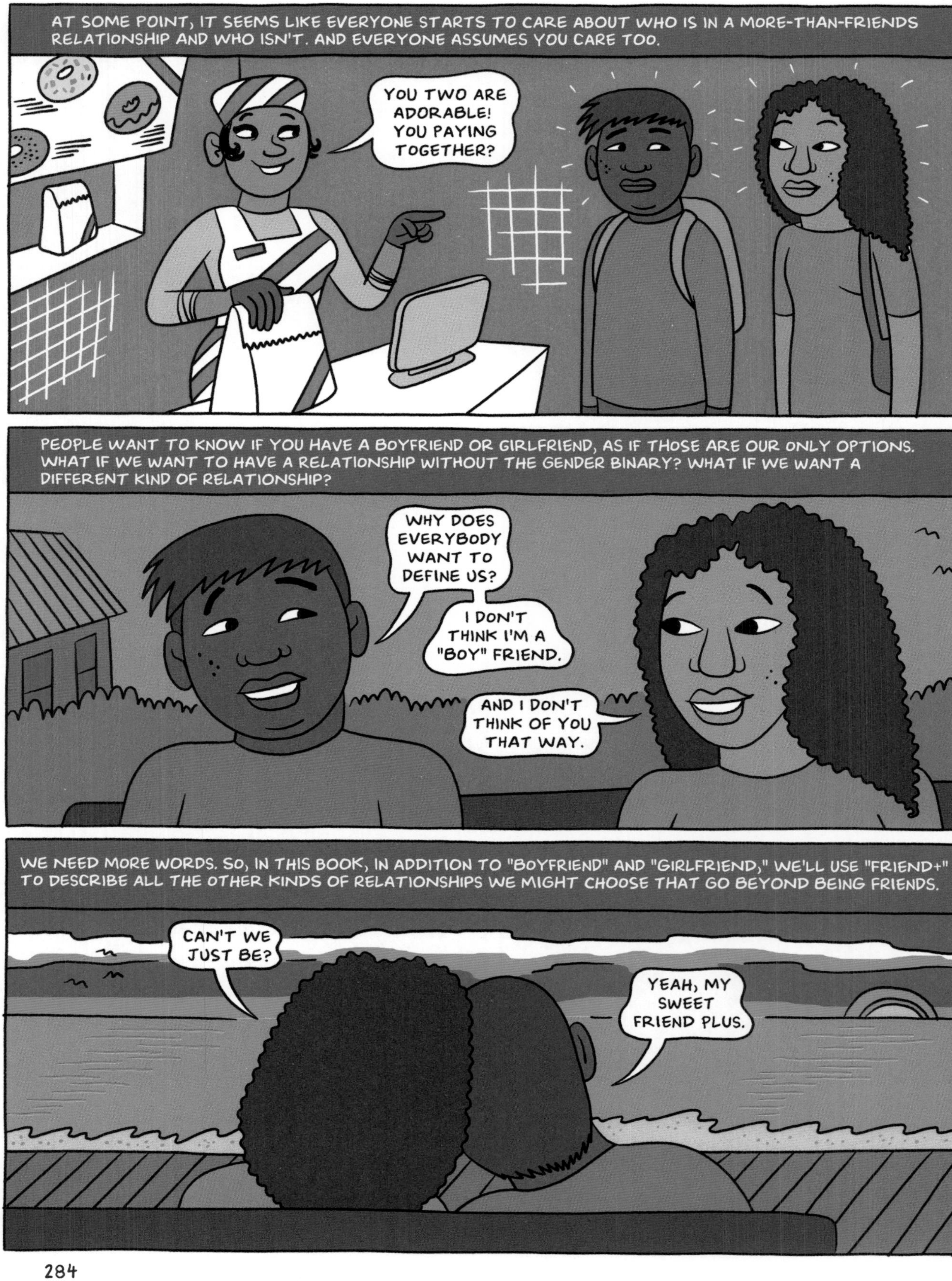
AT SOME POINT, IT SEEMS LIKE EVERYONE STARTS TO CARE ABOUT WHO IS IN A MORE-THAN-FRIENDS RELATIONSHIP AND WHO ISN'T. AND EVERYONE ASSUMES YOU CARE TOO.
YOU TWO ARE ADORABLE! YOU PAYING TOGETHER?
PEOPLE WANT TO KNOW IF YOU HAVE A BOYFRIEND OR GIRLFRIEND, AS IF THOSE ARE OUR ONLY OPTIONS. WHAT IF WE WANT TO HAVE A RELATIONSHIP WITHOUT THE GENDER BINARY? WHAT IF WE WANT A DIFFERENT KIND OF RELATIONSHIP?
WHY DOES EVERYBODY WANT TO DEFINE US?
I DON'T THINK I'M A "BOY" FRIEND.
AND I DON'T THINK OF YOU THAT WAY.
WE NEED MORE WORDS. SO, IN THIS BOOK, IN ADDITION TO "BOYFRIEND" AND "GIRLFRIEND," WE'LL USE "FRIEND+" TO DESCRIBE ALL THE OTHER KINDS OF RELATIONSHIPS WE MIGHT CHOOSE THAT GO BEYOND BEING FRIENDS.
CAN'T WE JUST BE?
YEAH, MY SWEET FRIEND PLUS.

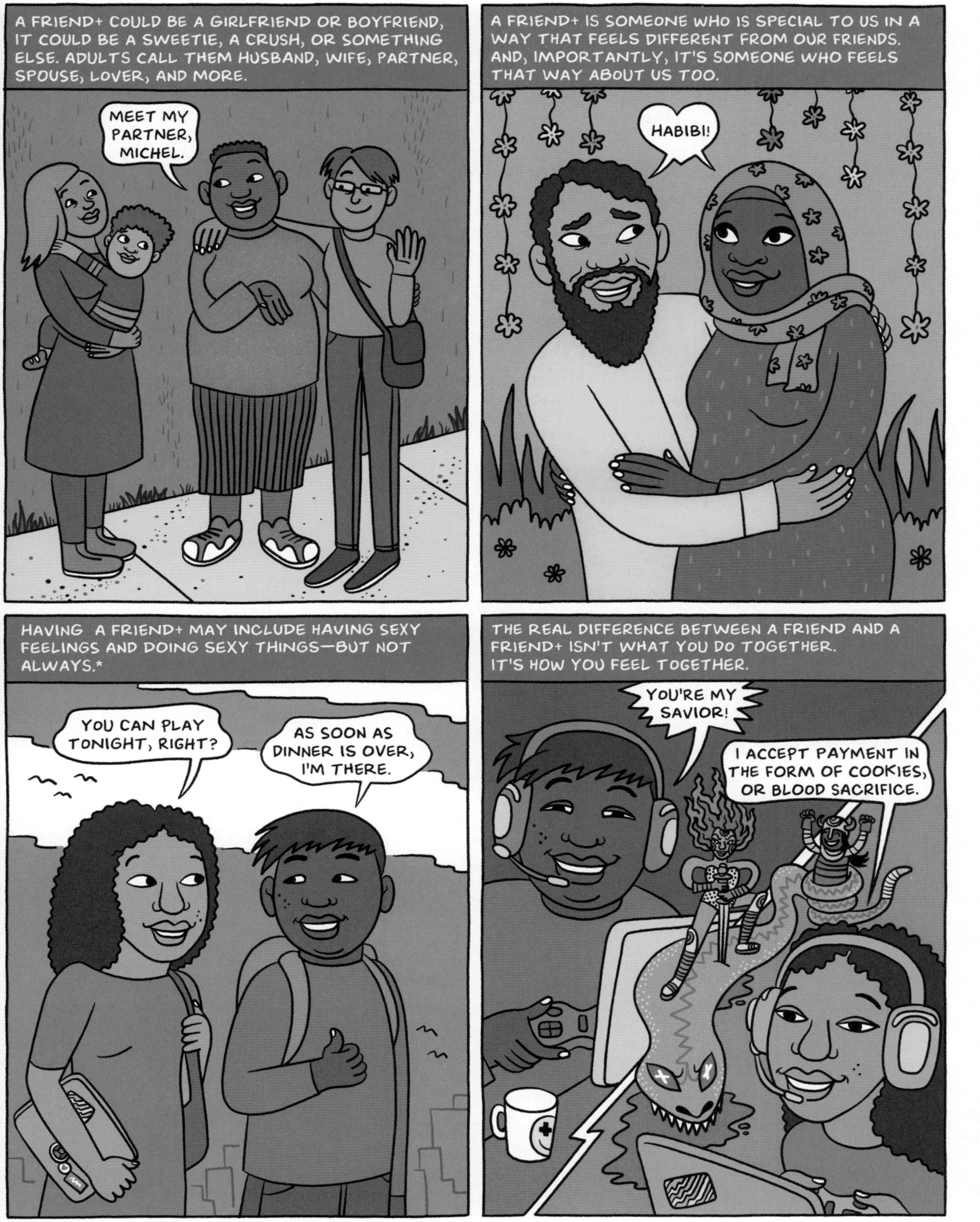
A FRIEND+ COULD BE A GIRLFRIEND OR BOYFRIEND, IT COULD BE A SWEETIE, A CRUSH, OR SOMETHING ELSE. ADULTS CALL THEM HUSBAND, WIFE, PARTNER, SPOUSE, LOVER, AND MORE.
MEET MY PARTNER, MICHEL.
A FRIEND+ IS SOMEONE WHO IS SPECIAL TO US IN A WAY THAT FEELS DIFFERENT FROM OUR FRIENDS. AND, IMPORTANTLY, IT'S SOMEONE WHO FEELS THAT WAY ABOUT US TOO.
HABIBI!
HAVING A FRIEND+ MAY INCLUDE HAVING SEXY FEELINGS AND DOING SEXY THINGS—BUT NOT ALWAYS.*
YOU CAN PLAY TONIGHT, RIGHT?
AS SOON AS DINNER IS OVER, I'M THERE.
THE REAL DIFFERENCE BETWEEN A FRIEND AND A FRIEND+ ISN'T WHAT YOU DO TOGETHER. IT'S HOW YOU FEEL TOGETHER.
YOU'RE MY SAVIOR!
I ACCEPT PAYMENT IN THE FORM OF COOKIES, OR BLOOD SACRIFICE.

* IF YOU MISSED THE PART ABOUT ASEXUALITY, FLIP BACK TO P. 201

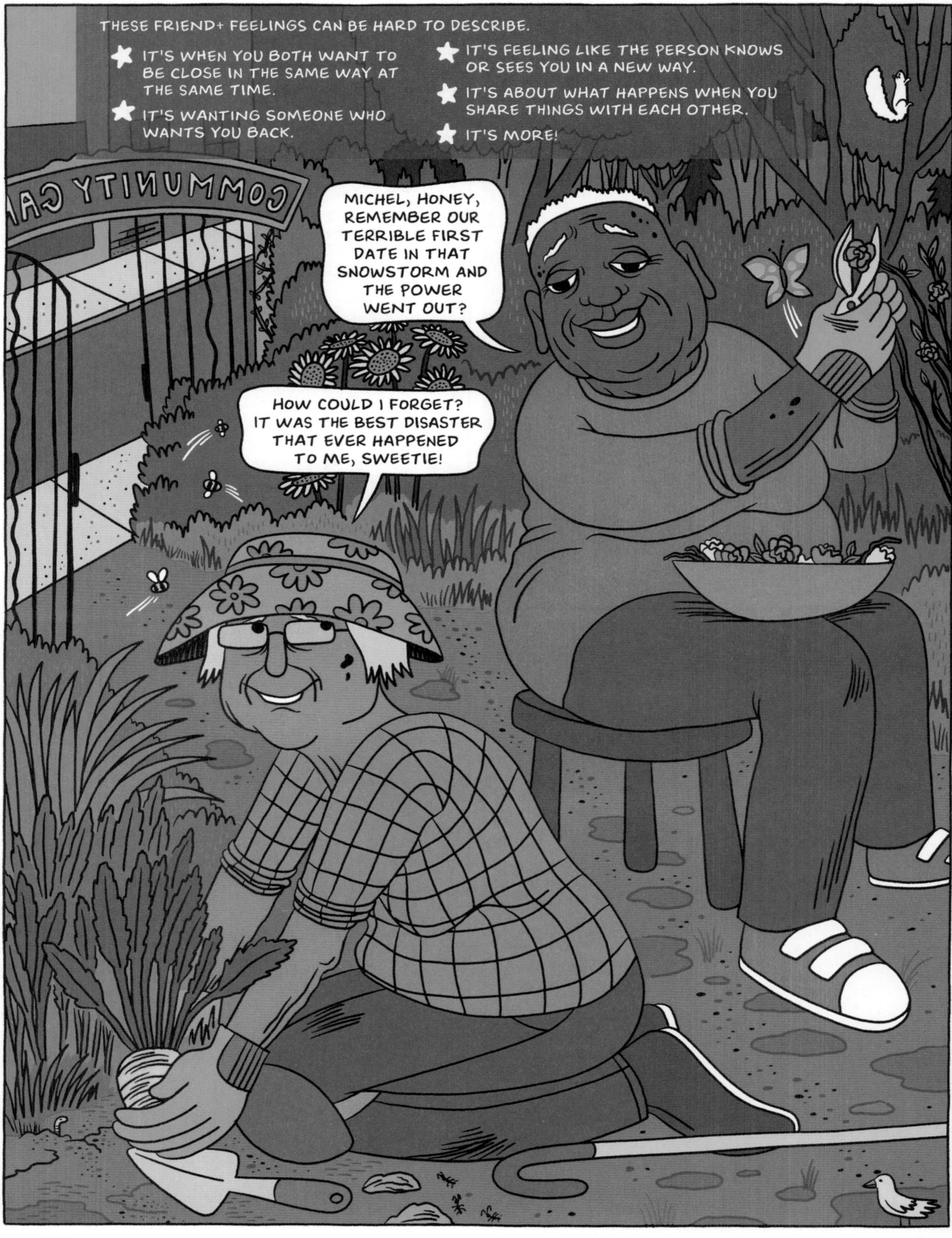
THESE FRIEND+ FEELINGS CAN BE HARD TO DESCRIBE.
IT'S WHEN YOU BOTH WANT TO BE CLOSE IN THE SAME WAY AT THE SAME TIME.
IT'S WANTING SOMEONE WHO WANTS YOU BACK.
IT'S FEELING LIKE THE PERSON KNOWS OR SEES YOU IN A NEW WAY.
IT'S ABOUT WHAT HAPPENS WHEN YOU SHARE THINGS WITH EACH OTHER.
IT'S MORE!
COMMUNITY GA
MICHEL, HONEY, REMEMBER OUR TERRIBLE FIRST DATE IN THAT SNOWSTORM AND THE POWER WENT OUT?
HOW COULD I FORGET? IT WAS THE BEST DISASTER THAT EVER HAPPENED TO ME, SWEETIE!

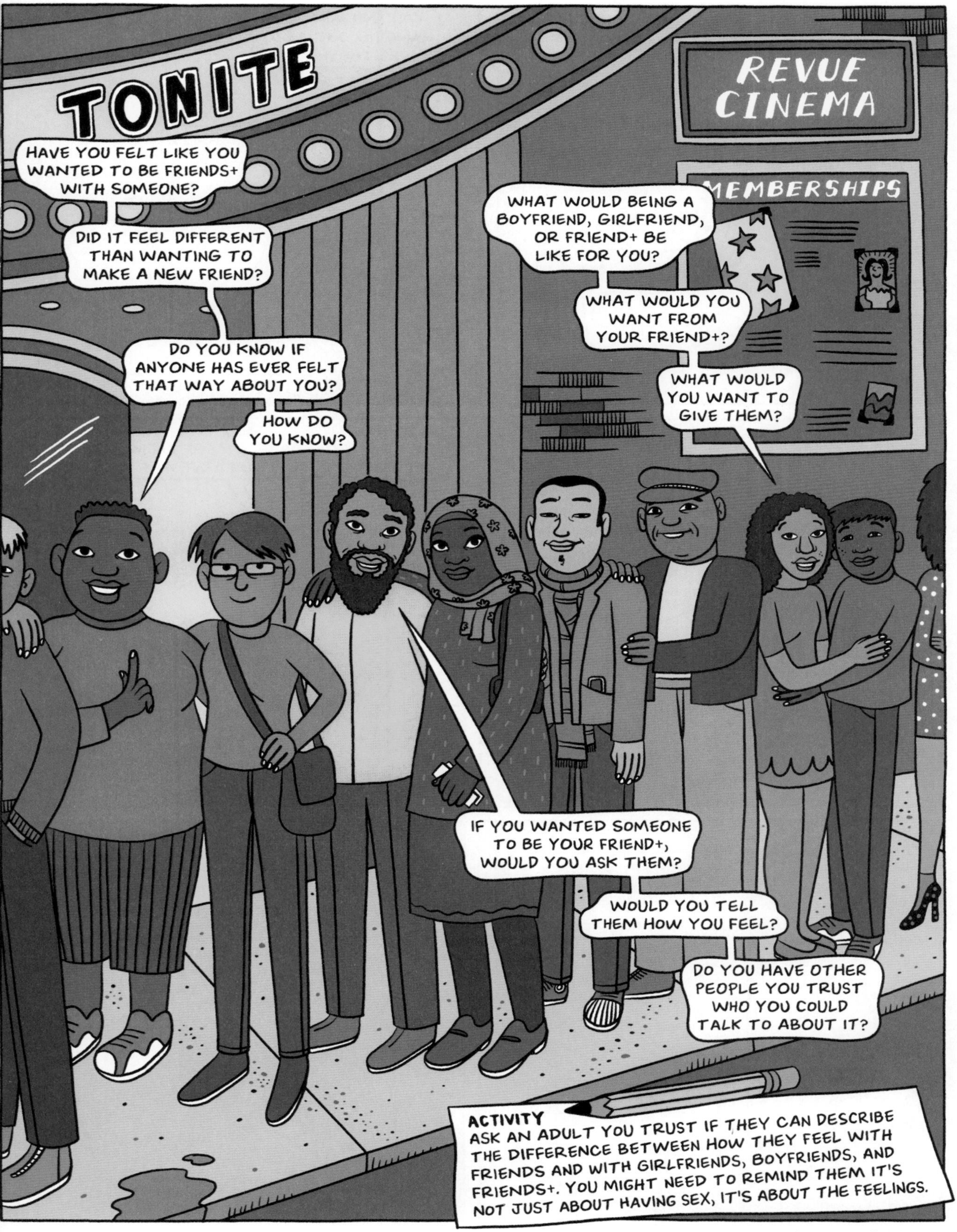
TONITE
REVUE CINEMA
MEMBERSHIPS
HAVE YOU FELT LIKE YOU WANTED TO BE FRIENDS+ WITH SOMEONE?
DID IT FEEL DIFFERENT THAN WANTING TO MAKE A NEW FRIEND?
DO YOU KNOW IF ANYONE HAS EVER FELT THAT WAY ABOUT YOU?
HOW DO YOU KNOW?
WHAT WOULD BEING A BOYFRIEND, GIRLFRIEND, OR FRIEND+ BE LIKE FOR YOU?
WHAT WOULD YOU WANT FROM YOUR FRIEND+?
WHAT WOULD YOU WANT TO GIVE THEM?
IF YOU WANTED SOMEONE TO BE YOUR FRIEND+, WOULD YOU ASK THEM?
WOULD YOU TELL THEM HOW YOU FEEL?
DO YOU HAVE OTHER PEOPLE YOU TRUST WHO YOU COULD TALK TO ABOUT IT?
ACTIVITY
ASK AN ADULT YOU TRUST IF THEY CAN DESCRIBE THE DIFFERENCE BETWEEN HOW THEY FEEL WITH FRIENDS AND WITH GIRLFRIENDS, BOYFRIENDS, AND FRIENDS+. YOU MIGHT NEED TO REMIND THEM IT'S NOT JUST ABOUT HAVING SEX, IT'S ABOUT THE FEELINGS.

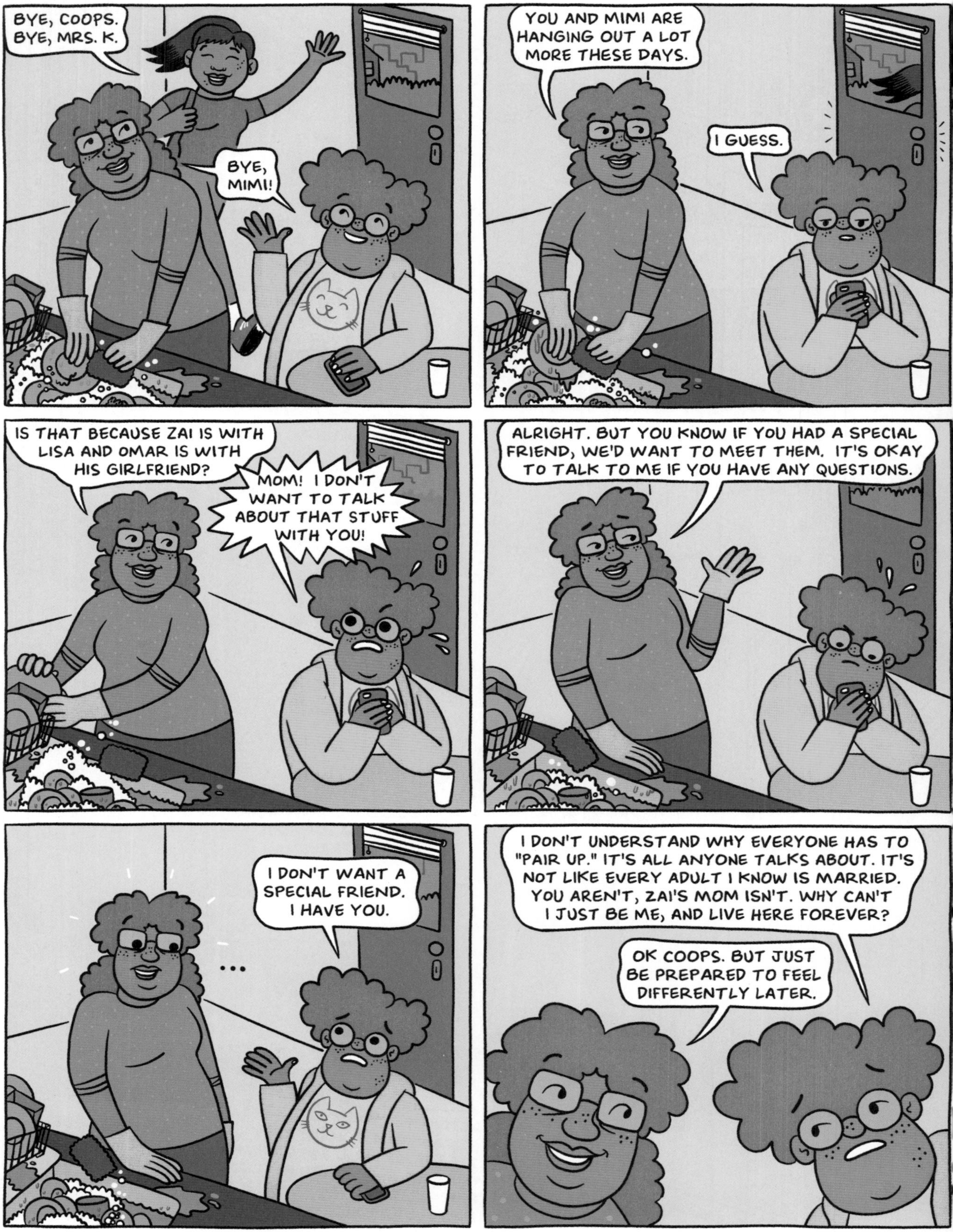
BYE, COOPS. BYE, MRS. K.
BYE, MIMI!
YOU AND MIMI ARE HANGING OUT A LOT MORE THESE DAYS.
I GUESS.
IS THAT BECAUSE ZAI IS WITH LISA AND OMAR IS WITH HIS GIRLFRIEND?
MOM! I DON'T WANT TO TALK ABOUT THAT STUFF WITH YOU!
ALRIGHT. BUT YOU KNOW IF YOU HAD A SPECIAL FRIEND, WE'D WANT TO MEET THEM. IT'S OKAY TO TALK TO ME IF YOU HAVE ANY QUESTIONS.
I DON'T WANT A SPECIAL FRIEND. I HAVE YOU.
...
I DON'T UNDERSTAND WHY EVERYONE HAS TO "PAIR UP." IT'S ALL ANYONE TALKS ABOUT. IT'S NOT LIKE EVERY ADULT I KNOW IS MARRIED. YOU AREN'T, ZAI'S MOM ISN'T. WHY CAN'T I JUST BE ME, AND LIVE HERE FOREVER?
OK COOPS. BUT JUST BE PREPARED TO FEEL DIFFERENTLY LATER.

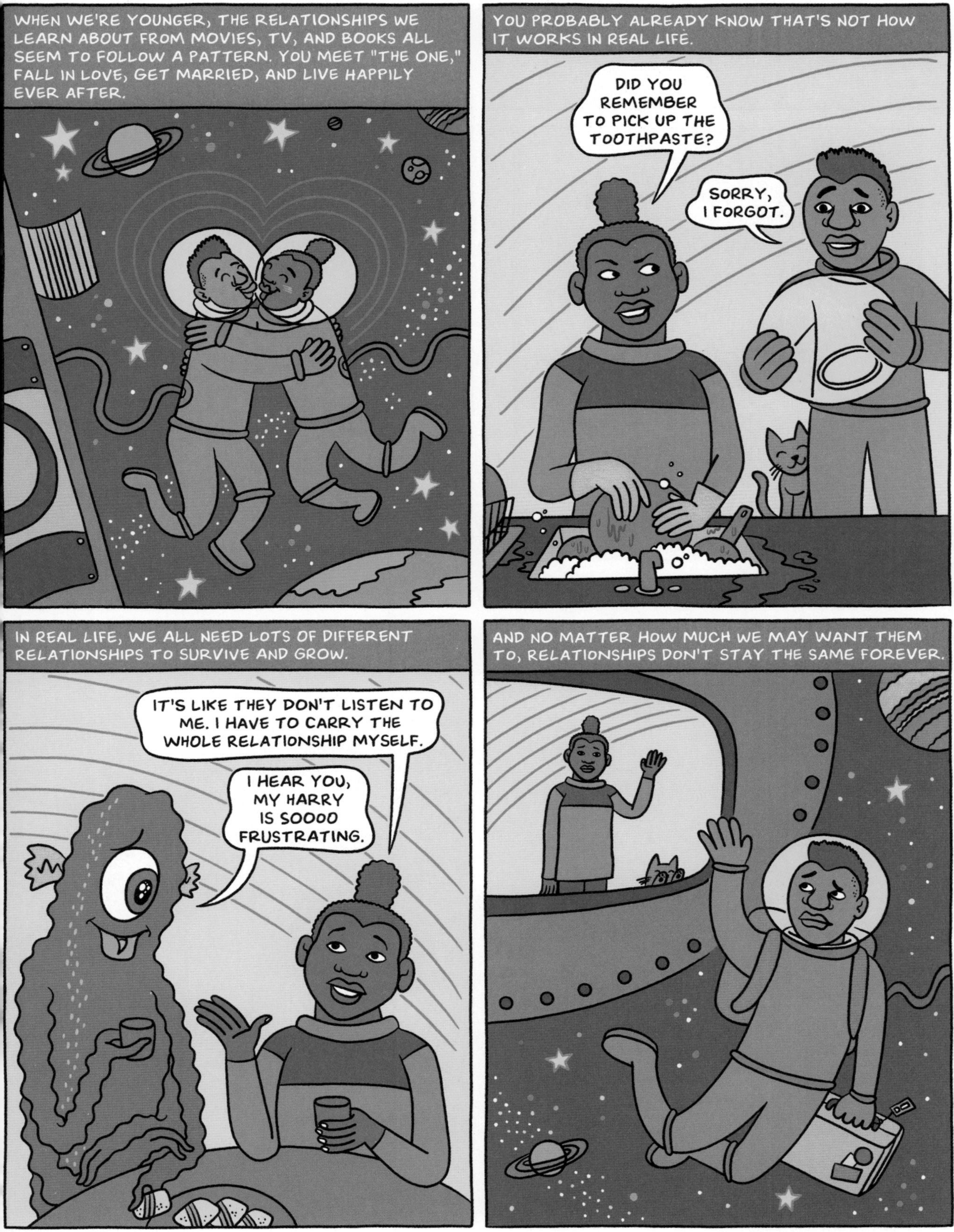
WHEN WE'RE YOUNGER, THE RELATIONSHIPS WE LEARN ABOUT FROM MOVIES, TV, AND BOOKS ALL SEEM TO FOLLOW A PATTERN. YOU MEET "THE ONE," FALL IN LOVE, GET MARRIED, AND LIVE HAPPILY EVER AFTER.
YOU PROBABLY ALREADY KNOW THAT'S NOT HOW IT WORKS IN REAL LIFE.
DID YOU REMEMBER TO PICK UP THE TOOTHPASTE?
SORRY, I FORGOT.
IN REAL LIFE, WE ALL NEED LOTS OF DIFFERENT RELATIONSHIPS TO SURVIVE AND GROW.
IT'S LIKE THEY DON'T LISTEN TO ME. I HAVE TO CARRY THE WHOLE RELATIONSHIP MYSELF.
I HEAR YOU, MY HARRY IS SOOOO FRUSTRATING.
AND NO MATTER HOW MUCH WE MAY WANT THEM TO, RELATIONSHIPS DON'T STAY THE SAME FOREVER.

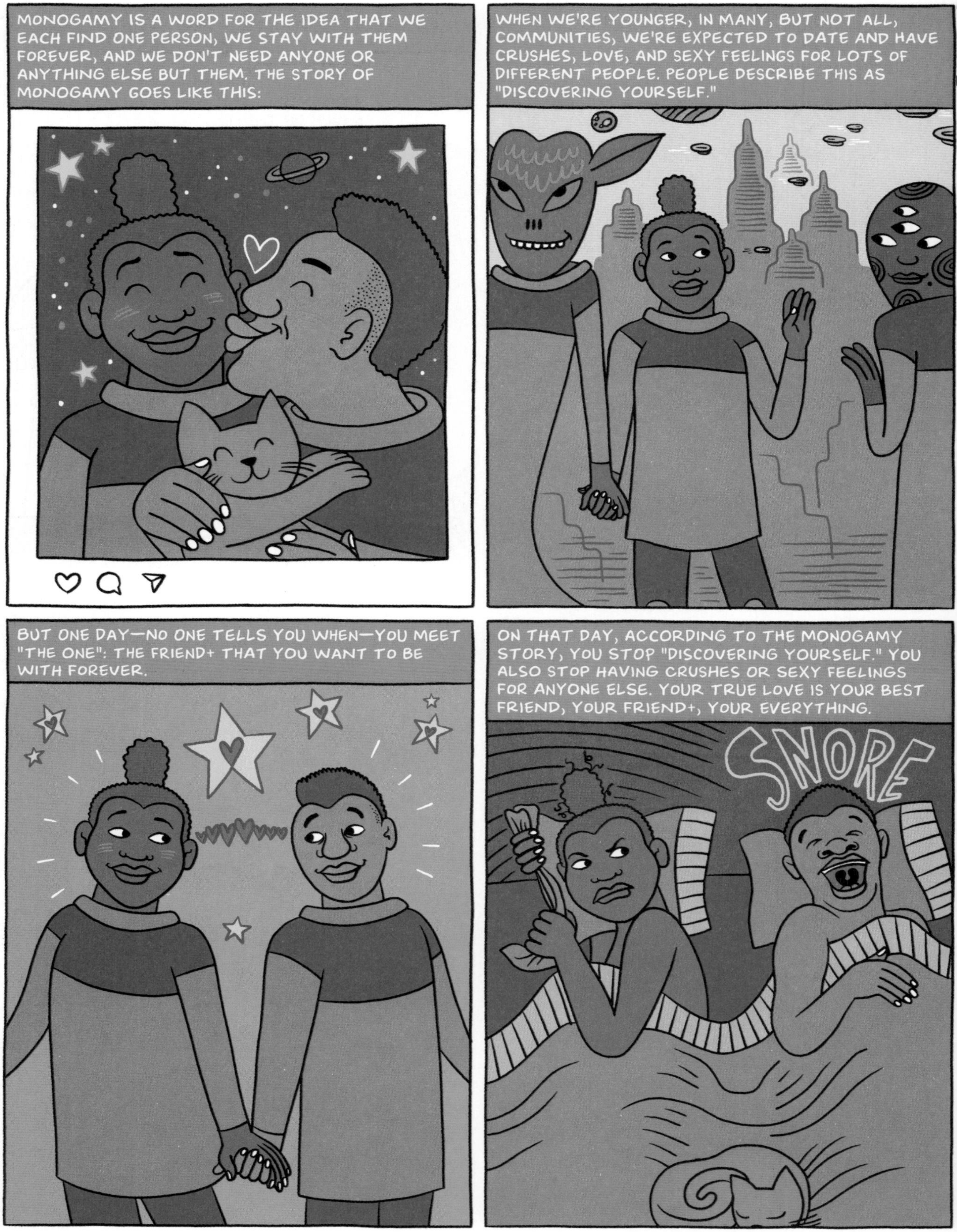
MONOGAMY IS A WORD FOR THE IDEA THAT WE EACH FIND ONE PERSON, WE STAY WITH THEM FOREVER, AND WE DON'T NEED ANYONE OR ANYTHING ELSE BUT THEM. THE STORY OF MONOGAMY GOES LIKE THIS:
WHEN WE'RE YOUNGER, IN MANY, BUT NOT ALL, COMMUNITIES, WE'RE EXPECTED TO DATE AND HAVE CRUSHES, LOVE, AND SEXY FEELINGS FOR LOTS OF DIFFERENT PEOPLE. PEOPLE DESCRIBE THIS AS "DISCOVERING YOURSELF."
BUT ONE DAY—NO ONE TELLS YOU WHEN—YOU MEET "THE ONE": THE FRIEND+ THAT YOU WANT TO BE WITH FOREVER.
ON THAT DAY, ACCORDING TO THE MONOGAMY STORY, YOU STOP "DISCOVERING YOURSELF." YOU ALSO STOP HAVING CRUSHES OR SEXY FEELINGS FOR ANYONE ELSE. YOUR TRUE LOVE IS YOUR BEST FRIEND, YOUR FRIEND+, YOUR EVERYTHING.
SNORE

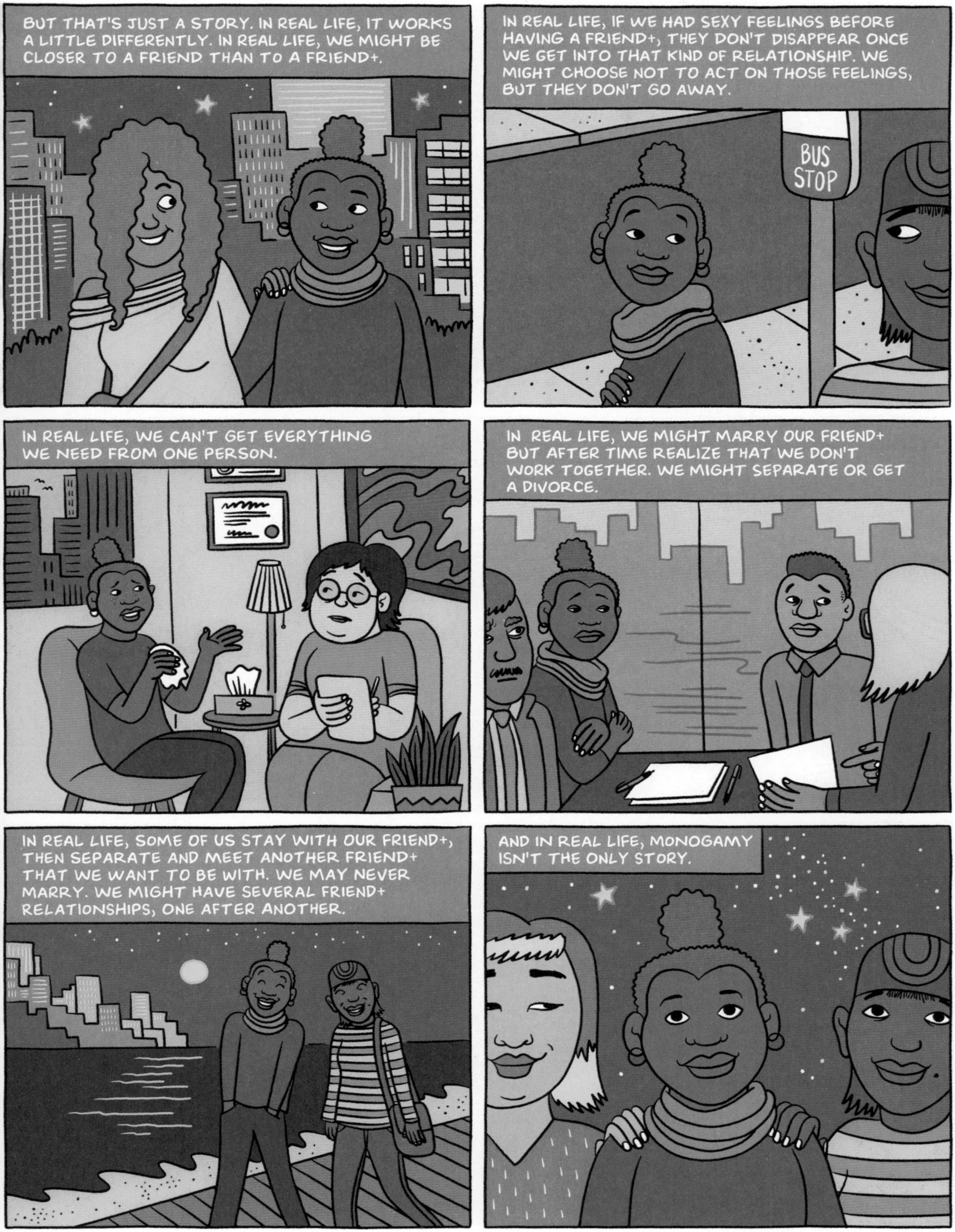
BUT THAT'S JUST A STORY. IN REAL LIFE, IT WORKS A LITTLE DIFFERENTLY. IN REAL LIFE, WE MIGHT BE CLOSER TO A FRIEND THAN TO A FRIEND+.
IN REAL LIFE, IF WE HAD SEXY FEELINGS BEFORE HAVING A FRIEND+, THEY DON'T DISAPPEAR ONCE WE GET INTO THAT KIND OF RELATIONSHIP. WE MIGHT CHOOSE NOT TO ACT ON THOSE FEELINGS, BUT THEY DON'T GO AWAY.
BUS STOP
IN REAL LIFE, WE CAN'T GET EVERYTHING WE NEED FROM ONE PERSON.
IN REAL LIFE, WE MIGHT MARRY OUR FRIEND+ BUT AFTER TIME REALIZE THAT WE DON'T WORK TOGETHER. WE MIGHT SEPARATE OR GET A DIVORCE.
IN REAL LIFE, SOME OF US STAY WITH OUR FRIEND+, THEN SEPARATE AND MEET ANOTHER FRIEND+ THAT WE WANT TO BE WITH. WE MAY NEVER MARRY. WE MIGHT HAVE SEVERAL FRIEND+ RELATIONSHIPS, ONE AFTER ANOTHER.
AND IN REAL LIFE, MONOGAMY ISN'T THE ONLY STORY.

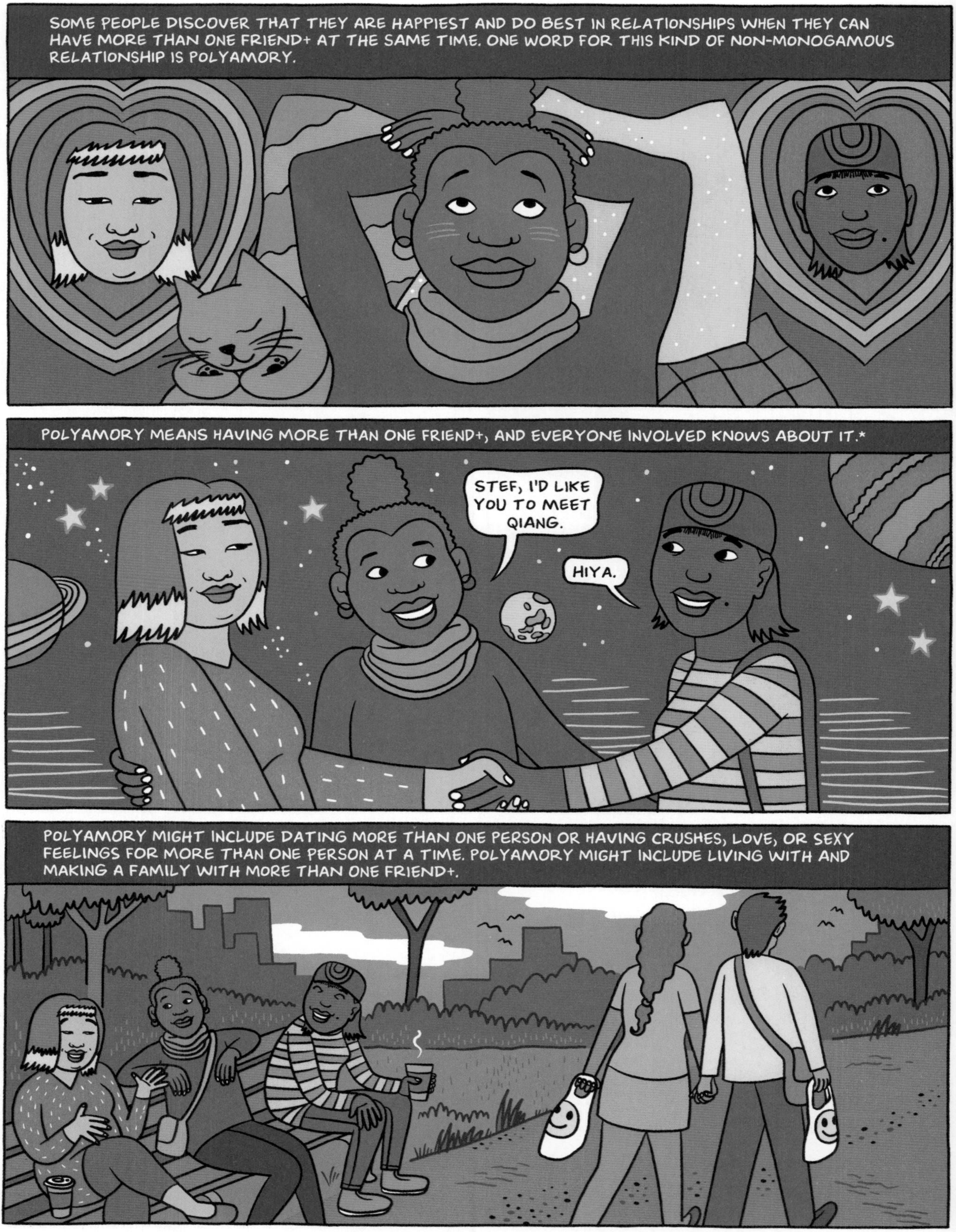
SOME PEOPLE DISCOVER THAT THEY ARE HAPPIEST AND DO BEST IN RELATIONSHIPS WHEN THEY CAN HAVE MORE THAN ONE FRIEND+ AT THE SAME TIME. ONE WORD FOR THIS KIND OF NON-MONOGAMOUS RELATIONSHIP IS POLYAMORY.
POLYAMORY MEANS HAVING MORE THAN ONE FRIEND+, AND EVERYONE INVOLVED KNOWS ABOUT IT.*
STEF, I'D LIKE YOU TO MEET QIANG.
HIYA.
POLYAMORY MIGHT INCLUDE DATING MORE THAN ONE PERSON OR HAVING CRUSHES, LOVE, OR SEXY FEELINGS FOR MORE THAN ONE PERSON AT A TIME. POLYAMORY MIGHT INCLUDE LIVING WITH AND MAKING A FAMILY WITH MORE THAN ONE FRIEND+.

* WHEN YOU HAVE MORE THAN ONE FRIEND+ AND DON'T TELL ANYONE, THAT'S USUALLY CALLED CHEATING

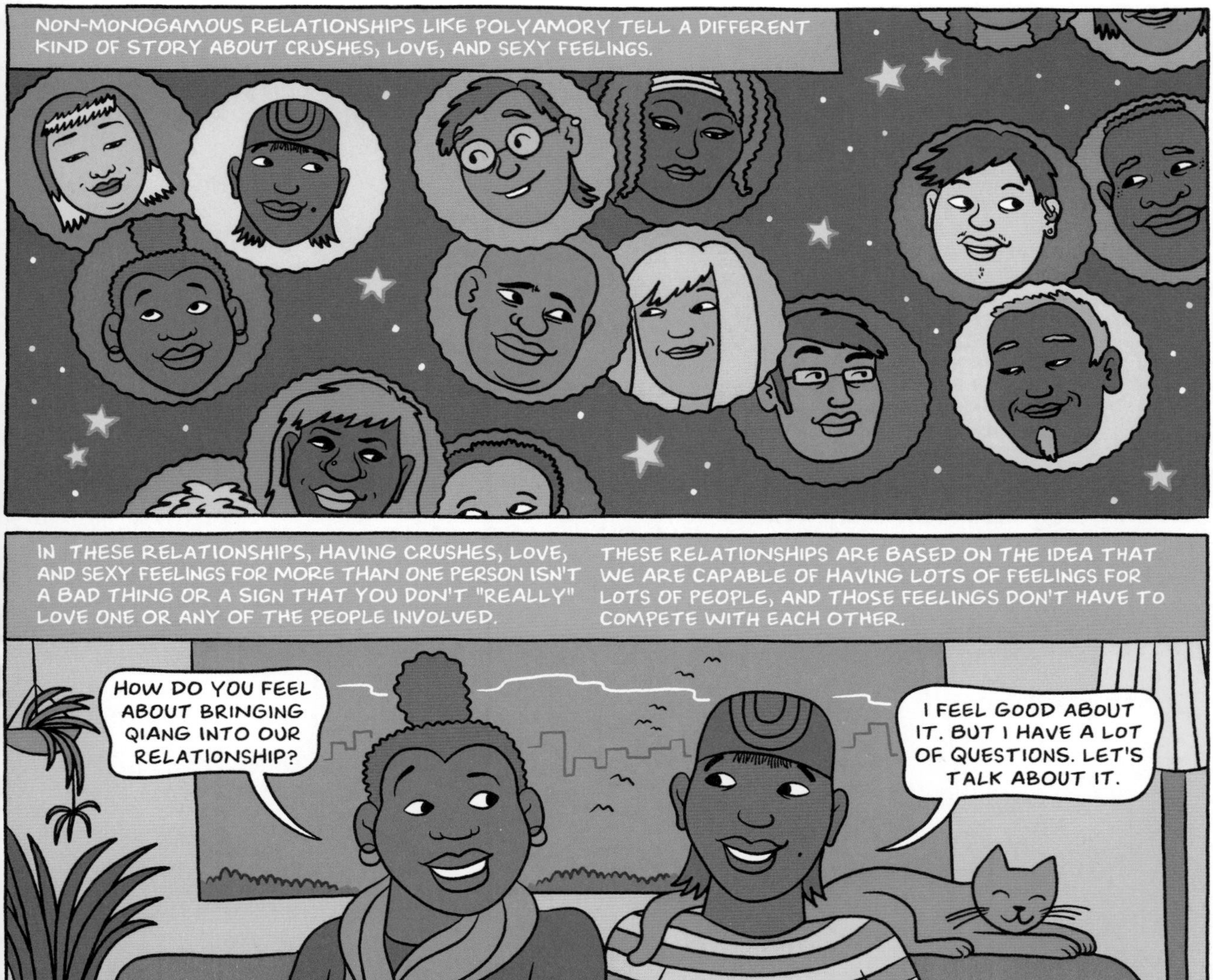
NON-MONOGAMOUS RELATIONSHIPS LIKE POLYAMORY TELL A DIFFERENT KIND OF STORY ABOUT CRUSHES, LOVE, AND SEXY FEELINGS.
IN THESE RELATIONSHIPS, HAVING CRUSHES, LOVE, AND SEXY FEELINGS FOR MORE THAN ONE PERSON ISN'T A BAD THING OR A SIGN THAT YOU DON'T "REALLY" LOVE ONE OR ANY OF THE PEOPLE INVOLVED.
THESE RELATIONSHIPS ARE BASED ON THE IDEA THAT WE ARE CAPABLE OF HAVING LOTS OF FEELINGS FOR LOTS OF PEOPLE, AND THOSE FEELINGS DON'T HAVE TO COMPETE WITH EACH OTHER.
HOW DO YOU FEEL ABOUT BRINGING QIANG INTO OUR RELATIONSHIP?
I FEEL GOOD ABOUT IT. BUT I HAVE A LOT OF QUESTIONS. LET'S TALK ABOUT IT.
LIKE ALL RELATIONSHIPS, NON-MONOGAMOUS RELATIONSHIPS TAKE WORK AND COMMITMENT. THIS INCLUDES A LOT OF TALKING ABOUT FEELINGS, BOTH THE WARM FUZZY KIND, AND THE HARDER KIND—
LIKE JEALOUSY, HURT, AND ANGER. IT MEANS EVERYONE INVOLVED TALKS ABOUT WHAT IS HAPPENING AND MAKES A CHOICE TO STAY IN THE RELATIONSHIP.
WELCOME

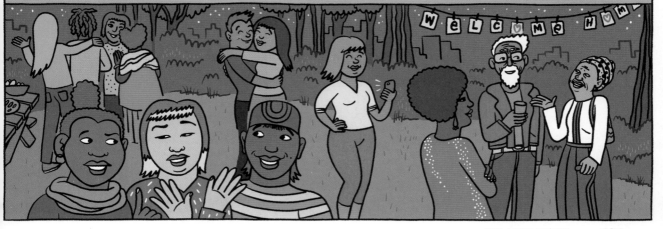

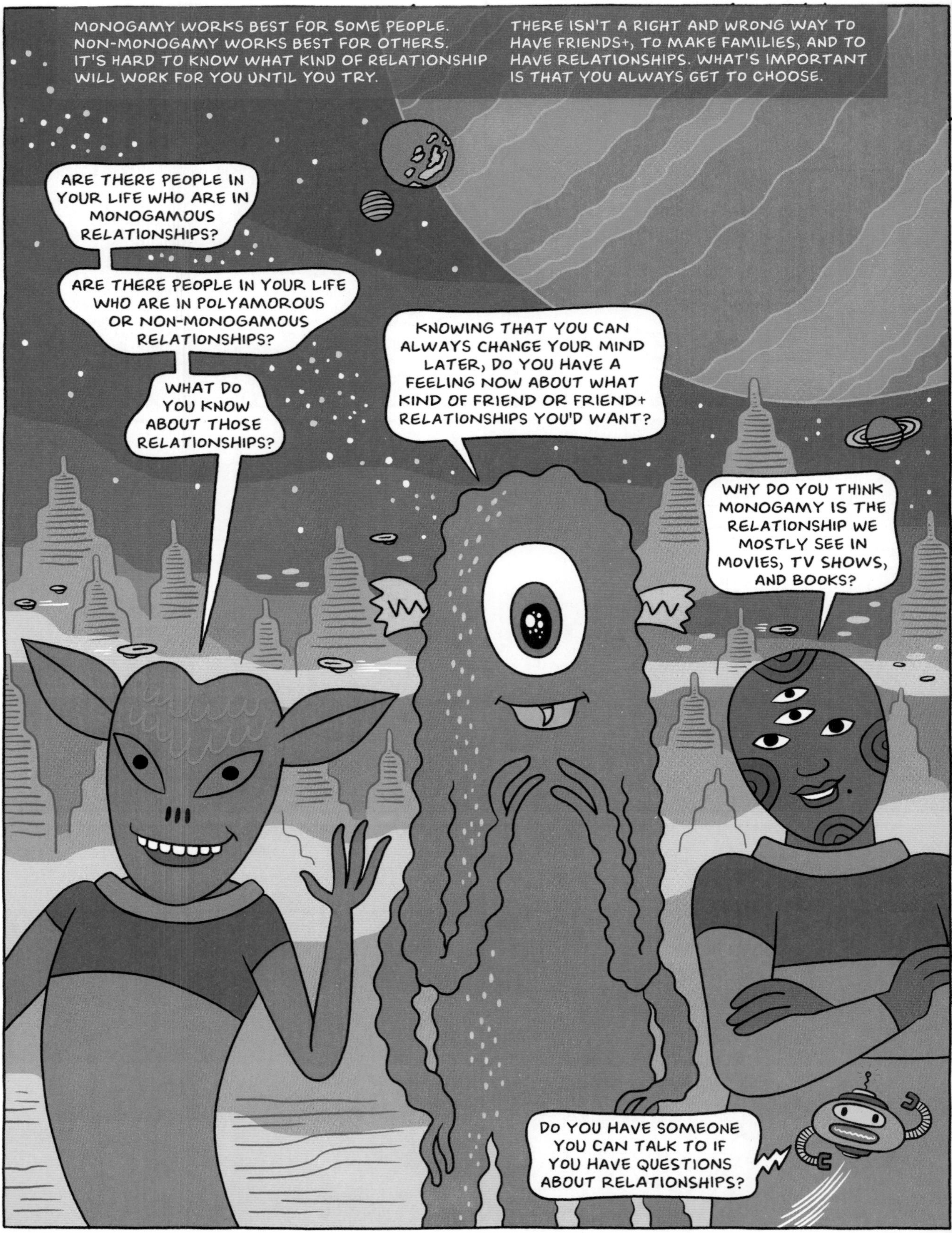
MONOGAMY WORKS BEST FOR SOME PEOPLE. NON-MONOGAMY WORKS BEST FOR OTHERS. IT'S HARD TO KNOW WHAT KIND OF RELATIONSHIP WILL WORK FOR YOU UNTIL YOU TRY.
THERE ISN'T A RIGHT AND WRONG WAY TO HAVE FRIENDS+, TO MAKE FAMILIES, AND TO HAVE RELATIONSHIPS. WHAT'S IMPORTANT IS THAT YOU ALWAYS GET TO CHOOSE.
ARE THERE PEOPLE IN YOUR LIFE WHO ARE IN MONOGAMOUS RELATIONSHIPS?
ARE THERE PEOPLE IN YOUR LIFE WHO ARE IN POLYAMOROUS OR NON-MONOGAMOUS RELATIONSHIPS?
WHAT DO YOU KNOW ABOUT THOSE RELATIONSHIPS?
KNOWING THAT YOU CAN ALWAYS CHANGE YOUR MIND LATER, DO YOU HAVE A FEELING NOW ABOUT WHAT KIND OF FRIEND OR FRIEND+ RELATIONSHIPS YOU'D WANT?
WHY DO YOU THINK MONOGAMY IS THE RELATIONSHIP WE MOSTLY SEE IN MOVIES, TV SHOWS, AND BOOKS?
DO YOU HAVE SOMEONE YOU CAN TALK TO IF YOU HAVE QUESTIONS ABOUT RELATIONSHIPS?

9

REPRODUCTION

REPRODUCTIVE JUSTICE FOR ALL
GET YOUR LAWS OFF MY BODY
SUPPO
ALL
WOME

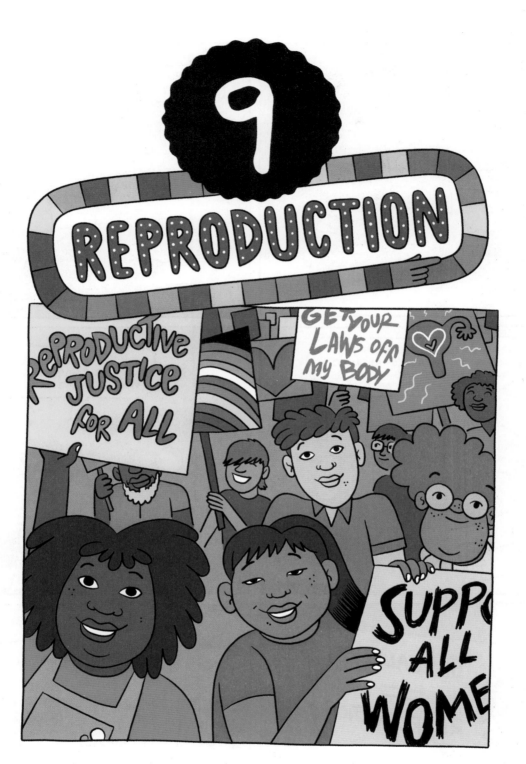

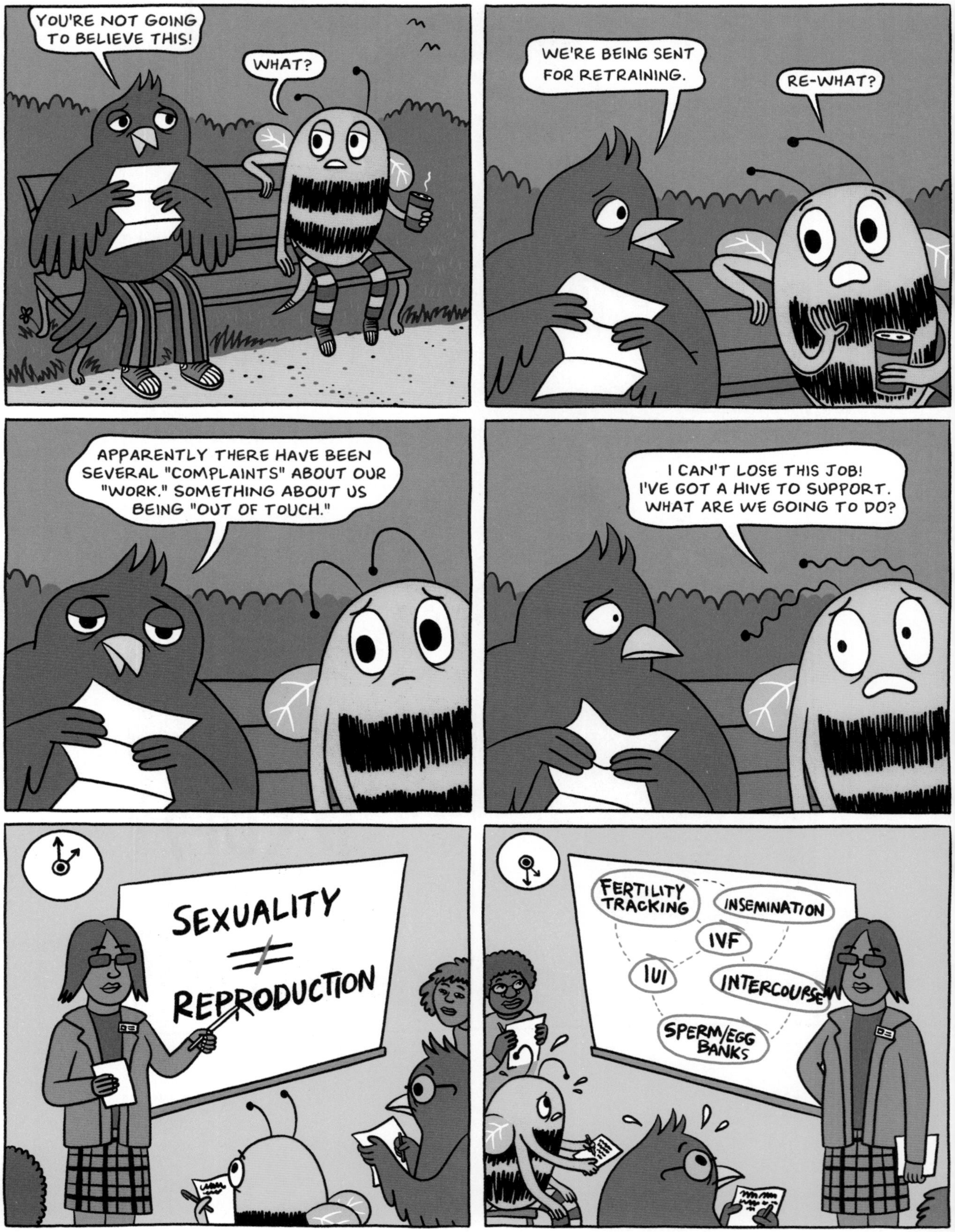
YOU'RE NOT GOING TO BELIEVE THIS!
WHAT?
WE'RE BEING SENT FOR RETRAINING.
RE-WHAT?
APPARENTLY THERE HAVE BEEN SEVERAL "COMPLAINTS" ABOUT OUR "WORK." SOMETHING ABOUT US BEING "OUT OF TOUCH."
I CAN'T LOSE THIS JOB! I'VE GOT A HIVE TO SUPPORT. WHAT ARE WE GOING TO DO?
SEXUALITY ≠ REPRODUCTION
FERTILITY TRACKING
INSEMINATION
IVF
IUI
INTERCOURSE
SPERM/EGG BANKS

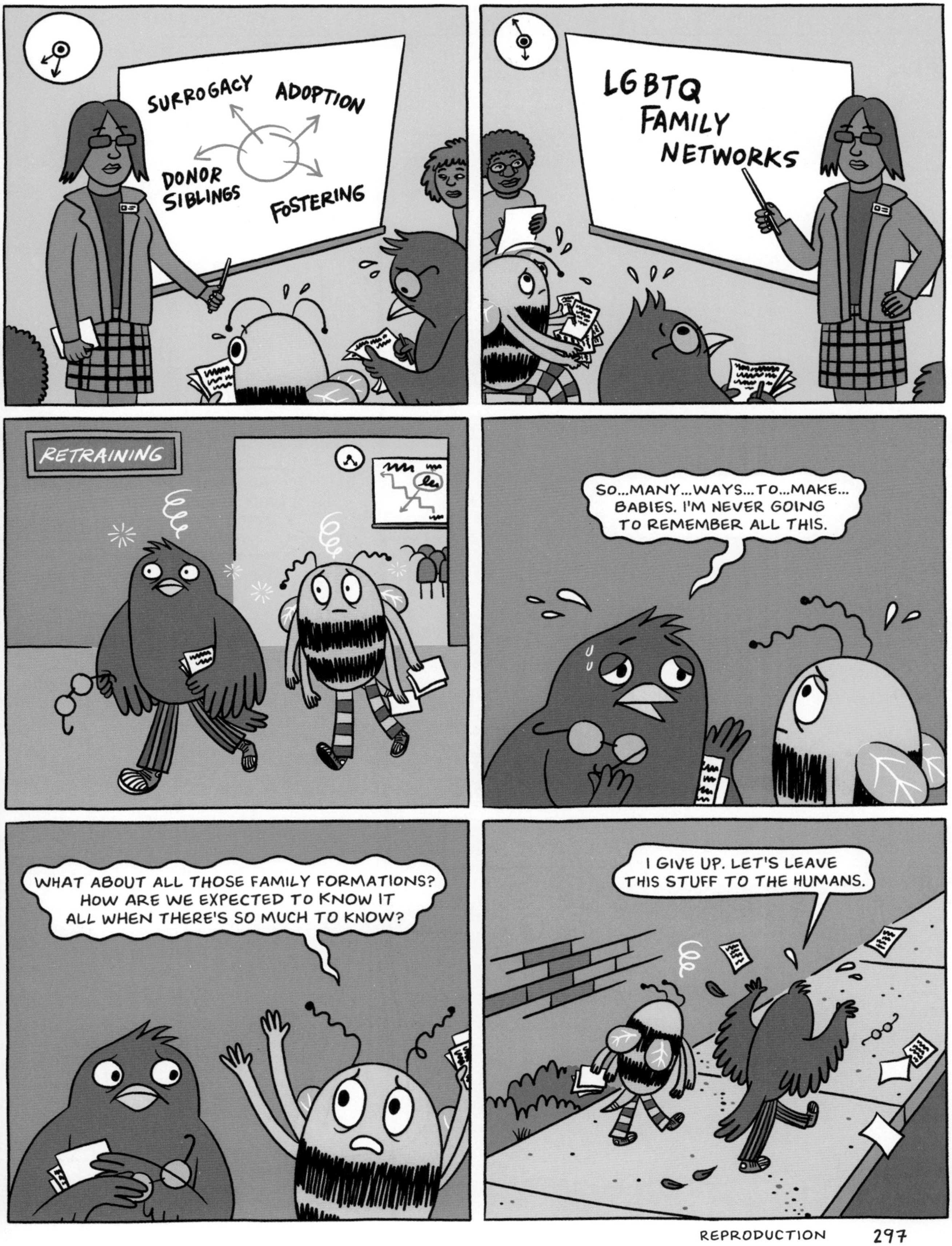
SURROGACY
ADOPTION
DONOR SIBLINGS
FOSTERING
LGBTQ FAMILY NETWORKS
RETRAINING
SO...MANY...WAYS...TO...MAKE... BABIES. I'M NEVER GOING TO REMEMBER ALL THIS.
WHAT ABOUT ALL THOSE FAMILY FORMATIONS? HOW ARE WE EXPECTED TO KNOW IT ALL WHEN THERE'S SO MUCH TO KNOW?
I GIVE UP. LET'S LEAVE THIS STUFF TO THE HUMANS.

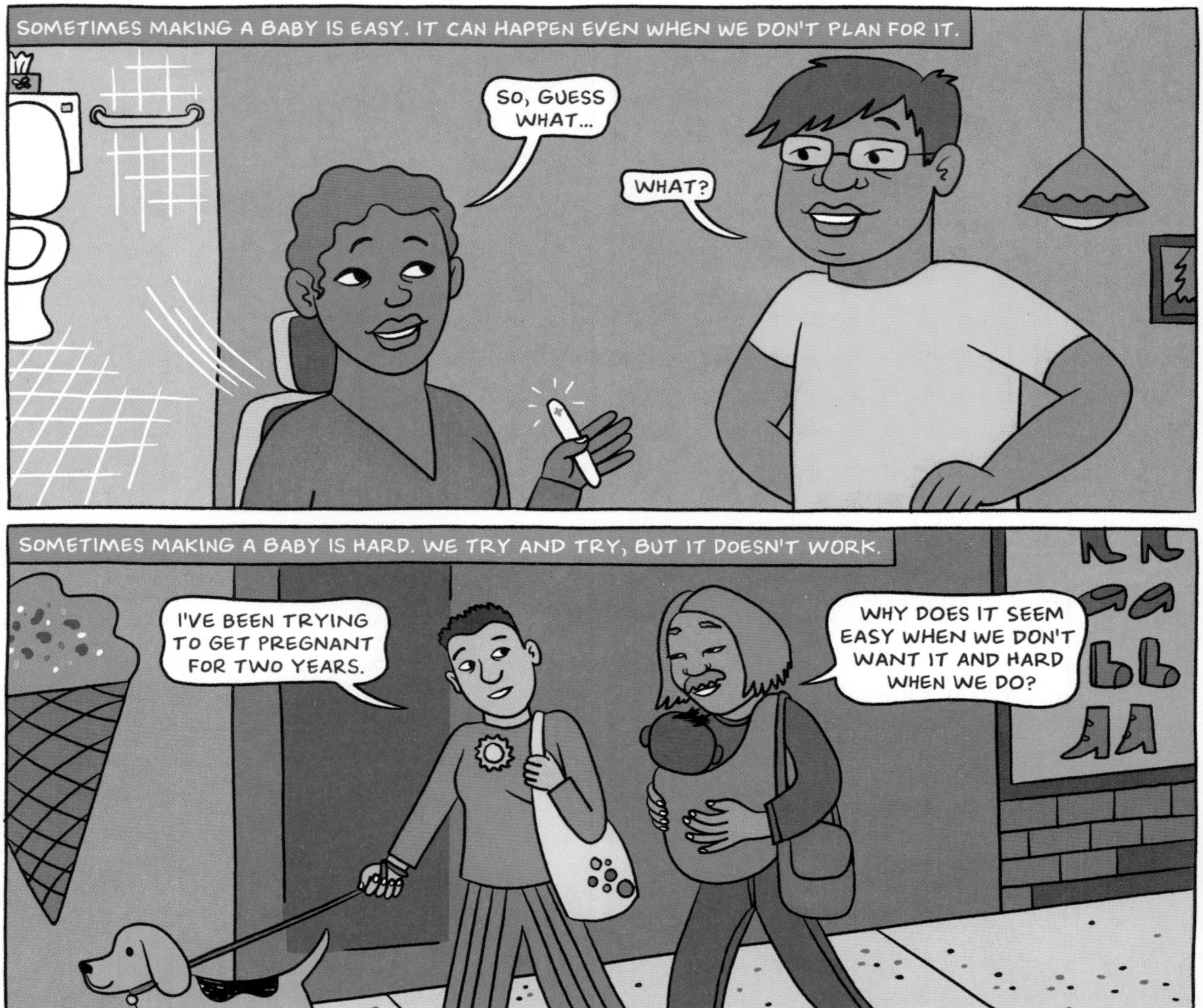
SOMETIMES MAKING A BABY IS EASY. IT CAN HAPPEN EVEN WHEN WE DON'T PLAN FOR IT.
SO, GUESS WHAT...
WHAT?
SOMETIMES MAKING A BABY IS HARD. WE TRY AND TRY, BUT IT DOESN'T WORK.
I'VE BEEN TRYING TO GET PREGNANT FOR TWO YEARS.
WHY DOES IT SEEM EASY WHEN WE DON'T WANT IT AND HARD WHEN WE DO?
THERE ARE LOTS OF DIFFERENT WAYS TO MAKE A BABY, BUT ALL BABIES START WITH THE SAME THREE THINGS.
IT DOESN'T HAPPEN THIS WAY!

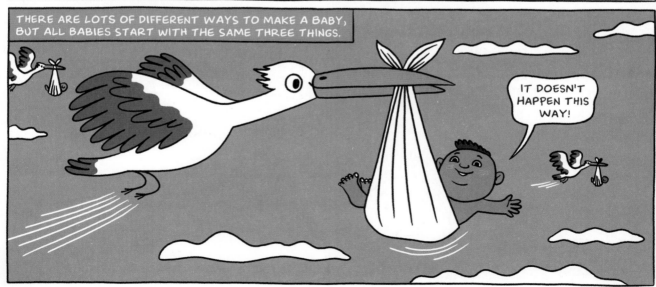

TO MAKE A BABY, YOU NEED AN EGG (OVUM). THIS IS AN EGG.

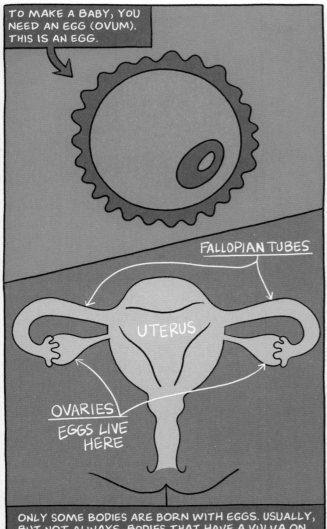

TO MAKE A BABY, YOU ALSO NEED SPERM. THIS IS SPERM.

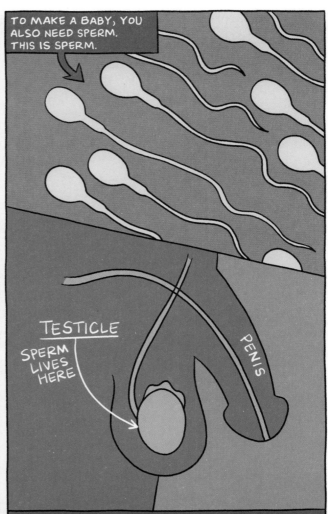

FALLOPIAN TUBES

UTERUS

OVARIES
EGGS LIVE HERE

TESTICLE
SPERM LIVES HERE

PENIS

ONLY SOME BODIES ARE BORN WITH EGGS. USUALLY, BUT NOT ALWAYS, BODIES THAT HAVE A VULVA ON THE OUTSIDE WILL HAVE EGGS ON THE INSIDE. IF A BODY HAS EGGS, THESE EGGS ARE MADE AND STORED IN THE OVARIES.

ONLY SOME BODIES HAVE SPERM. USUALLY, BUT NOT ALWAYS, BODIES THAT HAVE TESTICLES AND A PENIS ON THE OUTSIDE CAN MAKE SPERM ON THE INSIDE. IF A BODY CAN MAKE SPERM, IT'S MADE IN THE TESTICLES.

INSIDE THE SPERM AND THE EGG—JUST LIKE INSIDE EVERY CELL IN YOUR BODY—THERE IS DNA (SHORT FOR DEOXYRIBONUCLEIC ACID).

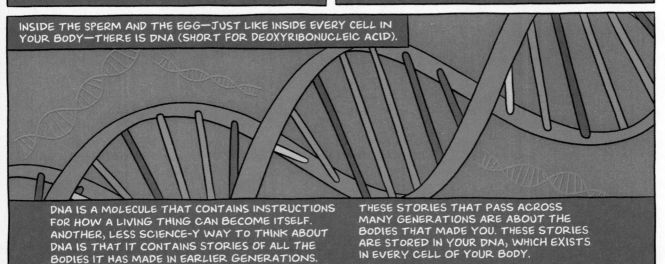

DNA IS A MOLECULE THAT CONTAINS INSTRUCTIONS FOR HOW A LIVING THING CAN BECOME ITSELF. ANOTHER, LESS SCIENCE-Y WAY TO THINK ABOUT DNA IS THAT IT CONTAINS STORIES OF ALL THE BODIES IT HAS MADE IN EARLIER GENERATIONS.

THESE STORIES THAT PASS ACROSS MANY GENERATIONS ARE ABOUT THE BODIES THAT MADE YOU. THESE STORIES ARE STORED IN YOUR DNA, WHICH EXISTS IN EVERY CELL OF YOUR BODY.

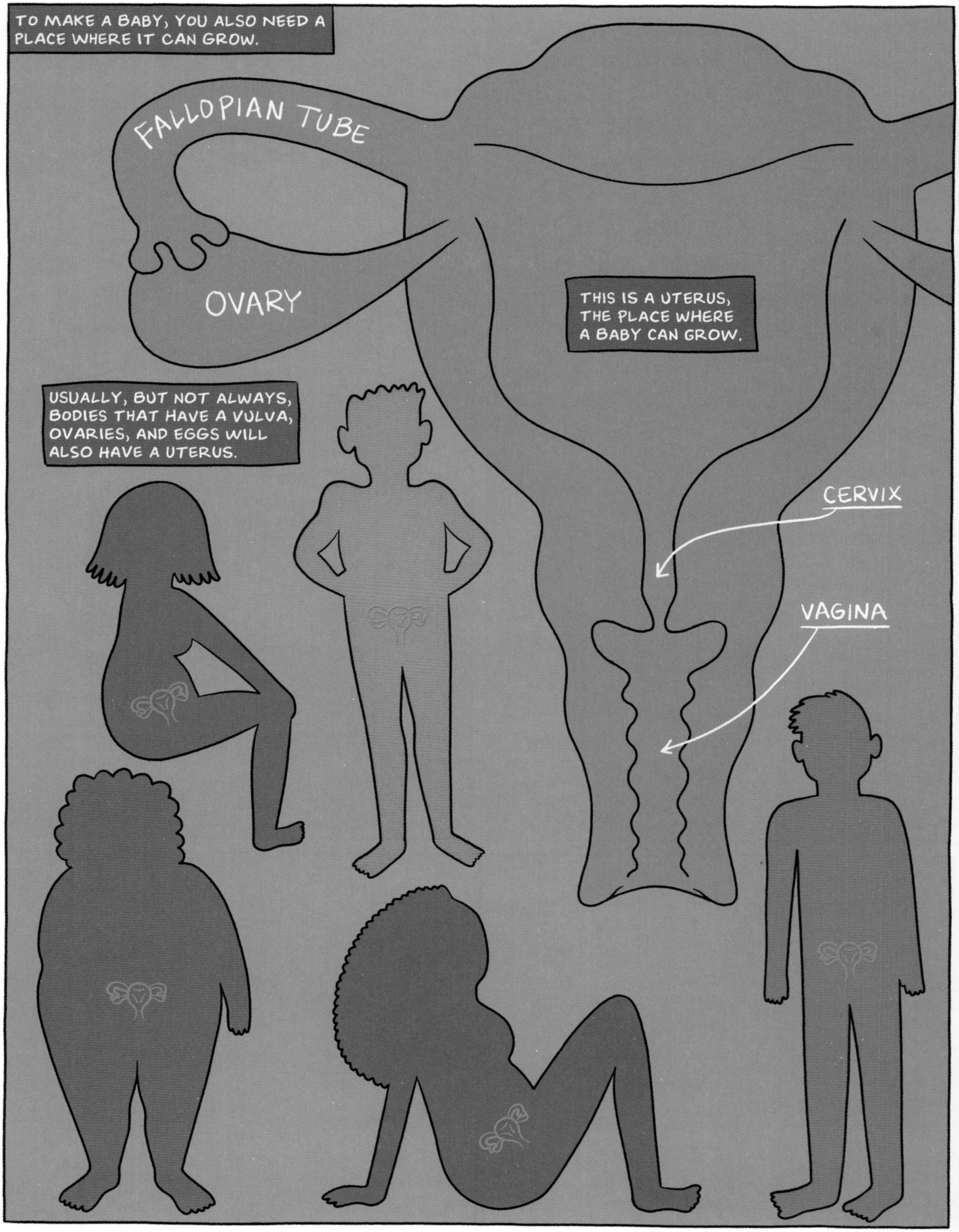
TO MAKE A BABY, YOU ALSO NEED A PLACE WHERE IT CAN GROW.
FALLOPIAN TUBE
OVARY
THIS IS A UTERUS, THE PLACE WHERE A BABY CAN GROW.
USUALLY, BUT NOT ALWAYS, BODIES THAT HAVE A VULVA, OVARIES, AND EGGS WILL ALSO HAVE A UTERUS.
CERVIX
VAGINA

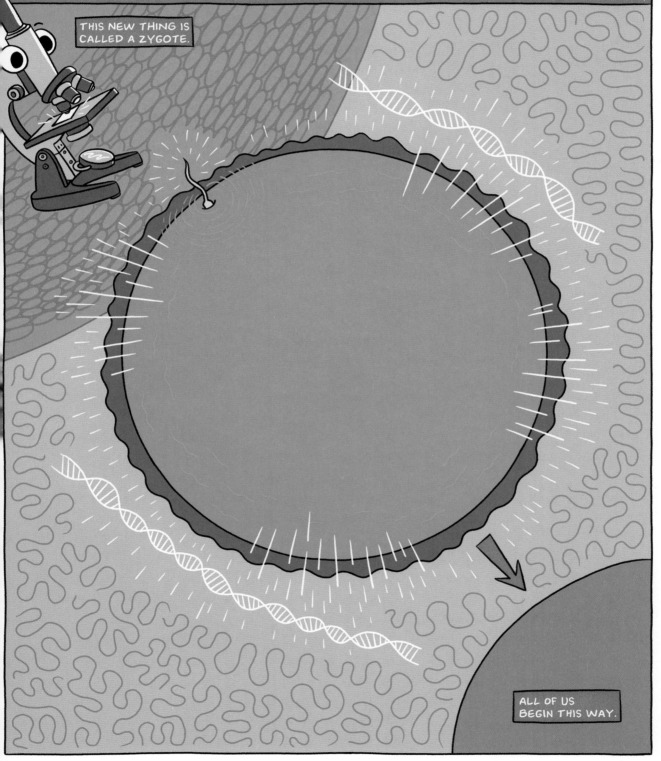

SOMETIMES WHEN AN EGG AND A SPERM MEET, THEY FUSE TOGETHER THROUGH A PROCESS CALLED FERTILIZATION. WHEN THEY FUSE, THESE TWO SEPARATE THINGS—SPERM AND EGG—ARE NOW ONE THING WITH A NEW NAME. THE DNA FROM THE EGG AND THE DNA FROM THE SPERM COMBINE INTO THIS NEW THING THAT HAS ITS OWN DNA. THIS DNA IS A SET OF INSTRUCTIONS DRAWN FROM THE STORIES OF ALL THE GENERATIONS THAT CAME BEFORE IT. IT ISN'T EXACTLY LIKE THE DNA IN THE SPERM OR THE DNA IN THE EGG THAT MADE IT.

THIS NEW THING IS CALLED A ZYGOTE.

ALL OF US BEGIN THIS WAY.

THE ZYGOTE IS ONE CELL, BUT IF IT'S GOING TO GROW AT ALL, IT QUICKLY SPLITS INTO TWO. THOSE TWO CELLS SPLIT INTO FOUR, FOUR INTO SIXTEEN, AND SO ON. AFTER ALMOST A WEEK OF DIVIDING AND DIVIDING AGAIN, IT'S A BALL OF CELLS CALLED AN EMBRYO. A NEW EMBRYO IS SO SMALL YOU CAN ONLY SEE IT WITH A SPECIAL MICROSCOPE. AFTER AROUND EIGHT WEEKS OF GROWING IT'S CALLED A FETUS.

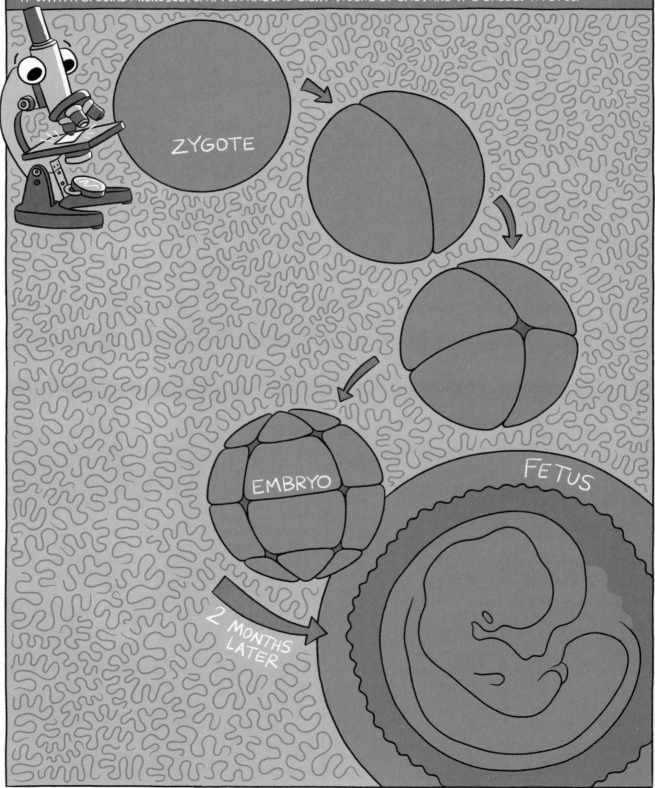

ZYGOTE

EMBRYO

2 MONTHS LATER

FETUS

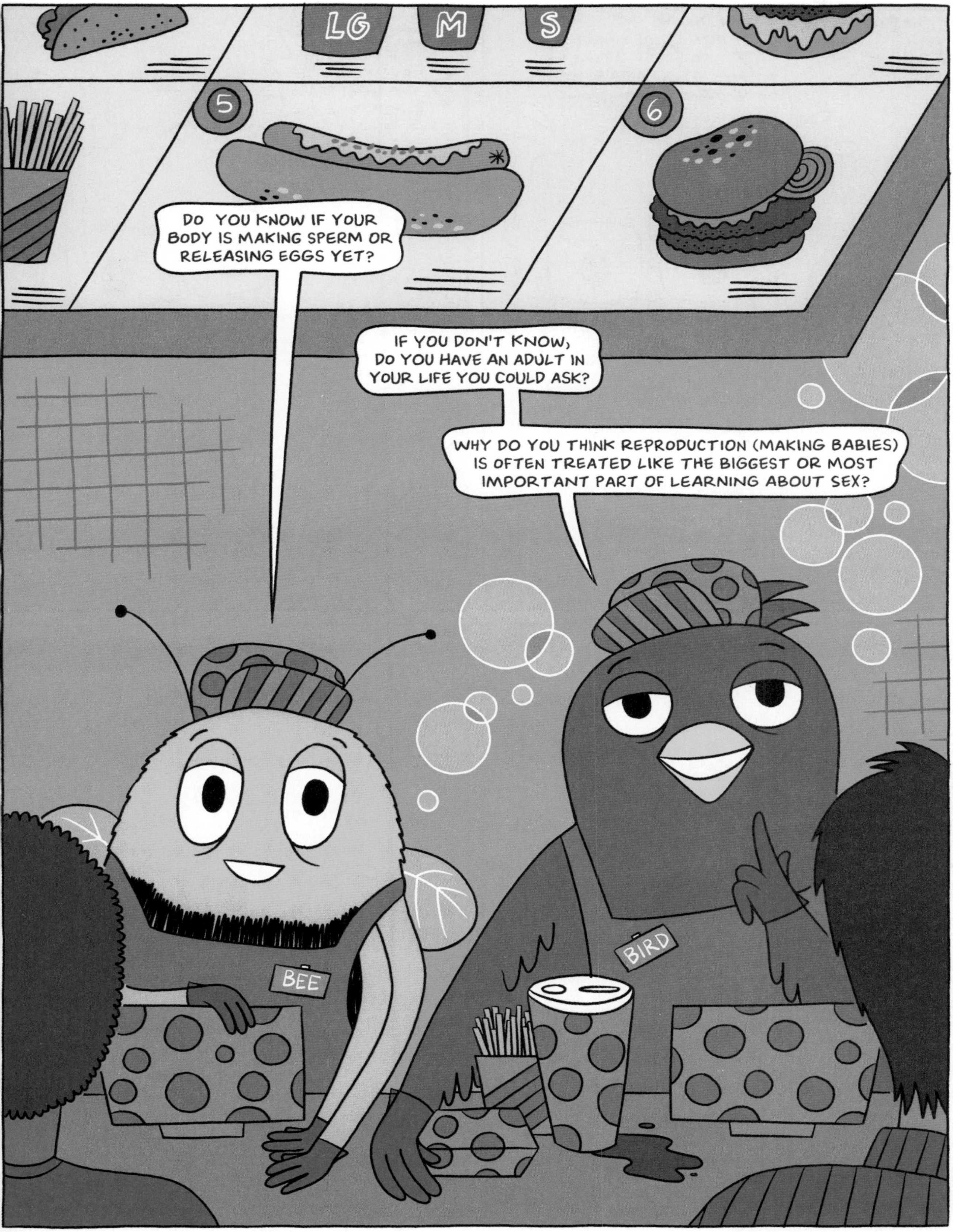
LG
M
S
5
6
DO YOU KNOW IF YOUR BODY IS MAKING SPERM OR RELEASING EGGS YET?
IF YOU DON'T KNOW, DO YOU HAVE AN ADULT IN YOUR LIFE YOU COULD ASK?
WHY DO YOU THINK REPRODUCTION (MAKING BABIES) IS OFTEN TREATED LIKE THE BIGGEST OR MOST IMPORTANT PART OF LEARNING ABOUT SEX?
BEE
BIRD

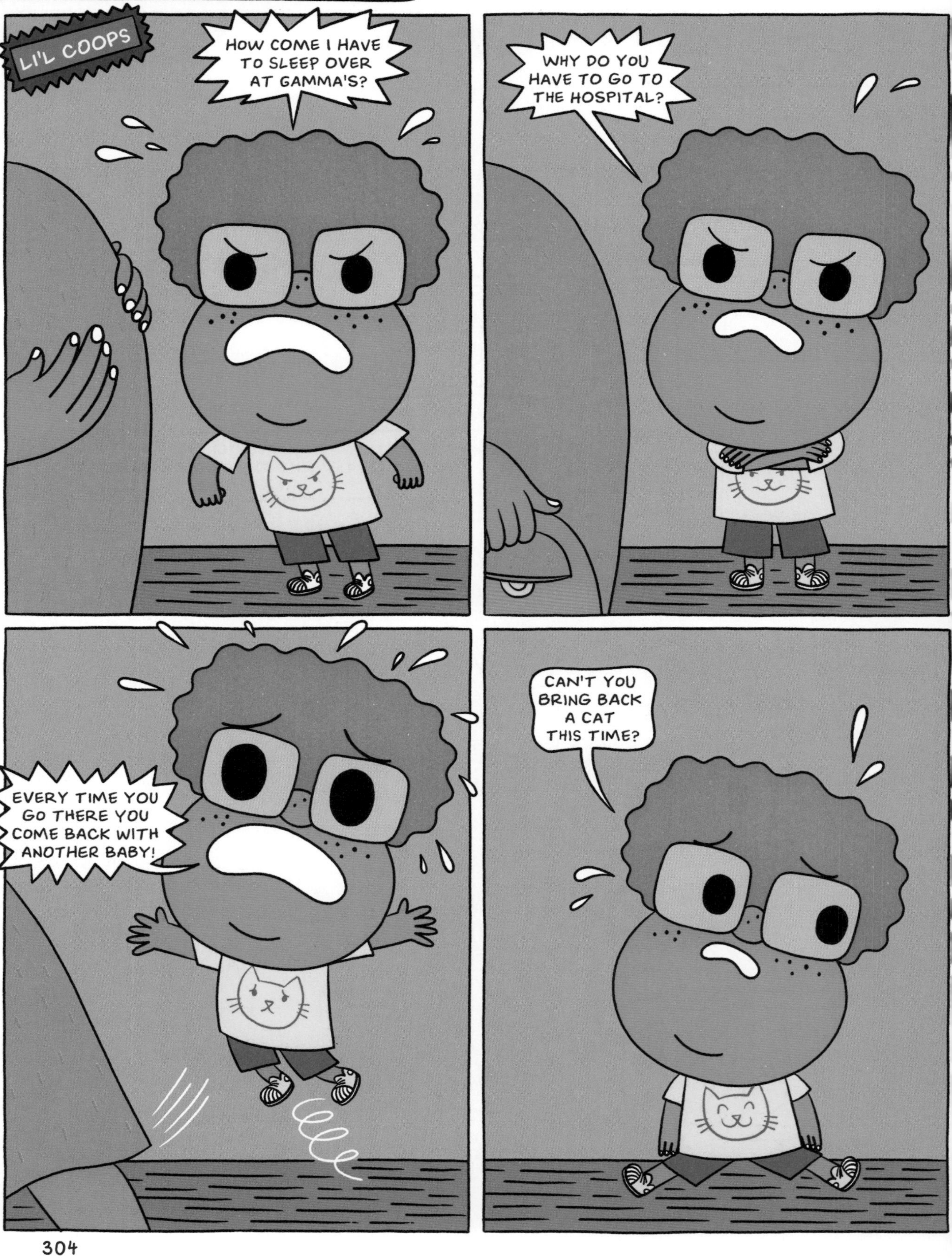
LI'L COOPS
HOW COME I HAVE TO SLEEP OVER AT GAMMA'S?
WHY DO YOU HAVE TO GO TO THE HOSPITAL?
EVERY TIME YOU GO THERE YOU COME BACK WITH ANOTHER BABY!
CAN'T YOU BRING BACK A CAT THIS TIME?

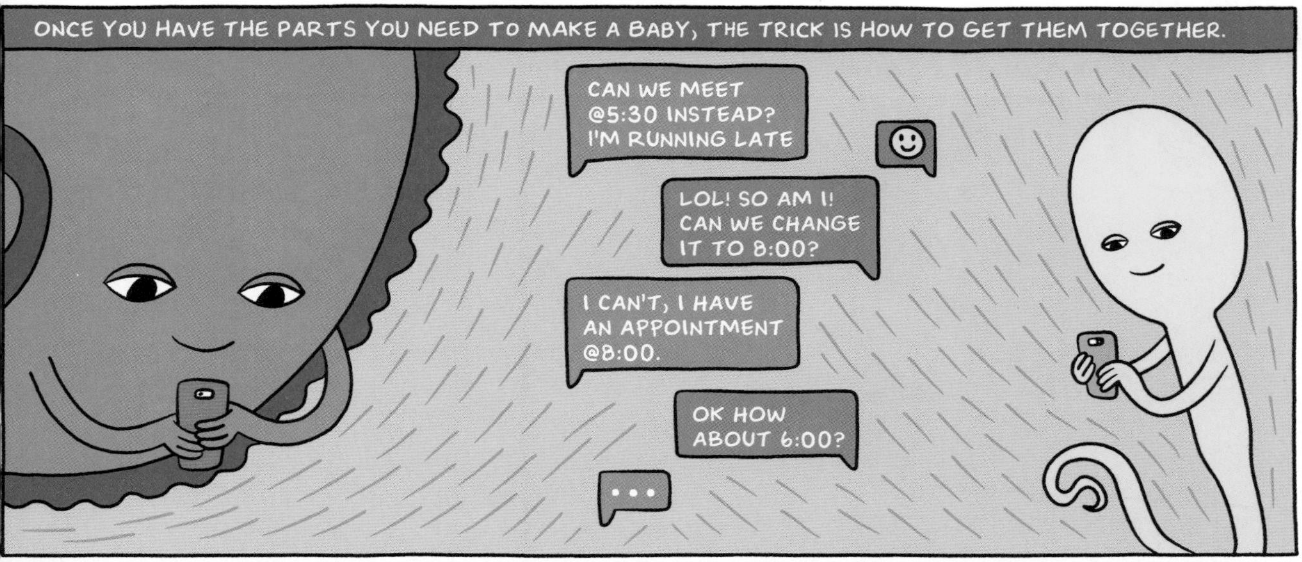
ONCE YOU HAVE THE PARTS YOU NEED TO MAKE A BABY, THE TRICK IS HOW TO GET THEM TOGETHER.
CAN WE MEET @5:30 INSTEAD? I'M RUNNING LATE
LOL! SO AM I! CAN WE CHANGE IT TO 8:00?
I CAN'T, I HAVE AN APPOINTMENT @8:00.
OK HOW ABOUT 6:00?

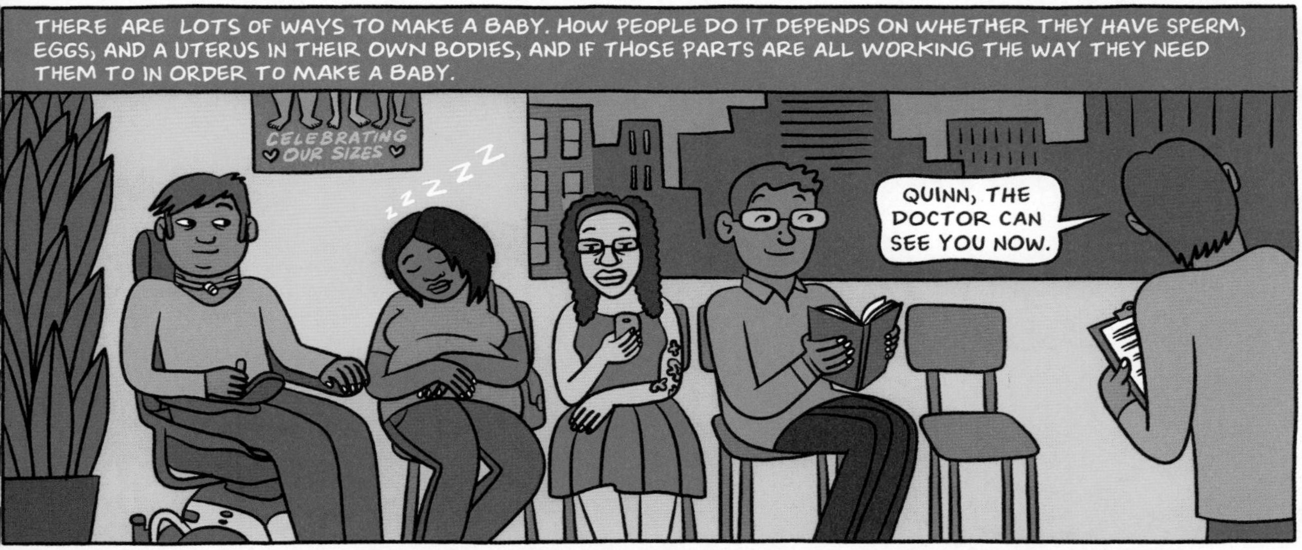
THERE ARE LOTS OF WAYS TO MAKE A BABY. HOW PEOPLE DO IT DEPENDS ON WHETHER THEY HAVE SPERM, EGGS, AND A UTERUS IN THEIR OWN BODIES, AND IF THOSE PARTS ARE ALL WORKING THE WAY THEY NEED THEM TO IN ORDER TO MAKE A BABY.
CELEBRATING OUR SIZES
ZZZZZ
QUINN, THE DOCTOR CAN SEE YOU NOW.

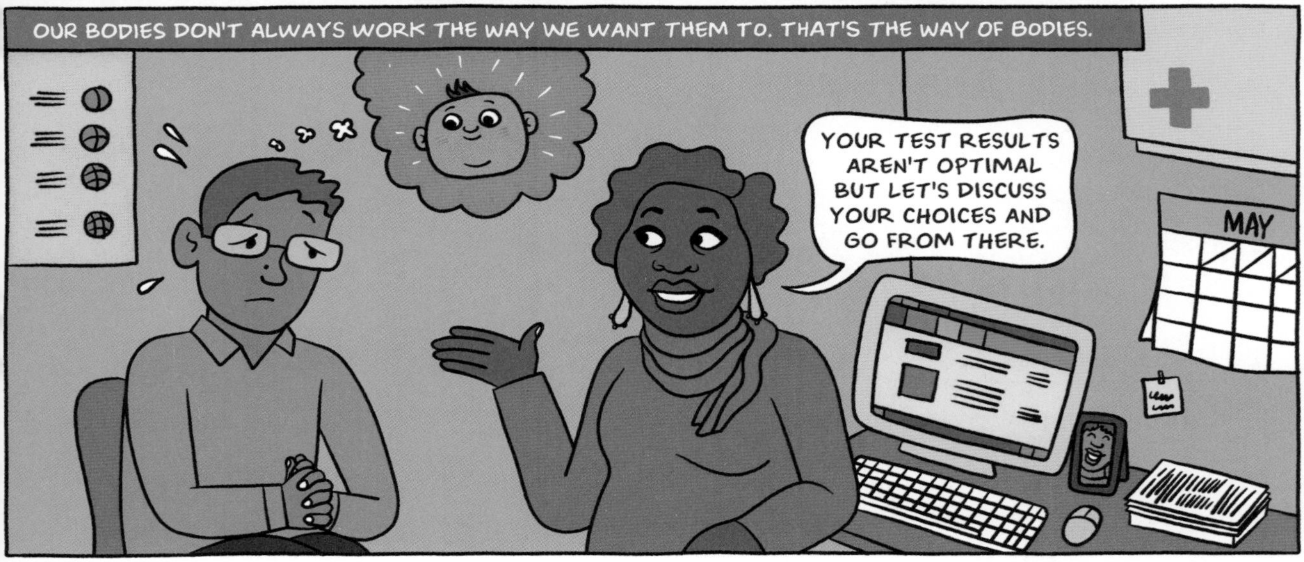
OUR BODIES DON'T ALWAYS WORK THE WAY WE WANT THEM TO. THAT'S THE WAY OF BODIES.
YOUR TEST RESULTS AREN'T OPTIMAL BUT LET'S DISCUSS YOUR CHOICES AND GO FROM THERE.
MAY

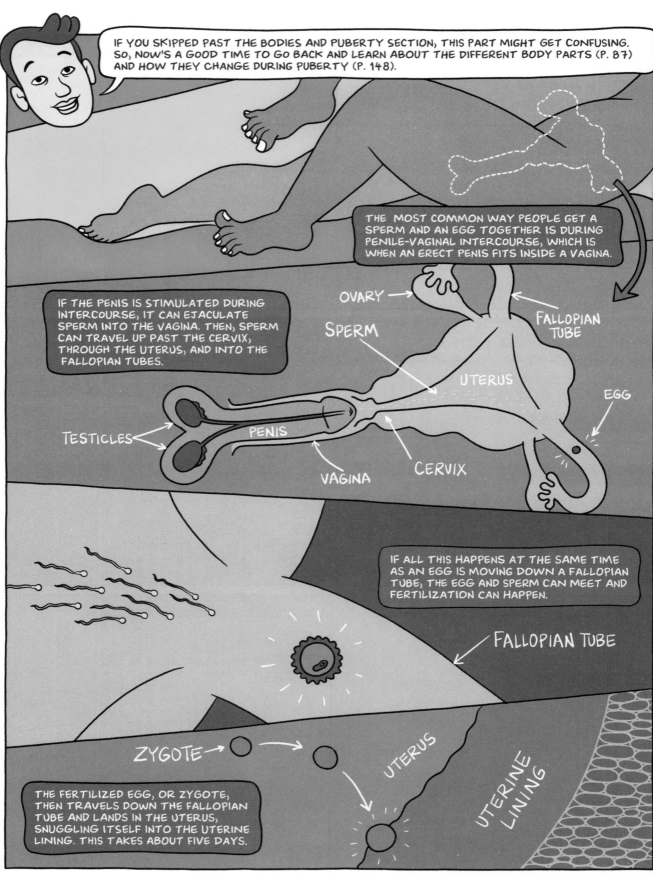

IF YOU SKIPPED PAST THE BODIES AND PUBERTY SECTION, THIS PART MIGHT GET CONFUSING. SO, NOW'S A GOOD TIME TO GO BACK AND LEARN ABOUT THE DIFFERENT BODY PARTS (P. 87) AND HOW THEY CHANGE DURING PUBERTY (P. 148).

THE MOST COMMON WAY PEOPLE GET A SPERM AND AN EGG TOGETHER IS DURING PENILE-VAGINAL INTERCOURSE, WHICH IS WHEN AN ERECT PENIS FITS INSIDE A VAGINA.

IF THE PENIS IS STIMULATED DURING INTERCOURSE, IT CAN EJACULATE SPERM INTO THE VAGINA. THEN, SPERM CAN TRAVEL UP PAST THE CERVIX, THROUGH THE UTERUS, AND INTO THE FALLOPIAN TUBES.

OVARY

FALLOPIAN TUBE

SPERM

UTERUS

EGG

TESTICLES

PENIS

VAGINA

CERVIX

IF ALL THIS HAPPENS AT THE SAME TIME AS AN EGG IS MOVING DOWN A FALLOPIAN TUBE, THE EGG AND SPERM CAN MEET AND FERTILIZATION CAN HAPPEN.

FALLOPIAN TUBE

ZYGOTE

UTERUS

UTERINE LINING

THE FERTILIZED EGG, OR ZYGOTE, THEN TRAVELS DOWN THE FALLOPIAN TUBE AND LANDS IN THE UTERUS, SNUGGLING ITSELF INTO THE UTERINE LINING. THIS TAKES ABOUT FIVE DAYS.

THERE ARE MANY OTHER WAYS PEOPLE GET SPERM AND EGG TO MEET. HERE ARE A FEW:

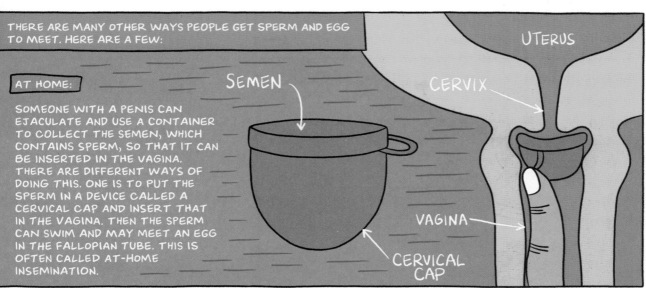

AT HOME:

SOMEONE WITH A PENIS CAN EJACULATE AND USE A CONTAINER TO COLLECT THE SEMEN, WHICH CONTAINS SPERM, SO THAT IT CAN BE INSERTED IN THE VAGINA. THERE ARE DIFFERENT WAYS OF DOING THIS. ONE IS TO PUT THE SPERM IN A DEVICE CALLED A CERVICAL CAP AND INSERT THAT IN THE VAGINA. THEN THE SPERM CAN SWIM AND MAY MEET AN EGG IN THE FALLOPIAN TUBE. THIS IS OFTEN CALLED AT-HOME INSEMINATION.

SEMEN

UTERUS

CERVIX

VAGINA

CERVICAL CAP

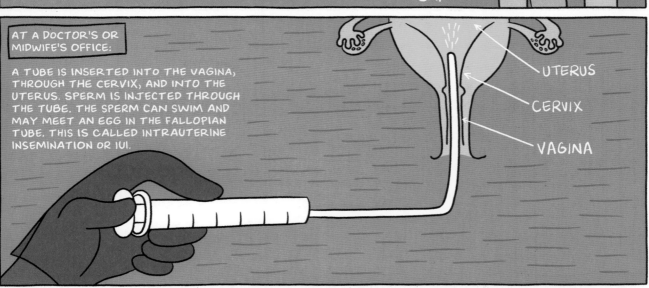

AT A DOCTOR'S OR MIDWIFE'S OFFICE:

A TUBE IS INSERTED INTO THE VAGINA, THROUGH THE CERVIX, AND INTO THE UTERUS. SPERM IS INJECTED THROUGH THE TUBE. THE SPERM CAN SWIM AND MAY MEET AN EGG IN THE FALLOPIAN TUBE. THIS IS CALLED INTRAUTERINE INSEMINATION OR IUI.

UTERUS

CERVIX

VAGINA

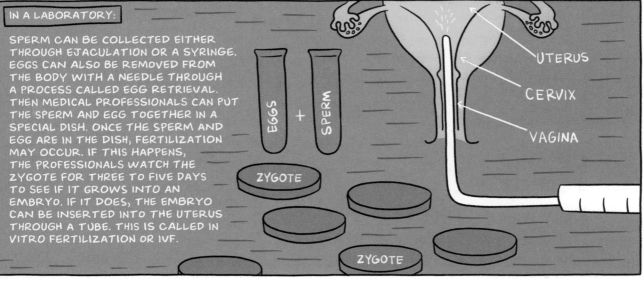

IN A LABORATORY:

SPERM CAN BE COLLECTED EITHER THROUGH EJACULATION OR A SYRINGE. EGGS CAN ALSO BE REMOVED FROM THE BODY WITH A NEEDLE THROUGH A PROCESS CALLED EGG RETRIEVAL. THEN MEDICAL PROFESSIONALS CAN PUT THE SPERM AND EGG TOGETHER IN A SPECIAL DISH. ONCE THE SPERM AND EGG ARE IN THE DISH, FERTILIZATION MAY OCCUR. IF THIS HAPPENS, THE PROFESSIONALS WATCH THE ZYGOTE FOR THREE TO FIVE DAYS TO SEE IF IT GROWS INTO AN EMBRYO. IF IT DOES, THE EMBRYO CAN BE INSERTED INTO THE UTERUS THROUGH A TUBE. THIS IS CALLED IN VITRO FERTILIZATION OR IVF.

EGGS + SPERM

ZYGOTE

UTERUS

CERVIX

VAGINA

ZYGOTE

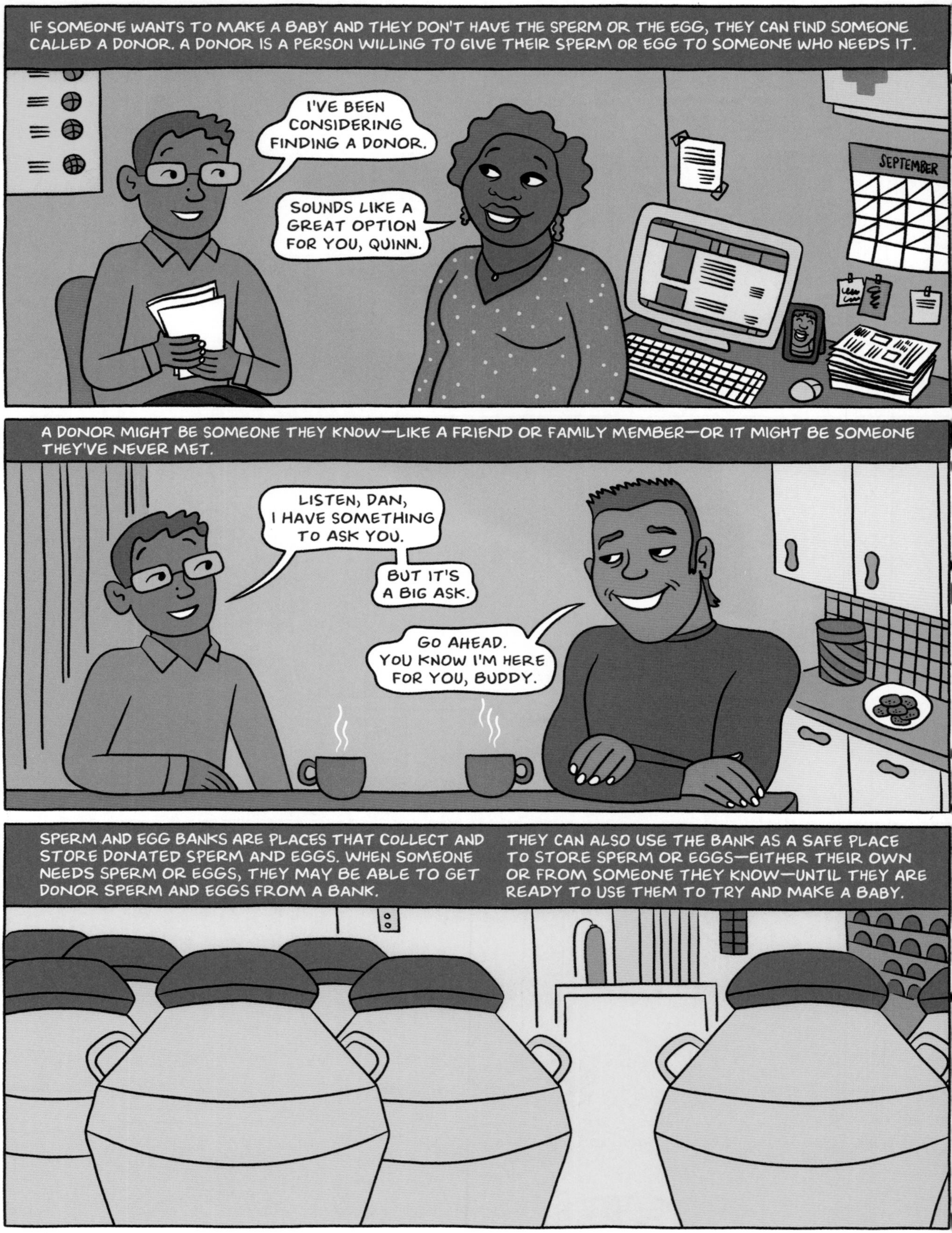
IF SOMEONE WANTS TO MAKE A BABY AND THEY DON'T HAVE THE SPERM OR THE EGG, THEY CAN FIND SOMEONE CALLED A DONOR. A DONOR IS A PERSON WILLING TO GIVE THEIR SPERM OR EGG TO SOMEONE WHO NEEDS IT.
I'VE BEEN CONSIDERING FINDING A DONOR.
SOUNDS LIKE A GREAT OPTION FOR YOU, QUINN.
SEPTEMBER
A DONOR MIGHT BE SOMEONE THEY KNOW—LIKE A FRIEND OR FAMILY MEMBER—OR IT MIGHT BE SOMEONE THEY'VE NEVER MET.
LISTEN, DAN, I HAVE SOMETHING TO ASK YOU.
BUT IT'S A BIG ASK.
GO AHEAD. YOU KNOW I'M HERE FOR YOU, BUDDY.
SPERM AND EGG BANKS ARE PLACES THAT COLLECT AND STORE DONATED SPERM AND EGGS. WHEN SOMEONE NEEDS SPERM OR EGGS, THEY MAY BE ABLE TO GET DONOR SPERM AND EGGS FROM A BANK.
THEY CAN ALSO USE THE BANK AS A SAFE PLACE TO STORE SPERM OR EGGS—EITHER THEIR OWN OR FROM SOMEONE THEY KNOW—UNTIL THEY ARE READY TO USE THEM TO TRY AND MAKE A BABY.

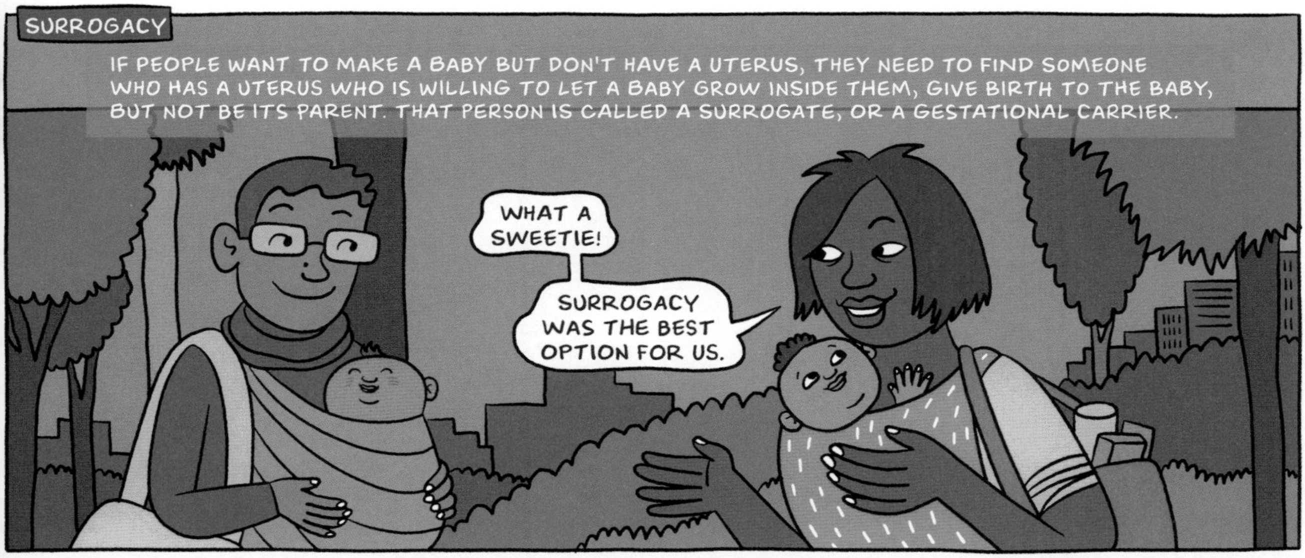
SURROGACY
IF PEOPLE WANT TO MAKE A BABY BUT DON'T HAVE A UTERUS, THEY NEED TO FIND SOMEONE WHO HAS A UTERUS WHO IS WILLING TO LET A BABY GROW INSIDE THEM, GIVE BIRTH TO THE BABY, BUT NOT BE ITS PARENT. THAT PERSON IS CALLED A SURROGATE, OR A GESTATIONAL CARRIER.
WHAT A SWEETIE!
SURROGACY WAS THE BEST OPTION FOR US.

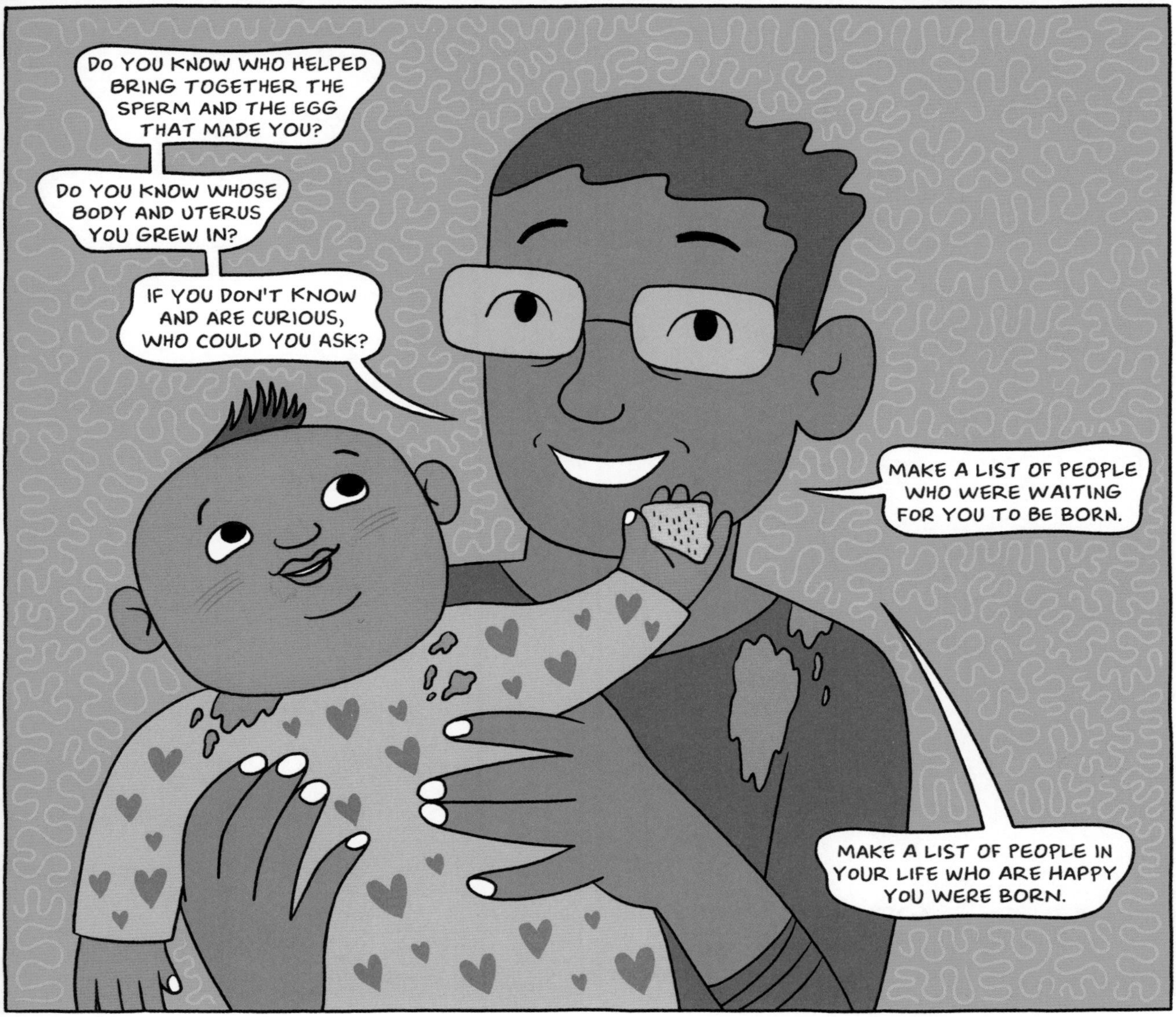
DO YOU KNOW WHO HELPED BRING TOGETHER THE SPERM AND THE EGG THAT MADE YOU?
DO YOU KNOW WHOSE BODY AND UTERUS YOU GREW IN?
IF YOU DON'T KNOW AND ARE CURIOUS, WHO COULD YOU ASK?
MAKE A LIST OF PEOPLE WHO WERE WAITING FOR YOU TO BE BORN.
MAKE A LIST OF PEOPLE IN YOUR LIFE WHO ARE HAPPY YOU WERE BORN.

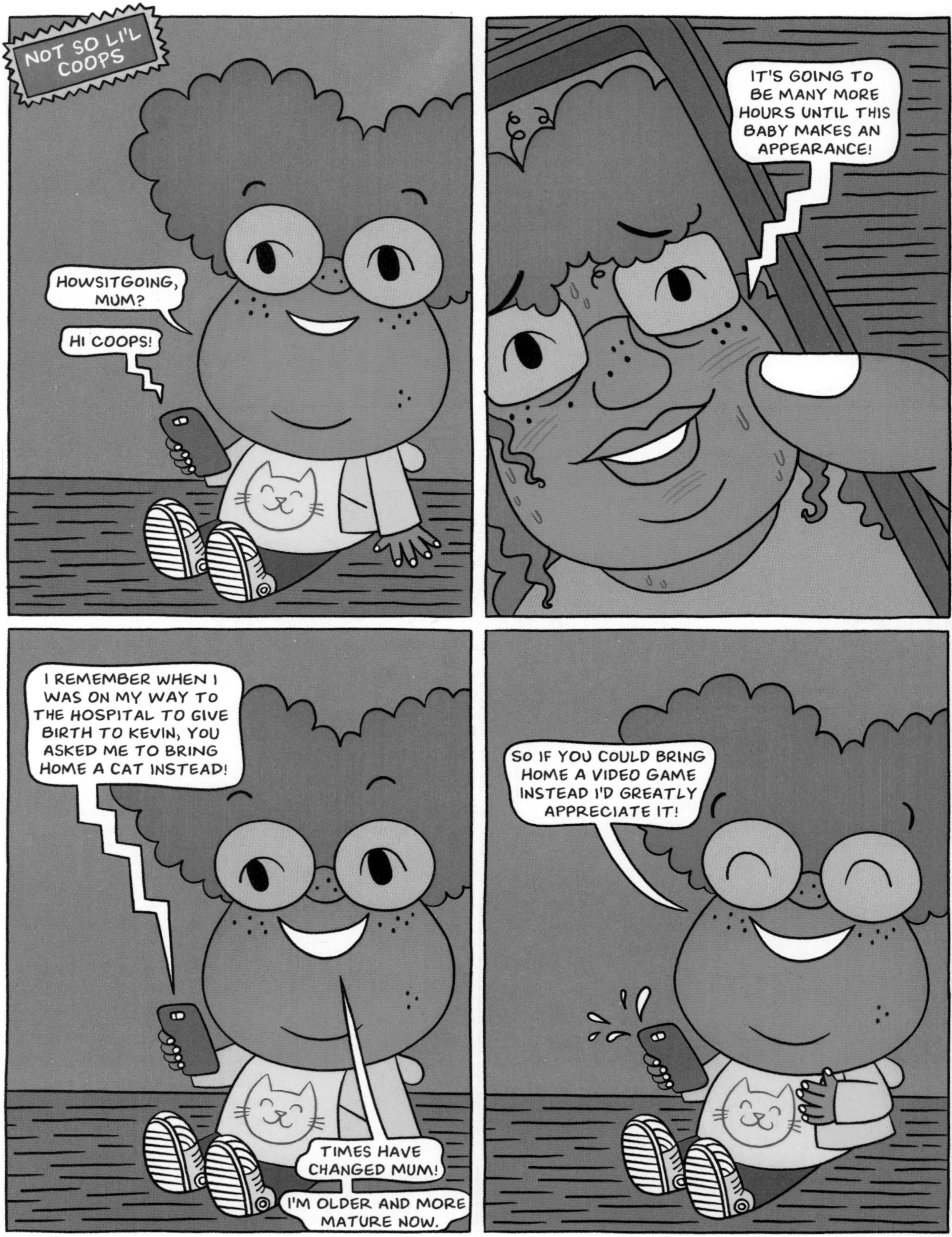
NOT SO LI'L COOPS
HOWSITGOING, MUM?
HI COOPS!
IT'S GOING TO BE MANY MORE HOURS UNTIL THIS BABY MAKES AN APPEARANCE!
I REMEMBER WHEN I WAS ON MY WAY TO THE HOSPITAL TO GIVE BIRTH TO KEVIN, YOU ASKED ME TO BRING HOME A CAT INSTEAD!
TIMES HAVE CHANGED MUM!
I'M OLDER AND MORE MATURE NOW.
SO IF YOU COULD BRING HOME A VIDEO GAME INSTEAD I'D GREATLY APPRECIATE IT!

MOST OF THE TIME, IF IT'S GOING TO WORK, ONE SPERM MEETS ONE EGG, THEY FERTILIZE, IMPLANT IN THE UTERUS, AND GROW INTO ONE BABY.

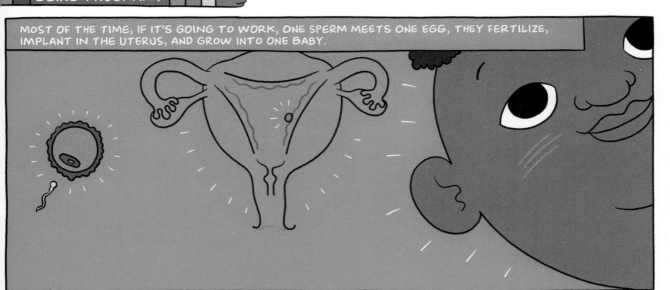

BUT SOMETIMES MORE THAN ONE BABY IS MADE. SOMETIMES YOU GET TWO (TWINS), OR THREE (TRIPLETS), OR MORE.

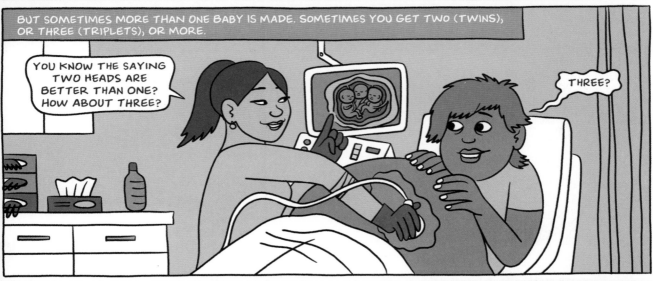

YOU KNOW THE SAYING TWO HEADS ARE BETTER THAN ONE? HOW ABOUT THREE?

THREE?

THESE ARE CALLED MULTIPLES. SOME MULTIPLES ARE IDENTICAL AND SOME ARE NOT. IT DEPENDS ON WHAT HAPPENS WHEN THE SPERM AND EGG FUSE.

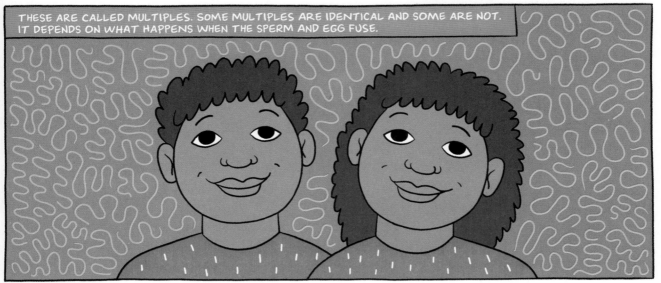

SOMETIMES, INSTEAD OF THE EGG AND SPERM FUSING INTO ONE ZYGOTE AND BEGINNING TO GROW, THE FIRST THING THAT HAPPENS IS THAT THEY DIVIDE INTO TWO (OR MORE) IDENTICAL ZYGOTES WITH IDENTICAL DNA.

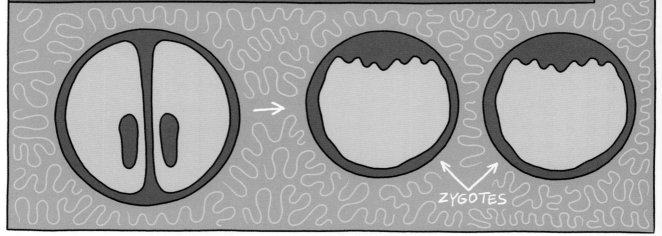

ZYGOTES

THE MULTIPLE ZYGOTES IMPLANT IN THE UTERUS AND DEVELOP INTO FETUSES THAT HAVE THE EXACT SAME DNA AND CAN BE BORN AS MORE OR LESS IDENTICAL BABIES. BUT EVEN IDENTICAL SIBLINGS AREN'T EXACTLY THE SAME.

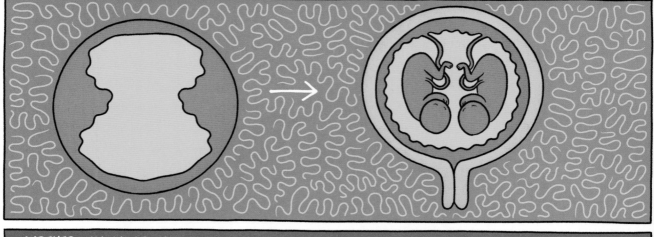

ANOTHER WAY MULTIPLES CAN OCCUR IS WHEN MORE THAN ONE EGG IS RELEASED FROM THE OVARIES. EACH EGG MEETS A SPERM AND MULTIPLE ZYGOTES ARE CREATED. IN THIS CASE, EACH ZYGOTE HAS ITS OWN UNIQUE MIX OF STORIES AND DNA, AND IF THEY GROW, THESE MULTIPLES WON'T BE IDENTICAL. THESE MULTIPLES ARE CALLED FRATERNAL INSTEAD OF IDENTICAL.

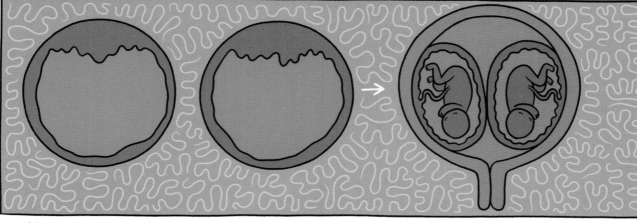

A NEW PART-TIME ORGAN

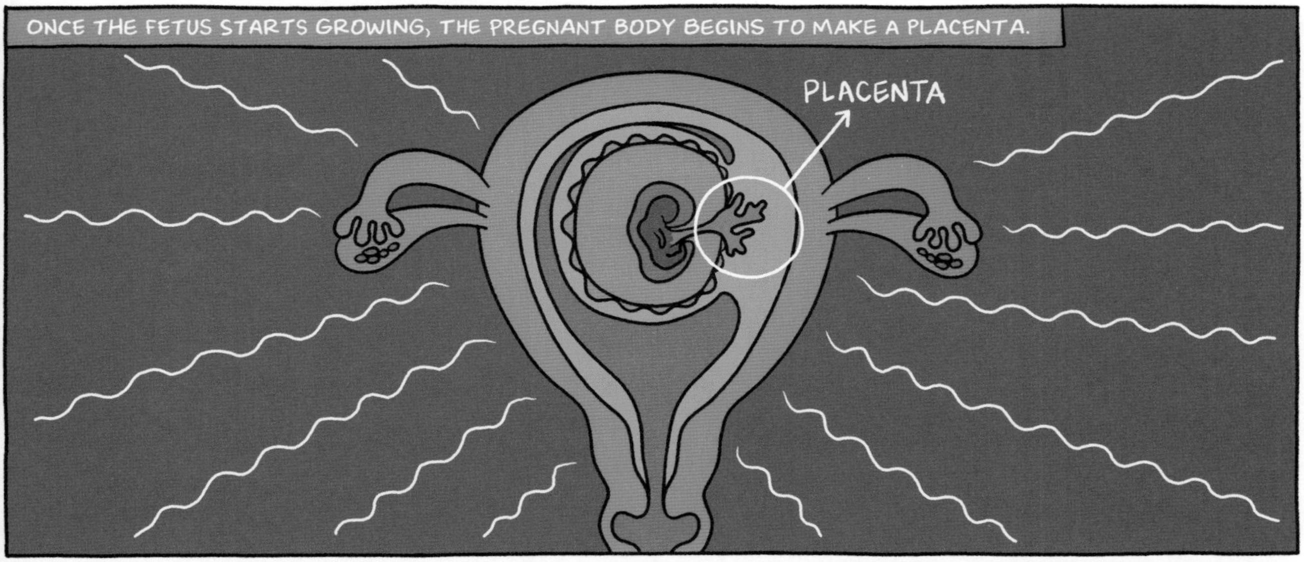
ONCE THE FETUS STARTS GROWING, THE PREGNANT BODY BEGINS TO MAKE A PLACENTA.
PLACENTA

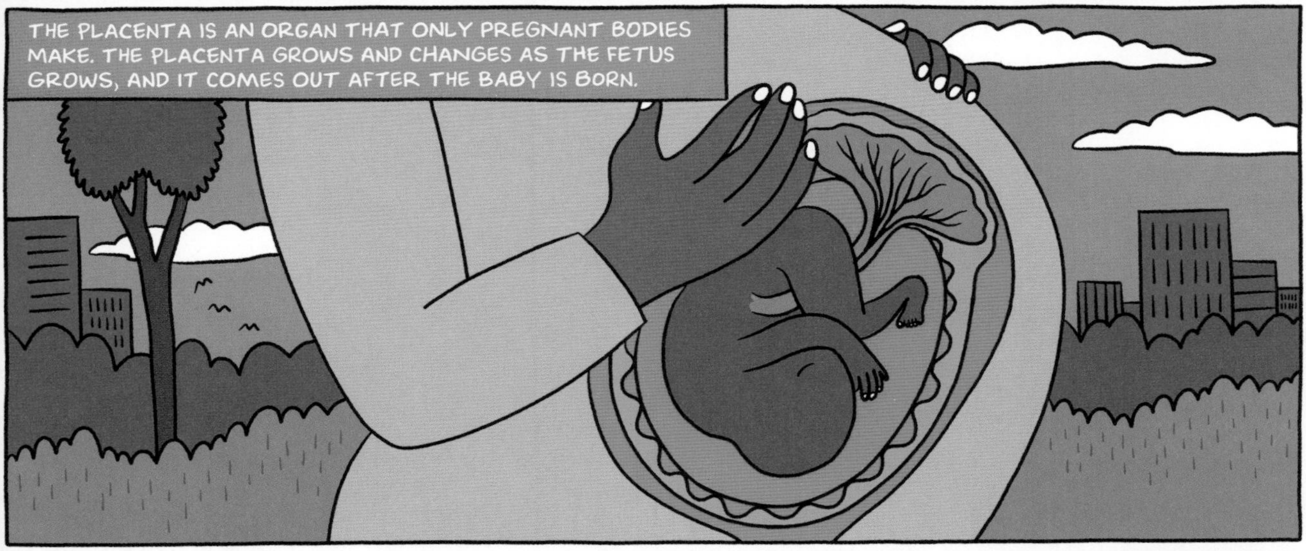
THE PLACENTA IS AN ORGAN THAT ONLY PREGNANT BODIES MAKE. THE PLACENTA GROWS AND CHANGES AS THE FETUS GROWS, AND IT COMES OUT AFTER THE BABY IS BORN.

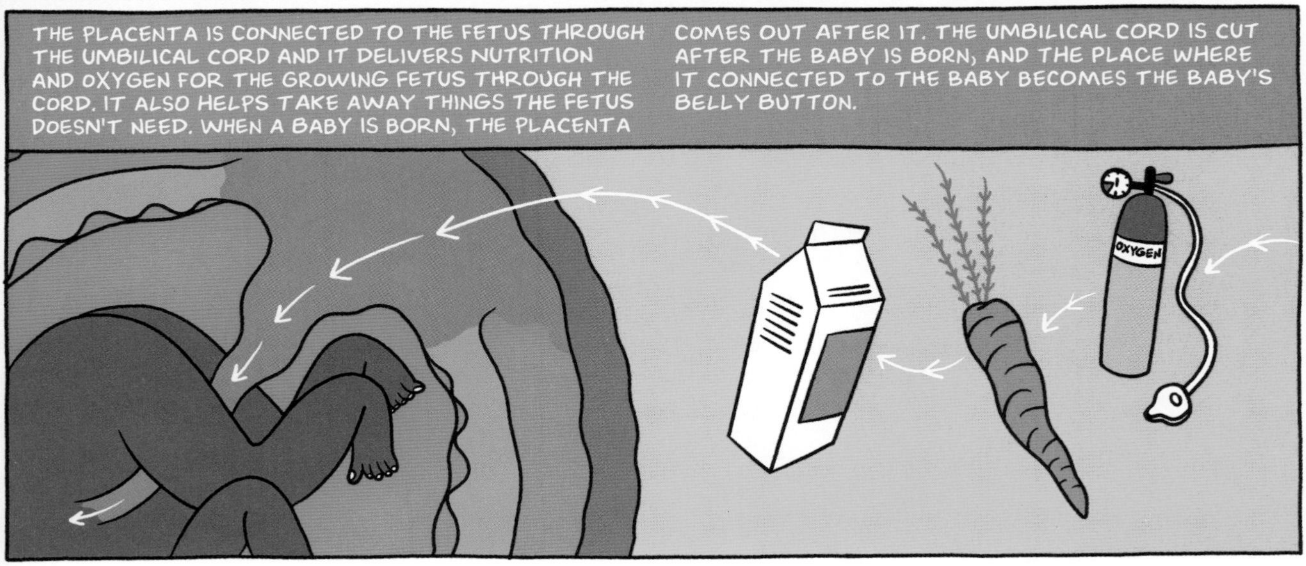
THE PLACENTA IS CONNECTED TO THE FETUS THROUGH THE UMBILICAL CORD AND IT DELIVERS NUTRITION AND OXYGEN FOR THE GROWING FETUS THROUGH THE CORD. IT ALSO HELPS TAKE AWAY THINGS THE FETUS DOESN'T NEED. WHEN A BABY IS BORN, THE PLACENTA COMES OUT AFTER IT. THE UMBILICAL CORD IS CUT AFTER THE BABY IS BORN, AND THE PLACE WHERE IT CONNECTED TO THE BABY BECOMES THE BABY'S BELLY BUTTON.
OXYGEN

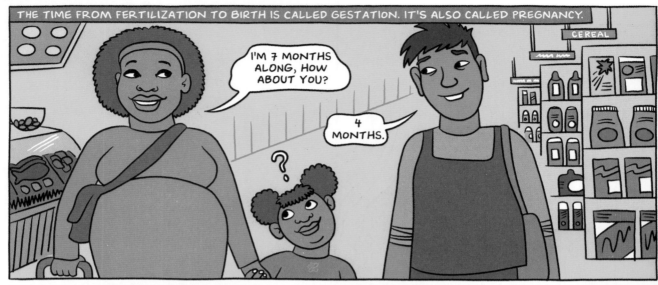

THE TIME FROM FERTILIZATION TO BIRTH IS CALLED GESTATION. IT'S ALSO CALLED PREGNANCY.

I'M 7 MONTHS ALONG, HOW ABOUT YOU?

4 MONTHS.

CEREAL

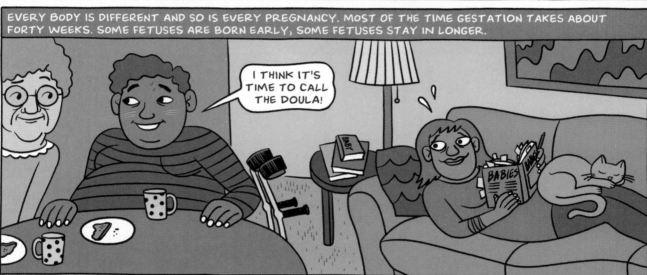

EVERY BODY IS DIFFERENT AND SO IS EVERY PREGNANCY. MOST OF THE TIME GESTATION TAKES ABOUT FORTY WEEKS. SOME FETUSES ARE BORN EARLY, SOME FETUSES STAY IN LONGER.

I THINK IT'S TIME TO CALL THE DOULA!

BABY

BABIES

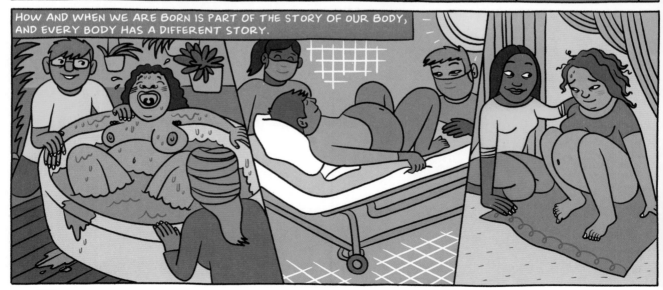

HOW AND WHEN WE ARE BORN IS PART OF THE STORY OF OUR BODY, AND EVERY BODY HAS A DIFFERENT STORY.

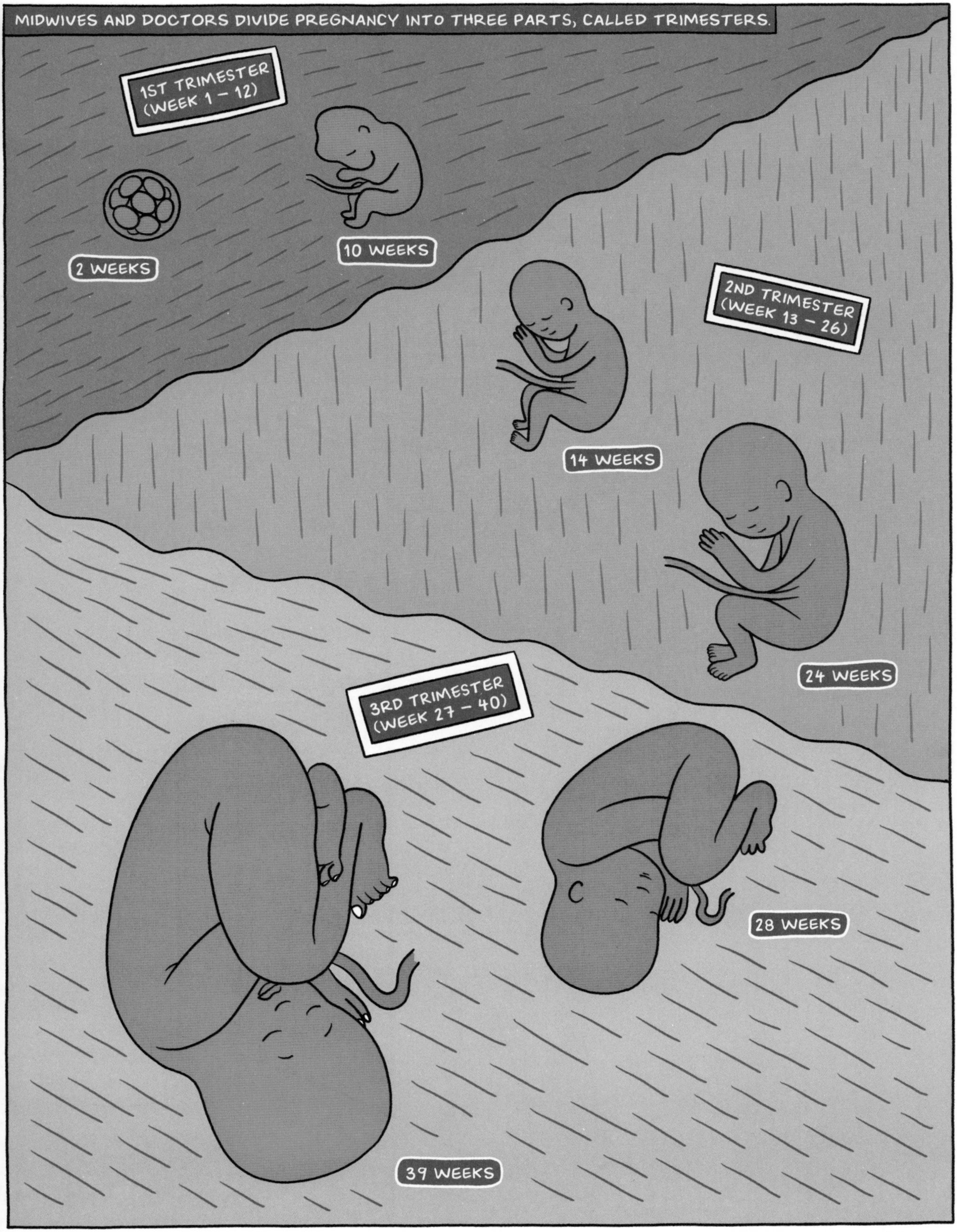
MIDWIVES AND DOCTORS DIVIDE PREGNANCY INTO THREE PARTS, CALLED TRIMESTERS.
1ST TRIMESTER (WEEK 1 – 12)
2 WEEKS
10 WEEKS
2ND TRIMESTER (WEEK 13 – 26)
14 WEEKS
24 WEEKS
3RD TRIMESTER (WEEK 27 – 40)
28 WEEKS
39 WEEKS

MAKING A BABY DOESN'T HAPPEN EVERY TIME A SPERM AND EGG HAVE A CHANCE TO MEET.

SOMETIMES THEY MEET, AND FERTILIZE. THE EMBRYO MAY GROW FOR A WHILE, BUT THEN STOPS GROWING. USUALLY, THIS IS BECAUSE THE CONDITIONS AREN'T RIGHT.

WHEN AN EMBRYO STOPS GROWING, IT LEAVES THE BODY THROUGH THE VAGINA. THIS IS CALLED HAVING A MISCARRIAGE.

LIKE WITH SEX, PEOPLE DON'T TALK ABOUT MISCARRIAGES EVEN THOUGH THEY HAPPEN ALL THE TIME. SOMETIMES A MISCARRIAGE IS PHYSICALLY PAINFUL. SOMETIMES IT ISN'T.

BUT IT USUALLY COMES WITH A LOT OF FEELINGS. PEOPLE MIGHT FEEL SAD, ANGRY, CONFUSED, ASHAMED, GUILTY, OR MORE. PEOPLE MIGHT THINK IT'S THEIR FAULT. BUT IT'S NOT.

THEY MIGHT WANT TO TALK ABOUT IT OR THEY MIGHT NOT.

MISCARRIAGES ARE ALSO CALLED SPONTANEOUS ABORTION BECAUSE THE GROWING STOPS BEFORE IT'S DONE. THE WORD ABORTION MEANS TO END SOMETHING BEFORE IT'S FINISHED.

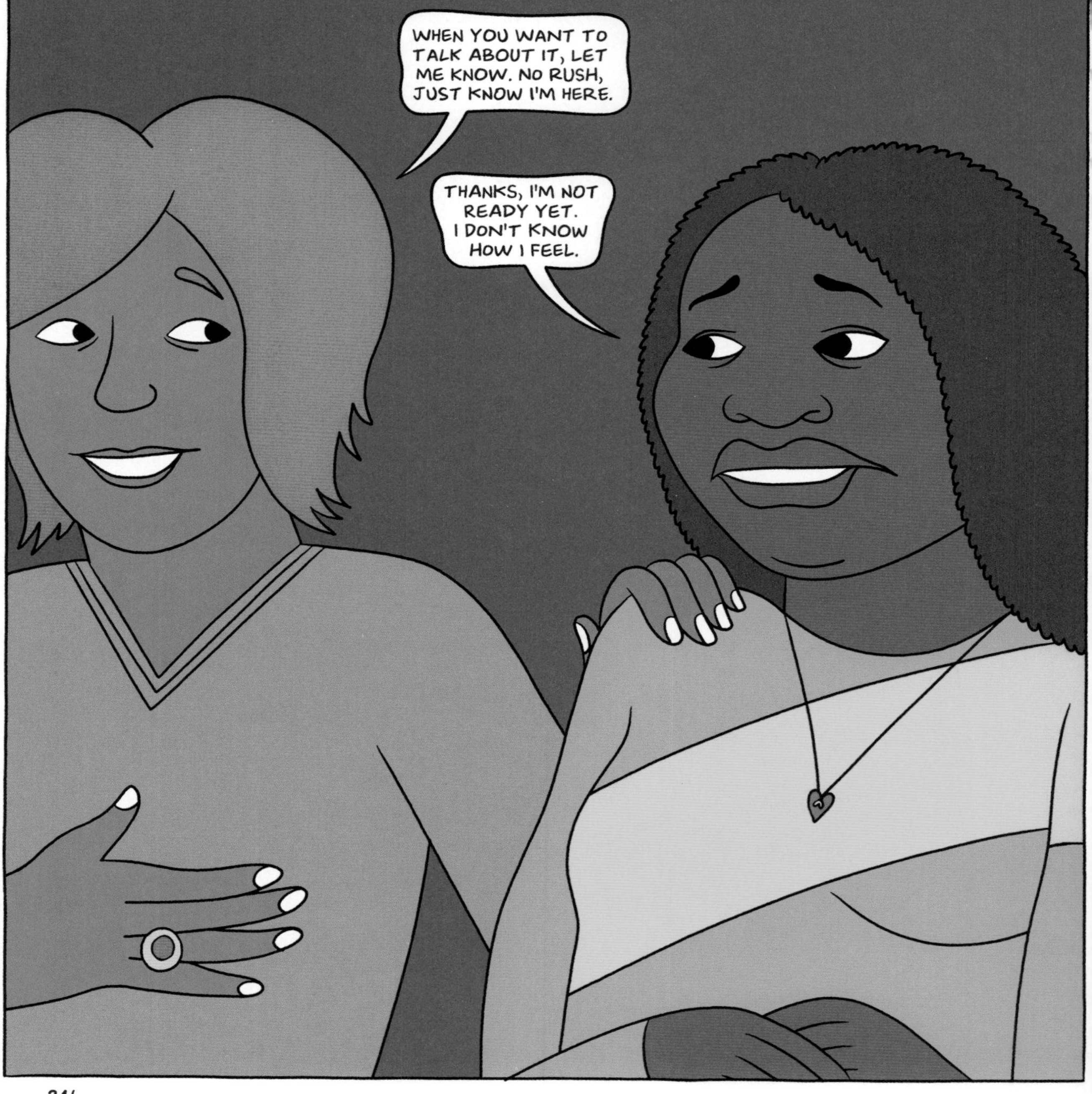
WHEN YOU WANT TO TALK ABOUT IT, LET ME KNOW. NO RUSH, JUST KNOW I'M HERE.
THANKS, I'M NOT READY YET. I DON'T KNOW HOW I FEEL.

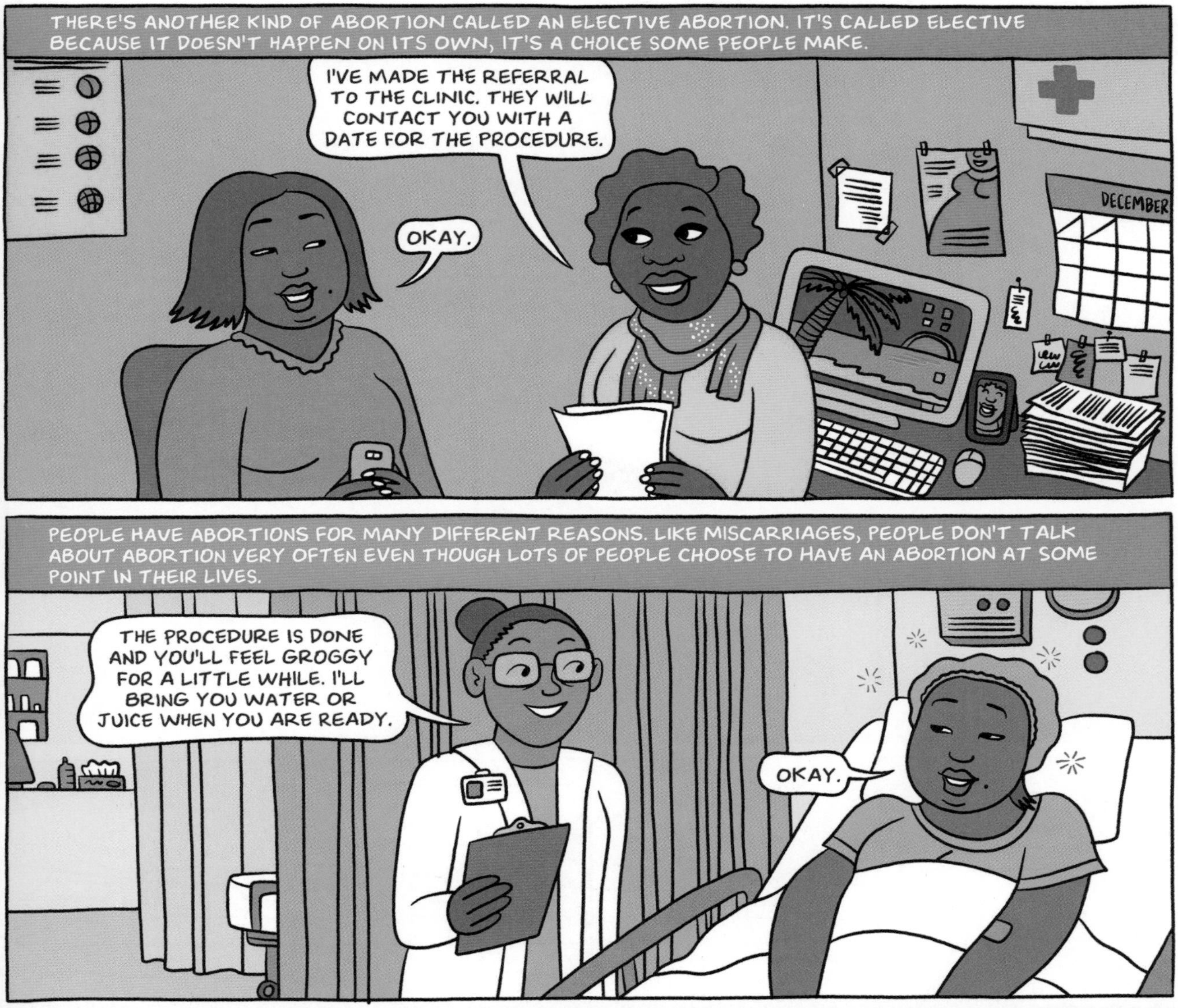
THERE'S ANOTHER KIND OF ABORTION CALLED AN ELECTIVE ABORTION. IT'S CALLED ELECTIVE BECAUSE IT DOESN'T HAPPEN ON ITS OWN, IT'S A CHOICE SOME PEOPLE MAKE.
I'VE MADE THE REFERRAL TO THE CLINIC. THEY WILL CONTACT YOU WITH A DATE FOR THE PROCEDURE.
OKAY.
DECEMBER
PEOPLE HAVE ABORTIONS FOR MANY DIFFERENT REASONS. LIKE MISCARRIAGES, PEOPLE DON'T TALK ABOUT ABORTION VERY OFTEN EVEN THOUGH LOTS OF PEOPLE CHOOSE TO HAVE AN ABORTION AT SOME POINT IN THEIR LIVES.
THE PROCEDURE IS DONE AND YOU'LL FEEL GROGGY FOR A LITTLE WHILE. I'LL BRING YOU WATER OR JUICE WHEN YOU ARE READY.
OKAY.
CHOOSING TO HAVE AN ABORTION MAY NOT BE AN EASY CHOICE, AND IT MIGHT NOT BE A CHOICE EVERYONE AGREES WITH, BUT THE CHOICE BELONGS TO THE PERSON WHO IS PREGNANT.
BODY AUTONOMY MEANS THAT WE MAKE DECISIONS FOR OUR OWN BODIES. NO ONE SHOULD GET TO TELL US WE MUST HAVE A BABY OR WE MUST NOT HAVE A BABY.
CLINIC
PRO CHOICE
PRO CHOICE
WE KNOW BETTER
NO ABORTION
NO ABORTION
CLINIC ESCORT

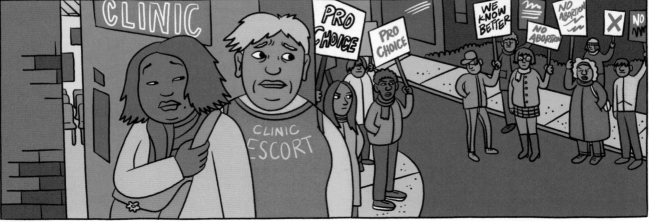

NERD ALERT MAKING A BABY AND BEING A PARENT

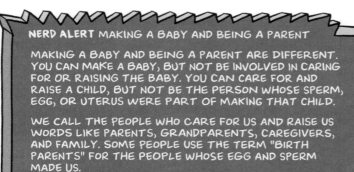

MAKING A BABY AND BEING A PARENT ARE DIFFERENT. YOU CAN MAKE A BABY, BUT NOT BE INVOLVED IN CARING FOR OR RAISING THE BABY. YOU CAN CARE FOR AND RAISE A CHILD, BUT NOT BE THE PERSON WHOSE SPERM, EGG, OR UTERUS WERE PART OF MAKING THAT CHILD.

WE CALL THE PEOPLE WHO CARE FOR US AND RAISE US WORDS LIKE PARENTS, GRANDPARENTS, CAREGIVERS, AND FAMILY. SOME PEOPLE USE THE TERM "BIRTH PARENTS" FOR THE PEOPLE WHOSE EGG AND SPERM MADE US.

LOTS OF PEOPLE ASSUME THAT IF YOU HAVE A PARENT, YOU WERE MADE FROM THEIR SPERM OR EGG, OR GREW IN THEIR UTERUS. BUT THAT ISN'T ALWAYS TRUE. WE MAY BE ADOPTED, OR FOSTERED, AND OUR BIRTH MAY HAVE BEEN HELPED BY DONORS OR SURROGATES. JUST LIKE EVERY BODY HAS ITS OWN STORY, SO DOES EVERY FAMILY. ONE KIND OF FAMILY IS NOT BETTER THAN ANOTHER.

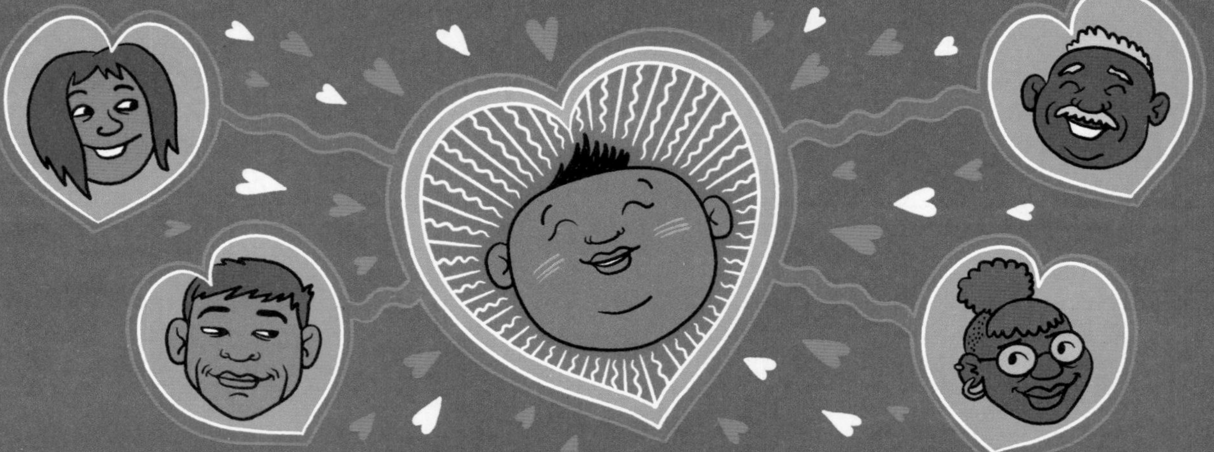

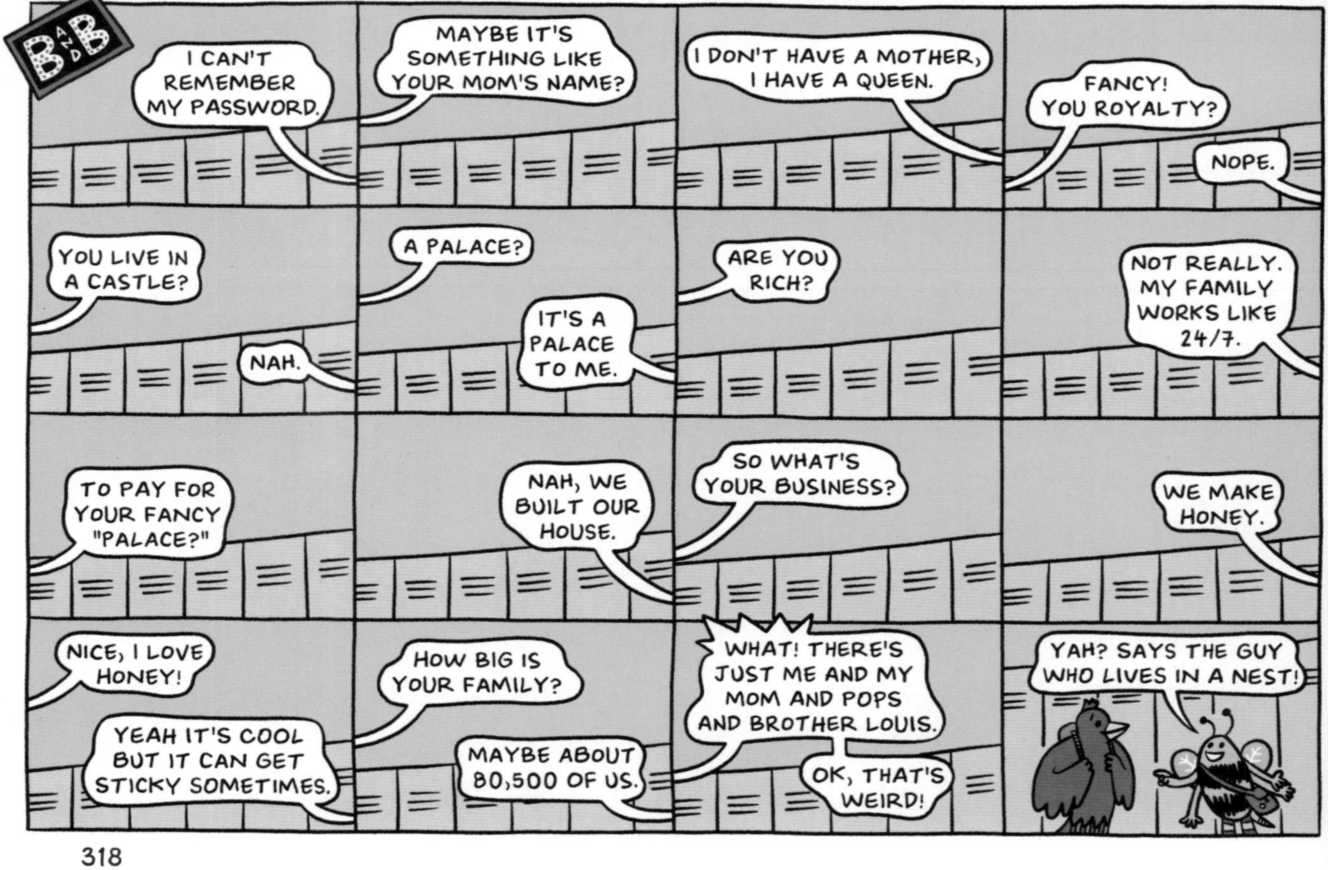
I CAN'T REMEMBER MY PASSWORD.
MAYBE IT'S SOMETHING LIKE YOUR MOM'S NAME?
I DON'T HAVE A MOTHER, I HAVE A QUEEN.
FANCY! YOU ROYALTY?
NOPE.
YOU LIVE IN A CASTLE?
NAH.
A PALACE?
IT'S A PALACE TO ME.
ARE YOU RICH?
NOT REALLY. MY FAMILY WORKS LIKE 24/7.
TO PAY FOR YOUR FANCY "PALACE?"
NAH, WE BUILT OUR HOUSE.
SO WHAT'S YOUR BUSINESS?
WE MAKE HONEY.
NICE, I LOVE HONEY!
YEAH IT'S COOL BUT IT CAN GET STICKY SOMETIMES.
HOW BIG IS YOUR FAMILY?
MAYBE ABOUT 80,500 OF US.
WHAT! THERE'S JUST ME AND MY MOM AND POPS AND BROTHER LOUIS.
OK, THAT'S WEIRD!
YAH? SAYS THE GUY WHO LIVES IN A NEST!

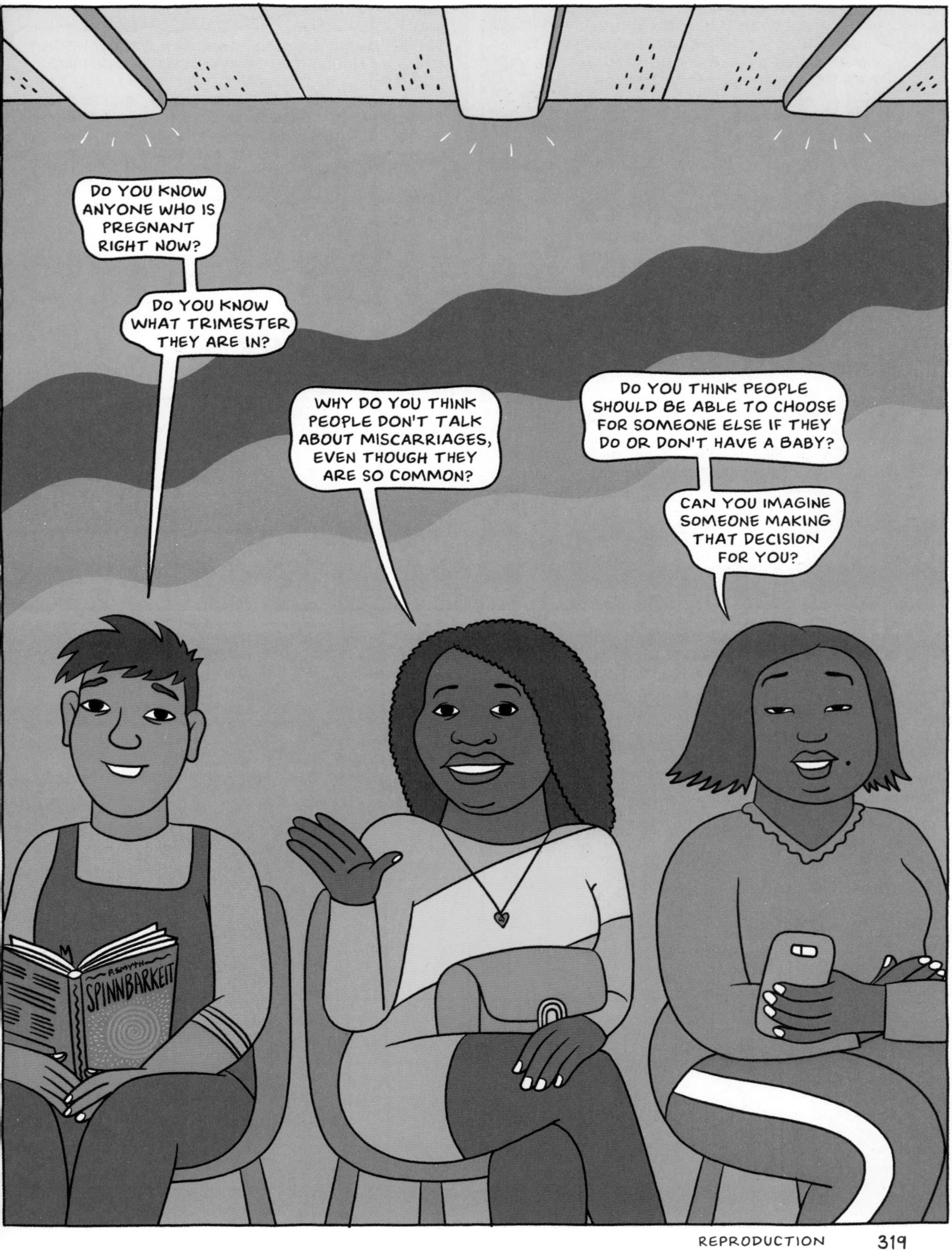
DO YOU KNOW ANYONE WHO IS PREGNANT RIGHT NOW?
DO YOU KNOW WHAT TRIMESTER THEY ARE IN?
WHY DO YOU THINK PEOPLE DON'T TALK ABOUT MISCARRIAGES, EVEN THOUGH THEY ARE SO COMMON?
DO YOU THINK PEOPLE SHOULD BE ABLE TO CHOOSE FOR SOMEONE ELSE IF THEY DO OR DON'T HAVE A BABY?
CAN YOU IMAGINE SOMEONE MAKING THAT DECISION FOR YOU?
P. SMYTH
SPINNBARKEIT

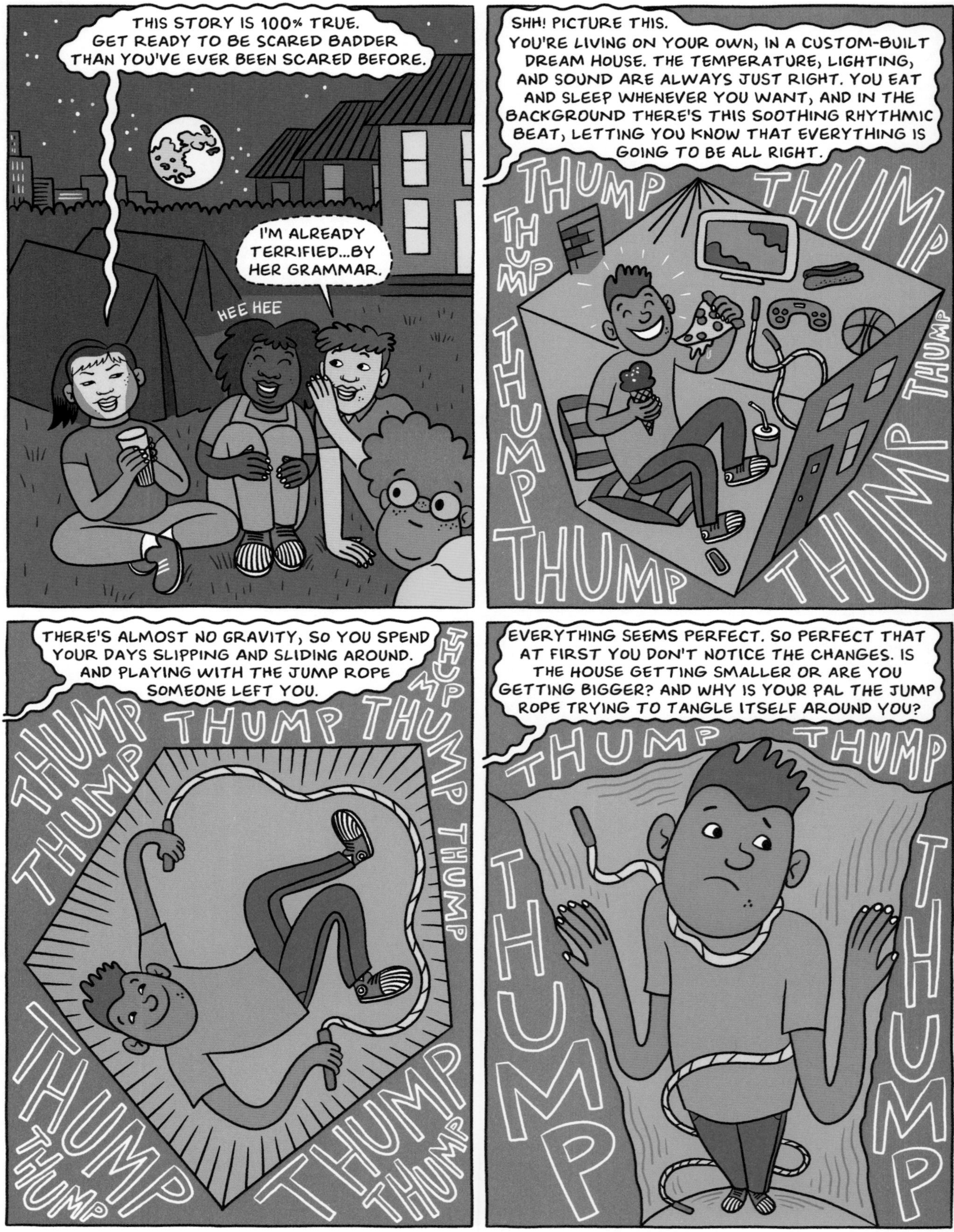
THIS STORY IS 100% TRUE. GET READY TO BE SCARED BADDER THAN YOU'VE EVER BEEN SCARED BEFORE.
HEE HEE
I'M ALREADY TERRIFIED...BY HER GRAMMAR.
SHH! PICTURE THIS. YOU'RE LIVING ON YOUR OWN, IN A CUSTOM-BUILT DREAM HOUSE. THE TEMPERATURE, LIGHTING, AND SOUND ARE ALWAYS JUST RIGHT. YOU EAT AND SLEEP WHENEVER YOU WANT, AND IN THE BACKGROUND THERE'S THIS SOOTHING RHYTHMIC BEAT, LETTING YOU KNOW THAT EVERYTHING IS GOING TO BE ALL RIGHT.
THUMP THUMP THUMP THUMP THUMP THUMP THUMP THUMP THUMP
THERE'S ALMOST NO GRAVITY, SO YOU SPEND YOUR DAYS SLIPPING AND SLIDING AROUND. AND PLAYING WITH THE JUMP ROPE SOMEONE LEFT YOU.
THUMP THUMP THUMP THUMP THUMP THUMP THUMP THUMP THUMP THUMP THUMP THUMP THUMP
EVERYTHING SEEMS PERFECT. SO PERFECT THAT AT FIRST YOU DON'T NOTICE THE CHANGES. IS THE HOUSE GETTING SMALLER OR ARE YOU GETTING BIGGER? AND WHY IS YOUR PAL THE JUMP ROPE TRYING TO TANGLE ITSELF AROUND YOU?
THUMP THUMP THUMP THUMP

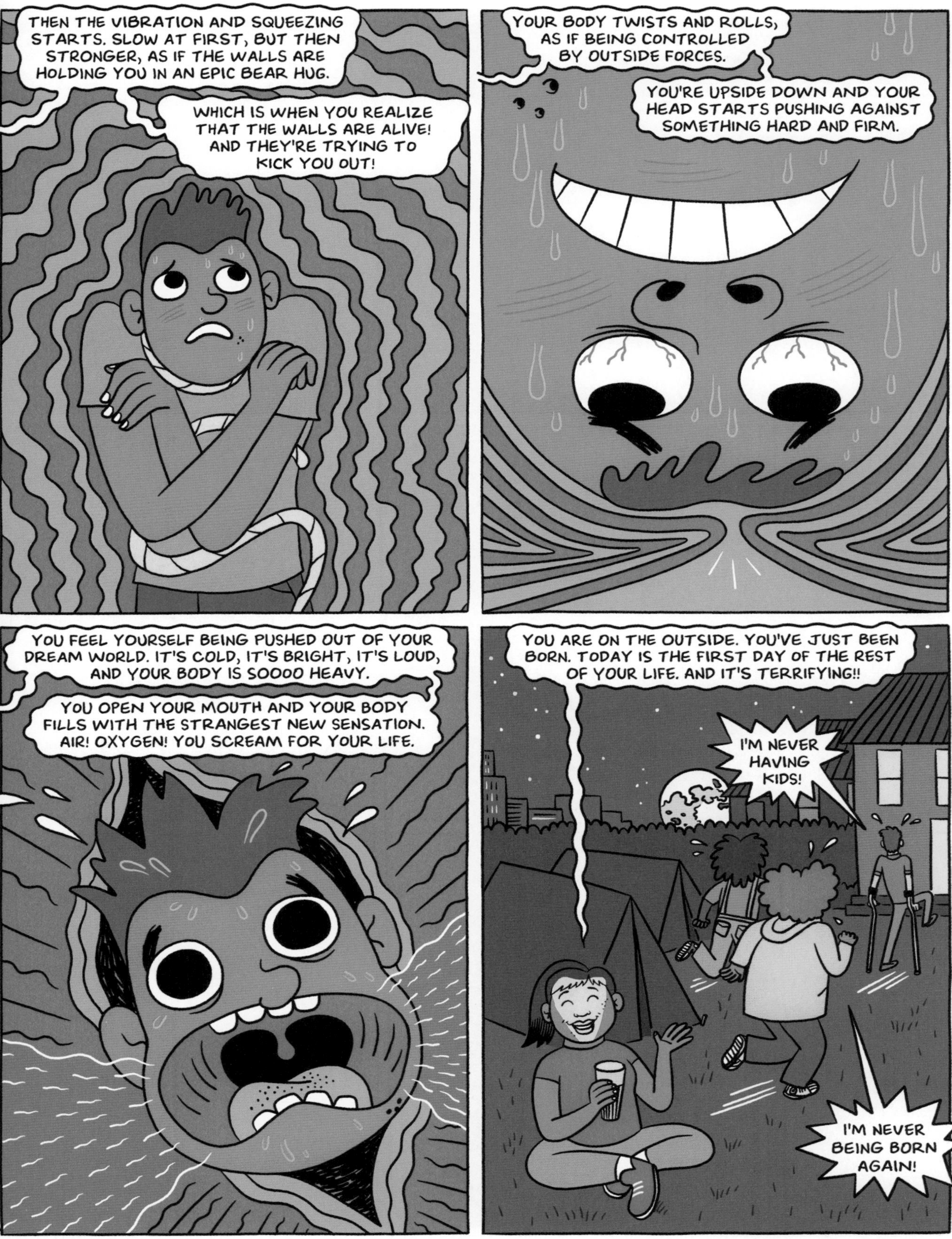
THEN THE VIBRATION AND SQUEEZING STARTS. SLOW AT FIRST, BUT THEN STRONGER, AS IF THE WALLS ARE HOLDING YOU IN AN EPIC BEAR HUG.
WHICH IS WHEN YOU REALIZE THAT THE WALLS ARE ALIVE! AND THEY'RE TRYING TO KICK YOU OUT!
YOUR BODY TWISTS AND ROLLS, AS IF BEING CONTROLLED BY OUTSIDE FORCES.
YOU'RE UPSIDE DOWN AND YOUR HEAD STARTS PUSHING AGAINST SOMETHING HARD AND FIRM.
YOU FEEL YOURSELF BEING PUSHED OUT OF YOUR DREAM WORLD. IT'S COLD, IT'S BRIGHT, IT'S LOUD, AND YOUR BODY IS SOOOO HEAVY.
YOU OPEN YOUR MOUTH AND YOUR BODY FILLS WITH THE STRANGEST NEW SENSATION. AIR! OXYGEN! YOU SCREAM FOR YOUR LIFE.
YOU ARE ON THE OUTSIDE. YOU'VE JUST BEEN BORN. TODAY IS THE FIRST DAY OF THE REST OF YOUR LIFE. AND IT'S TERRIFYING!!
I'M NEVER HAVING KIDS!
I'M NEVER BEING BORN AGAIN!

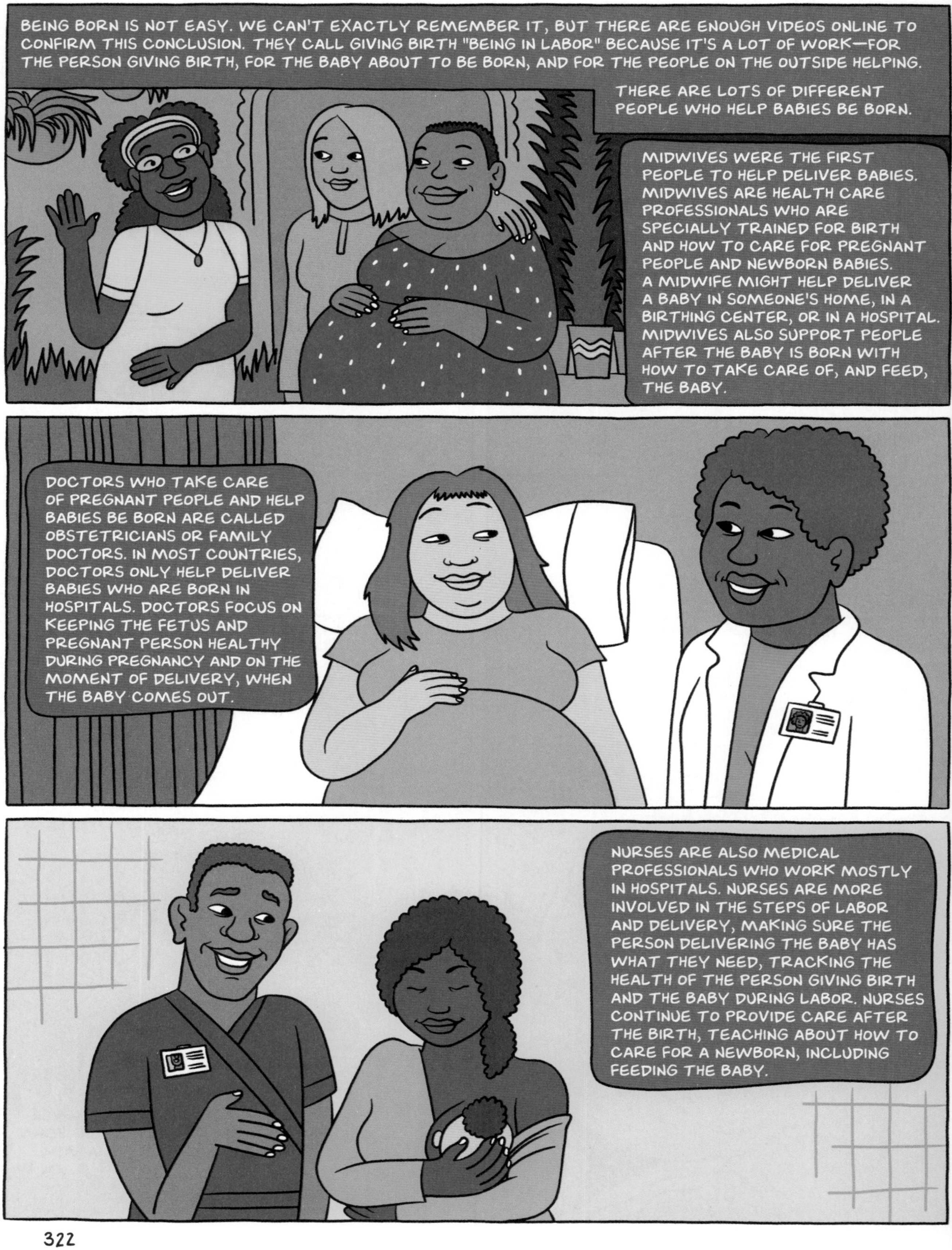
BEING BORN IS NOT EASY. WE CAN'T EXACTLY REMEMBER IT, BUT THERE ARE ENOUGH VIDEOS ONLINE TO CONFIRM THIS CONCLUSION. THEY CALL GIVING BIRTH "BEING IN LABOR" BECAUSE IT'S A LOT OF WORK—FOR THE PERSON GIVING BIRTH, FOR THE BABY ABOUT TO BE BORN, AND FOR THE PEOPLE ON THE OUTSIDE HELPING.
THERE ARE LOTS OF DIFFERENT PEOPLE WHO HELP BABIES BE BORN.
MIDWIVES WERE THE FIRST PEOPLE TO HELP DELIVER BABIES. MIDWIVES ARE HEALTH CARE PROFESSIONALS WHO ARE SPECIALLY TRAINED FOR BIRTH AND HOW TO CARE FOR PREGNANT PEOPLE AND NEWBORN BABIES. A MIDWIFE MIGHT HELP DELIVER A BABY IN SOMEONE'S HOME, IN A BIRTHING CENTER, OR IN A HOSPITAL. MIDWIVES ALSO SUPPORT PEOPLE AFTER THE BABY IS BORN WITH HOW TO TAKE CARE OF, AND FEED, THE BABY.
DOCTORS WHO TAKE CARE OF PREGNANT PEOPLE AND HELP BABIES BE BORN ARE CALLED OBSTETRICIANS OR FAMILY DOCTORS. IN MOST COUNTRIES, DOCTORS ONLY HELP DELIVER BABIES WHO ARE BORN IN HOSPITALS. DOCTORS FOCUS ON KEEPING THE FETUS AND PREGNANT PERSON HEALTHY DURING PREGNANCY AND ON THE MOMENT OF DELIVERY, WHEN THE BABY COMES OUT.
NURSES ARE ALSO MEDICAL PROFESSIONALS WHO WORK MOSTLY IN HOSPITALS. NURSES ARE MORE INVOLVED IN THE STEPS OF LABOR AND DELIVERY, MAKING SURE THE PERSON DELIVERING THE BABY HAS WHAT THEY NEED, TRACKING THE HEALTH OF THE PERSON GIVING BIRTH AND THE BABY DURING LABOR. NURSES CONTINUE TO PROVIDE CARE AFTER THE BIRTH, TEACHING ABOUT HOW TO CARE FOR A NEWBORN, INCLUDING FEEDING THE BABY.

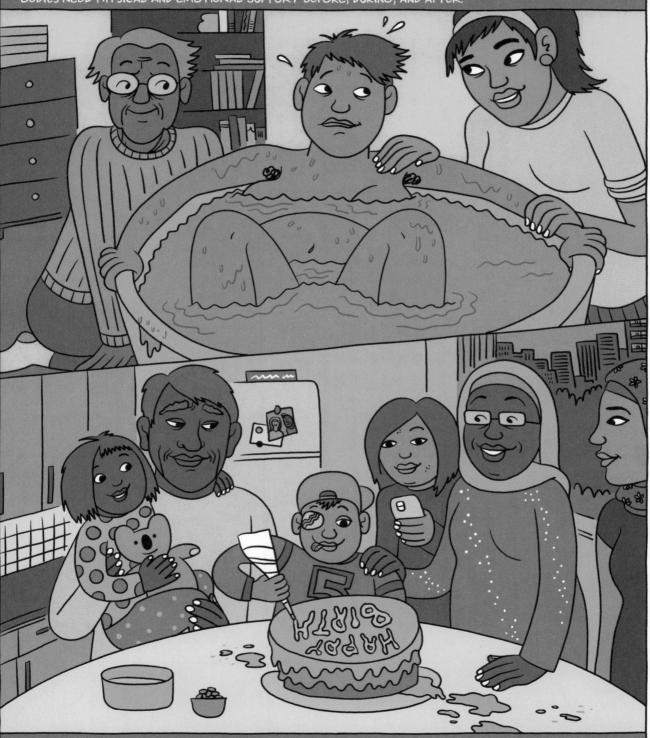

A BIRTH DOULA IS SOMEONE WHOSE JOB IS TO BE A COMPANION TO THE PERSON GIVING BIRTH. A BIRTH DOULA PROVIDES SUPPORT THROUGH LABOR AND BIRTH, AND AFTER THE BABY IS BORN. BIRTH DOULA IS A NEW TERM FOR A VERY OLD IDEA, WHICH IS THAT LABOR AND BIRTH ARE DIFFICULT AND POWERFUL, AND BODIES NEED PHYSICAL AND EMOTIONAL SUPPORT BEFORE, DURING, AND AFTER.

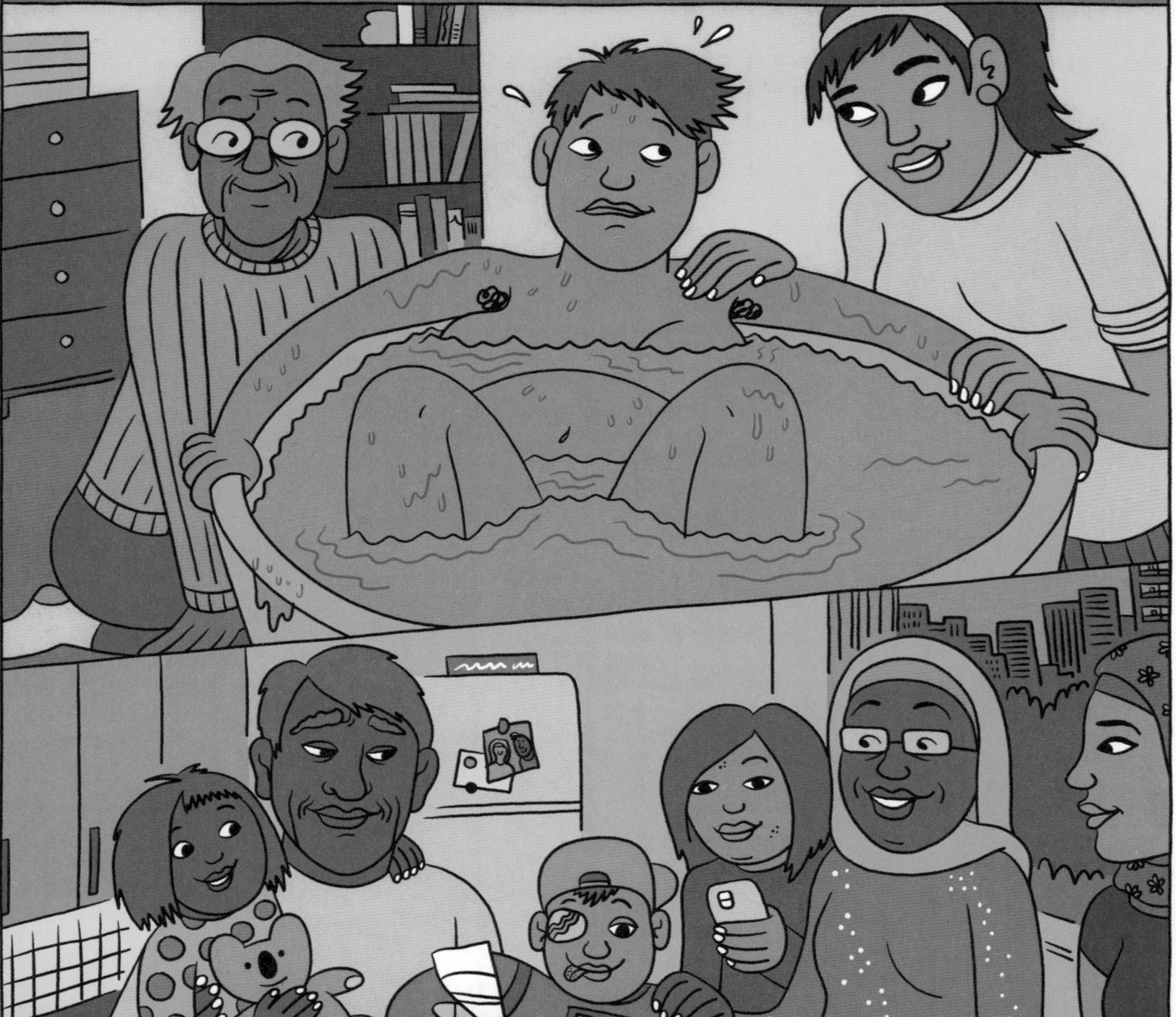
HAPPY BIRTH

SOMETIMES FAMILY AND FRIENDS WILL BE THERE TO HELP DURING LABOR AND BIRTH. SOMETIMES THEY HELP OUT BY OFFERING TO MAKE FOOD, HELP WITH HOUSEWORK, OR SPEND TIME WITH OTHER CHILDREN IN THE FAMILY, SINCE BOTH THE BABY AND THE PERSON WHO GAVE BIRTH USUALLY NEED TIME TO REST AND SETTLE IN AFTER THE JOURNEY.

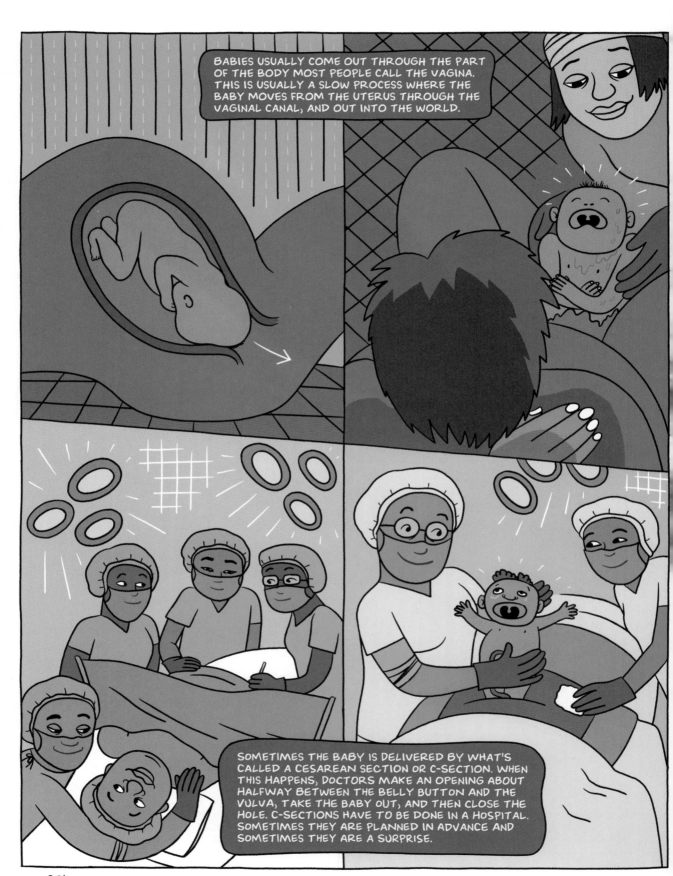

BABIES USUALLY COME OUT THROUGH THE PART OF THE BODY MOST PEOPLE CALL THE VAGINA. THIS IS USUALLY A SLOW PROCESS WHERE THE BABY MOVES FROM THE UTERUS THROUGH THE VAGINAL CANAL, AND OUT INTO THE WORLD.

SOMETIMES THE BABY IS DELIVERED BY WHAT'S CALLED A CESAREAN SECTION OR C-SECTION. WHEN THIS HAPPENS, DOCTORS MAKE AN OPENING ABOUT HALFWAY BETWEEN THE BELLY BUTTON AND THE VULVA, TAKE THE BABY OUT, AND THEN CLOSE THE HOLE. C-SECTIONS HAVE TO BE DONE IN A HOSPITAL. SOMETIMES THEY ARE PLANNED IN ADVANCE AND SOMETIMES THEY ARE A SURPRISE.

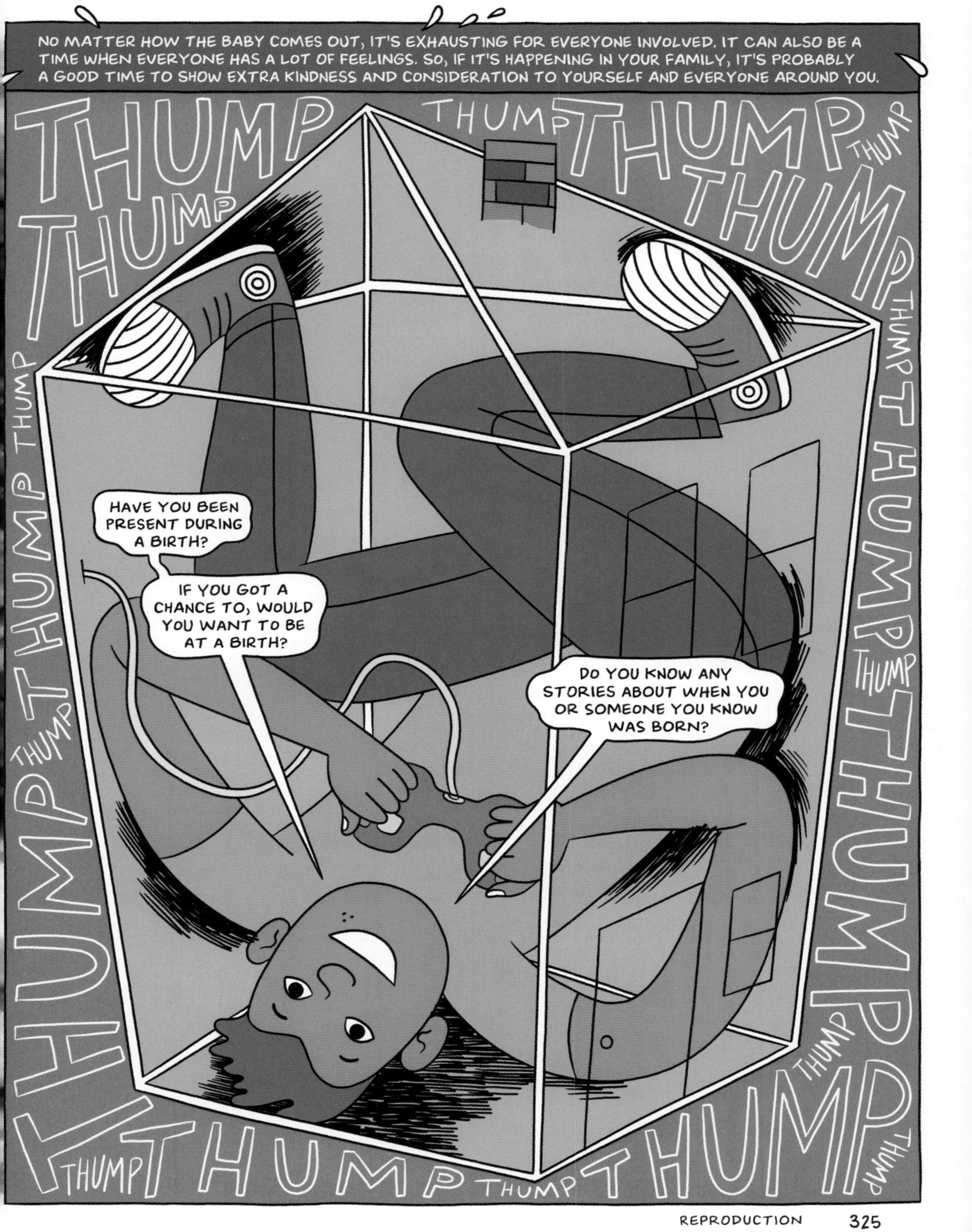
NO MATTER HOW THE BABY COMES OUT, IT'S EXHAUSTING FOR EVERYONE INVOLVED. IT CAN ALSO BE A TIME WHEN EVERYONE HAS A LOT OF FEELINGS. SO, IF IT'S HAPPENING IN YOUR FAMILY, IT'S PROBABLY A GOOD TIME TO SHOW EXTRA KINDNESS AND CONSIDERATION TO YOURSELF AND EVERYONE AROUND YOU.
THUMP
THUMP
THUMP
THUMP
THUMP
THUMP
HAVE YOU BEEN PRESENT DURING A BIRTH?
IF YOU GOT A CHANCE TO, WOULD YOU WANT TO BE AT A BIRTH?
DO YOU KNOW ANY STORIES ABOUT WHEN YOU OR SOMEONE YOU KNOW WAS BORN?
THUMP
THUMP
THUMP
THUMP
THUMP
THUMP
THUMP
THUMP

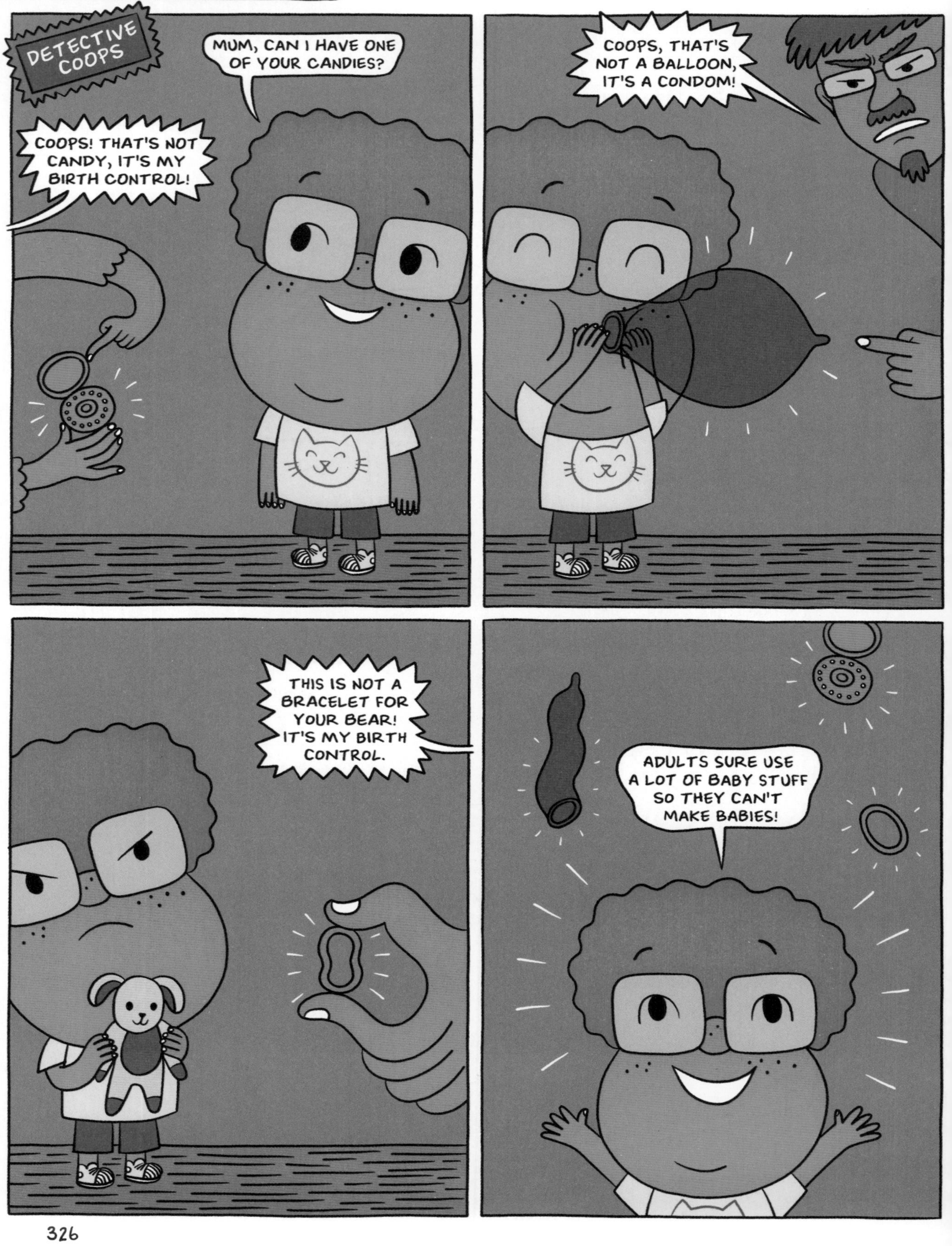
DETECTIVE COOPS
MUM, CAN I HAVE ONE OF YOUR CANDIES?
COOPS! THAT'S NOT CANDY, IT'S MY BIRTH CONTROL!
COOPS, THAT'S NOT A BALLOON, IT'S A CONDOM!
THIS IS NOT A BRACELET FOR YOUR BEAR! IT'S MY BIRTH CONTROL.
ADULTS SURE USE A LOT OF BABY STUFF SO THEY CAN'T MAKE BABIES!

MOST KINDS OF SEX CANNOT MAKE A BABY. BUT ONCE YOU'RE EXPERIENCING PUBERTY, YOU MIGHT BE ABLE TO MAKE A BABY IF YOU HAVE PENILE-VAGINAL INTERCOURSE.

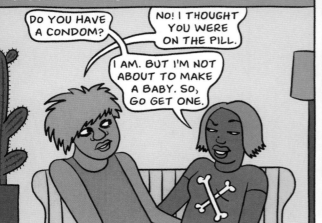

DO YOU HAVE A CONDOM?

NO! I THOUGHT YOU WERE ON THE PILL.

I AM. BUT I'M NOT ABOUT TO MAKE A BABY. SO, GO GET ONE.

MOST OF THE TIME, PEOPLE HAVE INTERCOURSE BECAUSE IT FEELS GOOD, NOT BECAUSE THEY WANT TO MAKE A BABY. WHICH IS WHERE BIRTH CONTROL COMES IN.

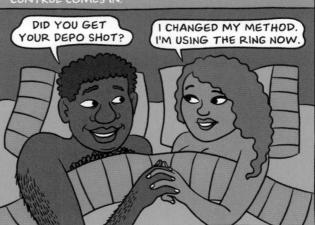

DID YOU GET YOUR DEPO SHOT?

I CHANGED MY METHOD. I'M USING THE RING NOW.

BIRTH CONTROL IS A WAY OF REDUCING THE CHANCES OF GETTING PREGNANT IF A PERSON HAS INTERCOURSE.

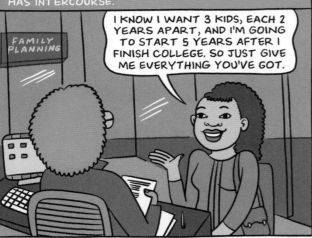

FAMILY PLANNING

I KNOW I WANT 3 KIDS, EACH 2 YEARS APART, AND I'M GOING TO START 5 YEARS AFTER I FINISH COLLEGE. SO JUST GIVE ME EVERYTHING YOU'VE GOT.

EVERYONE SHOULD KNOW SOMETHING ABOUT BIRTH CONTROL, EVEN IF THEY DON'T THINK THEY'LL EVER HAVE INTERCOURSE.

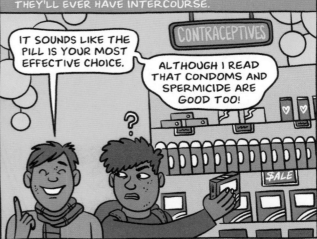

IT SOUNDS LIKE THE PILL IS YOUR MOST EFFECTIVE CHOICE.

CONTRACEPTIVES

ALTHOUGH I READ THAT CONDOMS AND SPERMICIDE ARE GOOD TOO!

$ALE

THERE ARE LOTS OF DIFFERENT KINDS OF BIRTH CONTROL. THEY VARY IN HOW MUCH THEY COST, HOW EASY THEY ARE TO USE, HOW PERMANENT THEY ARE, AND WHO USES THEM. WE'RE ONLY EXPLAINING A FEW OF THEM HERE.

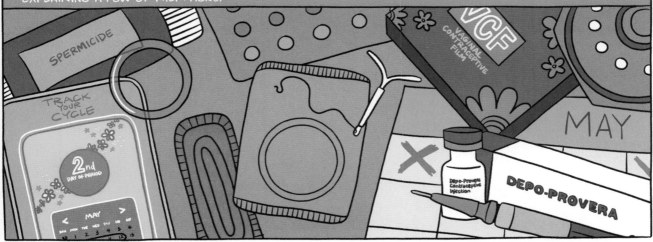

SPERMICIDE

VCF VAGINAL CONTRACEPTIVE FILM

TRACK YOUR CYCLE

2nd DAY OF PERIOD

MAY

Depo-Provera Contraceptive Injection

DEPO-PROVERA

CONDOMS

THERE ARE TWO KINDS OF CONDOMS. EXTERNAL CONDOMS GO OVER THE PENIS AND PREVENT SEMEN FROM GETTING INTO THE OTHER BODY DURING INTERCOURSE. SPERM IS IN SEMEN, SO NO SEMEN = NO SPERM = NO BABY MAKING.

INTERNAL CONDOMS ARE INSERTED INTO THE VAGINA TO CREATE A BARRIER SO NO SEMEN CAN GET INTO THE VAGINA.

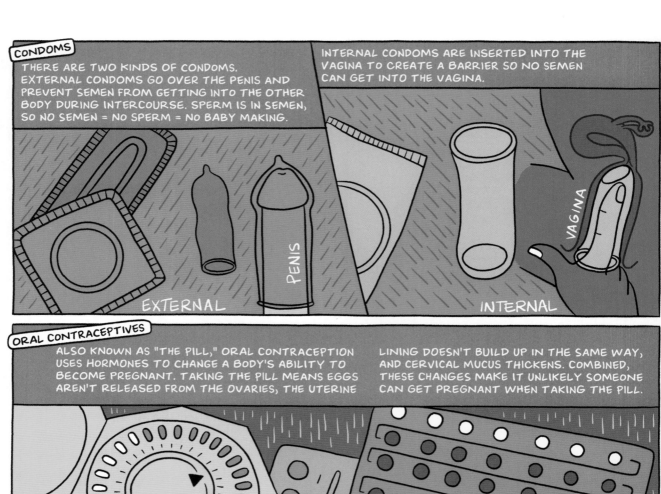

EXTERNAL

PENIS

INTERNAL

VAGINA

ORAL CONTRACEPTIVES

ALSO KNOWN AS "THE PILL," ORAL CONTRACEPTION USES HORMONES TO CHANGE A BODY'S ABILITY TO BECOME PREGNANT. TAKING THE PILL MEANS EGGS AREN'T RELEASED FROM THE OVARIES, THE UTERINE LINING DOESN'T BUILD UP IN THE SAME WAY, AND CERVICAL MUCUS THICKENS. COMBINED, THESE CHANGES MAKE IT UNLIKELY SOMEONE CAN GET PREGNANT WHEN TAKING THE PILL.

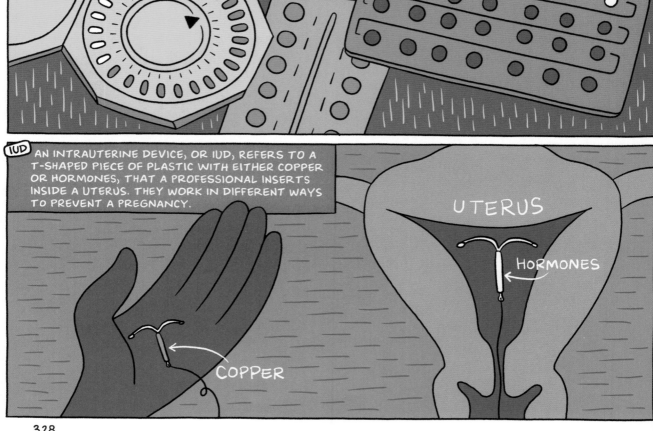

IUD

AN INTRAUTERINE DEVICE, OR IUD, REFERS TO A T-SHAPED PIECE OF PLASTIC WITH EITHER COPPER OR HORMONES, THAT A PROFESSIONAL INSERTS INSIDE A UTERUS. THEY WORK IN DIFFERENT WAYS TO PREVENT A PREGNANCY.

UTERUS

HORMONES

COPPER

VASECTOMY

A VASECTOMY IS CONSIDERED A FORM OF STERILIZATION* BECAUSE IT PREVENTS SOMEONE FROM BEING ABLE TO MAKE A BABY AND IS NOT EASY TO REVERSE. DURING A VASECTOMY, THE TUBE THAT CARRIES SPERM FROM THE SCROTUM TO THE TIP OF THE PENIS—CALLED THE VAS DEFERENS—IS CUT AND A SHORT PIECE IS REMOVED. THE TWO ENDS ARE THEN BLOCKED, SO THAT NO SPERM ARE RELEASED IN THE SEMEN.

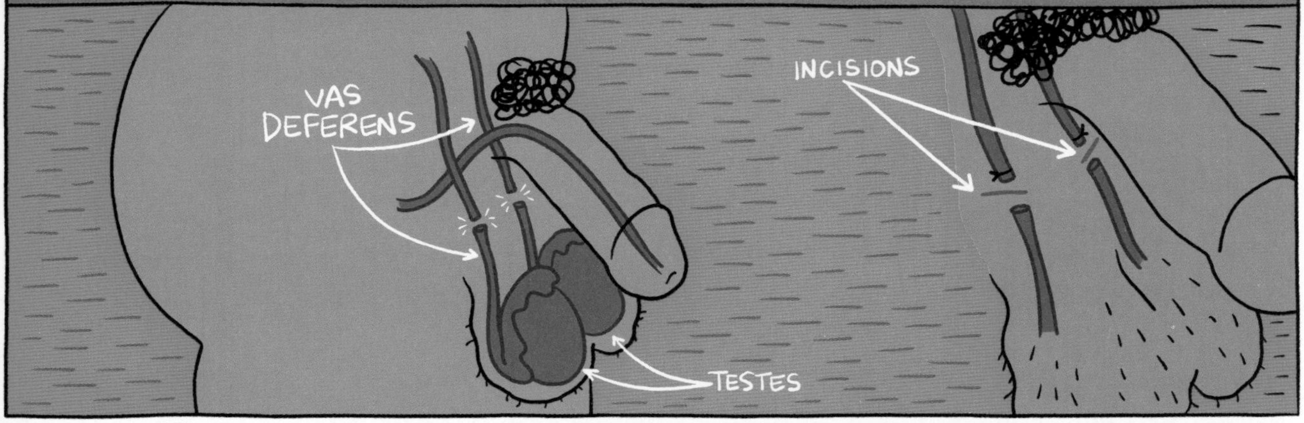
VAS DEFERENS
INCISIONS
TESTES

TUBAL LIGATION

ANOTHER FORM OF STERILIZATION IS CALLED TUBAL LIGATION. THIS CUTS, BLOCKS OFF, OR REMOVES THE FALLOPIAN TUBES, SO AN EGG IS NOT ABLE TO MEET WITH SPERM.

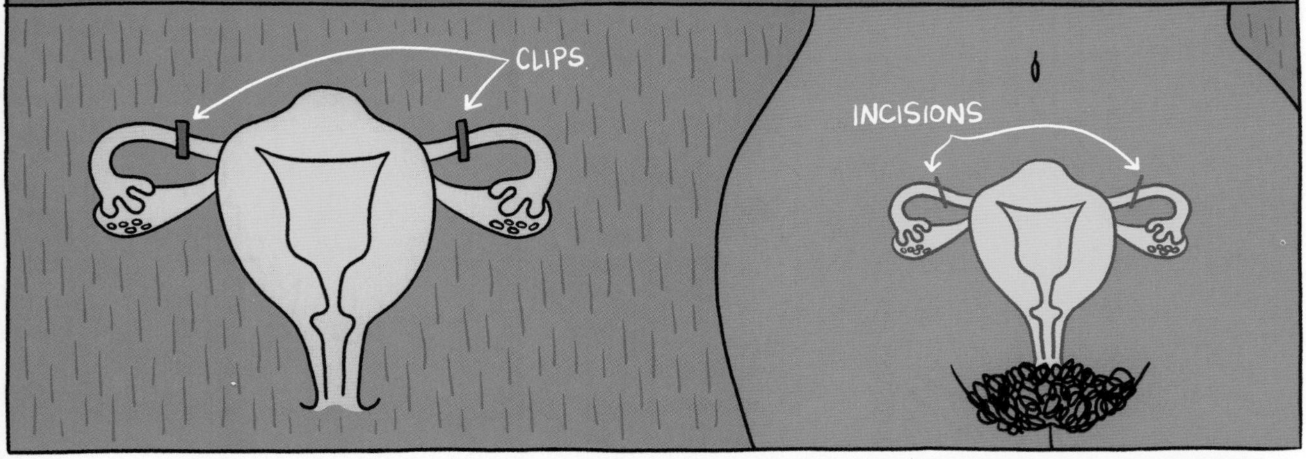
CLIPS
INCISIONS

ABSTINENCE

TO ABSTAIN FROM SOMETHING MEANS TO CHOOSE NOT TO DO IT. ABSTAINING FROM SEX MEANS CHOOSING NOT TO ENGAGE IN SEXUAL ACTIVITIES. IT MIGHT MEAN CHOOSING NOT TO ENGAGE IN ANY SEXUAL ACTIVITIES OR ENGAGING ONLY IN CERTAIN ONES. IF YOU CHOOSE NOT TO ENGAGE IN INTERCOURSE, THEN ABSTINENCE IS A FORM OF BIRTH CONTROL. YOU CAN READ MORE ABOUT ABSTINENCE ON P. 356.

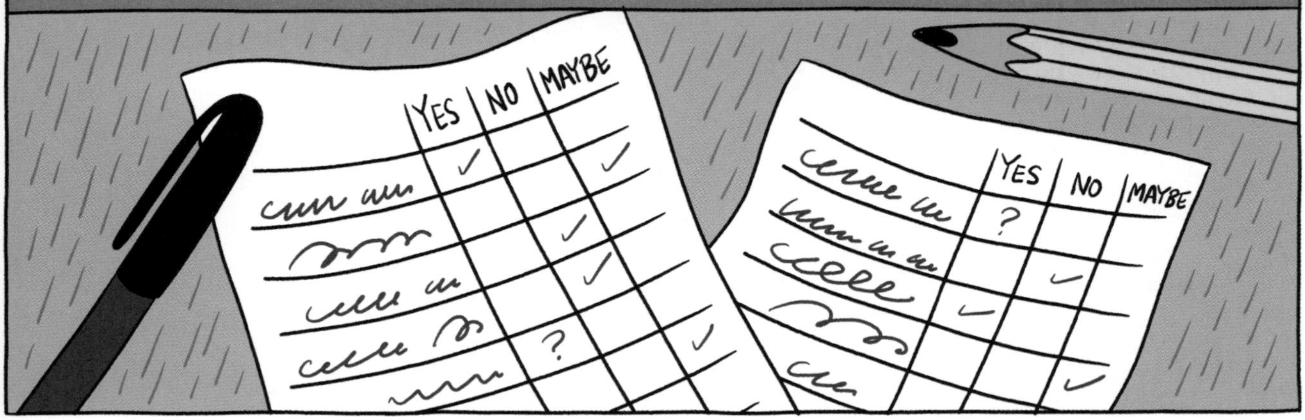
YES
NO
MAYBE
YES
NO
MAYBE

* FIND A DEFINITION OF STERILIZATION IN THE GLOSSARY ON P. 424

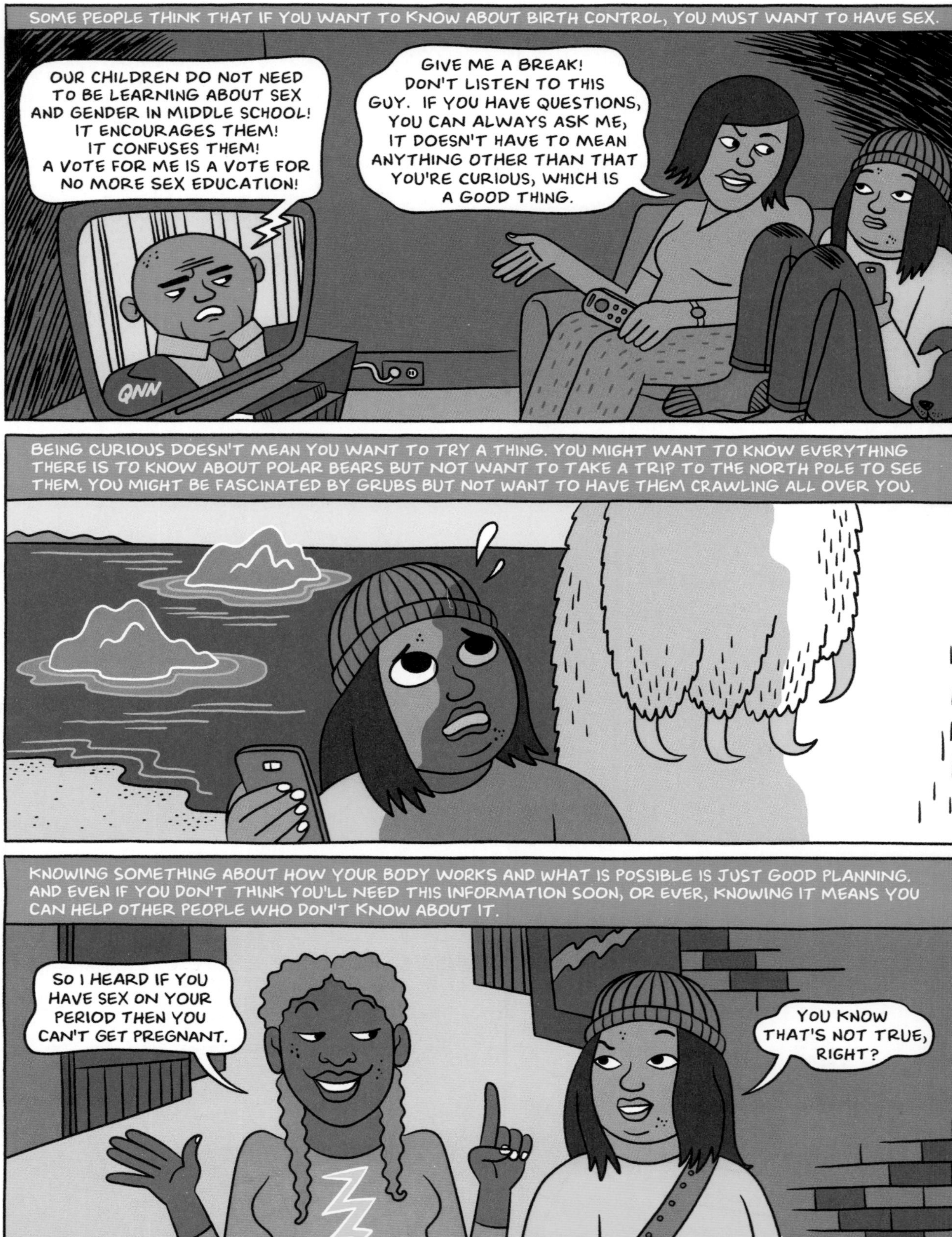
SOME PEOPLE THINK THAT IF YOU WANT TO KNOW ABOUT BIRTH CONTROL, YOU MUST WANT TO HAVE SEX.
OUR CHILDREN DO NOT NEED TO BE LEARNING ABOUT SEX AND GENDER IN MIDDLE SCHOOL! IT ENCOURAGES THEM! IT CONFUSES THEM! A VOTE FOR ME IS A VOTE FOR NO MORE SEX EDUCATION!
QNN
GIVE ME A BREAK! DON'T LISTEN TO THIS GUY. IF YOU HAVE QUESTIONS, YOU CAN ALWAYS ASK ME, IT DOESN'T HAVE TO MEAN ANYTHING OTHER THAN THAT YOU'RE CURIOUS, WHICH IS A GOOD THING.
BEING CURIOUS DOESN'T MEAN YOU WANT TO TRY A THING. YOU MIGHT WANT TO KNOW EVERYTHING THERE IS TO KNOW ABOUT POLAR BEARS BUT NOT WANT TO TAKE A TRIP TO THE NORTH POLE TO SEE THEM. YOU MIGHT BE FASCINATED BY GRUBS BUT NOT WANT TO HAVE THEM CRAWLING ALL OVER YOU.
KNOWING SOMETHING ABOUT HOW YOUR BODY WORKS AND WHAT IS POSSIBLE IS JUST GOOD PLANNING. AND EVEN IF YOU DON'T THINK YOU'LL NEED THIS INFORMATION SOON, OR EVER, KNOWING IT MEANS YOU CAN HELP OTHER PEOPLE WHO DON'T KNOW ABOUT IT.
SO I HEARD IF YOU HAVE SEX ON YOUR PERIOD THEN YOU CAN'T GET PREGNANT.
YOU KNOW THAT'S NOT TRUE, RIGHT?

MY BODY MY CHOICE
eugenics is still happening
MY BODY MY RIGHTS!
MY BIRTH CONTROL MY DECISION
KEEP YOUR LAWS OFF MY BODY
MINE

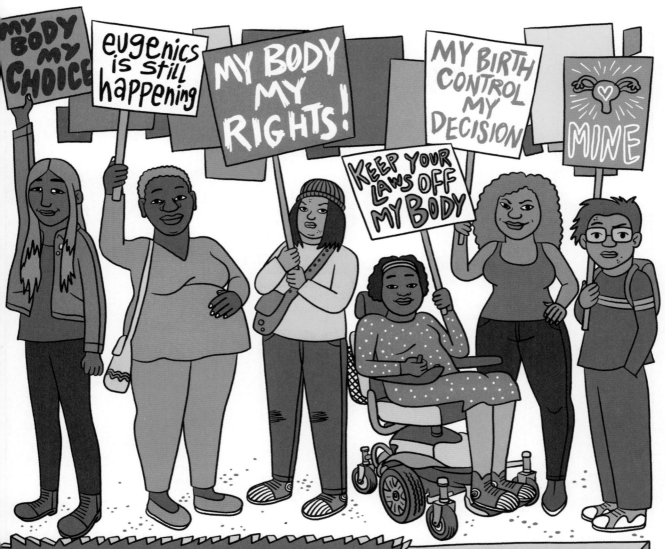

JUSTICE NERD ALERT BIRTH CONTROL SHOULD BE OUR CHOICE

BODY AUTONOMY MEANS THAT PEOPLE WHO HAVE BODIES THAT CAN MAKE BABIES GET TO CHOOSE WHETHER OR NOT TO TRY AND MAKE ONE. NO ONE SHOULD PRESSURE OR FORCE YOU INTO HAVING A BABY OR NOT. BUT SOMETIMES PEOPLE DO. SOMETIMES WE'RE IN RELATIONSHIPS WITH PEOPLE WHO TRY TO PRESSURE US. THEY MIGHT TELL US WE SHOULD GET BIRTH CONTROL, OR THEY MIGHT TELL US WE SHOULDN'T. EITHER WAY, THEY ARE TRYING TO DECIDE FOR US.

IT ISN'T JUST INDIVIDUALS THAT TRY TO TAKE OUR CHOICE AWAY. GOVERNMENTS CREATE LAWS THAT TAKE AWAY A PERSON'S RIGHT TO CHOOSE TO HAVE, OR NOT HAVE, A BABY. ONE WAY THEY DO THIS IS BY LIMITING PEOPLE'S ACCESS TO BIRTH CONTROL, ABORTION, AND HEALTH CARE. ANOTHER IS BY FORCIBLY STERILIZING SOME PEOPLE.

WHO GETS TARGETED? USUALLY WOMEN AND QUEER PEOPLE; DISABLED PEOPLE; PEOPLE WHO ARE BLACK, BROWN, OR INDIGENOUS; AND PEOPLE WHO BELONG TO MORE THAN ONE OF THOSE GROUPS.

FORCED STERILIZATION IS CONNECTED TO A FAKE SCIENCE CALLED EUGENICS. EUGENICISTS, WHO WERE MOSTLY WEALTHY WHITE PEOPLE, CLAIMED THAT THE HUMAN RACE WOULD BE BETTER IF WE ONLY LET SOME PEOPLE REPRODUCE. NOT SURPRISINGLY, THEY ONLY WANTED PEOPLE LIKE THEM TO REPRODUCE. PEOPLE WHO WEREN'T LIKE THEM WERE SUPPOSED TO BE STERILIZED, SO THEY COULDN'T HAVE BABIES EVEN IF THEY WANTED TO. THIS STILL HAPPENS TODAY, ALTHOUGH IN SOME COUNTRIES THE LAWS HAVE CHANGED TO MAKE IT HARDER TO TARGET AN ENTIRE GROUP OF PEOPLE.

BIRTH CONTROL IS GOOD WHEN IT IS SOMEONE'S CHOICE. BUT NO ONE SHOULD EVER BE ABLE TO MAKE THAT CHOICE FOR YOU. NO ONE SHOULD EVEN TRY.

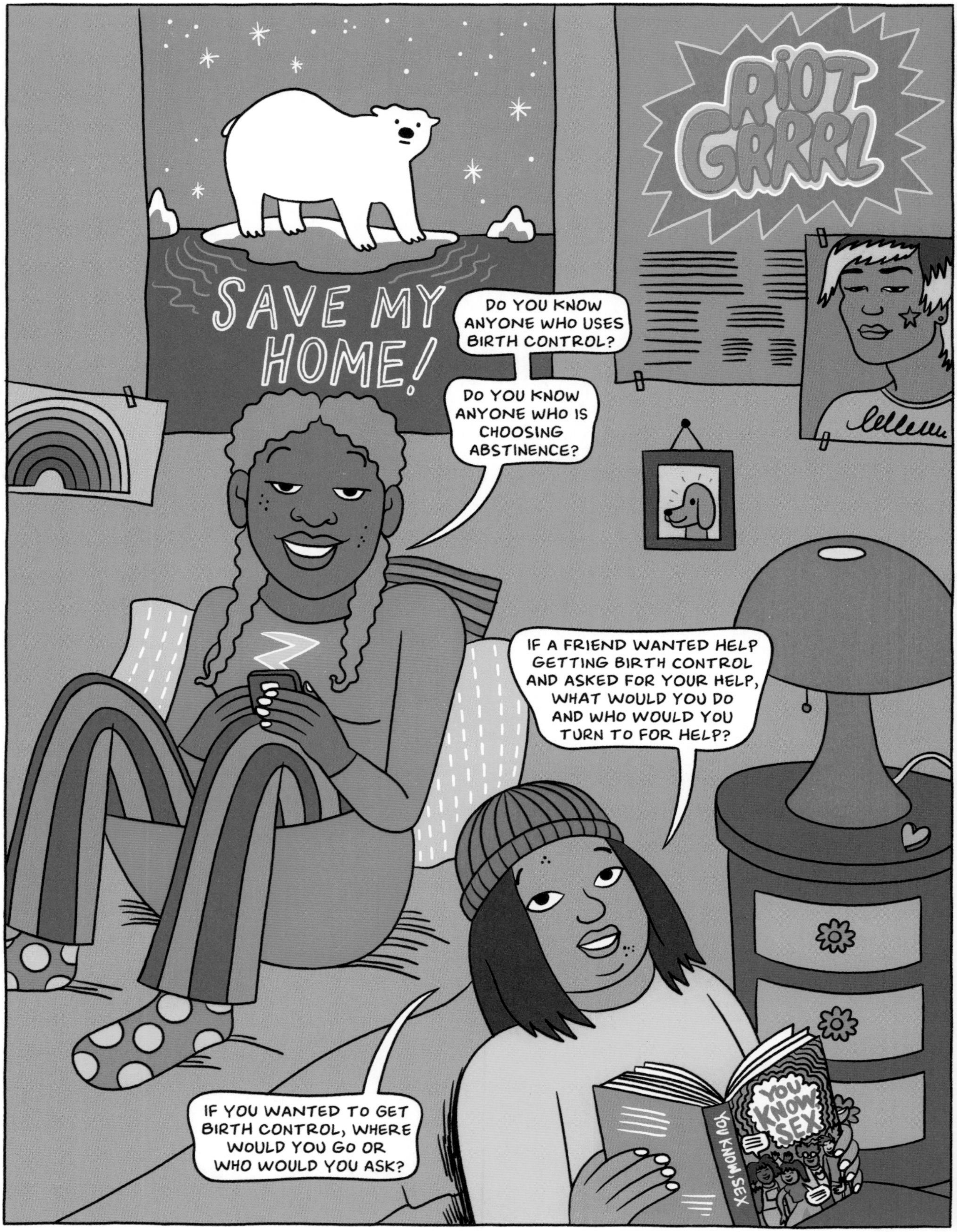
SAVE MY HOME!
RIOT GRRRL
DO YOU KNOW ANYONE WHO USES BIRTH CONTROL?
DO YOU KNOW ANYONE WHO IS CHOOSING ABSTINENCE?
IF A FRIEND WANTED HELP GETTING BIRTH CONTROL AND ASKED FOR YOUR HELP, WHAT WOULD YOU DO AND WHO WOULD YOU TURN TO FOR HELP?
IF YOU WANTED TO GET BIRTH CONTROL, WHERE WOULD YOU GO OR WHO WOULD YOU ASK?
YOU KNOW SEX
YOU KNOW, SEX

10 TOUCHING

HEY COOPS! WHO'S THE NAKED LADIES APPRECIATOR?
COOPER
1968

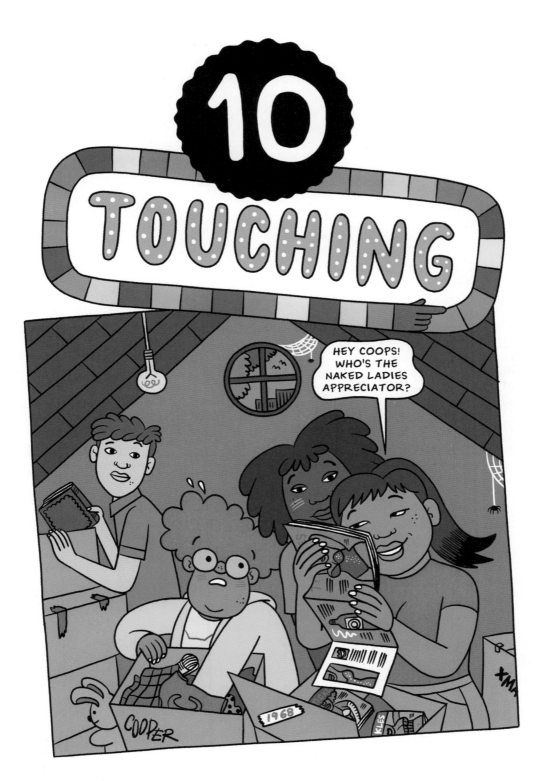

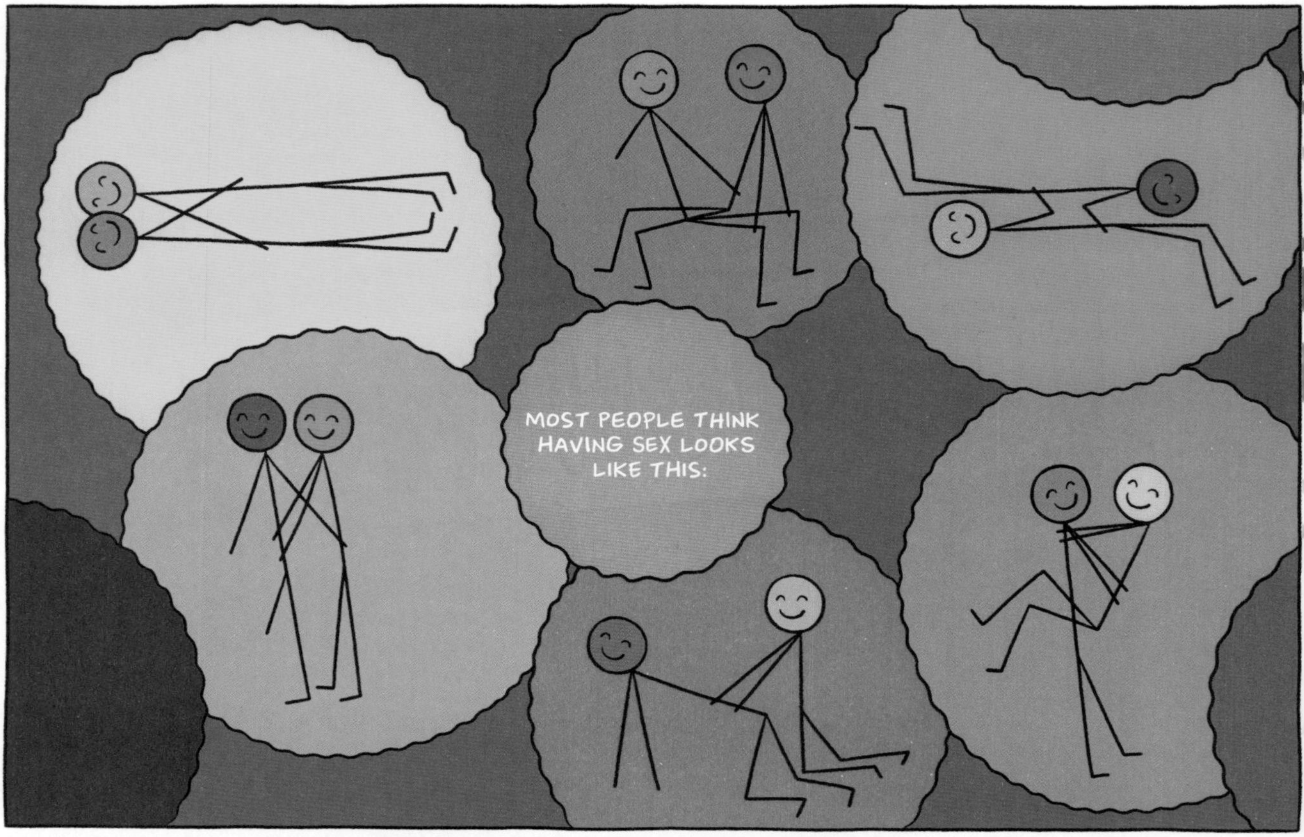
MOST PEOPLE THINK HAVING SEX LOOKS LIKE THIS:

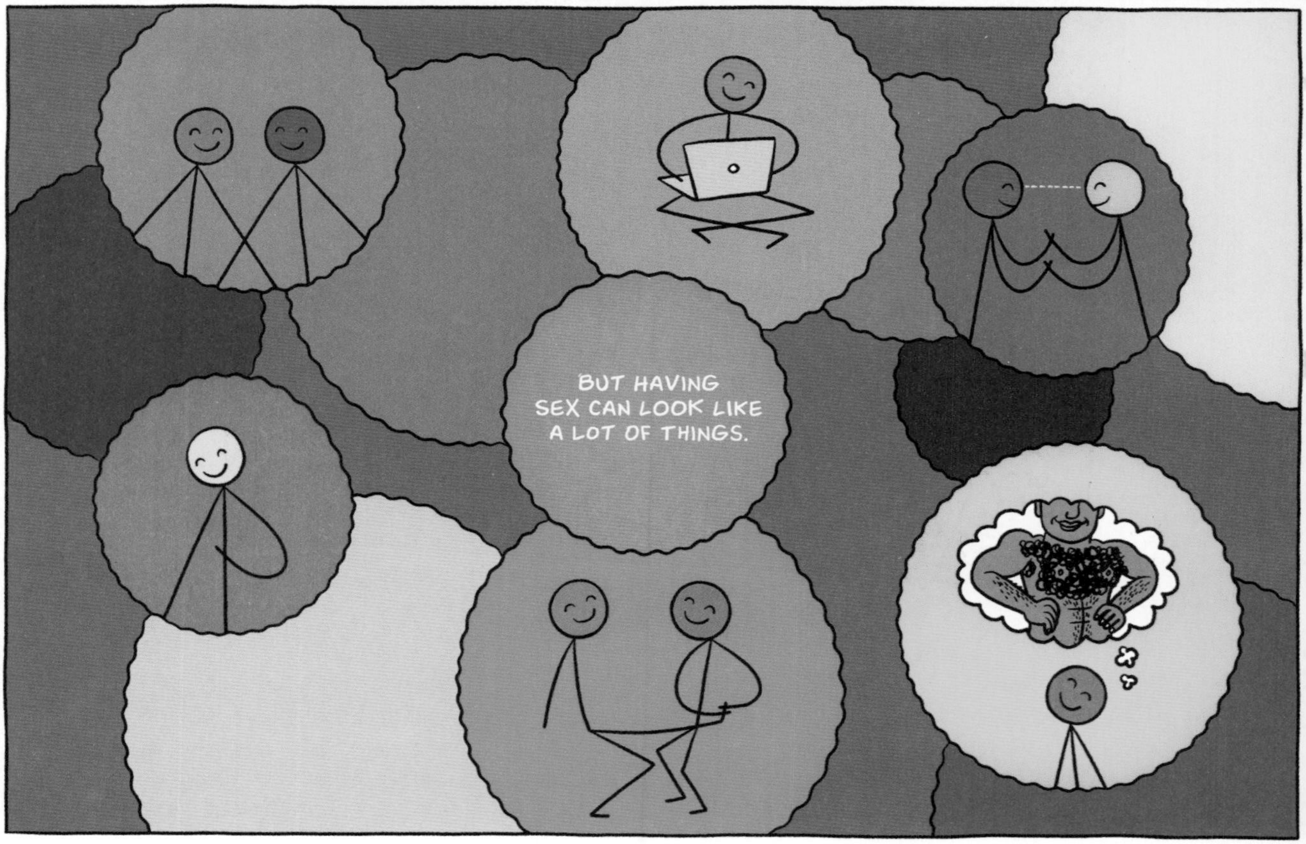
BUT HAVING SEX CAN LOOK LIKE A LOT OF THINGS.

UNTIL WE CHOOSE TO DO IT, MOST OF US DON'T KNOW WHAT HAVING SEX LOOKS OR FEELS LIKE. THE SEX IN PORNOGRAPHY* ISN'T THE SAME AS THE SEX MOST PEOPLE HAVE. AND IF WE CHOOSE TO HAVE SEX, MOST OF US DO IT IN PRIVATE. SO YOU DON'T USUALLY SEE IT UNTIL YOU'RE DOING IT.

THERE'S A LOT OF MISINFORMATION OUT THERE ABOUT WHAT HAVING SEX LOOKS AND FEELS LIKE. IN THIS SECTION WE TRY TO CLEAR UP SOME OF THE MYSTERY BY TALKING ABOUT HAVING SEX WITHOUT FILTERS OR SPECIAL EFFECTS.

BUT FIRST, THERE ARE A FEW THINGS THAT WE THINK YOU SHOULD KNOW, WHETHER OR NOT YOU EVER PLAN TO HAVE SEX.

★ HAVING SEX CAN FEEL DIFFERENT EVERY TIME WE DO IT. EVEN IF WE'RE DOING THE SAME THING, WITH THE SAME PERSON, IT CAN FEEL DIFFERENT BECAUSE SEX ISN'T JUST SOMETHING THAT HAPPENS TO US, IT'S SOMETHING WE DO. AND WE ARE ALWAYS CHANGING.

★ SEX ISN'T ALWAYS GREAT, OR EVEN GOOD. SEX CAN BE AWKWARD AND UNCOMFORTABLE, IT CAN BE BORING OR PAINFUL. IT CAN ALSO BE BEAUTIFUL AND AMAZING.

★ SEX IS NOT USUALLY GREAT THE FIRST TIME WE TRY IT. IT TAKES A WHILE TO FIGURE OUT WHAT WE LIKE AND WHO WE LIKE IT WITH. ALSO, WE'RE USUALLY NERVOUS THE FIRST TIME, WHICH CAN MAKE IT DIFFICULT TO FEEL RELAXED AND SAFE.

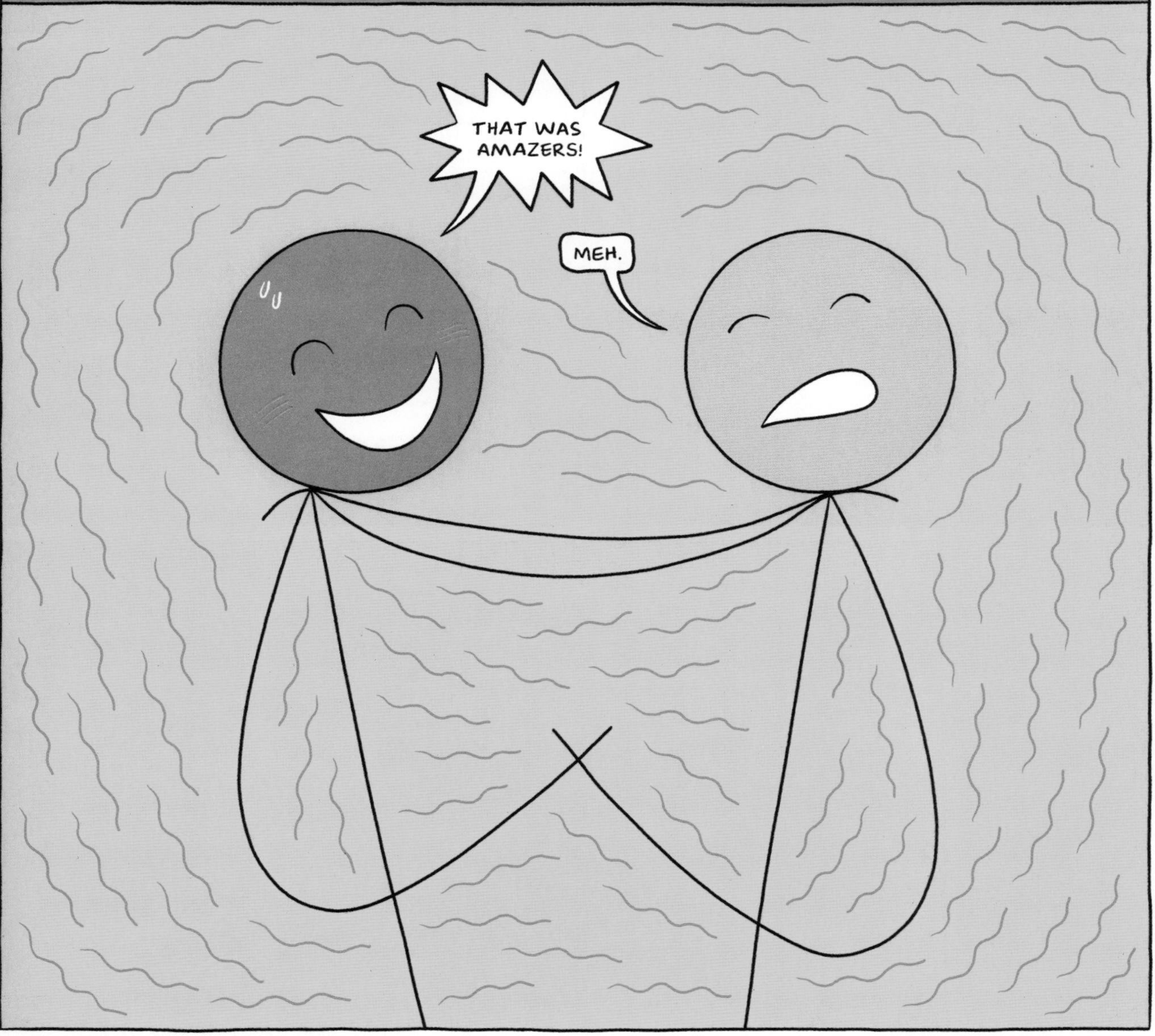
THAT WAS AMAZERS!
MEH.

* READ MORE ABOUT PORNOGRAPHY ON P. 357

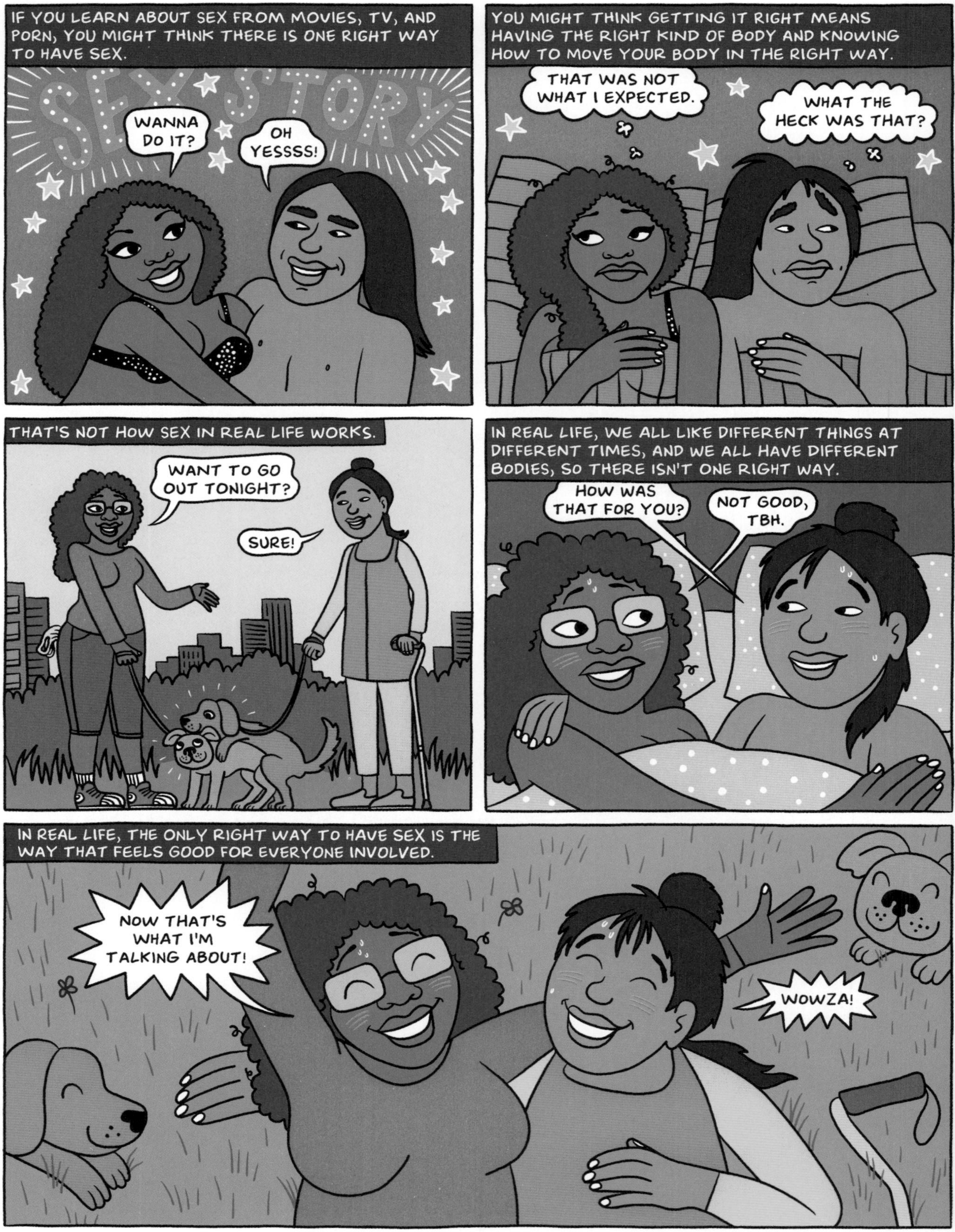
IF YOU LEARN ABOUT SEX FROM MOVIES, TV, AND PORN, YOU MIGHT THINK THERE IS ONE RIGHT WAY TO HAVE SEX.
SEX STORY
WANNA DO IT?
OH YESSSS!
YOU MIGHT THINK GETTING IT RIGHT MEANS HAVING THE RIGHT KIND OF BODY AND KNOWING HOW TO MOVE YOUR BODY IN THE RIGHT WAY.
THAT WAS NOT WHAT I EXPECTED.
WHAT THE HECK WAS THAT?
THAT'S NOT HOW SEX IN REAL LIFE WORKS.
WANT TO GO OUT TONIGHT?
SURE!
IN REAL LIFE, WE ALL LIKE DIFFERENT THINGS AT DIFFERENT TIMES, AND WE ALL HAVE DIFFERENT BODIES, SO THERE ISN'T ONE RIGHT WAY.
HOW WAS THAT FOR YOU?
NOT GOOD, TBH.
IN REAL LIFE, THE ONLY RIGHT WAY TO HAVE SEX IS THE WAY THAT FEELS GOOD FOR EVERYONE INVOLVED.
NOW THAT'S WHAT I'M TALKING ABOUT!
WOWZA!

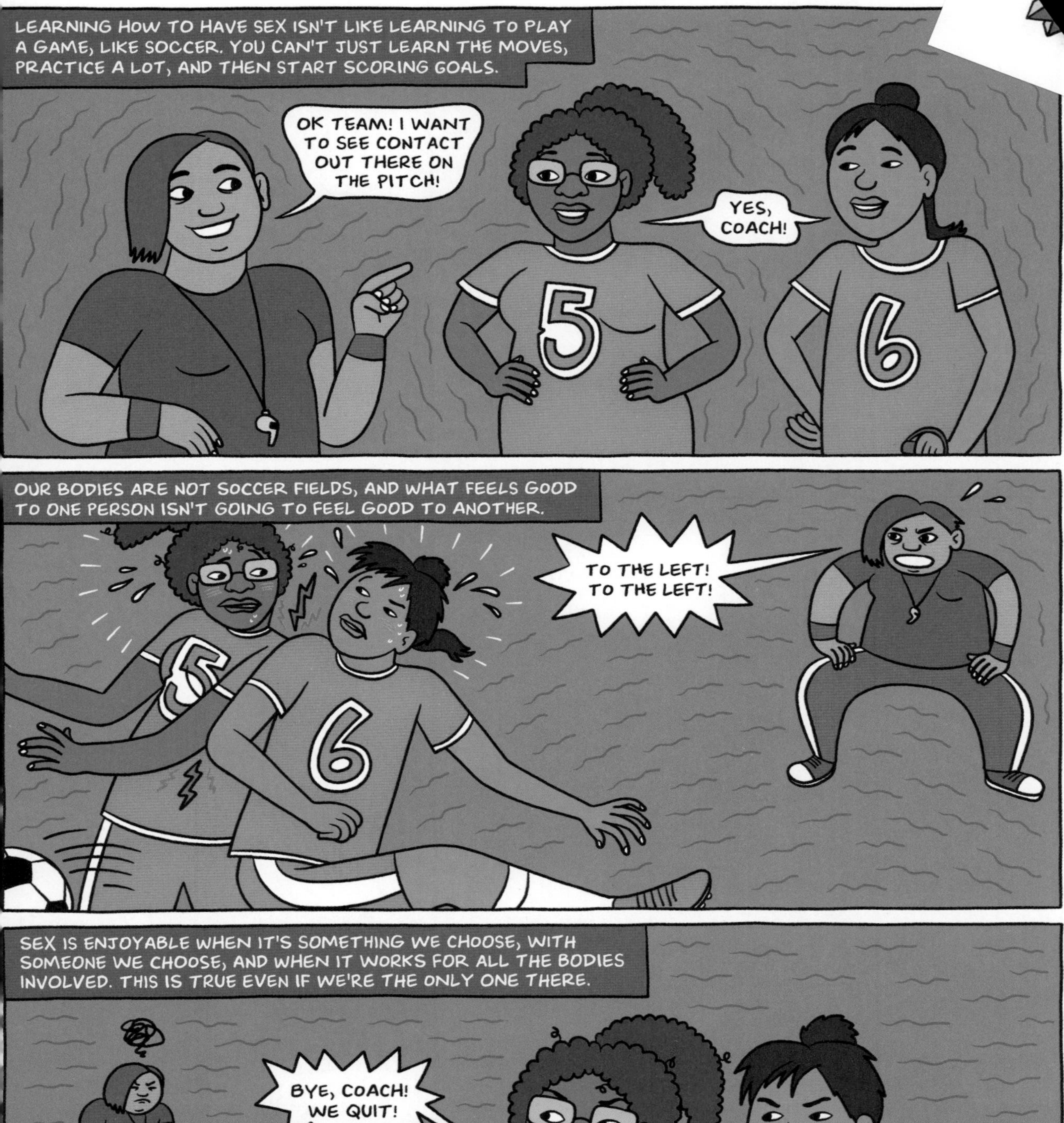
LEARNING HOW TO HAVE SEX ISN'T LIKE LEARNING TO PLAY A GAME, LIKE SOCCER. YOU CAN'T JUST LEARN THE MOVES, PRACTICE A LOT, AND THEN START SCORING GOALS.
OK TEAM! I WANT TO SEE CONTACT OUT THERE ON THE PITCH!
YES, COACH!
5
6
OUR BODIES ARE NOT SOCCER FIELDS, AND WHAT FEELS GOOD TO ONE PERSON ISN'T GOING TO FEEL GOOD TO ANOTHER.
TO THE LEFT! TO THE LEFT!
5
6
SEX IS ENJOYABLE WHEN IT'S SOMETHING WE CHOOSE, WITH SOMEONE WE CHOOSE, AND WHEN IT WORKS FOR ALL THE BODIES INVOLVED. THIS IS TRUE EVEN IF WE'RE THE ONLY ONE THERE.
BYE, COACH! WE QUIT!
5
6

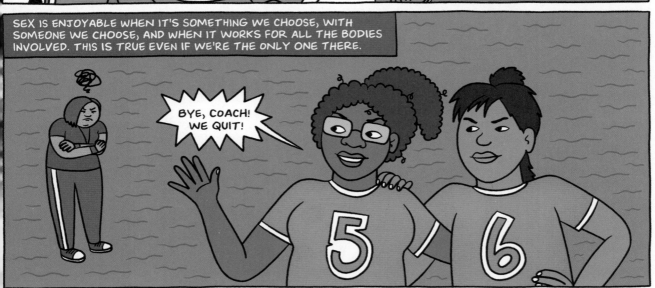

NERD ALERT IS SEX A GAME?

SOME PEOPLE ACT LIKE SEX IS A GAME WITH WINNERS AND LOSERS. THEY TALK ABOUT HOW FAR THEY GOT. THEY TALK ABOUT "SCORING." THEY TALK ABOUT SEX LIKE IT'S A COMPETITION, AND THE PERSON WITH THE MOST POINTS WINS.

TREATING SEX LIKE IT'S A COMPETITION CREATES A LOT OF PRESSURE: PRESSURE TO KNOW THE RULES, AND PRESSURE TO WIN. ALL THAT PRESSURE MAKES GETTING AND GIVING CONSENT HARDER.*

WHEN WE'RE YOUNGER IT CAN FEEL LIKE EVERYONE THINKS THIS WAY, AND THE ONLY CHOICE YOU HAVE IS TO PLAY OR BE LEFT OUT.

AS WE GET OLDER, WE DISCOVER THAT NOT EVERYONE TREATS SEX LIKE A GAME. FOR SOME PEOPLE SEX IS MORE LIKE A DANCE, OR A RELATIONSHIP, OR A CEREMONY.

BUT IF WE DO THINK OF SEX AS A GAME, IT'S IMPORTANT TO REMEMBER THAT WE SHOULD ONLY PLAY WITH PEOPLE WHO WANT TO PLAY WITH US, AND WE SHOULD COME UP WITH THE RULES TOGETHER. WE SHOULDN'T TRY TO TRICK PEOPLE INTO EXPLORING SEX.

IF WE WANT TO EXPLORE IT, WE CAN FIND SOMEONE WHO WANTS TO EXPLORE IT WITH US.

IF SOMEONE DOESN'T WANT TO PLAY WITH YOU, DON'T TRY TO PLAY WITH THEM.

HAVING SEX THAT INCLUDES TRUST, RESPECT, JUSTICE, JOY, AND CHOICE MEANS FINDING OUT HOW THE PERSON YOU WANT TO DO IT WITH FEELS ABOUT IT. IF THEY THINK IT'S A GAME, WHAT ARE THEIR RULES FOR PLAYING?

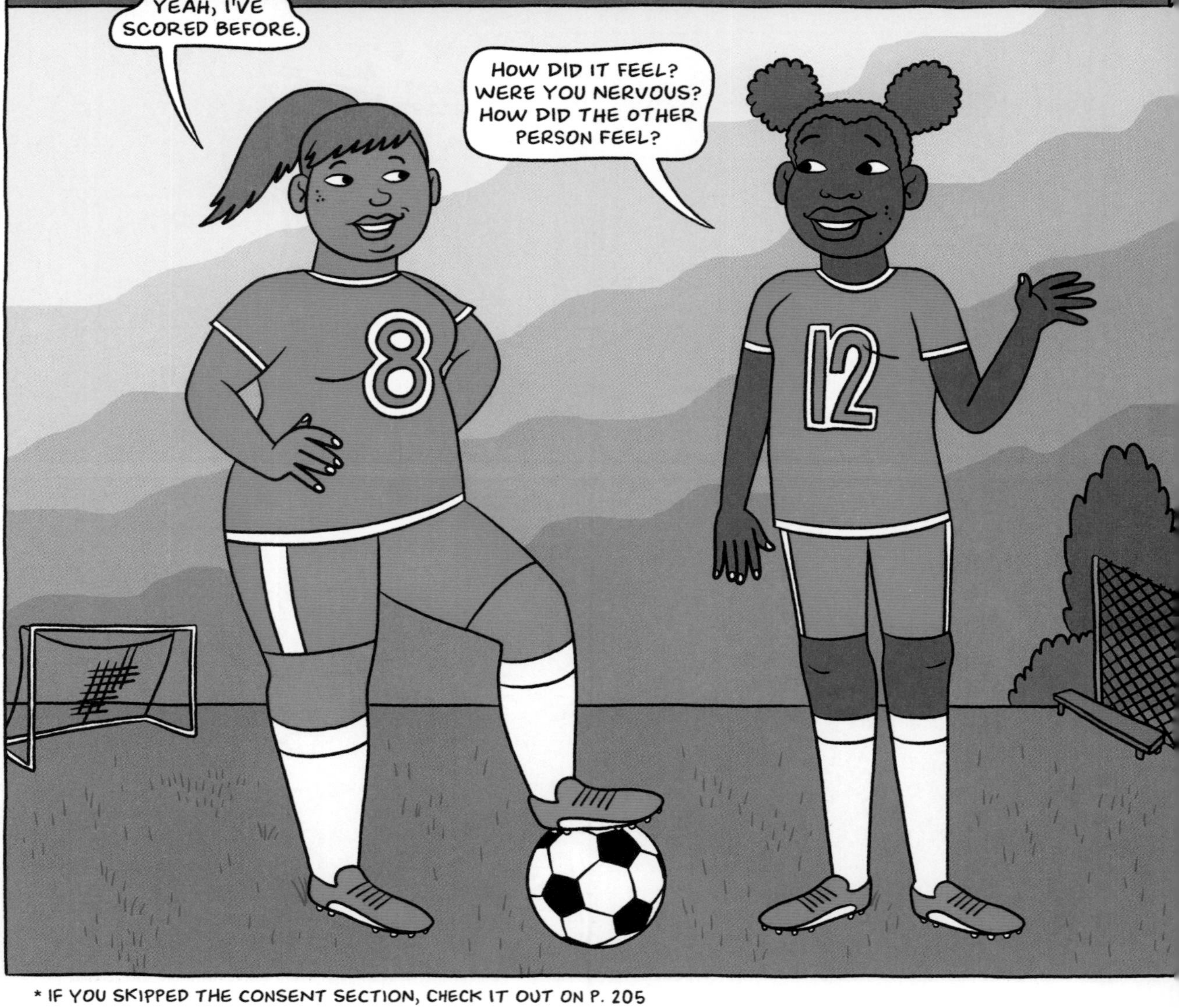
YEAH, I'VE SCORED BEFORE.
HOW DID IT FEEL? WERE YOU NERVOUS? HOW DID THE OTHER PERSON FEEL?

* IF YOU SKIPPED THE CONSENT SECTION, CHECK IT OUT ON P. 205

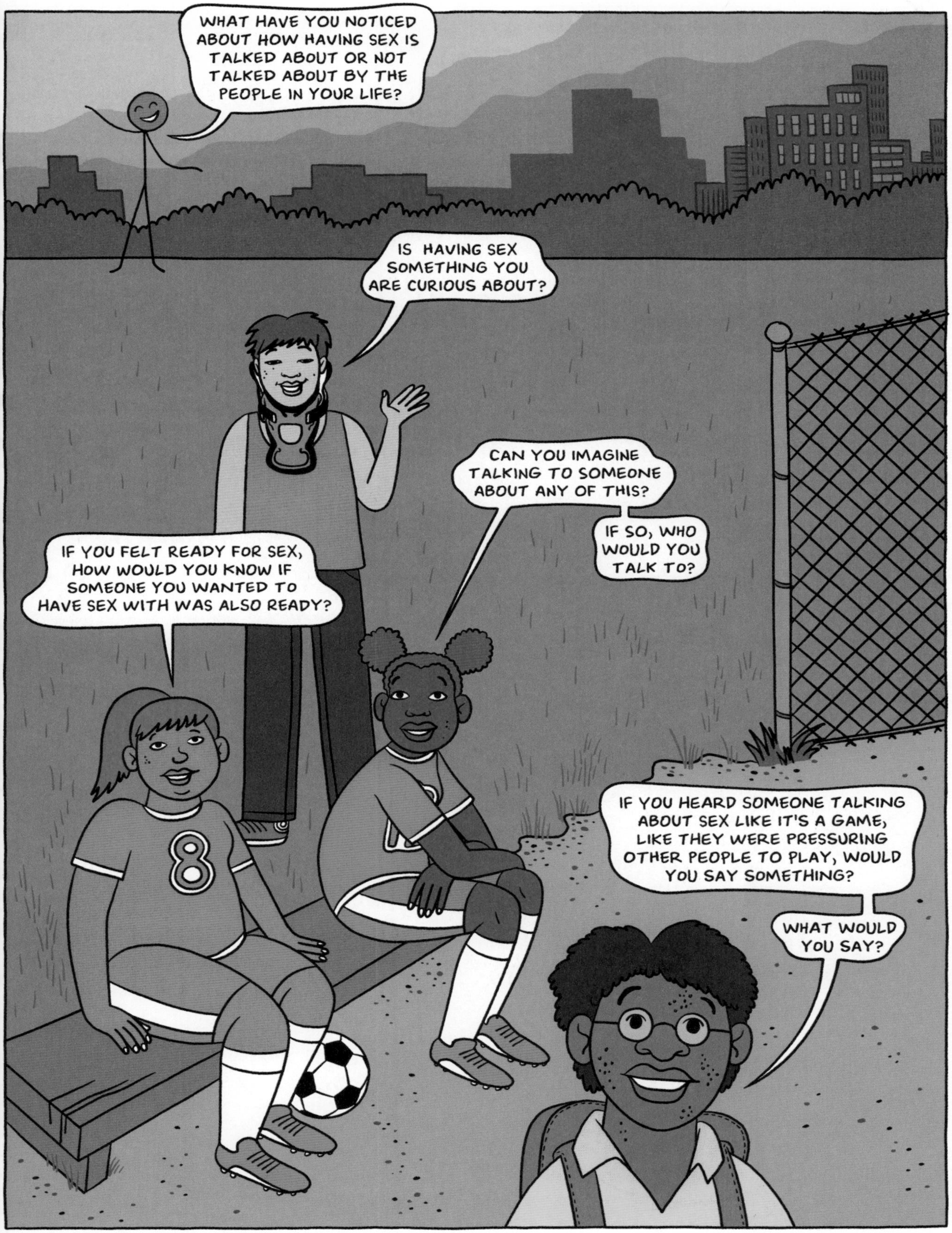
WHAT HAVE YOU NOTICED ABOUT HOW HAVING SEX IS TALKED ABOUT OR NOT TALKED ABOUT BY THE PEOPLE IN YOUR LIFE?
IS HAVING SEX SOMETHING YOU ARE CURIOUS ABOUT?
CAN YOU IMAGINE TALKING TO SOMEONE ABOUT ANY OF THIS?
IF SO, WHO WOULD YOU TALK TO?
IF YOU FELT READY FOR SEX, HOW WOULD YOU KNOW IF SOMEONE YOU WANTED TO HAVE SEX WITH WAS ALSO READY?
IF YOU HEARD SOMEONE TALKING ABOUT SEX LIKE IT'S A GAME, LIKE THEY WERE PRESSURING OTHER PEOPLE TO PLAY, WOULD YOU SAY SOMETHING?
WHAT WOULD YOU SAY?

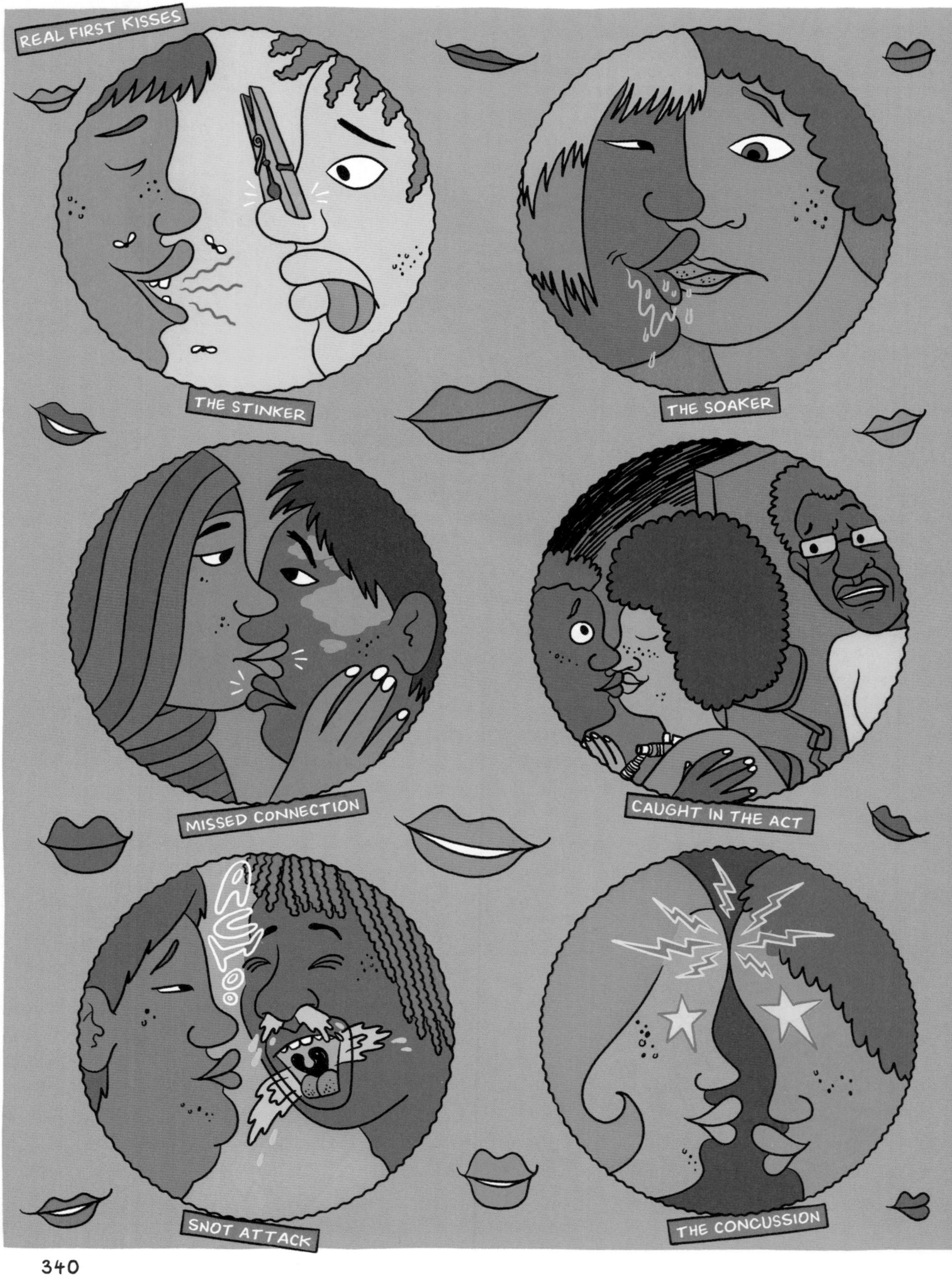
REAL FIRST KISSES
THE STINKER
THE SOAKER
MISSED CONNECTION
CAUGHT IN THE ACT
ACHOO
SNOT ATTACK
THE CONCUSSION

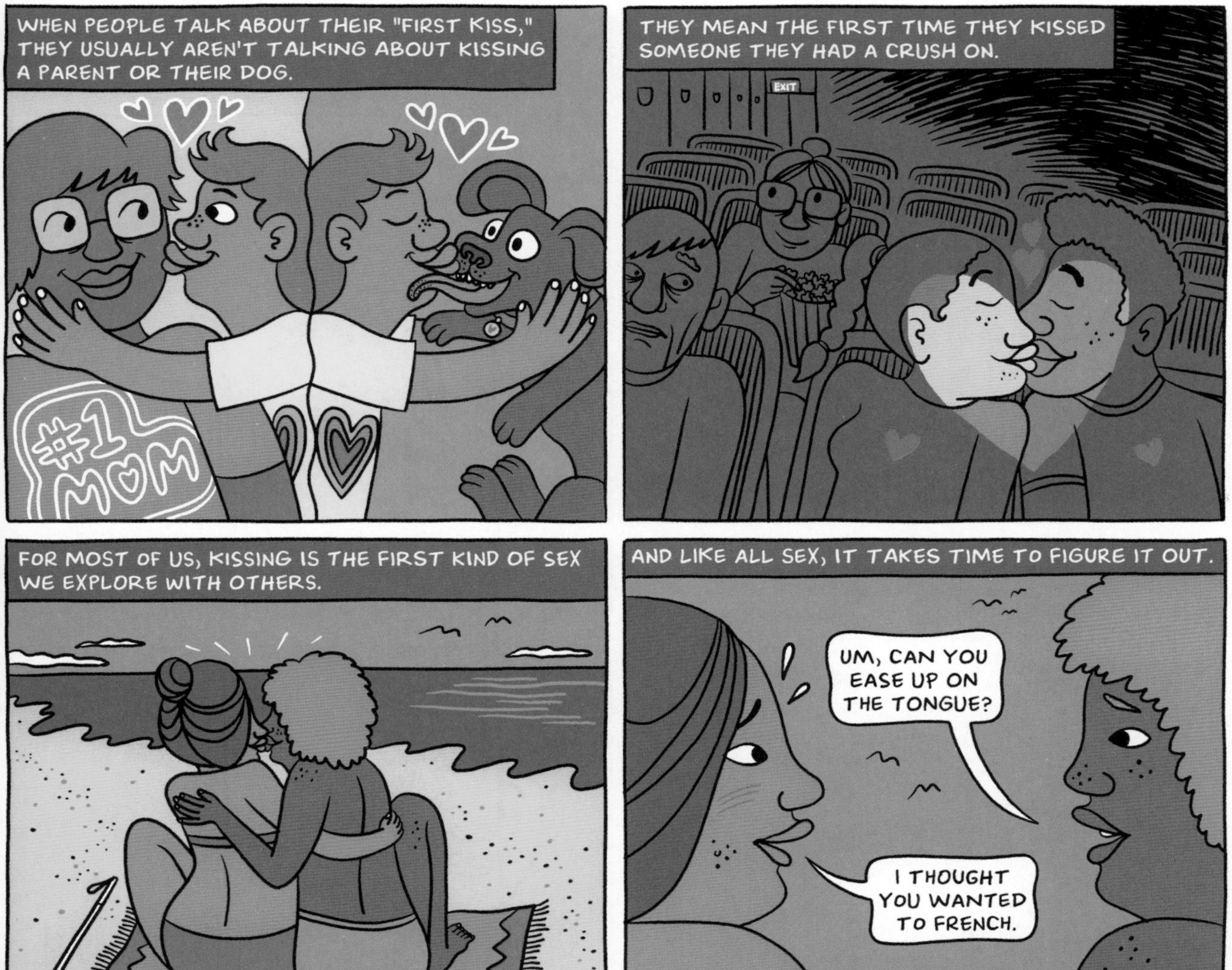
WHEN PEOPLE TALK ABOUT THEIR "FIRST KISS," THEY USUALLY AREN'T TALKING ABOUT KISSING A PARENT OR THEIR DOG.
#1 MOM
THEY MEAN THE FIRST TIME THEY KISSED SOMEONE THEY HAD A CRUSH ON.
EXIT
FOR MOST OF US, KISSING IS THE FIRST KIND OF SEX WE EXPLORE WITH OTHERS.
AND LIKE ALL SEX, IT TAKES TIME TO FIGURE IT OUT.
UM, CAN YOU EASE UP ON THE TONGUE?
I THOUGHT YOU WANTED TO FRENCH.
SOME PEOPLE PRACTICE KISSING ON THEMSELVES, SOME PEOPLE PRACTICE WITH A FRIEND.
SMACK
EXCEPT ONCE YOU START "PRACTICING" WITH SOMEONE, THEN AREN'T YOU BASICALLY DOING IT?
SO, ARE WE LIKE DATING NOW?

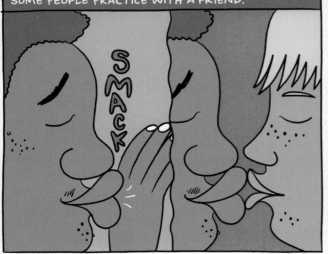

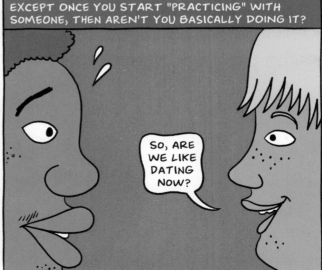

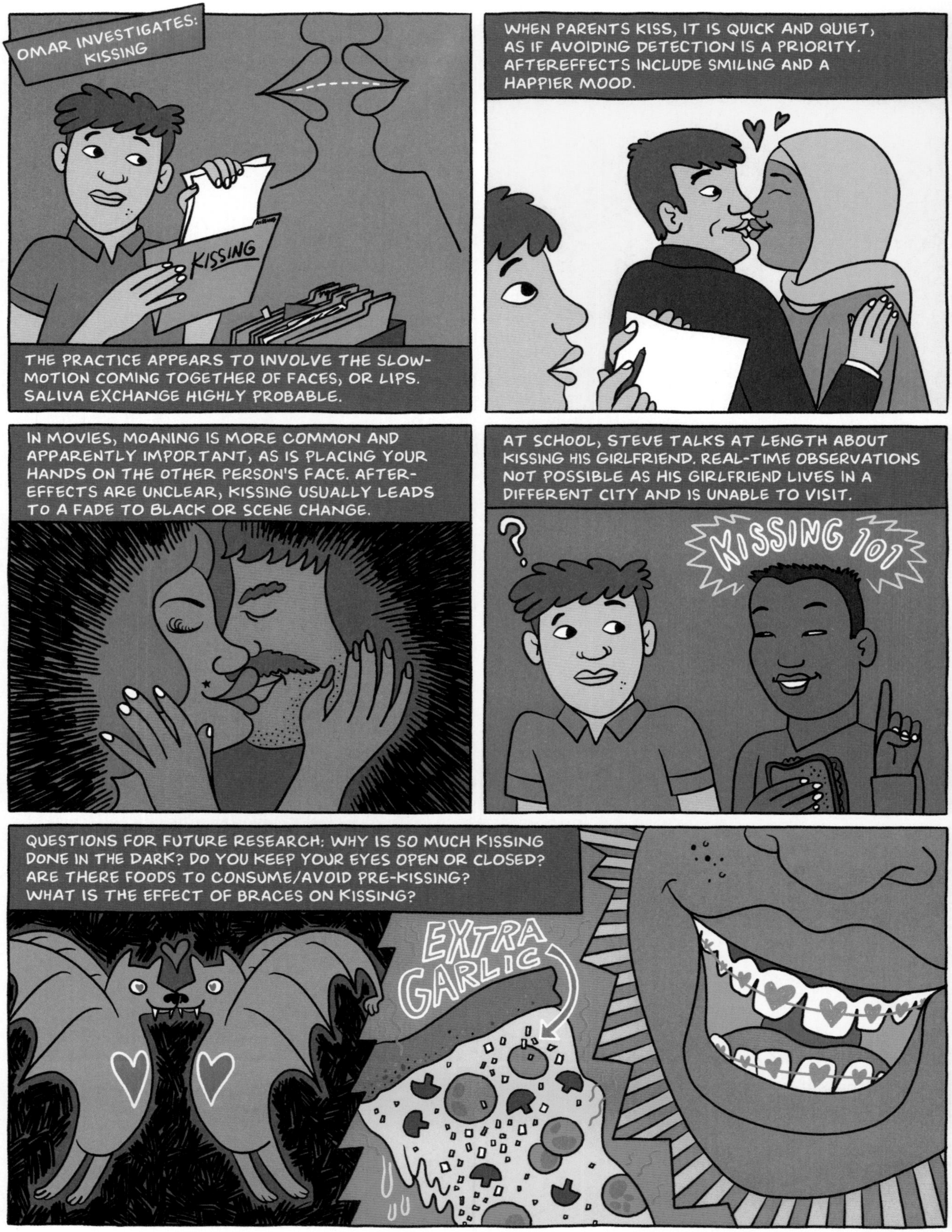
OMAR INVESTIGATES: KISSING
KISSING
THE PRACTICE APPEARS TO INVOLVE THE SLOW-MOTION COMING TOGETHER OF FACES, OR LIPS. SALIVA EXCHANGE HIGHLY PROBABLE.
WHEN PARENTS KISS, IT IS QUICK AND QUIET, AS IF AVOIDING DETECTION IS A PRIORITY. AFTEREFFECTS INCLUDE SMILING AND A HAPPIER MOOD.
IN MOVIES, MOANING IS MORE COMMON AND APPARENTLY IMPORTANT, AS IS PLACING YOUR HANDS ON THE OTHER PERSON'S FACE. AFTER-EFFECTS ARE UNCLEAR, KISSING USUALLY LEADS TO A FADE TO BLACK OR SCENE CHANGE.
AT SCHOOL, STEVE TALKS AT LENGTH ABOUT KISSING HIS GIRLFRIEND. REAL-TIME OBSERVATIONS NOT POSSIBLE AS HIS GIRLFRIEND LIVES IN A DIFFERENT CITY AND IS UNABLE TO VISIT.
?
KISSING 101
QUESTIONS FOR FUTURE RESEARCH: WHY IS SO MUCH KISSING DONE IN THE DARK? DO YOU KEEP YOUR EYES OPEN OR CLOSED? ARE THERE FOODS TO CONSUME/AVOID PRE-KISSING? WHAT IS THE EFFECT OF BRACES ON KISSING?
EXTRA GARLIC

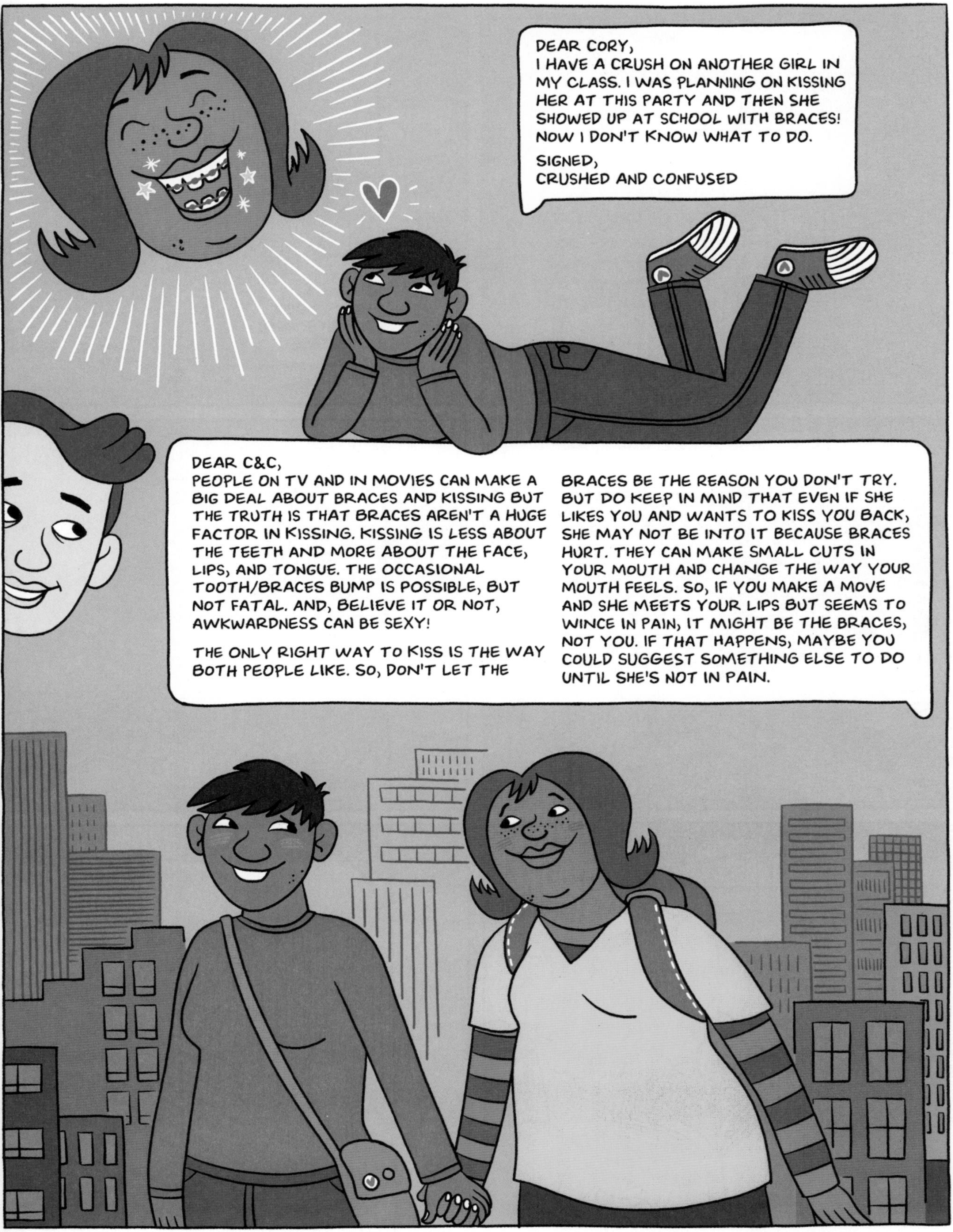
DEAR CORY,
I HAVE A CRUSH ON ANOTHER GIRL IN MY CLASS. I WAS PLANNING ON KISSING HER AT THIS PARTY AND THEN SHE SHOWED UP AT SCHOOL WITH BRACES! NOW I DON'T KNOW WHAT TO DO.
SIGNED,
CRUSHED AND CONFUSED
DEAR C&C,
PEOPLE ON TV AND IN MOVIES CAN MAKE A BIG DEAL ABOUT BRACES AND KISSING BUT THE TRUTH IS THAT BRACES AREN'T A HUGE FACTOR IN KISSING. KISSING IS LESS ABOUT THE TEETH AND MORE ABOUT THE FACE, LIPS, AND TONGUE. THE OCCASIONAL TOOTH/BRACES BUMP IS POSSIBLE, BUT NOT FATAL. AND, BELIEVE IT OR NOT, AWKWARDNESS CAN BE SEXY!
THE ONLY RIGHT WAY TO KISS IS THE WAY BOTH PEOPLE LIKE. SO, DON'T LET THE BRACES BE THE REASON YOU DON'T TRY. BUT DO KEEP IN MIND THAT EVEN IF SHE LIKES YOU AND WANTS TO KISS YOU BACK, SHE MAY NOT BE INTO IT BECAUSE BRACES HURT. THEY CAN MAKE SMALL CUTS IN YOUR MOUTH AND CHANGE THE WAY YOUR MOUTH FEELS. SO, IF YOU MAKE A MOVE AND SHE MEETS YOUR LIPS BUT SEEMS TO WINCE IN PAIN, IT MIGHT BE THE BRACES, NOT YOU. IF THAT HAPPENS, MAYBE YOU COULD SUGGEST SOMETHING ELSE TO DO UNTIL SHE'S NOT IN PAIN.

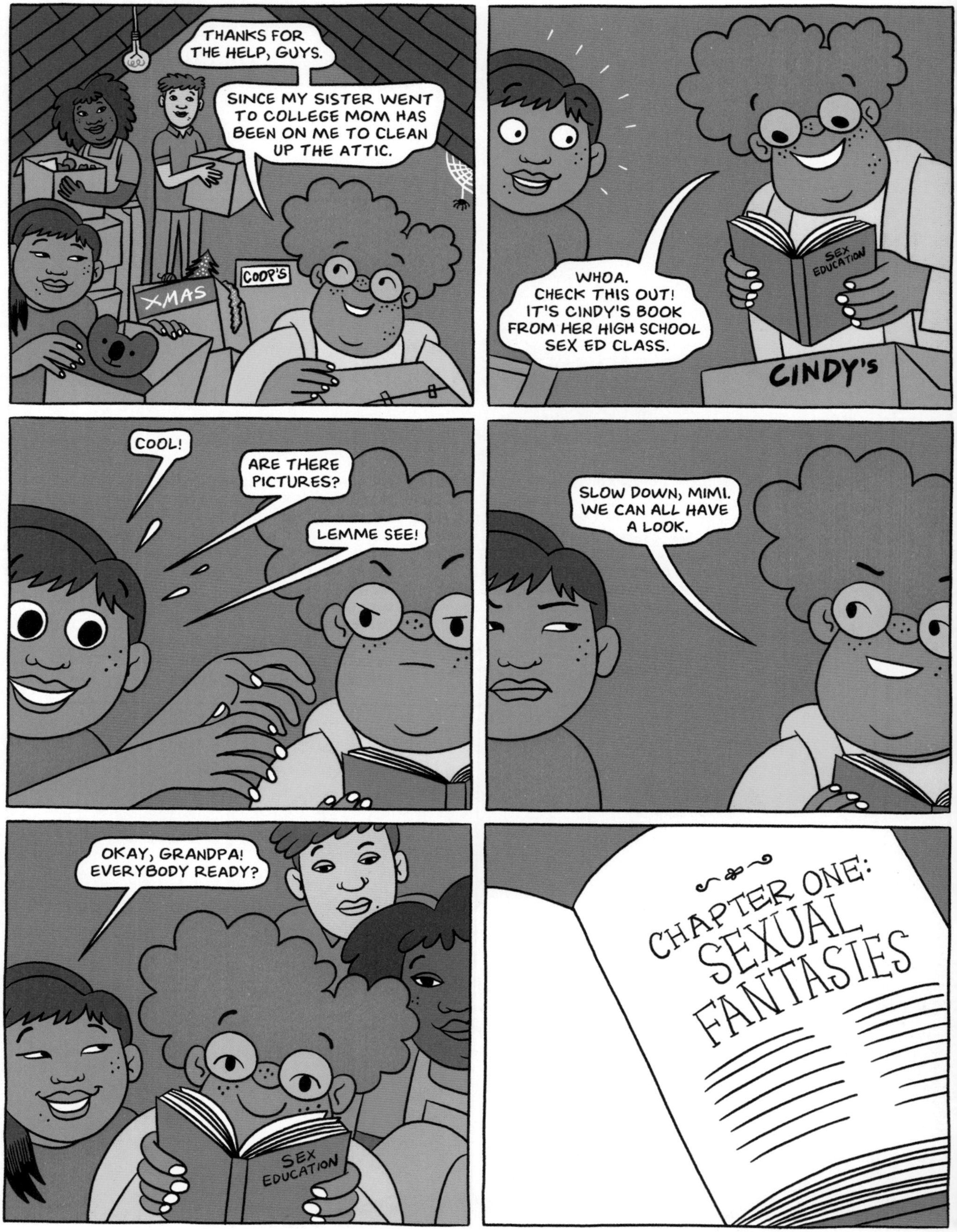
THANKS FOR THE HELP, GUYS.
SINCE MY SISTER WENT TO COLLEGE MOM HAS BEEN ON ME TO CLEAN UP THE ATTIC.
XMAS
COOP'S
WHOA. CHECK THIS OUT! IT'S CINDY'S BOOK FROM HER HIGH SCHOOL SEX ED CLASS.
SEX EDUCATION
CINDY's
COOL!
ARE THERE PICTURES?
LEMME SEE!
SLOW DOWN, MIMI. WE CAN ALL HAVE A LOOK.
OKAY, GRANDPA! EVERYBODY READY?
SEX EDUCATION
CHAPTER ONE: SEXUAL FANTASIES

SEXUAL FANTASIES

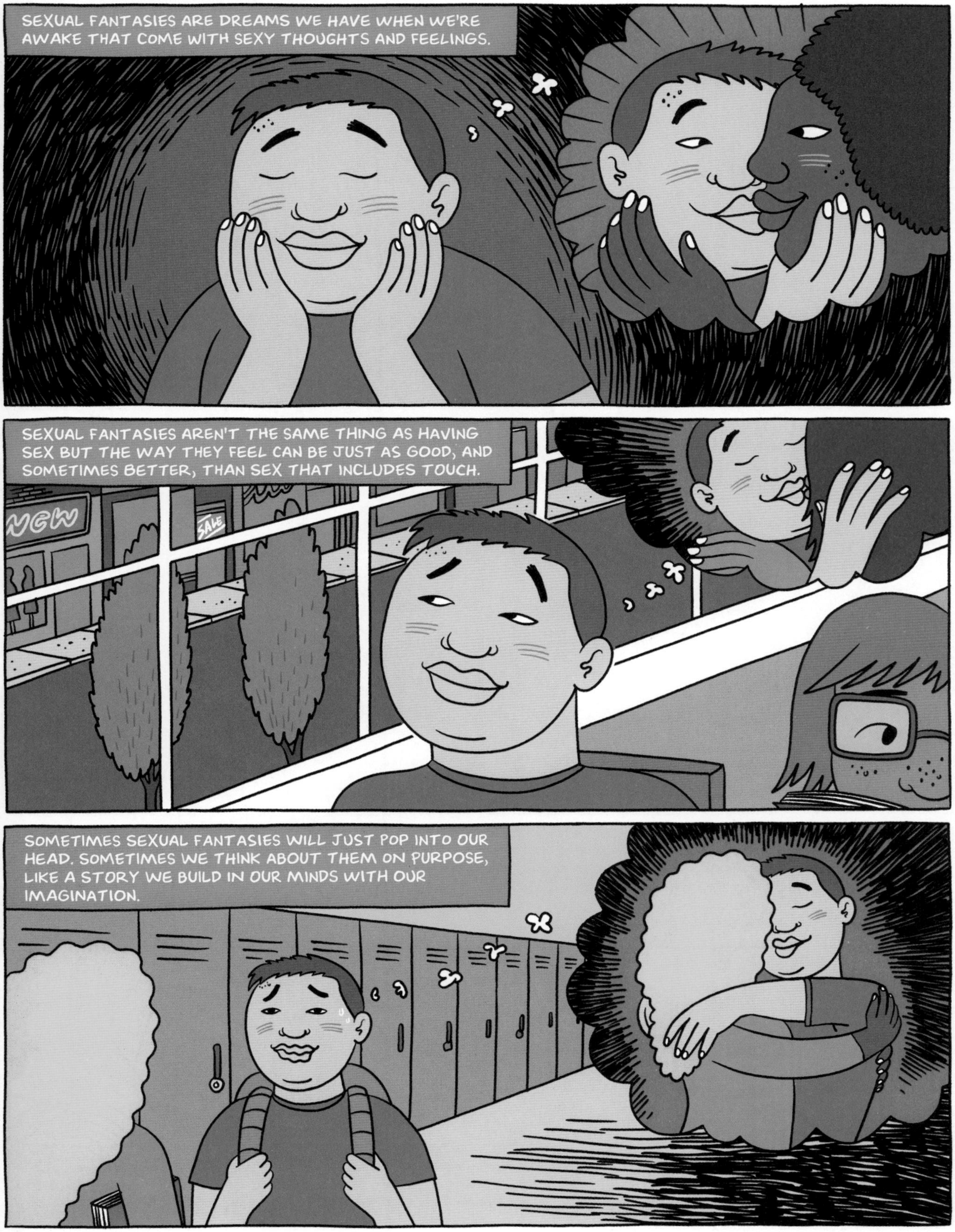

SEXUAL FANTASIES ARE DREAMS WE HAVE WHEN WE'RE AWAKE THAT COME WITH SEXY THOUGHTS AND FEELINGS.
SEXUAL FANTASIES AREN'T THE SAME THING AS HAVING SEX BUT THE WAY THEY FEEL CAN BE JUST AS GOOD, AND SOMETIMES BETTER, THAN SEX THAT INCLUDES TOUCH.
NEW
SALE
SOMETIMES SEXUAL FANTASIES WILL JUST POP INTO OUR HEAD. SOMETIMES WE THINK ABOUT THEM ON PURPOSE, LIKE A STORY WE BUILD IN OUR MINDS WITH OUR IMAGINATION.

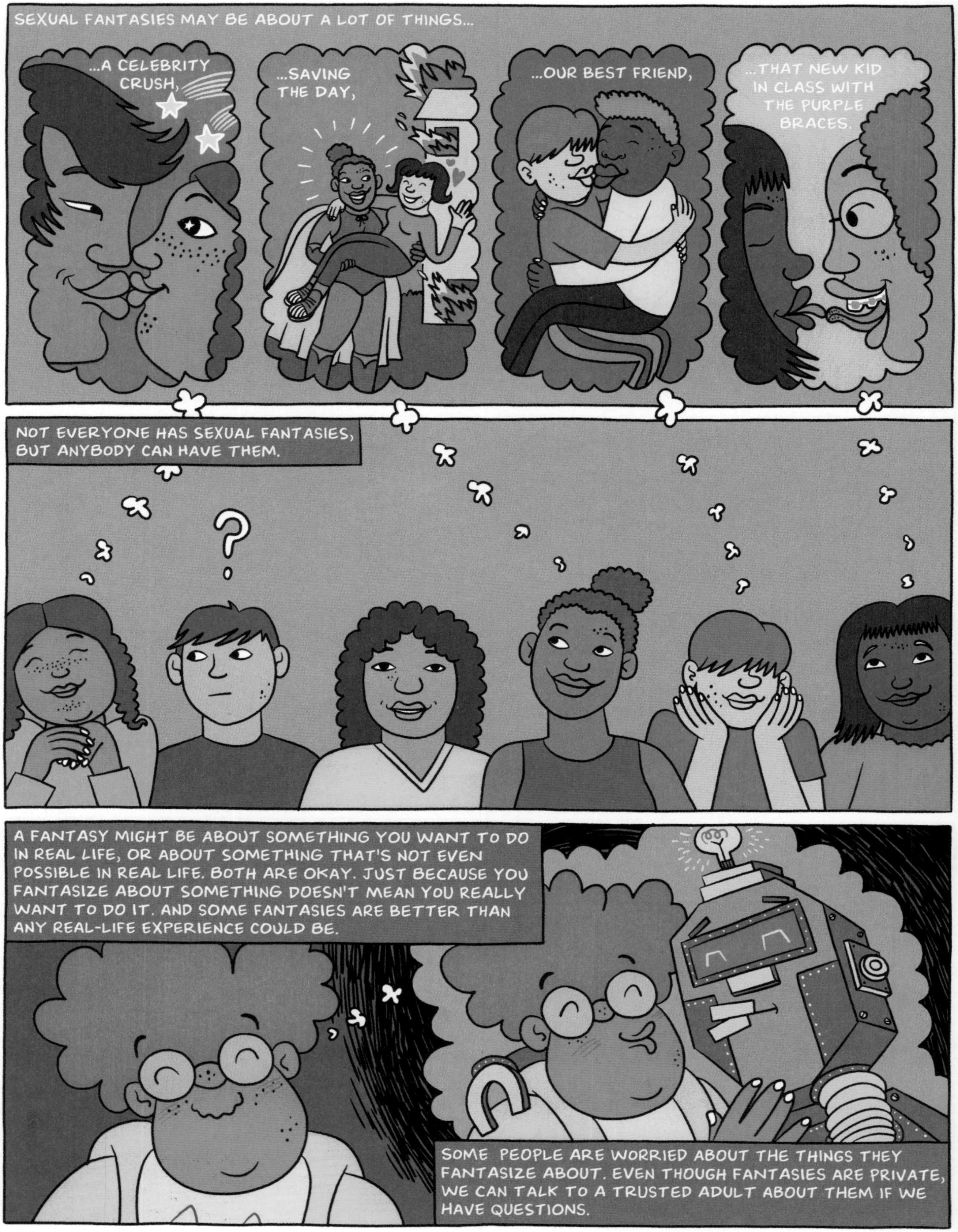
SEXUAL FANTASIES MAY BE ABOUT A LOT OF THINGS...
...A CELEBRITY CRUSH,
...SAVING THE DAY,
...OUR BEST FRIEND,
...THAT NEW KID IN CLASS WITH THE PURPLE BRACES.
NOT EVERYONE HAS SEXUAL FANTASIES, BUT ANYBODY CAN HAVE THEM.
A FANTASY MIGHT BE ABOUT SOMETHING YOU WANT TO DO IN REAL LIFE, OR ABOUT SOMETHING THAT'S NOT EVEN POSSIBLE IN REAL LIFE. BOTH ARE OKAY. JUST BECAUSE YOU FANTASIZE ABOUT SOMETHING DOESN'T MEAN YOU REALLY WANT TO DO IT. AND SOME FANTASIES ARE BETTER THAN ANY REAL-LIFE EXPERIENCE COULD BE.
SOME PEOPLE ARE WORRIED ABOUT THE THINGS THEY FANTASIZE ABOUT. EVEN THOUGH FANTASIES ARE PRIVATE, WE CAN TALK TO A TRUSTED ADULT ABOUT THEM IF WE HAVE QUESTIONS.

MASTURBATION

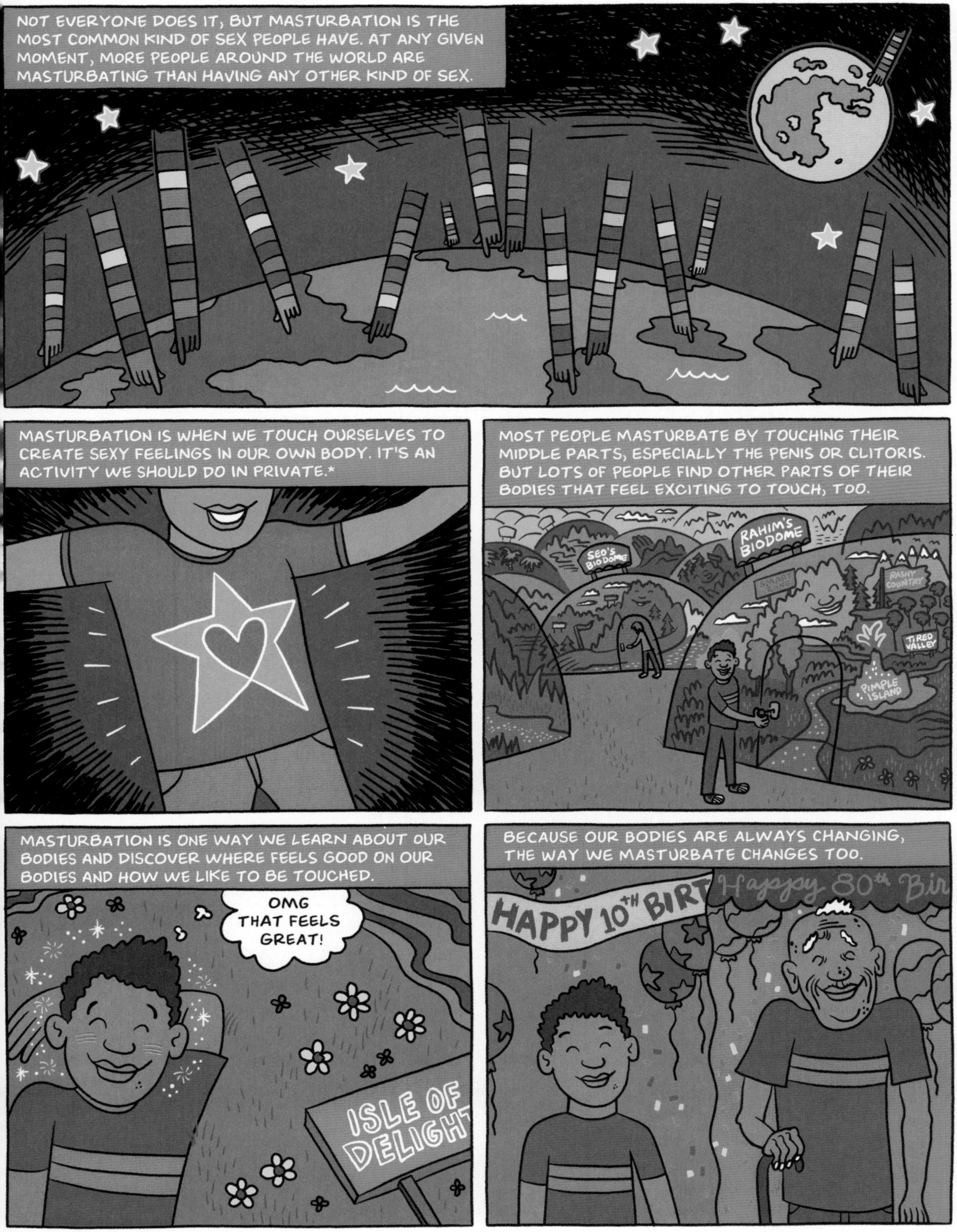
NOT EVERYONE DOES IT, BUT MASTURBATION IS THE MOST COMMON KIND OF SEX PEOPLE HAVE. AT ANY GIVEN MOMENT, MORE PEOPLE AROUND THE WORLD ARE MASTURBATING THAN HAVING ANY OTHER KIND OF SEX.
MASTURBATION IS WHEN WE TOUCH OURSELVES TO CREATE SEXY FEELINGS IN OUR OWN BODY. IT'S AN ACTIVITY WE SHOULD DO IN PRIVATE.*
MOST PEOPLE MASTURBATE BY TOUCHING THEIR MIDDLE PARTS, ESPECIALLY THE PENIS OR CLITORIS. BUT LOTS OF PEOPLE FIND OTHER PARTS OF THEIR BODIES THAT FEEL EXCITING TO TOUCH, TOO.
SEO'S BIODOME
RAHIM'S BIODOME
RASHY COUNTRY
TIRED VALLEY
PIMPLE ISLAND
MASTURBATION IS ONE WAY WE LEARN ABOUT OUR BODIES AND DISCOVER WHERE FEELS GOOD ON OUR BODIES AND HOW WE LIKE TO BE TOUCHED.
OMG THAT FEELS GREAT!
ISLE OF DELIGHT
BECAUSE OUR BODIES ARE ALWAYS CHANGING, THE WAY WE MASTURBATE CHANGES TOO.
HAPPY 10TH BIRT
Happy 80th Bir

* READ MORE ABOUT PRIVACY ON P. 80

SEX THROUGH TEXTS (AND MORE)

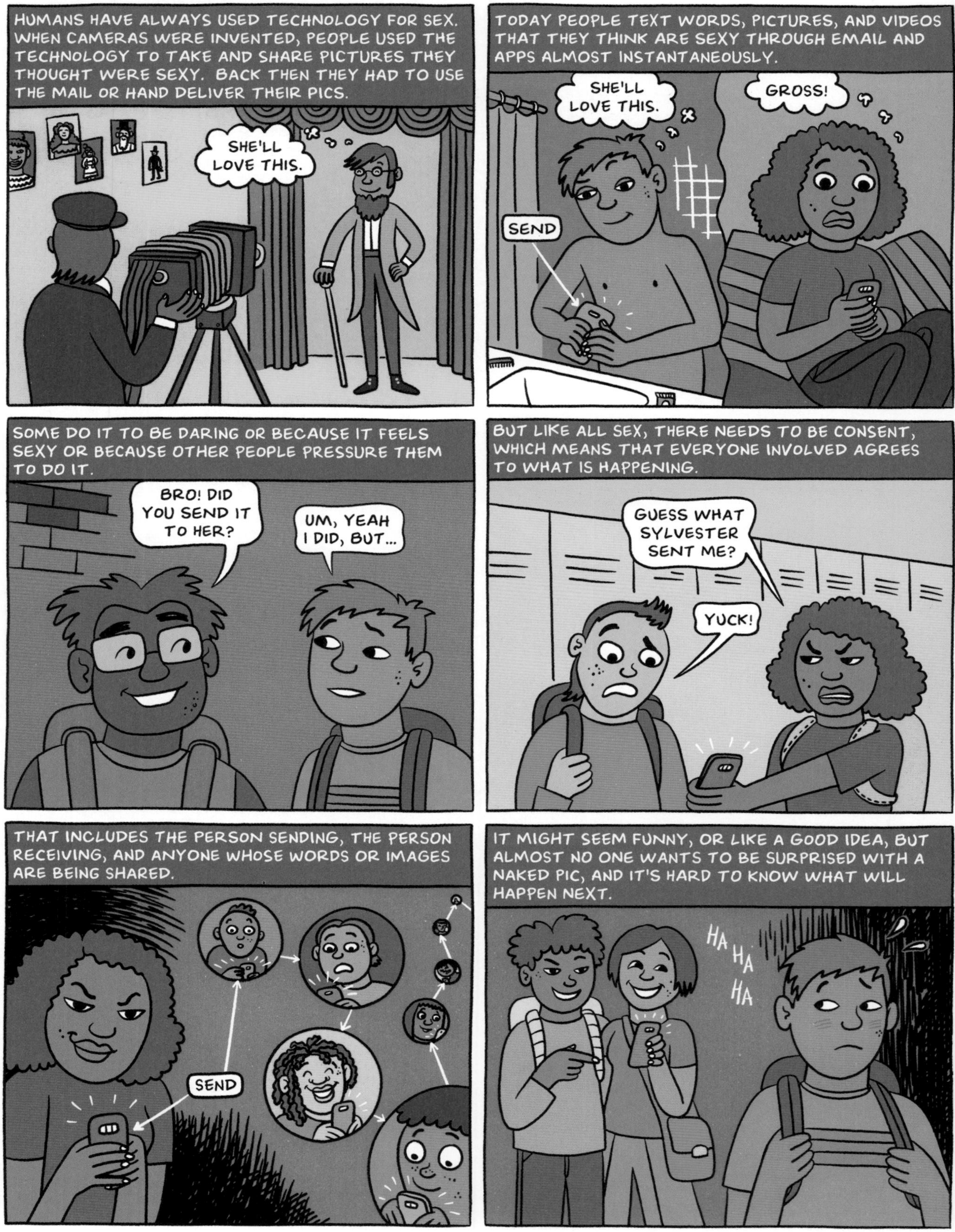
HUMANS HAVE ALWAYS USED TECHNOLOGY FOR SEX. WHEN CAMERAS WERE INVENTED, PEOPLE USED THE TECHNOLOGY TO TAKE AND SHARE PICTURES THEY THOUGHT WERE SEXY. BACK THEN THEY HAD TO USE THE MAIL OR HAND DELIVER THEIR PICS.
SHE'LL LOVE THIS.
TODAY PEOPLE TEXT WORDS, PICTURES, AND VIDEOS THAT THEY THINK ARE SEXY THROUGH EMAIL AND APPS ALMOST INSTANTANEOUSLY.
SHE'LL LOVE THIS.
SEND
GROSS!
SOME DO IT TO BE DARING OR BECAUSE IT FEELS SEXY OR BECAUSE OTHER PEOPLE PRESSURE THEM TO DO IT.
BRO! DID YOU SEND IT TO HER?
UM, YEAH I DID, BUT...
BUT LIKE ALL SEX, THERE NEEDS TO BE CONSENT, WHICH MEANS THAT EVERYONE INVOLVED AGREES TO WHAT IS HAPPENING.
GUESS WHAT SYLVESTER SENT ME?
YUCK!
THAT INCLUDES THE PERSON SENDING, THE PERSON RECEIVING, AND ANYONE WHOSE WORDS OR IMAGES ARE BEING SHARED.
SEND
IT MIGHT SEEM FUNNY, OR LIKE A GOOD IDEA, BUT ALMOST NO ONE WANTS TO BE SURPRISED WITH A NAKED PIC, AND IT'S HARD TO KNOW WHAT WILL HAPPEN NEXT.
HA HA HA HA

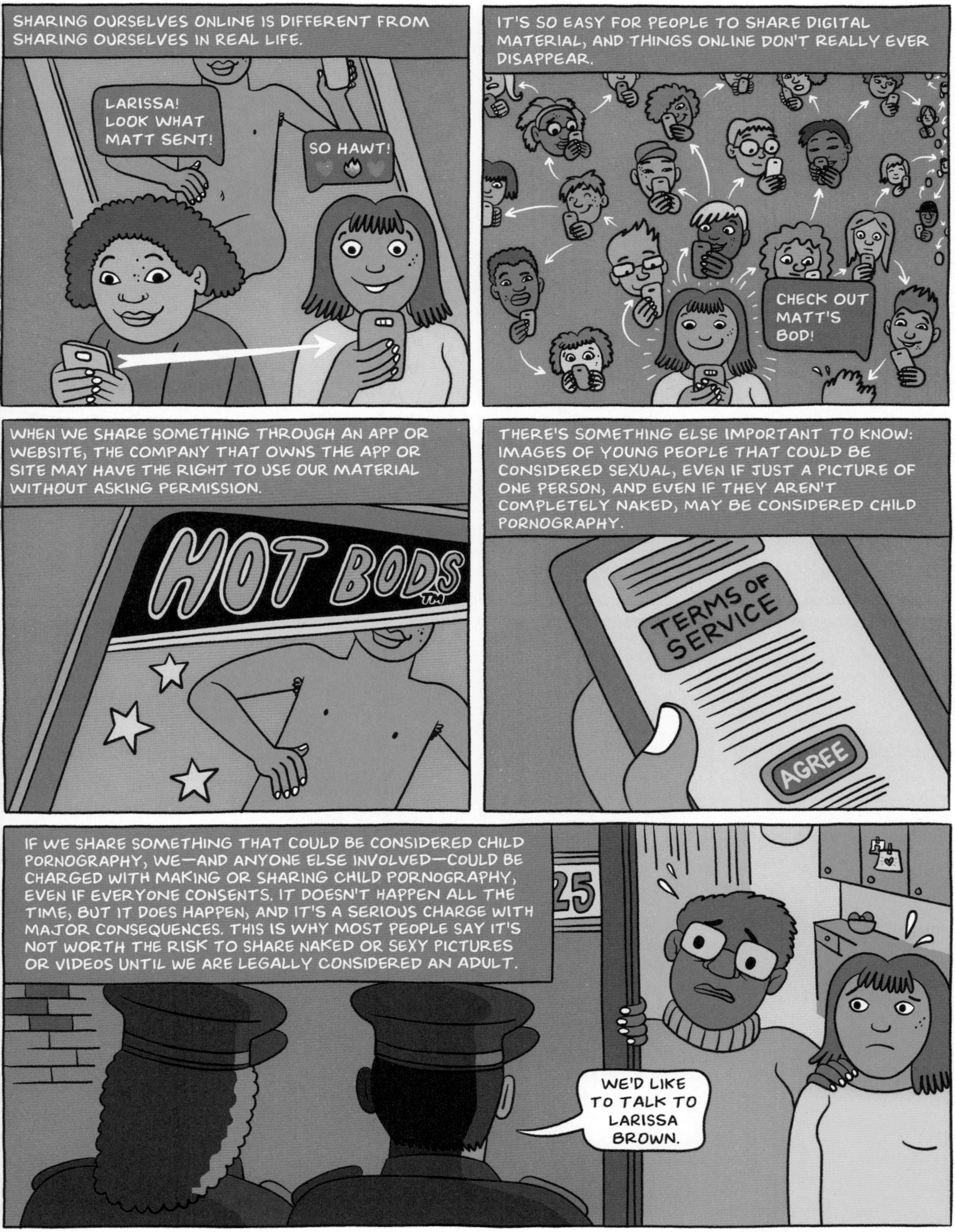
SHARING OURSELVES ONLINE IS DIFFERENT FROM SHARING OURSELVES IN REAL LIFE.
LARISSA! LOOK WHAT MATT SENT!
SO HAWT!
IT'S SO EASY FOR PEOPLE TO SHARE DIGITAL MATERIAL, AND THINGS ONLINE DON'T REALLY EVER DISAPPEAR.
CHECK OUT MATT'S BOD!
WHEN WE SHARE SOMETHING THROUGH AN APP OR WEBSITE, THE COMPANY THAT OWNS THE APP OR SITE MAY HAVE THE RIGHT TO USE OUR MATERIAL WITHOUT ASKING PERMISSION.
HOT BODS TM
THERE'S SOMETHING ELSE IMPORTANT TO KNOW: IMAGES OF YOUNG PEOPLE THAT COULD BE CONSIDERED SEXUAL, EVEN IF JUST A PICTURE OF ONE PERSON, AND EVEN IF THEY AREN'T COMPLETELY NAKED, MAY BE CONSIDERED CHILD PORNOGRAPHY.
TERMS OF SERVICE
AGREE
IF WE SHARE SOMETHING THAT COULD BE CONSIDERED CHILD PORNOGRAPHY, WE—AND ANYONE ELSE INVOLVED—COULD BE CHARGED WITH MAKING OR SHARING CHILD PORNOGRAPHY, EVEN IF EVERYONE CONSENTS. IT DOESN'T HAPPEN ALL THE TIME, BUT IT DOES HAPPEN, AND IT'S A SERIOUS CHARGE WITH MAJOR CONSEQUENCES. THIS IS WHY MOST PEOPLE SAY IT'S NOT WORTH THE RISK TO SHARE NAKED OR SEXY PICTURES OR VIDEOS UNTIL WE ARE LEGALLY CONSIDERED AN ADULT.
25
WE'D LIKE TO TALK TO LARISSA BROWN.

THERE ARE LOTS OF WAYS PEOPLE DESCRIBE AND CATEGORIZE DIFFERENT KINDS OF SEX.

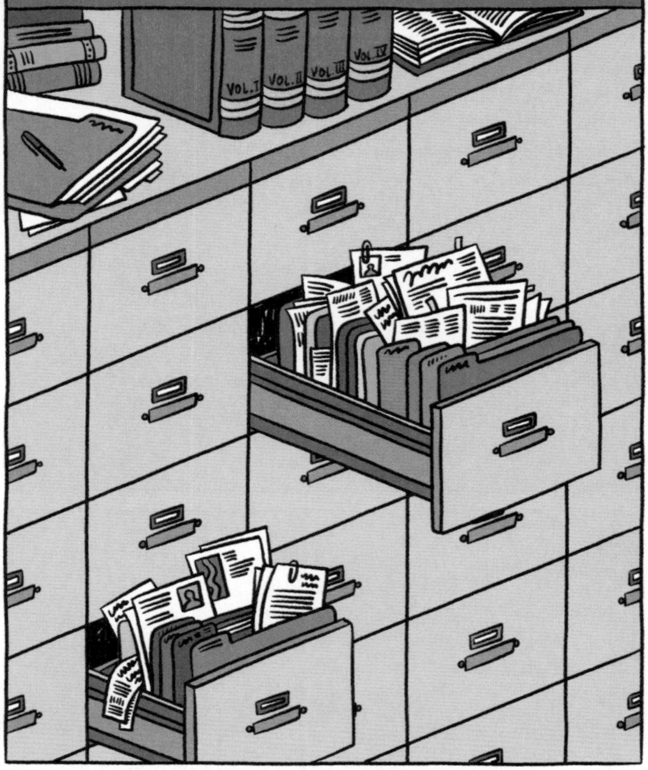
VOL. I
VOL. II
VOL. III
VOL. IV

ONE WAY IS BASED ON WHAT PARTS OF THE BODY ARE DOING MOST OF THE TOUCHING.

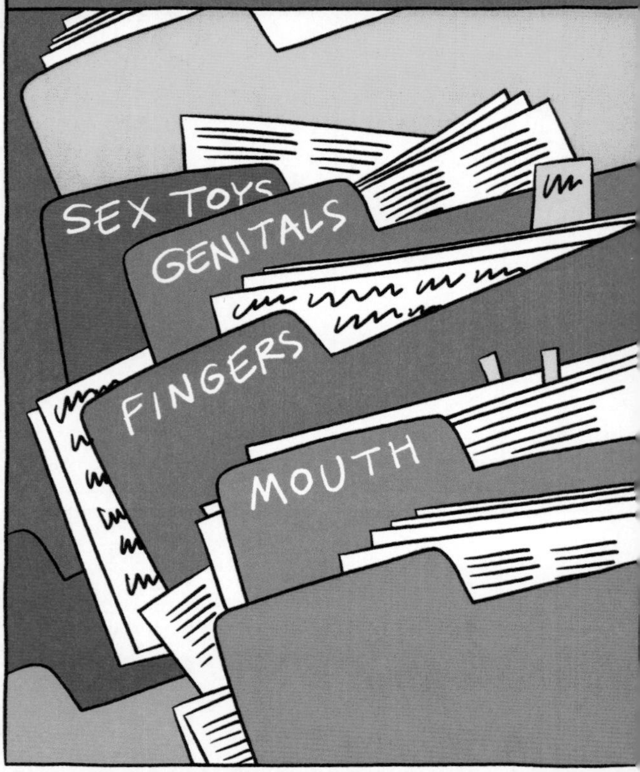
SEX TOYS
GENITALS
FINGERS
MOUTH

DIGITAL SEX INVOLVES USING FINGERS (A.K.A. DIGITS) AND HANDS TO TOUCH SOMEONE ELSE IN SEXY WAYS. SOME PEOPLE LIKE THE FEELING OF FINGERS GOING INSIDE A BODY PART—LIKE INSIDE THE VAGINA, OR INSIDE THE ANUS—AND MANY LIKE THE FEELING OF HANDS AND FINGERS TOUCHING THE OUTSIDE PARTS OF OUR BODIES.

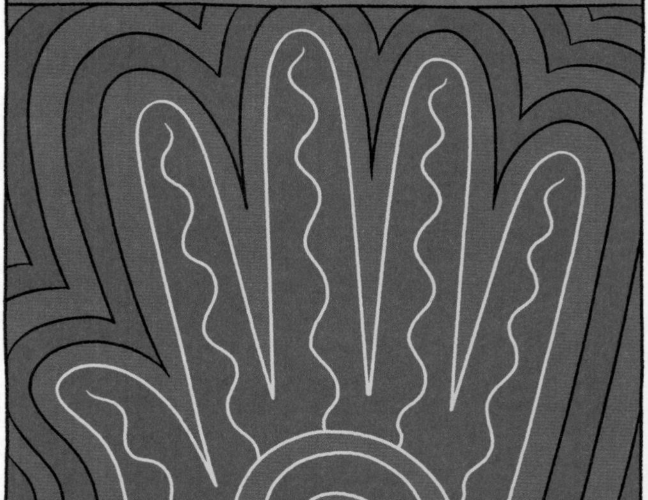

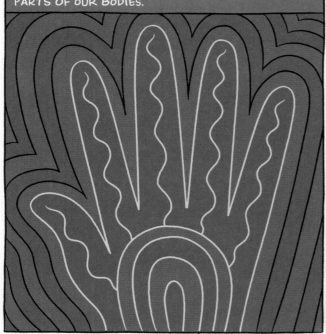

ORAL SEX INVOLVES USING MOUTHS AND TONGUES TO TOUCH AND STIMULATE SOMEONE ELSE'S BODY WHERE THEY FEEL MOST SENSITIVITY AND PLEASURE. USUALLY, ORAL SEX INCLUDES STIMULATING MIDDLE PARTS LIKE THE VULVA, CLITORIS, AND PENIS. BUT IT CAN INCLUDE ANY PART OF THE BODY THAT FEELS GOOD.

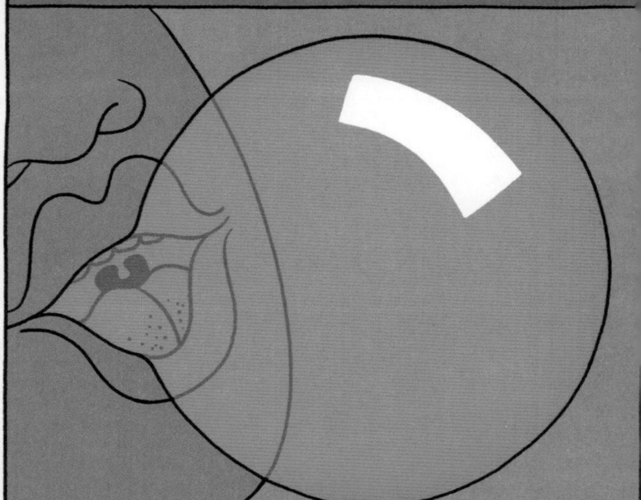

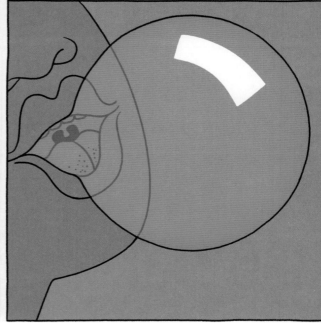

INTERCOURSE DESCRIBES SEX DURING WHICH PEOPLE FIT THEIR MIDDLE PARTS TOGETHER AND THEN MOVE AROUND IN WAYS THAT FEEL GOOD. THE KIND OF INTERCOURSE MOST PEOPLE LEARN ABOUT IS PENILE-VAGINAL INTERCOURSE, WHERE A PENIS AND VAGINA FIT TOGETHER. THIS IS ALSO THE KIND OF SEX THAT CAN LEAD TO MAKING A BABY (MORE ON THAT ON P. 295).

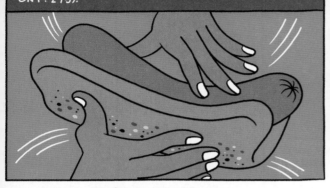

ANAL INTERCOURSE (ALSO CALLED ANAL SEX) IS SEX THAT INVOLVES FITTING MIDDLE PARTS AND AN ANUS TOGETHER, AND THEN MOVING BOTH BODIES IN WAYS THAT FEEL GOOD. EVEN THOUGH IT'S CALLED INTERCOURSE, THIS KIND OF SEX, ON ITS OWN, CANNOT LEAD TO MAKING A BABY.

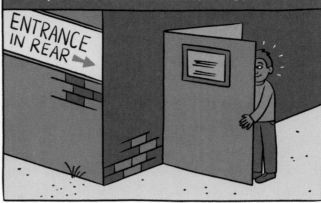

ENTRANCE IN REAR →

NERD ALERT SEXUALLY TRANSMITTED INFECTIONS

WHENEVER TWO BODIES ARE CLOSE TOGETHER IT'S POSSIBLE THAT IF ONE BODY HAS AN INFECTION IT CAN BE SHARED WITH ANOTHER BODY. FOR EXAMPLE, IF YOU HAVE A COLD AND SNEEZE ON SOMEONE NEAR YOU, OR SHARE THEIR WATER BOTTLE, IT'S POSSIBLE TO TRANSMIT THE COLD TO THE OTHER PERSON.

WHEN WE HAVE AN INFECTION AND WE SHARE IT WITH SOMEONE DURING SEX, IT'S CALLED A SEXUALLY TRANSMITTED INFECTION (STI FOR SHORT). STIS ARE NOT BETTER OR WORSE THAN OTHER INFECTIONS BUT THEY ARE TREATED LIKE THEY ARE WORSE. THIS IS BECAUSE OF STIGMA.*

BECAUSE SOME KINDS OF SEX INCLUDE PUTTING BODIES VERY CLOSE TOGETHER, IT CAN BE EASIER TO SHARE AN INFECTION, ESPECIALLY IF THEY ARE SHARING FLUIDS. TAKING CARE OF YOURSELF MEANS LEARNING ABOUT STIS. BEING TRUSTWORTHY AND SHOWING RESPECT FOR OTHERS MEANS KNOWING HOW TO REDUCE THE CHANCES OF SHARING AN STI. FIND OUT MORE IN THE STI CHAPTER ON P. 410.

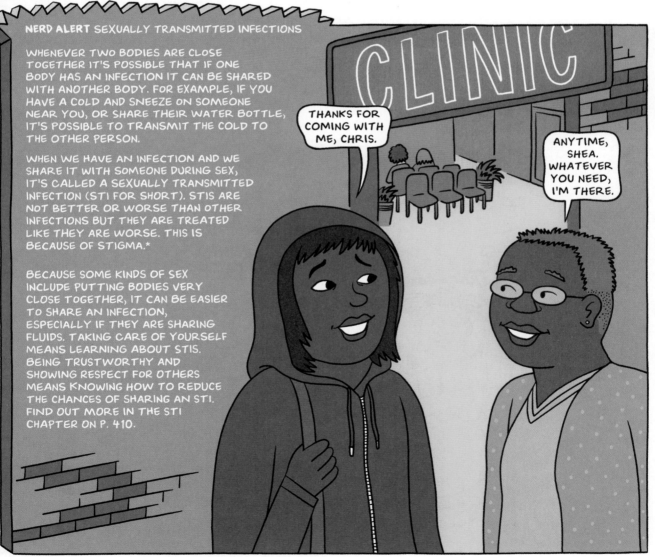

CLINIC

THANKS FOR COMING WITH ME, CHRIS.

ANYTIME, SHEA. WHATEVER YOU NEED, I'M THERE.

* IF YOU MISSED IT, CHECK OUT THE STIGMA CHAPTER ON P. 243

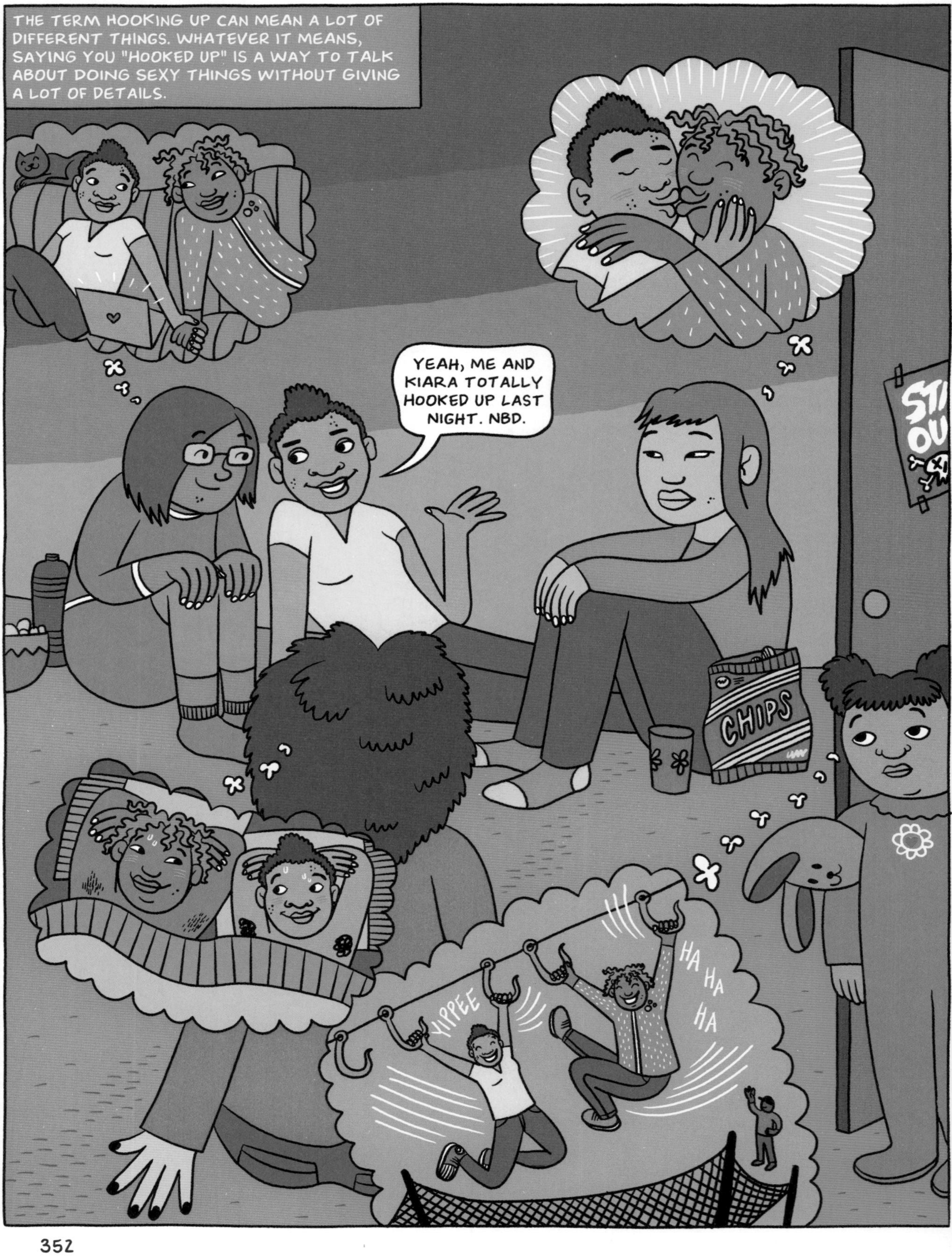
THE TERM HOOKING UP CAN MEAN A LOT OF DIFFERENT THINGS. WHATEVER IT MEANS, SAYING YOU "HOOKED UP" IS A WAY TO TALK ABOUT DOING SEXY THINGS WITHOUT GIVING A LOT OF DETAILS.
YEAH, ME AND KIARA TOTALLY HOOKED UP LAST NIGHT. NBD.
CHIPS
YIPPEE
HA HA HA

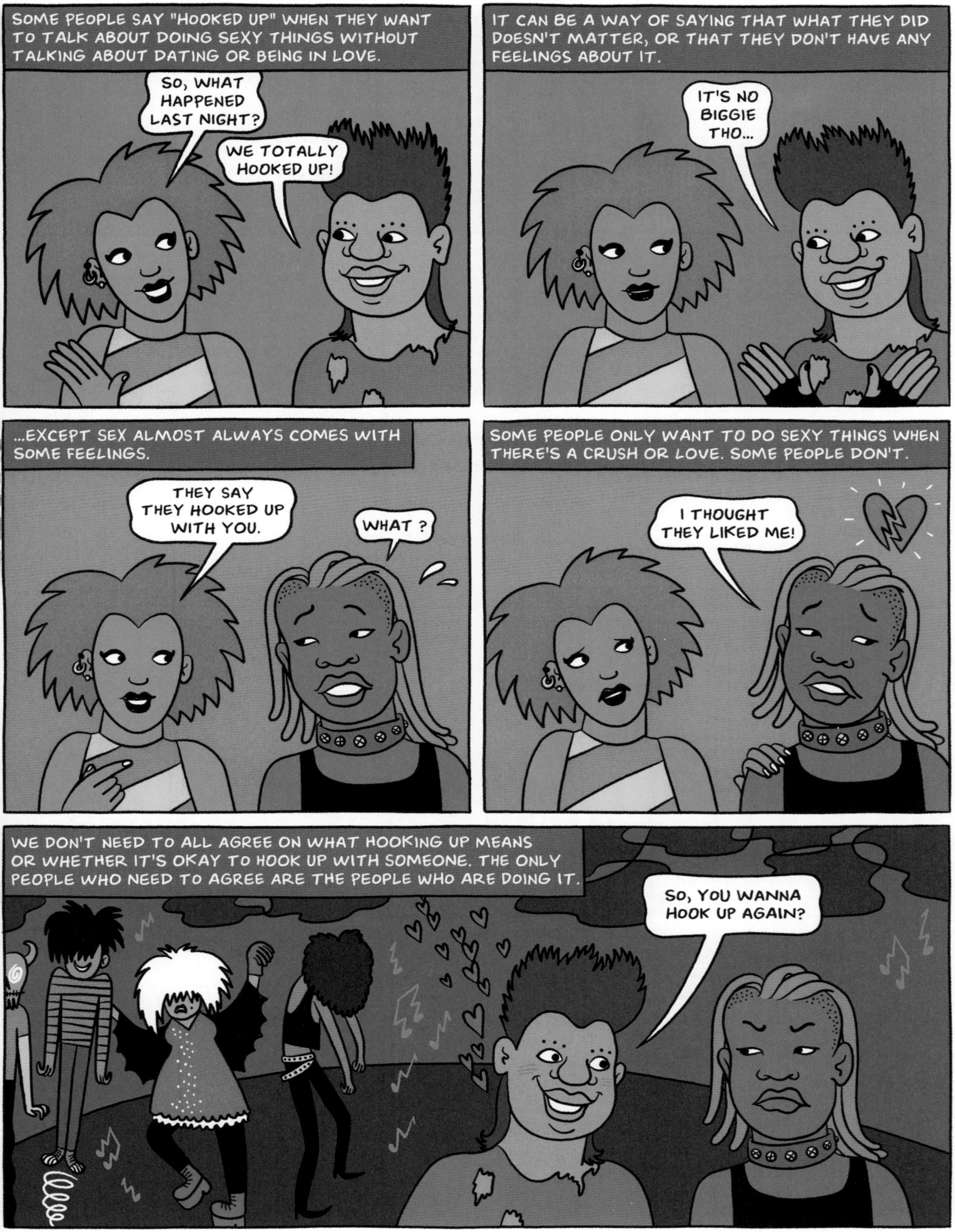
SOME PEOPLE SAY "HOOKED UP" WHEN THEY WANT TO TALK ABOUT DOING SEXY THINGS WITHOUT TALKING ABOUT DATING OR BEING IN LOVE.
SO, WHAT HAPPENED LAST NIGHT?
WE TOTALLY HOOKED UP!
IT CAN BE A WAY OF SAYING THAT WHAT THEY DID DOESN'T MATTER, OR THAT THEY DON'T HAVE ANY FEELINGS ABOUT IT.
IT'S NO BIGGIE THO...
...EXCEPT SEX ALMOST ALWAYS COMES WITH SOME FEELINGS.
THEY SAY THEY HOOKED UP WITH YOU.
WHAT ?
SOME PEOPLE ONLY WANT TO DO SEXY THINGS WHEN THERE'S A CRUSH OR LOVE. SOME PEOPLE DON'T.
I THOUGHT THEY LIKED ME!
WE DON'T NEED TO ALL AGREE ON WHAT HOOKING UP MEANS OR WHETHER IT'S OKAY TO HOOK UP WITH SOMEONE. THE ONLY PEOPLE WHO NEED TO AGREE ARE THE PEOPLE WHO ARE DOING IT.
SO, YOU WANNA HOOK UP AGAIN?

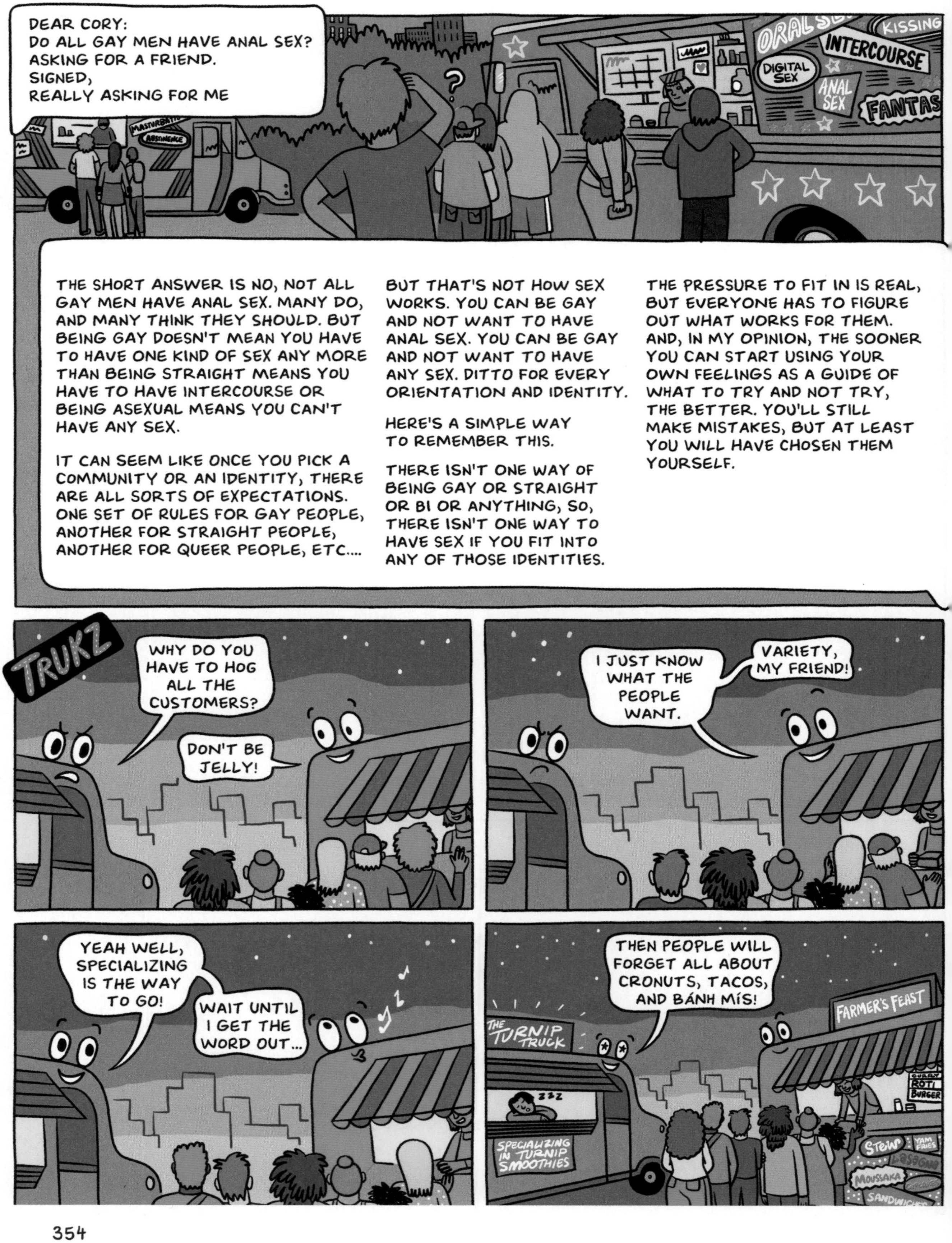
DEAR CORY:
DO ALL GAY MEN HAVE ANAL SEX? ASKING FOR A FRIEND.
SIGNED,
REALLY ASKING FOR ME
KISSING
INTERCOURSE
DIGITAL SEX
ANAL SEX
ABSTINENCE
THE SHORT ANSWER IS NO, NOT ALL GAY MEN HAVE ANAL SEX. MANY DO, AND MANY THINK THEY SHOULD. BUT BEING GAY DOESN'T MEAN YOU HAVE TO HAVE ONE KIND OF SEX ANY MORE THAN BEING STRAIGHT MEANS YOU HAVE TO HAVE INTERCOURSE OR BEING ASEXUAL MEANS YOU CAN'T HAVE ANY SEX.
IT CAN SEEM LIKE ONCE YOU PICK A COMMUNITY OR AN IDENTITY, THERE ARE ALL SORTS OF EXPECTATIONS. ONE SET OF RULES FOR GAY PEOPLE, ANOTHER FOR STRAIGHT PEOPLE, ANOTHER FOR QUEER PEOPLE, ETC....
BUT THAT'S NOT HOW SEX WORKS. YOU CAN BE GAY AND NOT WANT TO HAVE ANAL SEX. YOU CAN BE GAY AND NOT WANT TO HAVE ANY SEX. DITTO FOR EVERY ORIENTATION AND IDENTITY.
HERE'S A SIMPLE WAY TO REMEMBER THIS.
THERE ISN'T ONE WAY OF BEING GAY OR STRAIGHT OR BI OR ANYTHING, SO, THERE ISN'T ONE WAY TO HAVE SEX IF YOU FIT INTO ANY OF THOSE IDENTITIES.
THE PRESSURE TO FIT IN IS REAL, BUT EVERYONE HAS TO FIGURE OUT WHAT WORKS FOR THEM. AND, IN MY OPINION, THE SOONER YOU CAN START USING YOUR OWN FEELINGS AS A GUIDE OF WHAT TO TRY AND NOT TRY, THE BETTER. YOU'LL STILL MAKE MISTAKES, BUT AT LEAST YOU WILL HAVE CHOSEN THEM YOURSELF.
TRUKZ
WHY DO YOU HAVE TO HOG ALL THE CUSTOMERS?
DON'T BE JELLY!
I JUST KNOW WHAT THE PEOPLE WANT.
VARIETY, MY FRIEND!
YEAH WELL, SPECIALIZING IS THE WAY TO GO!
WAIT UNTIL I GET THE WORD OUT...
THE TURNIP TRUCK
THEN PEOPLE WILL FORGET ALL ABOUT CRONUTS, TACOS, AND BÁNH MÍS!
SPECIALIZING IN TURNIP SMOOTHIES
FARMER'S FEAST
ROTI BURGER
STEW
YAM FRIES
MOUSSAKA

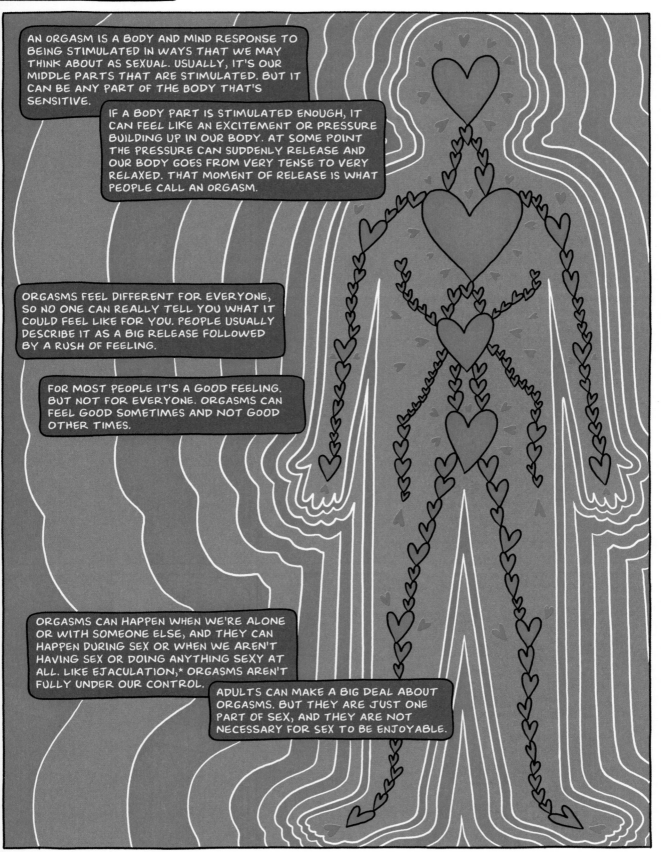

AN ORGASM IS A BODY AND MIND RESPONSE TO BEING STIMULATED IN WAYS THAT WE MAY THINK ABOUT AS SEXUAL. USUALLY, IT'S OUR MIDDLE PARTS THAT ARE STIMULATED. BUT IT CAN BE ANY PART OF THE BODY THAT'S SENSITIVE.

IF A BODY PART IS STIMULATED ENOUGH, IT CAN FEEL LIKE AN EXCITEMENT OR PRESSURE BUILDING UP IN OUR BODY. AT SOME POINT THE PRESSURE CAN SUDDENLY RELEASE AND OUR BODY GOES FROM VERY TENSE TO VERY RELAXED. THAT MOMENT OF RELEASE IS WHAT PEOPLE CALL AN ORGASM.

ORGASMS FEEL DIFFERENT FOR EVERYONE, SO NO ONE CAN REALLY TELL YOU WHAT IT COULD FEEL LIKE FOR YOU. PEOPLE USUALLY DESCRIBE IT AS A BIG RELEASE FOLLOWED BY A RUSH OF FEELING.

FOR MOST PEOPLE IT'S A GOOD FEELING. BUT NOT FOR EVERYONE. ORGASMS CAN FEEL GOOD SOMETIMES AND NOT GOOD OTHER TIMES.

ORGASMS CAN HAPPEN WHEN WE'RE ALONE OR WITH SOMEONE ELSE, AND THEY CAN HAPPEN DURING SEX OR WHEN WE AREN'T HAVING SEX OR DOING ANYTHING SEXY AT ALL. LIKE EJACULATION,* ORGASMS AREN'T FULLY UNDER OUR CONTROL.

ADULTS CAN MAKE A BIG DEAL ABOUT ORGASMS. BUT THEY ARE JUST ONE PART OF SEX, AND THEY ARE NOT NECESSARY FOR SEX TO BE ENJOYABLE.

* YOU CAN READ ABOUT EJACULATION ON P. 170

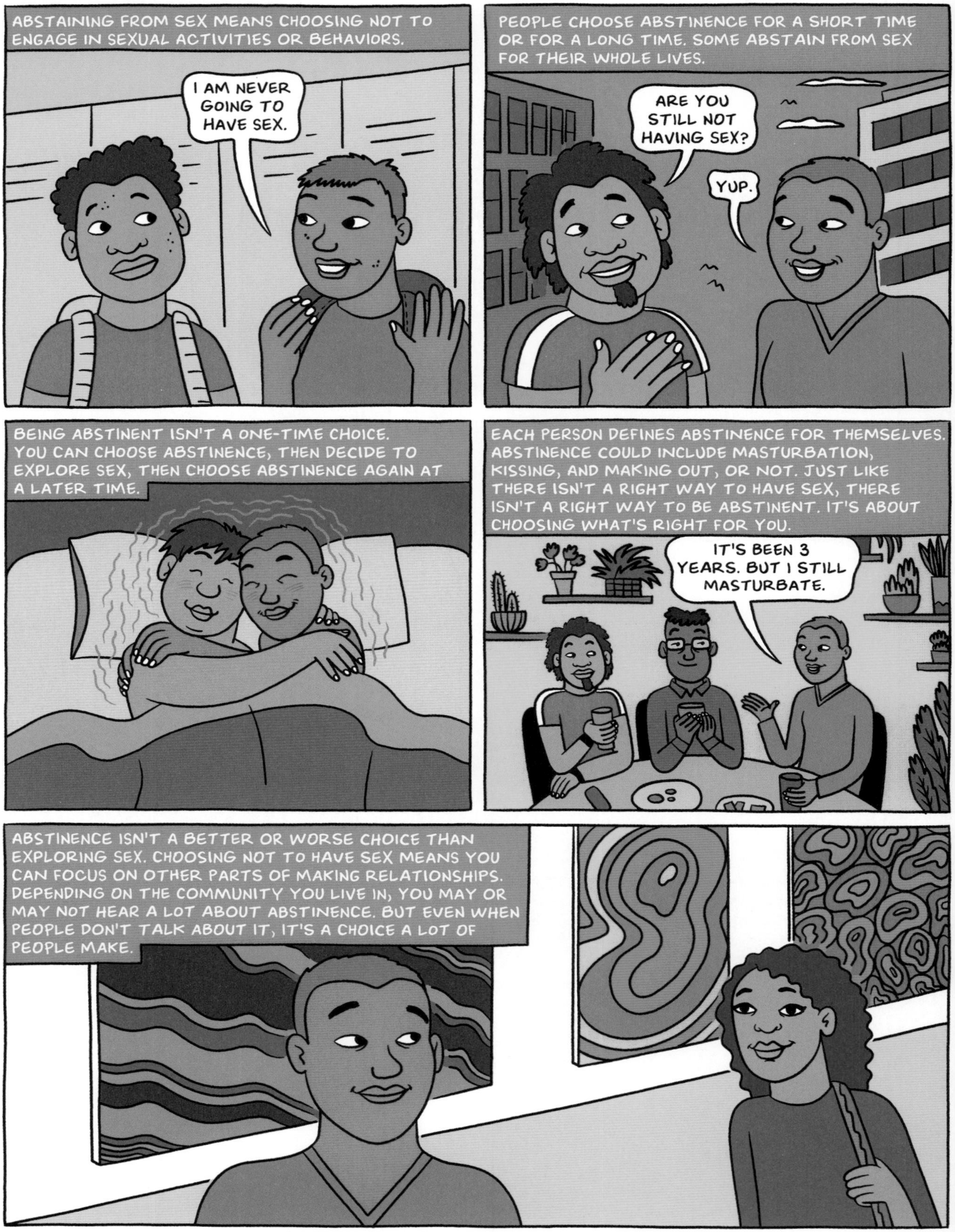
ABSTAINING FROM SEX MEANS CHOOSING NOT TO ENGAGE IN SEXUAL ACTIVITIES OR BEHAVIORS.
I AM NEVER GOING TO HAVE SEX.
PEOPLE CHOOSE ABSTINENCE FOR A SHORT TIME OR FOR A LONG TIME. SOME ABSTAIN FROM SEX FOR THEIR WHOLE LIVES.
ARE YOU STILL NOT HAVING SEX?
YUP.
BEING ABSTINENT ISN'T A ONE-TIME CHOICE. YOU CAN CHOOSE ABSTINENCE, THEN DECIDE TO EXPLORE SEX, THEN CHOOSE ABSTINENCE AGAIN AT A LATER TIME.
EACH PERSON DEFINES ABSTINENCE FOR THEMSELVES. ABSTINENCE COULD INCLUDE MASTURBATION, KISSING, AND MAKING OUT, OR NOT. JUST LIKE THERE ISN'T A RIGHT WAY TO HAVE SEX, THERE ISN'T A RIGHT WAY TO BE ABSTINENT. IT'S ABOUT CHOOSING WHAT'S RIGHT FOR YOU.
IT'S BEEN 3 YEARS. BUT I STILL MASTURBATE.
ABSTINENCE ISN'T A BETTER OR WORSE CHOICE THAN EXPLORING SEX. CHOOSING NOT TO HAVE SEX MEANS YOU CAN FOCUS ON OTHER PARTS OF MAKING RELATIONSHIPS. DEPENDING ON THE COMMUNITY YOU LIVE IN, YOU MAY OR MAY NOT HEAR A LOT ABOUT ABSTINENCE. BUT EVEN WHEN PEOPLE DON'T TALK ABOUT IT, IT'S A CHOICE A LOT OF PEOPLE MAKE.

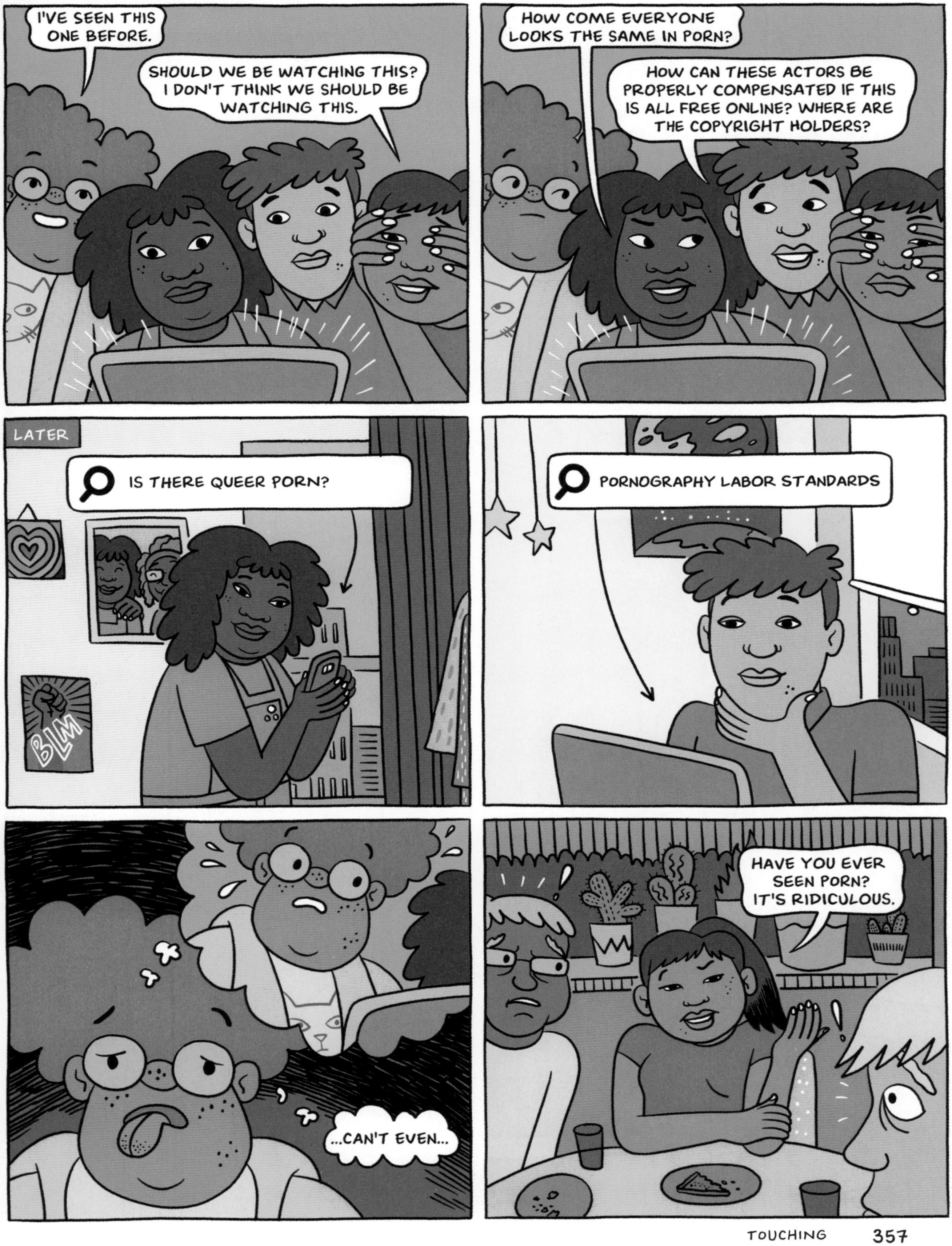
I'VE SEEN THIS ONE BEFORE.
SHOULD WE BE WATCHING THIS? I DON'T THINK WE SHOULD BE WATCHING THIS.
HOW COME EVERYONE LOOKS THE SAME IN PORN?
HOW CAN THESE ACTORS BE PROPERLY COMPENSATED IF THIS IS ALL FREE ONLINE? WHERE ARE THE COPYRIGHT HOLDERS?
LATER
IS THERE QUEER PORN?
BLM
PORNOGRAPHY LABOR STANDARDS
...CAN'T EVEN...
HAVE YOU EVER SEEN PORN? IT'S RIDICULOUS.

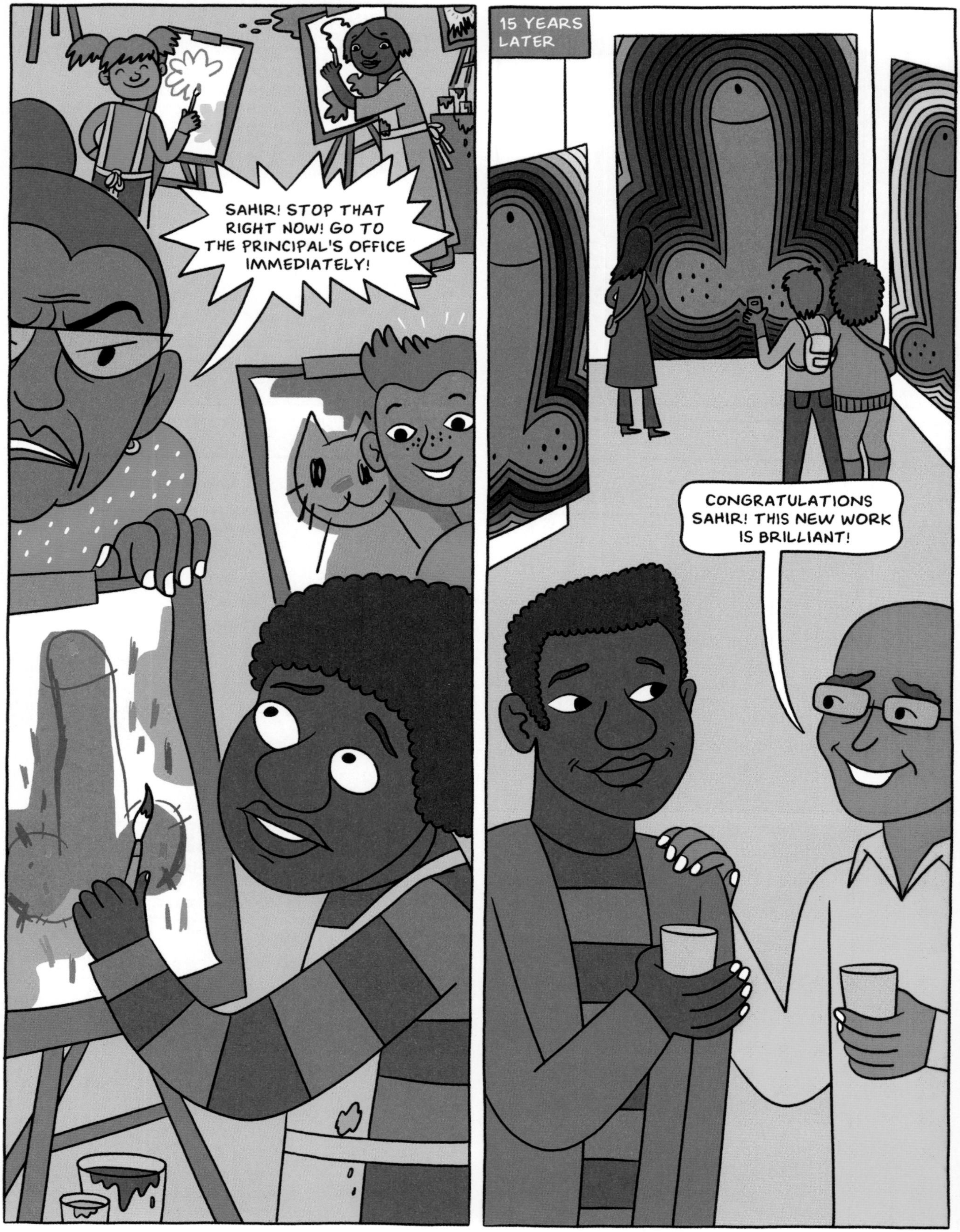
SAHIR! STOP THAT RIGHT NOW! GO TO THE PRINCIPAL'S OFFICE IMMEDIATELY!
15 YEARS LATER
CONGRATULATIONS SAHIR! THIS NEW WORK IS BRILLIANT!

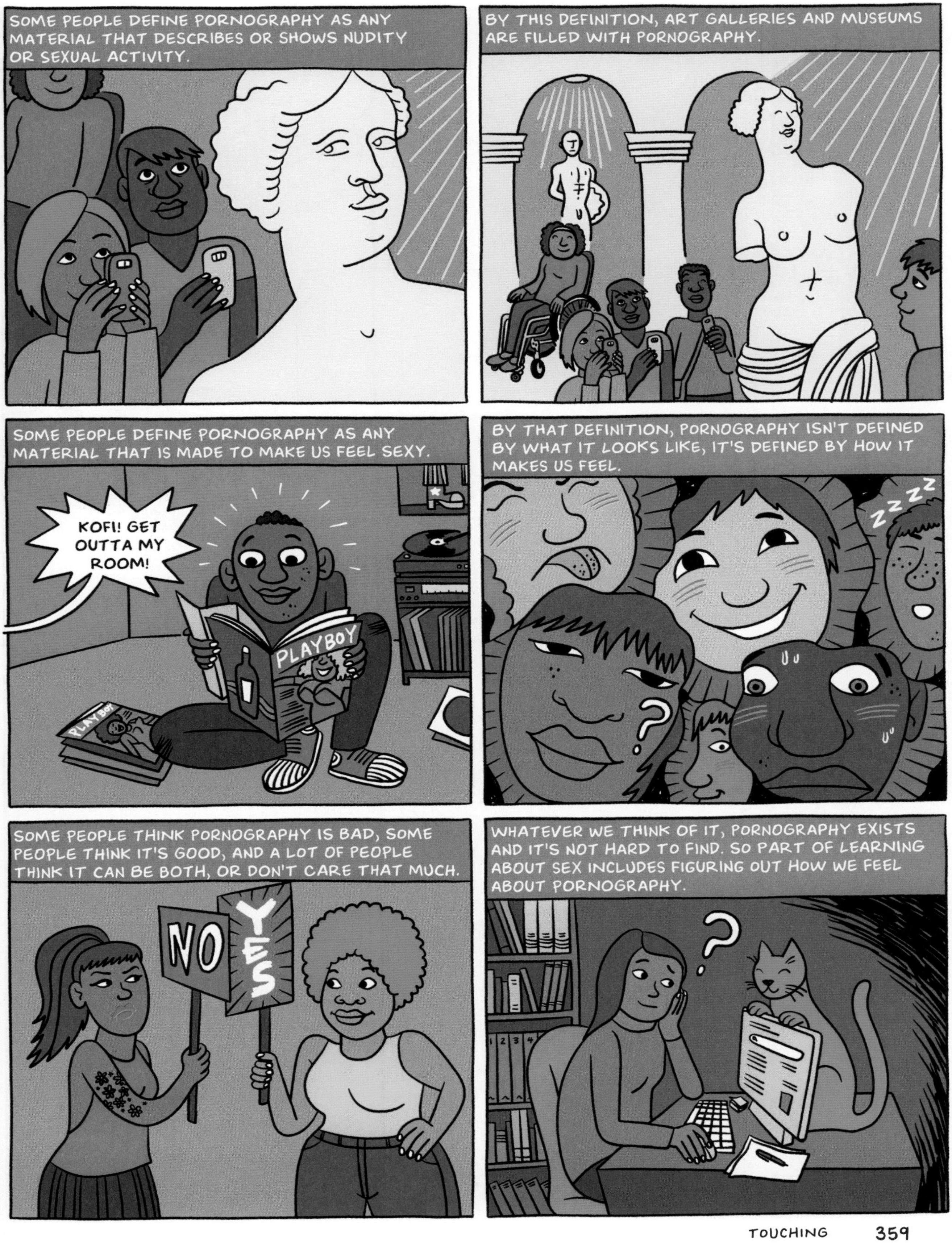
SOME PEOPLE DEFINE PORNOGRAPHY AS ANY MATERIAL THAT DESCRIBES OR SHOWS NUDITY OR SEXUAL ACTIVITY.
BY THIS DEFINITION, ART GALLERIES AND MUSEUMS ARE FILLED WITH PORNOGRAPHY.
SOME PEOPLE DEFINE PORNOGRAPHY AS ANY MATERIAL THAT IS MADE TO MAKE US FEEL SEXY.
KOFI! GET OUTTA MY ROOM!
PLAYBOY
PLAYBOY
BY THAT DEFINITION, PORNOGRAPHY ISN'T DEFINED BY WHAT IT LOOKS LIKE, IT'S DEFINED BY HOW IT MAKES US FEEL.
ZZZZ
SOME PEOPLE THINK PORNOGRAPHY IS BAD, SOME PEOPLE THINK IT'S GOOD, AND A LOT OF PEOPLE THINK IT CAN BE BOTH, OR DON'T CARE THAT MUCH.
NO
YES
WHATEVER WE THINK OF IT, PORNOGRAPHY EXISTS AND IT'S NOT HARD TO FIND. SO PART OF LEARNING ABOUT SEX INCLUDES FIGURING OUT HOW WE FEEL ABOUT PORNOGRAPHY.

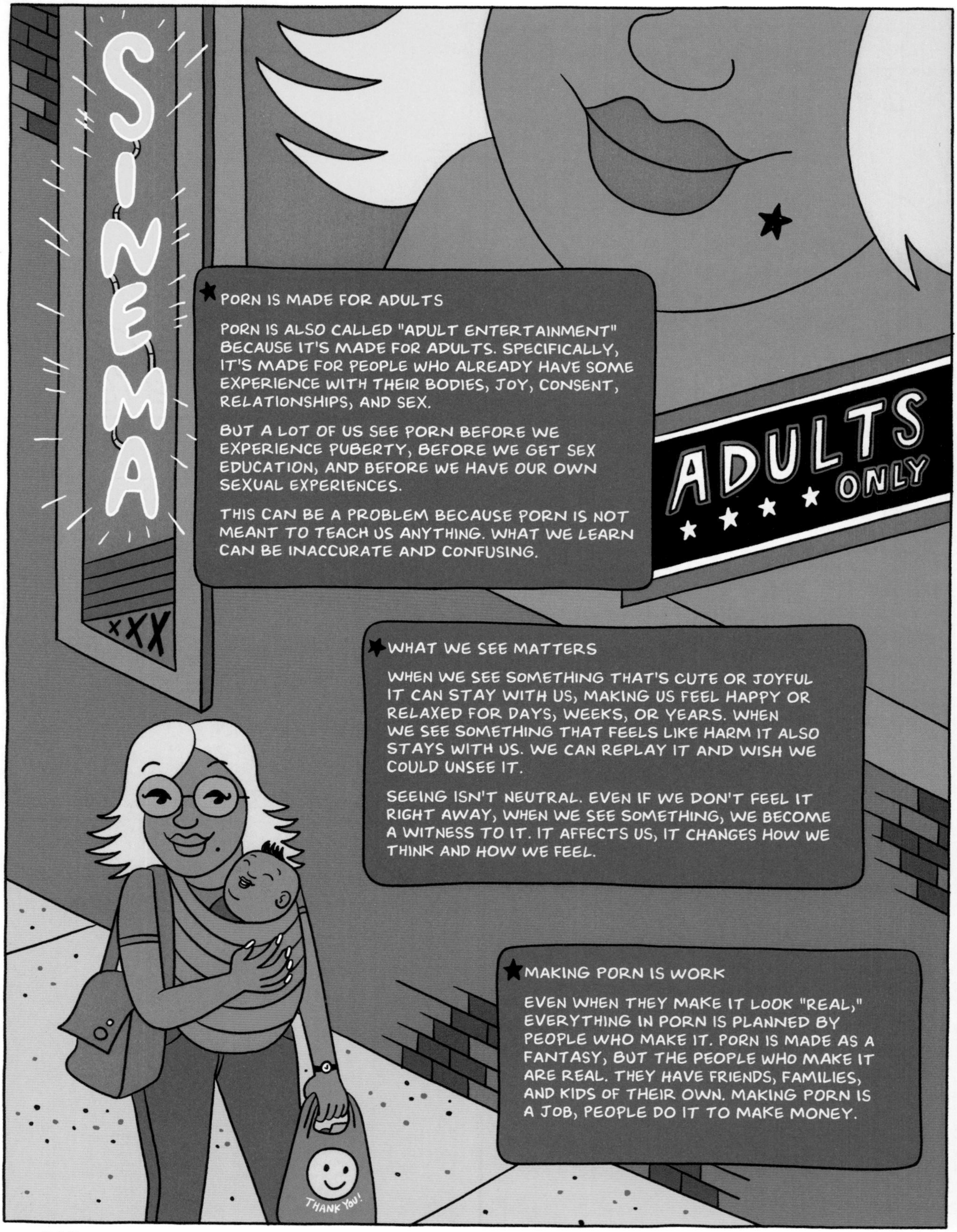
SINEMA
XXX
ADULTS ONLY
THANK YOU!

PORN IS MADE FOR ADULTS

PORN IS ALSO CALLED "ADULT ENTERTAINMENT" BECAUSE IT'S MADE FOR ADULTS. SPECIFICALLY, IT'S MADE FOR PEOPLE WHO ALREADY HAVE SOME EXPERIENCE WITH THEIR BODIES, JOY, CONSENT, RELATIONSHIPS, AND SEX.

BUT A LOT OF US SEE PORN BEFORE WE EXPERIENCE PUBERTY, BEFORE WE GET SEX EDUCATION, AND BEFORE WE HAVE OUR OWN SEXUAL EXPERIENCES.

THIS CAN BE A PROBLEM BECAUSE PORN IS NOT MEANT TO TEACH US ANYTHING. WHAT WE LEARN CAN BE INACCURATE AND CONFUSING.

WHAT WE SEE MATTERS

WHEN WE SEE SOMETHING THAT'S CUTE OR JOYFUL IT CAN STAY WITH US, MAKING US FEEL HAPPY OR RELAXED FOR DAYS, WEEKS, OR YEARS. WHEN WE SEE SOMETHING THAT FEELS LIKE HARM IT ALSO STAYS WITH US. WE CAN REPLAY IT AND WISH WE COULD UNSEE IT.

SEEING ISN'T NEUTRAL. EVEN IF WE DON'T FEEL IT RIGHT AWAY, WHEN WE SEE SOMETHING, WE BECOME A WITNESS TO IT. IT AFFECTS US, IT CHANGES HOW WE THINK AND HOW WE FEEL.

MAKING PORN IS WORK

EVEN WHEN THEY MAKE IT LOOK "REAL," EVERYTHING IN PORN IS PLANNED BY PEOPLE WHO MAKE IT. PORN IS MADE AS A FANTASY, BUT THE PEOPLE WHO MAKE IT ARE REAL. THEY HAVE FRIENDS, FAMILIES, AND KIDS OF THEIR OWN. MAKING PORN IS A JOB, PEOPLE DO IT TO MAKE MONEY.

WHAT'S REAL AND FAKE IN PORN

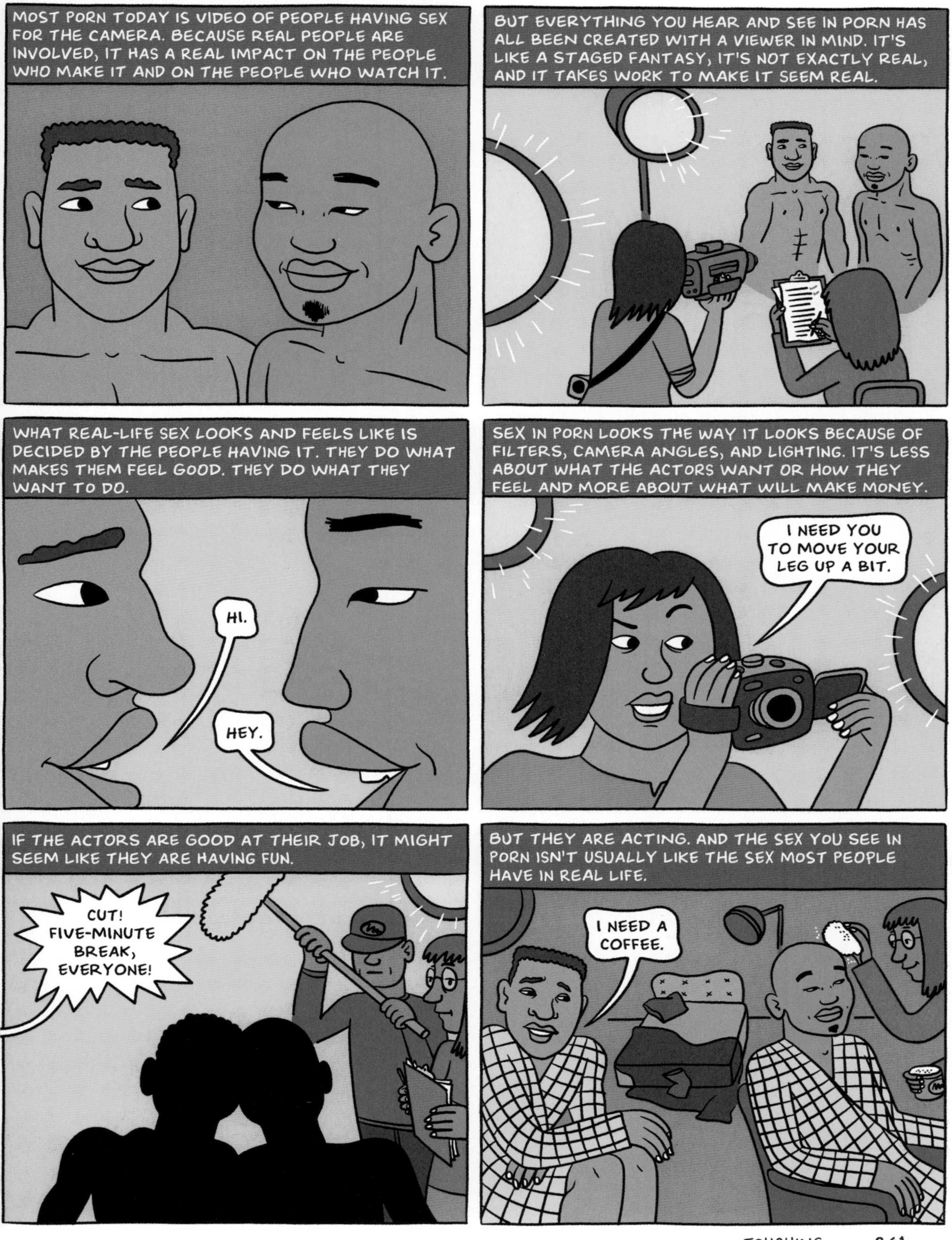
MOST PORN TODAY IS VIDEO OF PEOPLE HAVING SEX FOR THE CAMERA. BECAUSE REAL PEOPLE ARE INVOLVED, IT HAS A REAL IMPACT ON THE PEOPLE WHO MAKE IT AND ON THE PEOPLE WHO WATCH IT.
BUT EVERYTHING YOU HEAR AND SEE IN PORN HAS ALL BEEN CREATED WITH A VIEWER IN MIND. IT'S LIKE A STAGED FANTASY, IT'S NOT EXACTLY REAL, AND IT TAKES WORK TO MAKE IT SEEM REAL.
WHAT REAL-LIFE SEX LOOKS AND FEELS LIKE IS DECIDED BY THE PEOPLE HAVING IT. THEY DO WHAT MAKES THEM FEEL GOOD. THEY DO WHAT THEY WANT TO DO.
HI.
HEY.
SEX IN PORN LOOKS THE WAY IT LOOKS BECAUSE OF FILTERS, CAMERA ANGLES, AND LIGHTING. IT'S LESS ABOUT WHAT THE ACTORS WANT OR HOW THEY FEEL AND MORE ABOUT WHAT WILL MAKE MONEY.
I NEED YOU TO MOVE YOUR LEG UP A BIT.
IF THE ACTORS ARE GOOD AT THEIR JOB, IT MIGHT SEEM LIKE THEY ARE HAVING FUN.
CUT! FIVE-MINUTE BREAK, EVERYONE!
BUT THEY ARE ACTING. AND THE SEX YOU SEE IN PORN ISN'T USUALLY LIKE THE SEX MOST PEOPLE HAVE IN REAL LIFE.
I NEED A COFFEE.

PORN IS MADE TO MAKE YOU LOOK

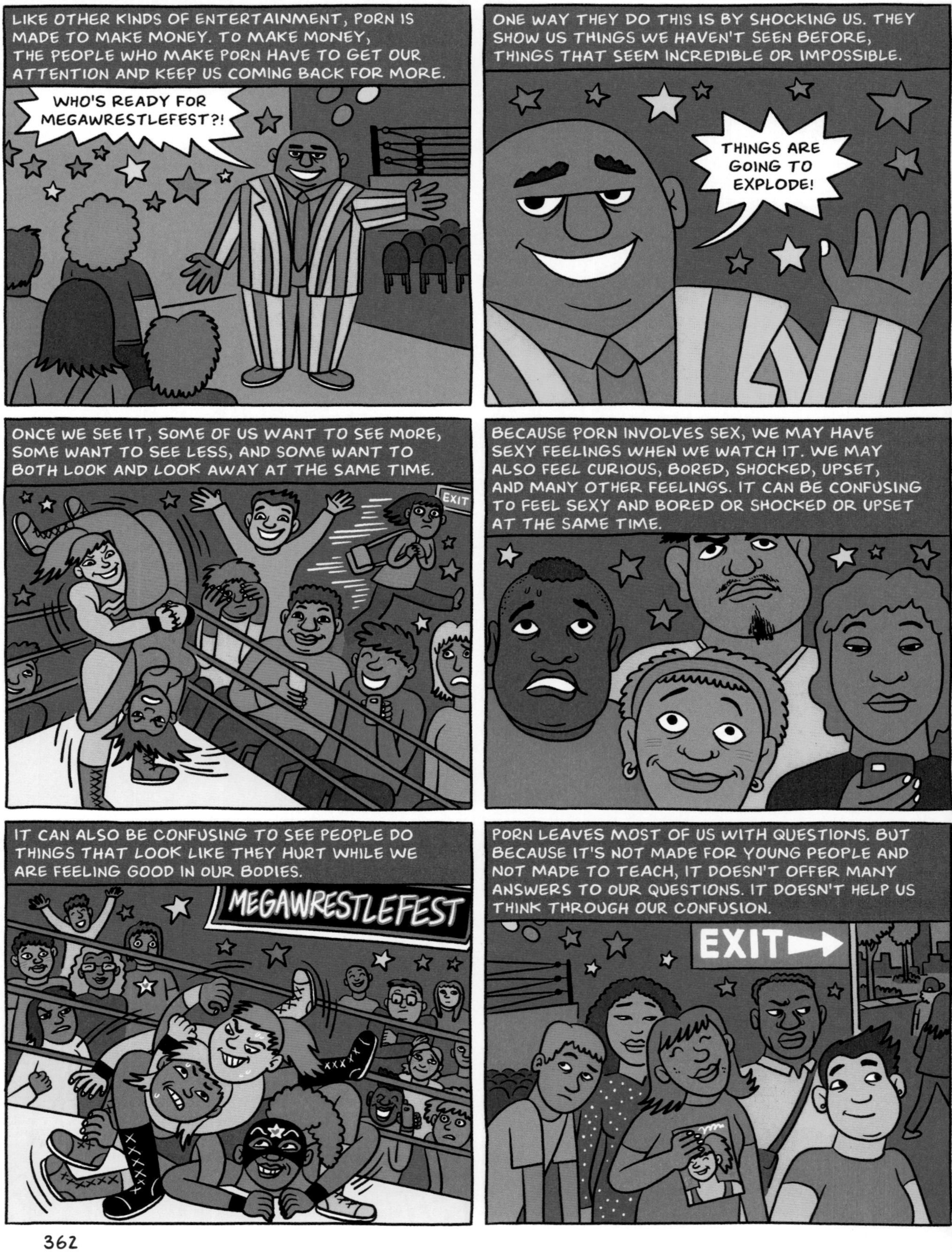

LIKE OTHER KINDS OF ENTERTAINMENT, PORN IS MADE TO MAKE MONEY. TO MAKE MONEY, THE PEOPLE WHO MAKE PORN HAVE TO GET OUR ATTENTION AND KEEP US COMING BACK FOR MORE.
WHO'S READY FOR MEGAWRESTLEFEST?!
ONE WAY THEY DO THIS IS BY SHOCKING US. THEY SHOW US THINGS WE HAVEN'T SEEN BEFORE, THINGS THAT SEEM INCREDIBLE OR IMPOSSIBLE.
THINGS ARE GOING TO EXPLODE!
ONCE WE SEE IT, SOME OF US WANT TO SEE MORE, SOME WANT TO SEE LESS, AND SOME WANT TO BOTH LOOK AND LOOK AWAY AT THE SAME TIME.
EXIT
BECAUSE PORN INVOLVES SEX, WE MAY HAVE SEXY FEELINGS WHEN WE WATCH IT. WE MAY ALSO FEEL CURIOUS, BORED, SHOCKED, UPSET, AND MANY OTHER FEELINGS. IT CAN BE CONFUSING TO FEEL SEXY AND BORED OR SHOCKED OR UPSET AT THE SAME TIME.
IT CAN ALSO BE CONFUSING TO SEE PEOPLE DO THINGS THAT LOOK LIKE THEY HURT WHILE WE ARE FEELING GOOD IN OUR BODIES.
MEGAWRESTLEFEST
PORN LEAVES MOST OF US WITH QUESTIONS. BUT BECAUSE IT'S NOT MADE FOR YOUNG PEOPLE AND NOT MADE TO TEACH, IT DOESN'T OFFER MANY ANSWERS TO OUR QUESTIONS. IT DOESN'T HELP US THINK THROUGH OUR CONFUSION.
EXIT

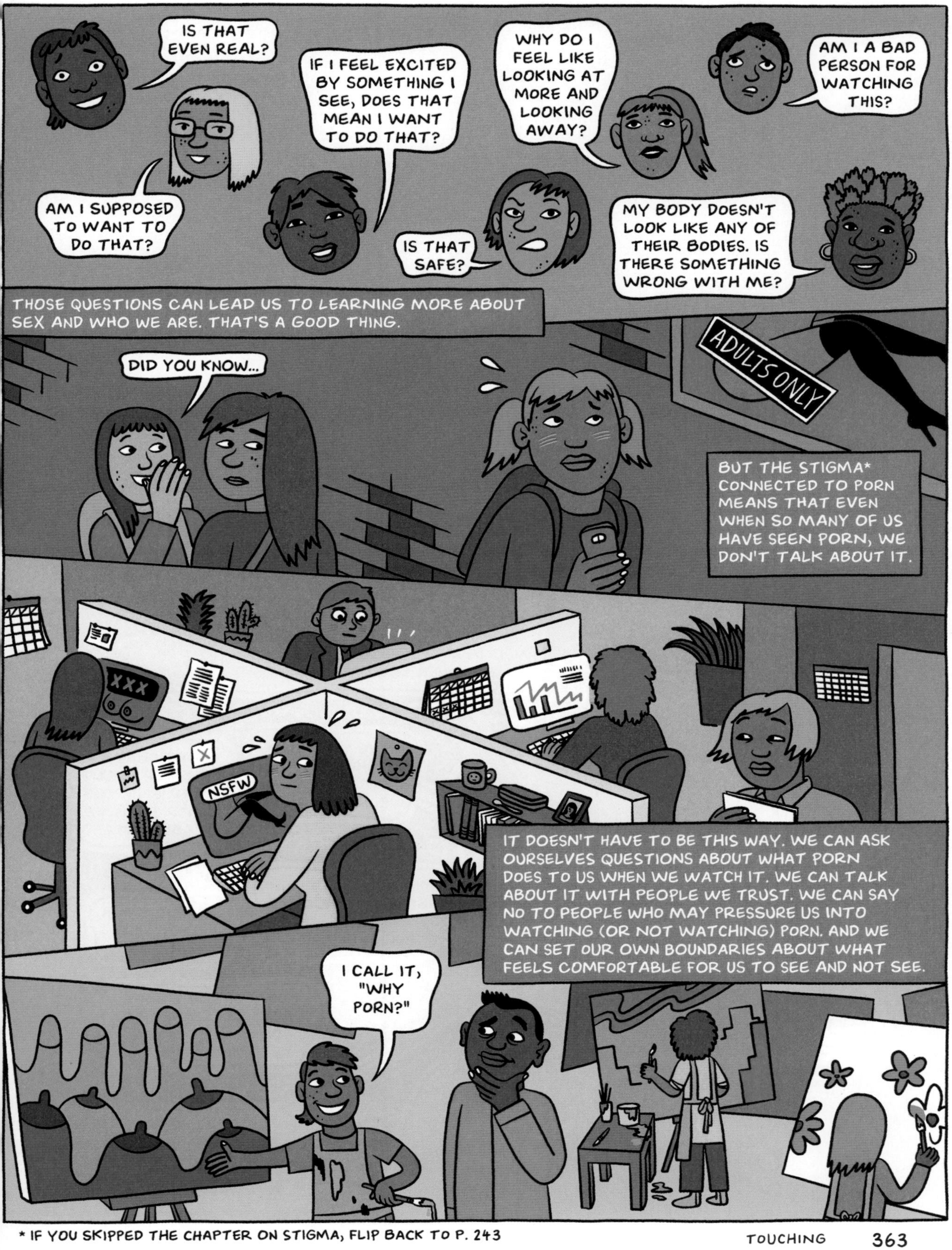
IS THAT EVEN REAL?
AM I SUPPOSED TO WANT TO DO THAT?
IF I FEEL EXCITED BY SOMETHING I SEE, DOES THAT MEAN I WANT TO DO THAT?
IS THAT SAFE?
WHY DO I FEEL LIKE LOOKING AT MORE AND LOOKING AWAY?
AM I A BAD PERSON FOR WATCHING THIS?
MY BODY DOESN'T LOOK LIKE ANY OF THEIR BODIES. IS THERE SOMETHING WRONG WITH ME?
THOSE QUESTIONS CAN LEAD US TO LEARNING MORE ABOUT SEX AND WHO WE ARE. THAT'S A GOOD THING.
DID YOU KNOW...
ADULTS ONLY
BUT THE STIGMA* CONNECTED TO PORN MEANS THAT EVEN WHEN SO MANY OF US HAVE SEEN PORN, WE DON'T TALK ABOUT IT.
XXX
NSFW
IT DOESN'T HAVE TO BE THIS WAY. WE CAN ASK OURSELVES QUESTIONS ABOUT WHAT PORN DOES TO US WHEN WE WATCH IT. WE CAN TALK ABOUT IT WITH PEOPLE WE TRUST. WE CAN SAY NO TO PEOPLE WHO MAY PRESSURE US INTO WATCHING (OR NOT WATCHING) PORN. AND WE CAN SET OUR OWN BOUNDARIES ABOUT WHAT FEELS COMFORTABLE FOR US TO SEE AND NOT SEE.
I CALL IT, "WHY PORN?"

* IF YOU SKIPPED THE CHAPTER ON STIGMA, FLIP BACK TO P. 243

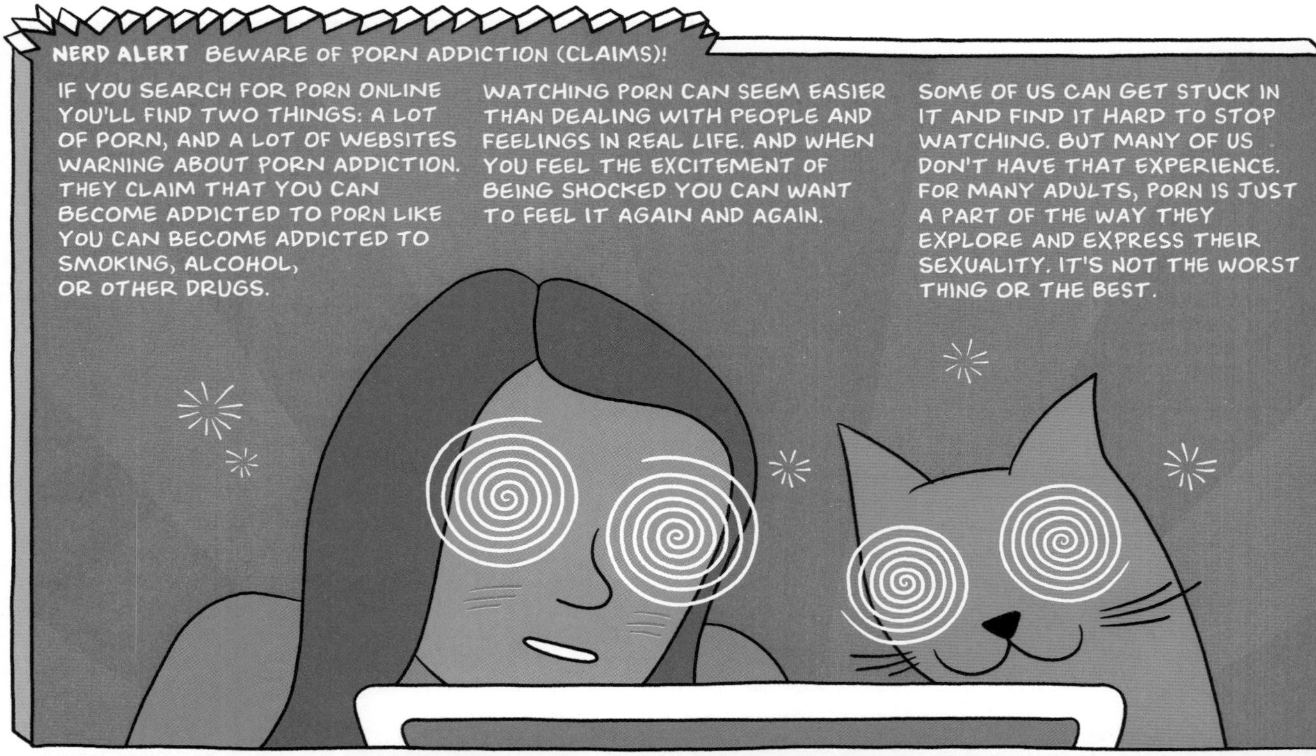
NERD ALERT BEWARE OF PORN ADDICTION (CLAIMS)!
IF YOU SEARCH FOR PORN ONLINE YOU'LL FIND TWO THINGS: A LOT OF PORN, AND A LOT OF WEBSITES WARNING ABOUT PORN ADDICTION. THEY CLAIM THAT YOU CAN BECOME ADDICTED TO PORN LIKE YOU CAN BECOME ADDICTED TO SMOKING, ALCOHOL, OR OTHER DRUGS.
WATCHING PORN CAN SEEM EASIER THAN DEALING WITH PEOPLE AND FEELINGS IN REAL LIFE. AND WHEN YOU FEEL THE EXCITEMENT OF BEING SHOCKED YOU CAN WANT TO FEEL IT AGAIN AND AGAIN.
SOME OF US CAN GET STUCK IN IT AND FIND IT HARD TO STOP WATCHING. BUT MANY OF US DON'T HAVE THAT EXPERIENCE. FOR MANY ADULTS, PORN IS JUST A PART OF THE WAY THEY EXPLORE AND EXPRESS THEIR SEXUALITY. IT'S NOT THE WORST THING OR THE BEST.

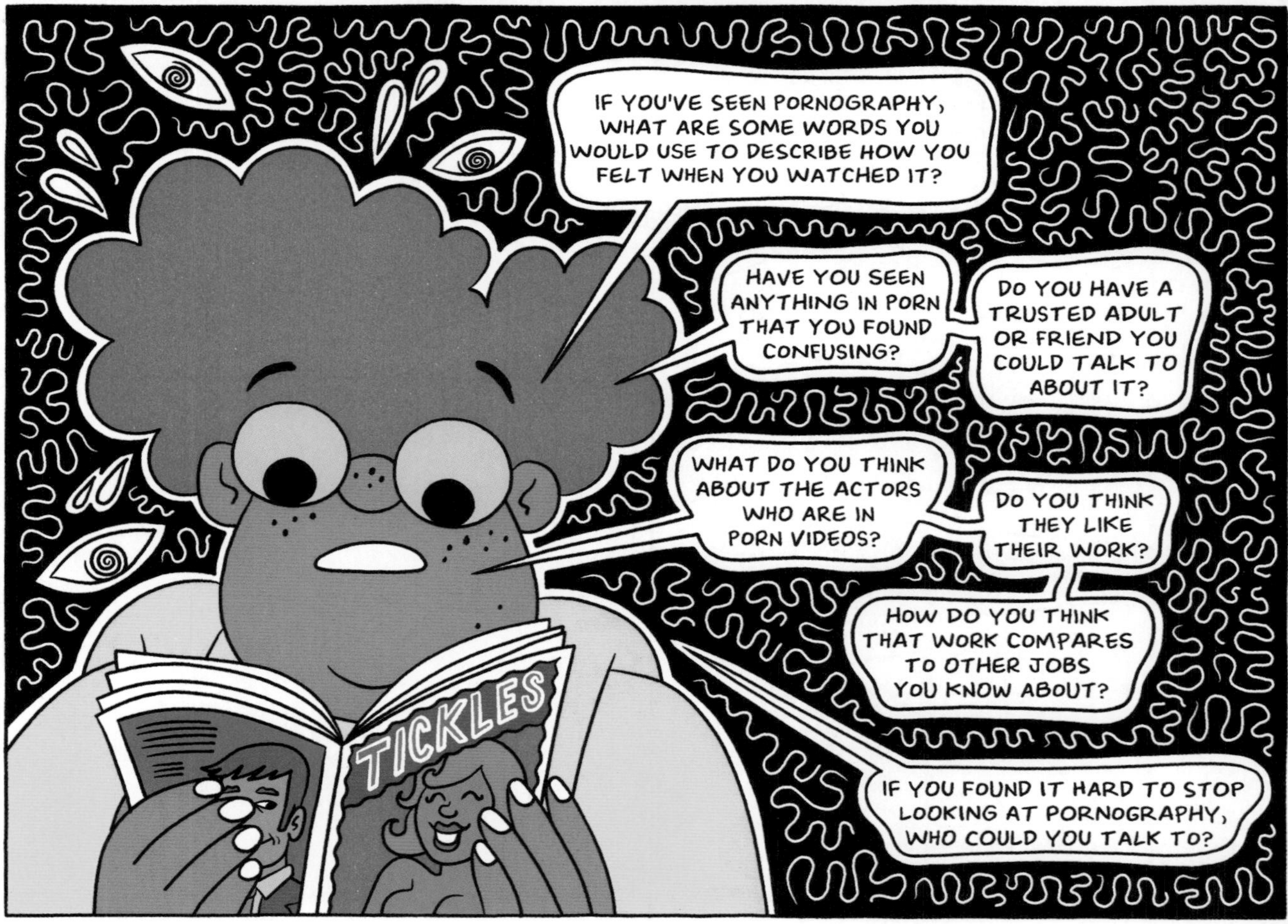
IF YOU'VE SEEN PORNOGRAPHY, WHAT ARE SOME WORDS YOU WOULD USE TO DESCRIBE HOW YOU FELT WHEN YOU WATCHED IT?
HAVE YOU SEEN ANYTHING IN PORN THAT YOU FOUND CONFUSING?
DO YOU HAVE A TRUSTED ADULT OR FRIEND YOU COULD TALK TO ABOUT IT?
WHAT DO YOU THINK ABOUT THE ACTORS WHO ARE IN PORN VIDEOS?
DO YOU THINK THEY LIKE THEIR WORK?
HOW DO YOU THINK THAT WORK COMPARES TO OTHER JOBS YOU KNOW ABOUT?
IF YOU FOUND IT HARD TO STOP LOOKING AT PORNOGRAPHY, WHO COULD YOU TALK TO?
TICKLES

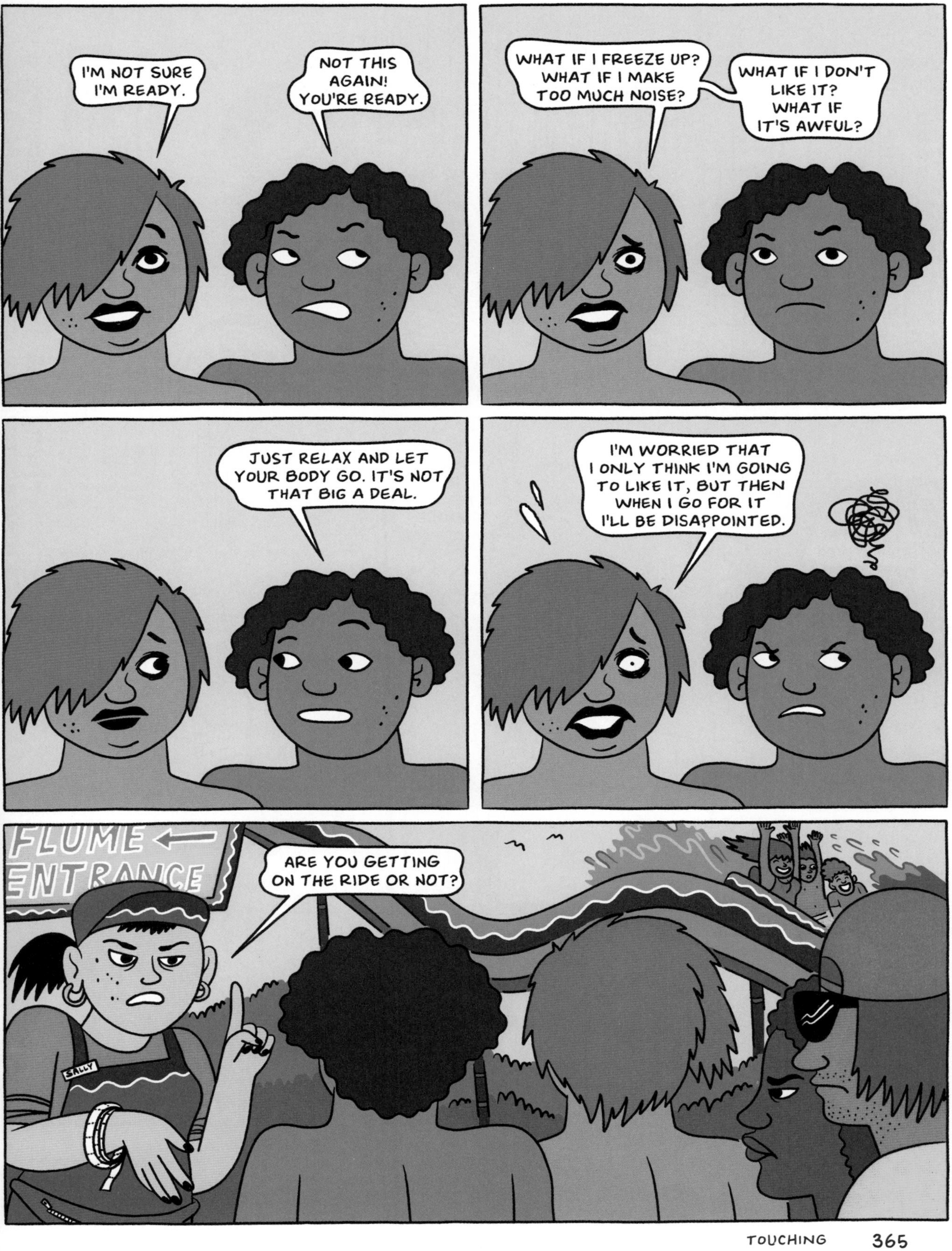
I'M NOT SURE I'M READY.
NOT THIS AGAIN! YOU'RE READY.
WHAT IF I FREEZE UP? WHAT IF I MAKE TOO MUCH NOISE?
WHAT IF I DON'T LIKE IT? WHAT IF IT'S AWFUL?
JUST RELAX AND LET YOUR BODY GO. IT'S NOT THAT BIG A DEAL.
I'M WORRIED THAT I ONLY THINK I'M GOING TO LIKE IT, BUT THEN WHEN I GO FOR IT I'LL BE DISAPPOINTED.
FLUME ← ENTRANCE
ARE YOU GETTING ON THE RIDE OR NOT?
SALLY

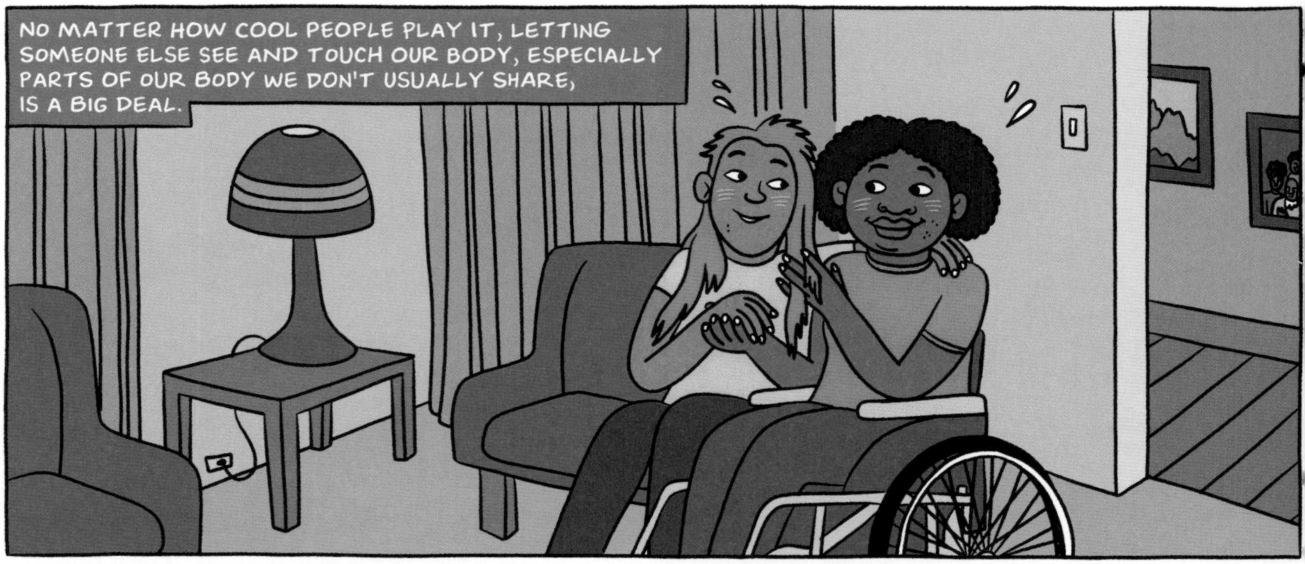
NO MATTER HOW COOL PEOPLE PLAY IT, LETTING SOMEONE ELSE SEE AND TOUCH OUR BODY, ESPECIALLY PARTS OF OUR BODY WE DON'T USUALLY SHARE, IS A BIG DEAL.

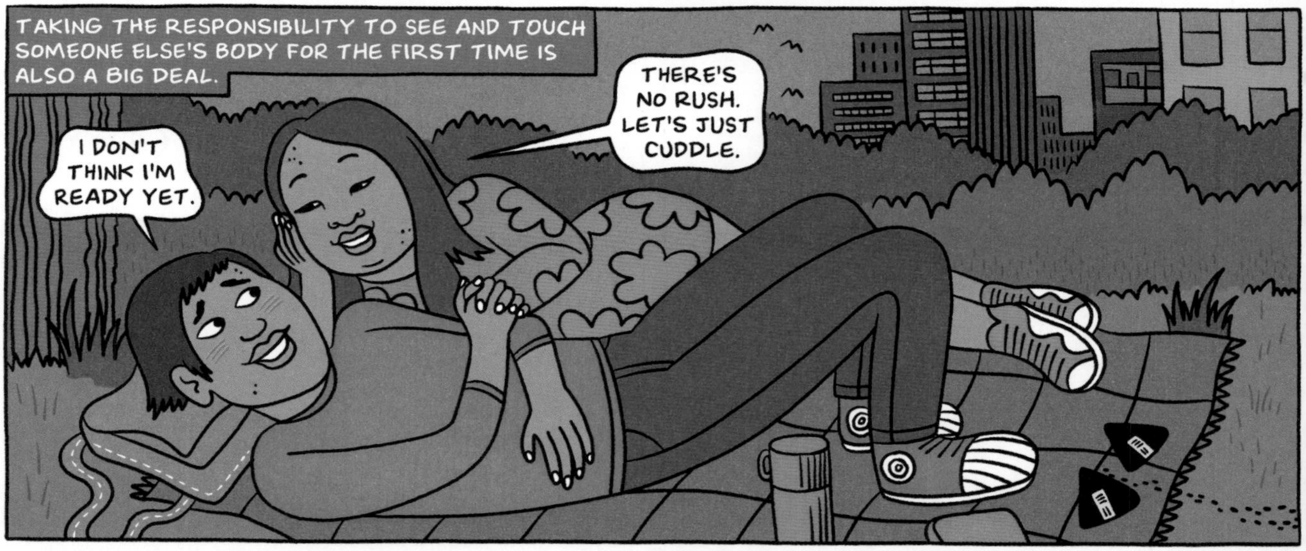
TAKING THE RESPONSIBILITY TO SEE AND TOUCH SOMEONE ELSE'S BODY FOR THE FIRST TIME IS ALSO A BIG DEAL.
I DON'T THINK I'M READY YET.
THERE'S NO RUSH. LET'S JUST CUDDLE.

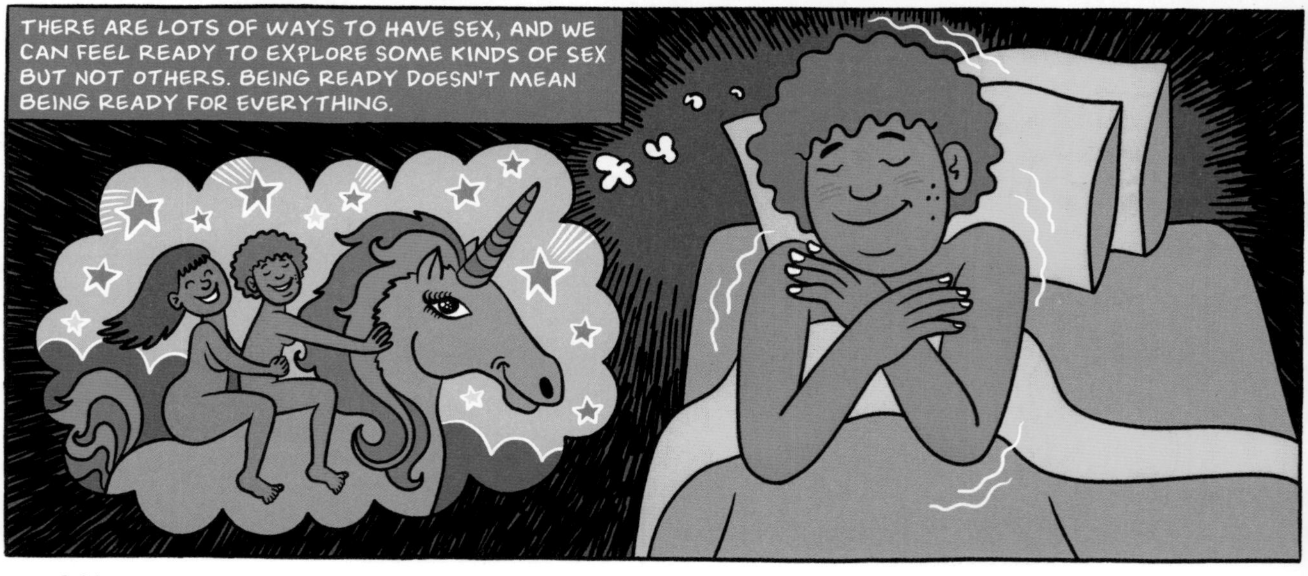
THERE ARE LOTS OF WAYS TO HAVE SEX, AND WE CAN FEEL READY TO EXPLORE SOME KINDS OF SEX BUT NOT OTHERS. BEING READY DOESN'T MEAN BEING READY FOR EVERYTHING.

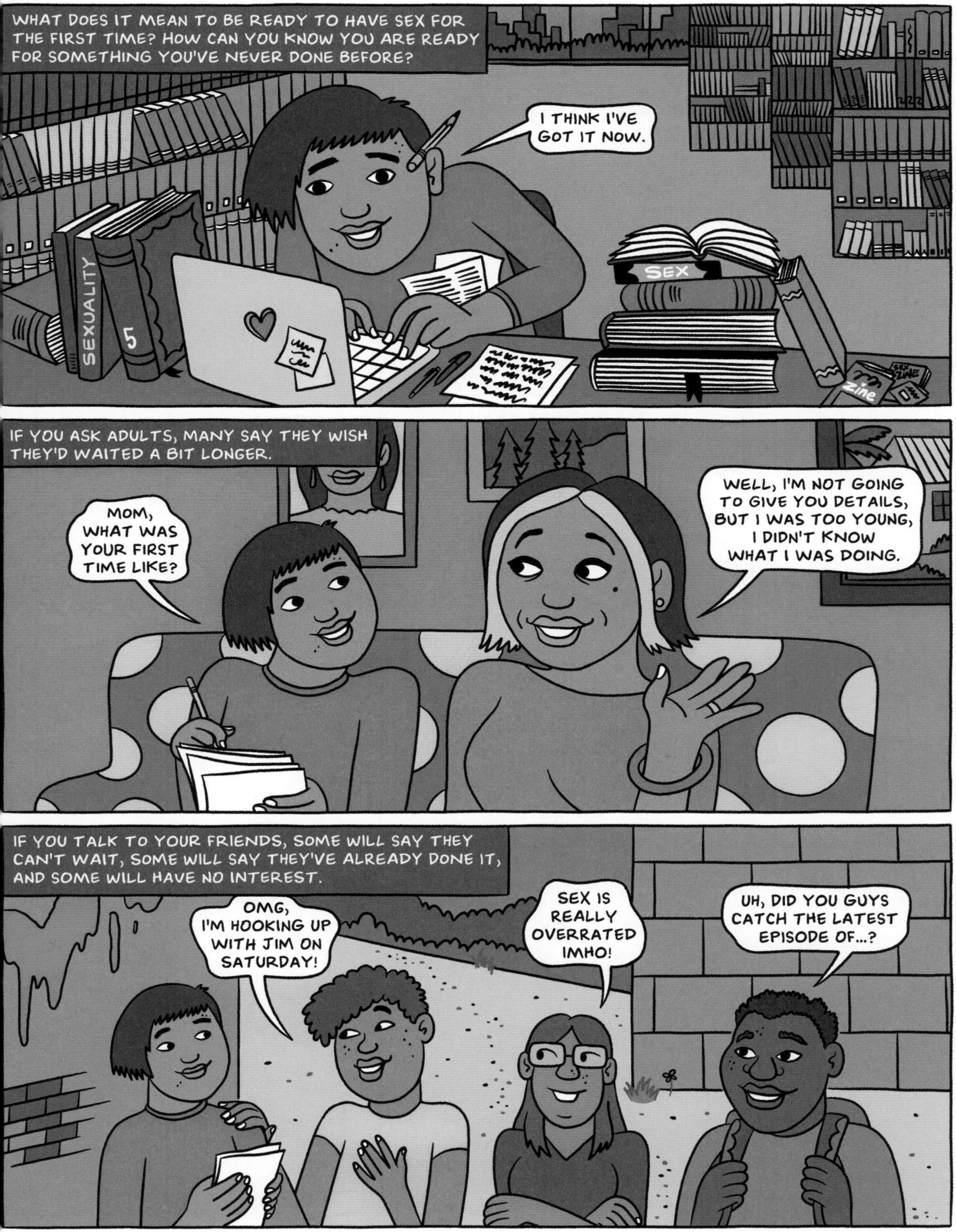
WHAT DOES IT MEAN TO BE READY TO HAVE SEX FOR THE FIRST TIME? HOW CAN YOU KNOW YOU ARE READY FOR SOMETHING YOU'VE NEVER DONE BEFORE?
I THINK I'VE GOT IT NOW.
SEXUALITY
5
SEX
ZINE
IF YOU ASK ADULTS, MANY SAY THEY WISH THEY'D WAITED A BIT LONGER.
MOM, WHAT WAS YOUR FIRST TIME LIKE?
WELL, I'M NOT GOING TO GIVE YOU DETAILS, BUT I WAS TOO YOUNG, I DIDN'T KNOW WHAT I WAS DOING.
IF YOU TALK TO YOUR FRIENDS, SOME WILL SAY THEY CAN'T WAIT, SOME WILL SAY THEY'VE ALREADY DONE IT, AND SOME WILL HAVE NO INTEREST.
OMG, I'M HOOKING UP WITH JIM ON SATURDAY!
SEX IS REALLY OVERRATED IMHO!
UH, DID YOU GUYS CATCH THE LATEST EPISODE OF...?

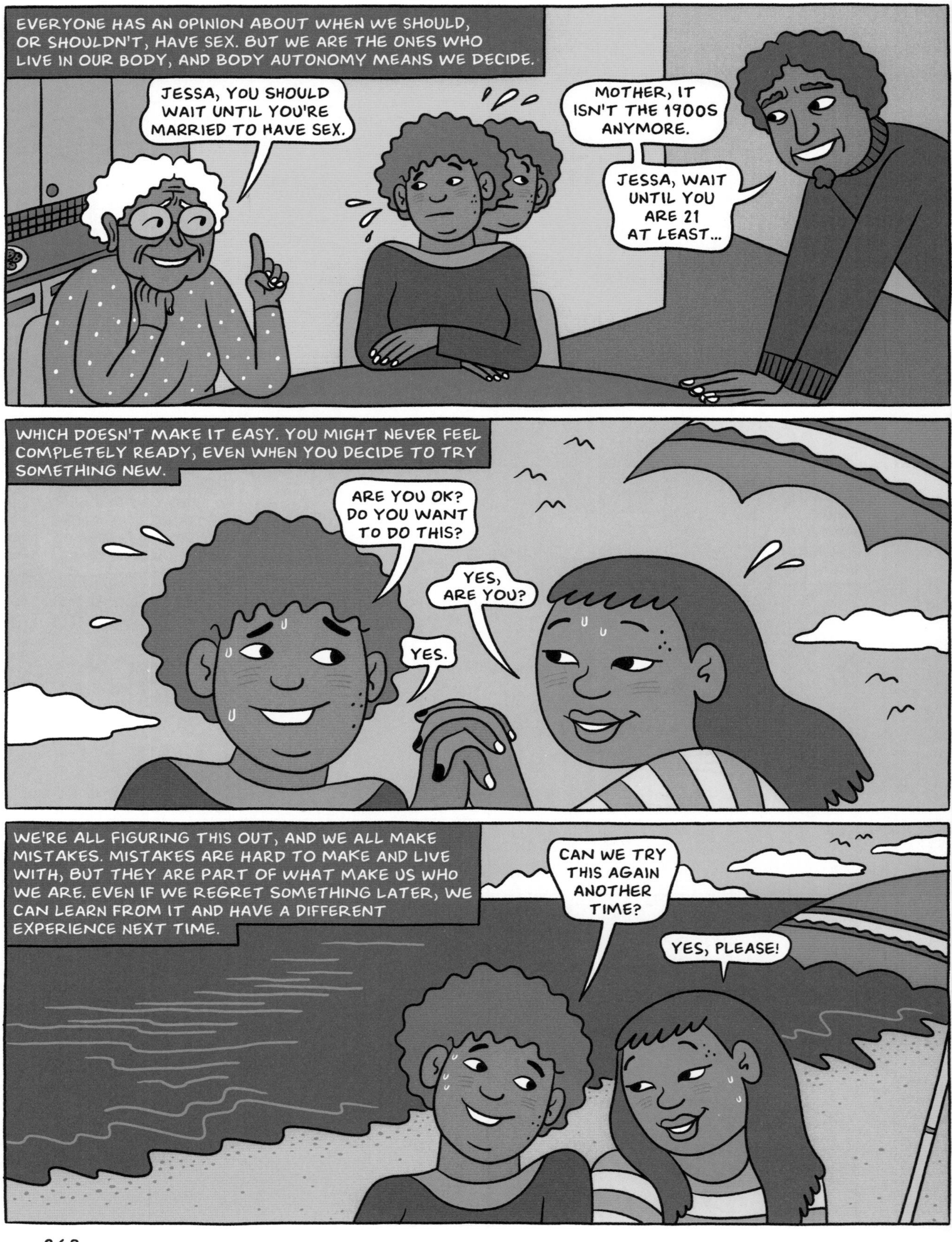
EVERYONE HAS AN OPINION ABOUT WHEN WE SHOULD, OR SHOULDN'T, HAVE SEX. BUT WE ARE THE ONES WHO LIVE IN OUR BODY, AND BODY AUTONOMY MEANS WE DECIDE.
JESSA, YOU SHOULD WAIT UNTIL YOU'RE MARRIED TO HAVE SEX.
MOTHER, IT ISN'T THE 1900S ANYMORE.
JESSA, WAIT UNTIL YOU ARE 21 AT LEAST...
WHICH DOESN'T MAKE IT EASY. YOU MIGHT NEVER FEEL COMPLETELY READY, EVEN WHEN YOU DECIDE TO TRY SOMETHING NEW.
ARE YOU OK? DO YOU WANT TO DO THIS?
YES, ARE YOU?
YES.
WE'RE ALL FIGURING THIS OUT, AND WE ALL MAKE MISTAKES. MISTAKES ARE HARD TO MAKE AND LIVE WITH, BUT THEY ARE PART OF WHAT MAKE US WHO WE ARE. EVEN IF WE REGRET SOMETHING LATER, WE CAN LEARN FROM IT AND HAVE A DIFFERENT EXPERIENCE NEXT TIME.
CAN WE TRY THIS AGAIN ANOTHER TIME?
YES, PLEASE!

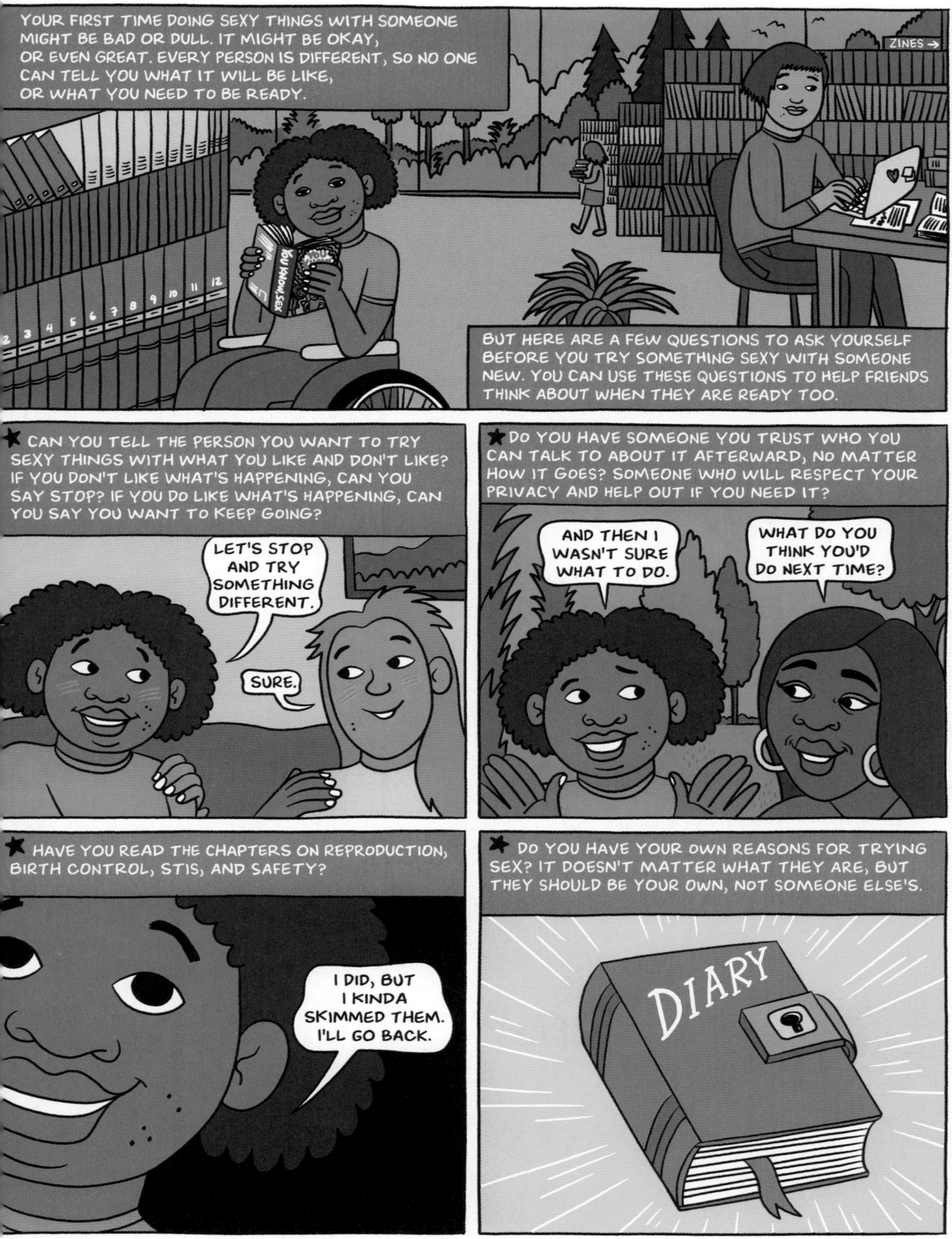

YOUR FIRST TIME DOING SEXY THINGS WITH SOMEONE MIGHT BE BAD OR DULL. IT MIGHT BE OKAY, OR EVEN GREAT. EVERY PERSON IS DIFFERENT, SO NO ONE CAN TELL YOU WHAT IT WILL BE LIKE, OR WHAT YOU NEED TO BE READY.
ZINES →
YOU KNOW, SEX
BUT HERE ARE A FEW QUESTIONS TO ASK YOURSELF BEFORE YOU TRY SOMETHING SEXY WITH SOMEONE NEW. YOU CAN USE THESE QUESTIONS TO HELP FRIENDS THINK ABOUT WHEN THEY ARE READY TOO.
★ CAN YOU TELL THE PERSON YOU WANT TO TRY SEXY THINGS WITH WHAT YOU LIKE AND DON'T LIKE? IF YOU DON'T LIKE WHAT'S HAPPENING, CAN YOU SAY STOP? IF YOU DO LIKE WHAT'S HAPPENING, CAN YOU SAY YOU WANT TO KEEP GOING?
LET'S STOP AND TRY SOMETHING DIFFERENT.
SURE.
★ DO YOU HAVE SOMEONE YOU TRUST WHO YOU CAN TALK TO ABOUT IT AFTERWARD, NO MATTER HOW IT GOES? SOMEONE WHO WILL RESPECT YOUR PRIVACY AND HELP OUT IF YOU NEED IT?
AND THEN I WASN'T SURE WHAT TO DO.
WHAT DO YOU THINK YOU'D DO NEXT TIME?
★ HAVE YOU READ THE CHAPTERS ON REPRODUCTION, BIRTH CONTROL, STIS, AND SAFETY?
I DID, BUT I KINDA SKIMMED THEM. I'LL GO BACK.
★ DO YOU HAVE YOUR OWN REASONS FOR TRYING SEX? IT DOESN'T MATTER WHAT THEY ARE, BUT THEY SHOULD BE YOUR OWN, NOT SOMEONE ELSE'S.
DIARY

NERD ALERT VIRGINITY IS A SCAM

A SCAM IS A TRICK OR A LIE.

CHOOSING TO NOT HAVE SEX OR TO WAIT TO HAVE SEX UNTIL LATER IS NOT A SCAM. IT'S A CHOICE WE MAKE AND A FORM OF USING OUR OWN POWER.

BUT THE IDEA OF VIRGINITY IS A BIG SCAM. HERE ARE THREE SIGNS VIRGINITY IS SCAMMING US ALL:

1. NO ONE AGREES ON WHAT IT MEANS TO BE A VIRGIN. ARE WE A VIRGIN AFTER MAKING OUT WITH SOMEONE? WHAT ABOUT GETTING NAKED WITH SOMEONE? IF THE ONLY WAY WE AREN'T A VIRGIN ANYMORE IS IF WE HAVE INTERCOURSE, DOES THAT MEAN WE CAN DO EVERYTHING BUT INTERCOURSE, AND STILL BE A VIRGIN?

2. VIRGINITY IS ABOUT OTHER PEOPLE'S POWER BEING MORE IMPORTANT THAN OUR OWN. HOW COME WE SAY PEOPLE "LOSE" THEIR VIRGINITY, AS IF IT'S TAKEN FROM US? SEX REQUIRES CONSENT, SO IF IT'S SEX, AND NOT ASSAULT, THEN NO ONE TAKES ANYTHING FROM US; WE CHOOSE TO SHARE IT.

3. VIRGINITY IS ALL ABOUT THE GENDER BINARY. GIRLS ARE SUPPOSED TO BE VIRGINS, BOYS ARE SUPPOSED TO BE EMBARRASSED IF THEY ARE VIRGINS. WHY? AND WHAT ABOUT THE REST OF US?

THE BIG LIE OF VIRGINITY IS THAT IT DEFINES US. IF USING THE WORD VIRGIN FOR OURSELVES IS HELPFUL, THAT'S GREAT. BUT IF WE USE IT TO MAKE OTHER PEOPLE FEEL LIKE THERE IS SOMETHING WRONG WITH THEM, THAT'S NOT OKAY.

CHOOSING TO HAVE SEX OR NOT IS JUST ONE PART OF WHO WE ARE. AND PEOPLE WHO CHOOSE TO WAIT OR NEVER HAVE SEX AREN'T BETTER OR CLEANER OR PURER THAN PEOPLE WHO DON'T WAIT.

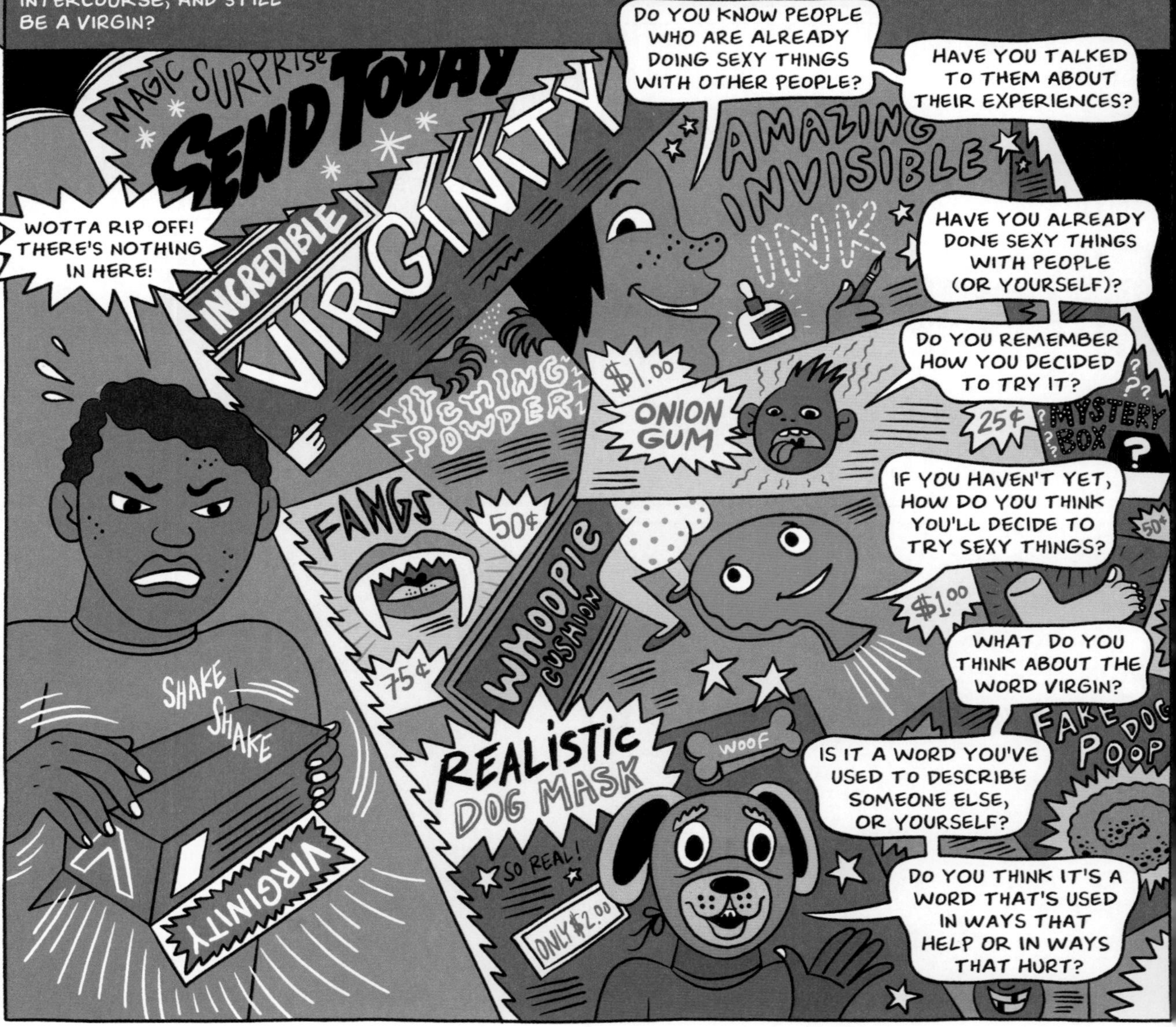

DO YOU KNOW PEOPLE WHO ARE ALREADY DOING SEXY THINGS WITH OTHER PEOPLE?
HAVE YOU TALKED TO THEM ABOUT THEIR EXPERIENCES?
MAGIC SURPRISE
SEND TODAY
INCREDIBLE VIRGINITY
AMAZING INVISIBLE INK
WOTTA RIP OFF! THERE'S NOTHING IN HERE!
HAVE YOU ALREADY DONE SEXY THINGS WITH PEOPLE (OR YOURSELF)?
DO YOU REMEMBER HOW YOU DECIDED TO TRY IT?
ITCHING POWDER
$1.00
ONION GUM
25¢
MYSTERY BOX
FANGS
50¢
WHOOPIE CUSHION
IF YOU HAVEN'T YET, HOW DO YOU THINK YOU'LL DECIDE TO TRY SEXY THINGS?
$1.00
75¢
SHAKE SHAKE
WHAT DO YOU THINK ABOUT THE WORD VIRGIN?
FAKE DOG POOP
REALISTIC DOG MASK
WOOF
IS IT A WORD YOU'VE USED TO DESCRIBE SOMEONE ELSE, OR YOURSELF?
SO REAL!
VIRGINITY
ONLY $2.00
DO YOU THINK IT'S A WORD THAT'S USED IN WAYS THAT HELP OR IN WAYS THAT HURT?

11

SAFETY

JUSTICE
POWER
JOY
CHOICE
RESPECT
TRUST

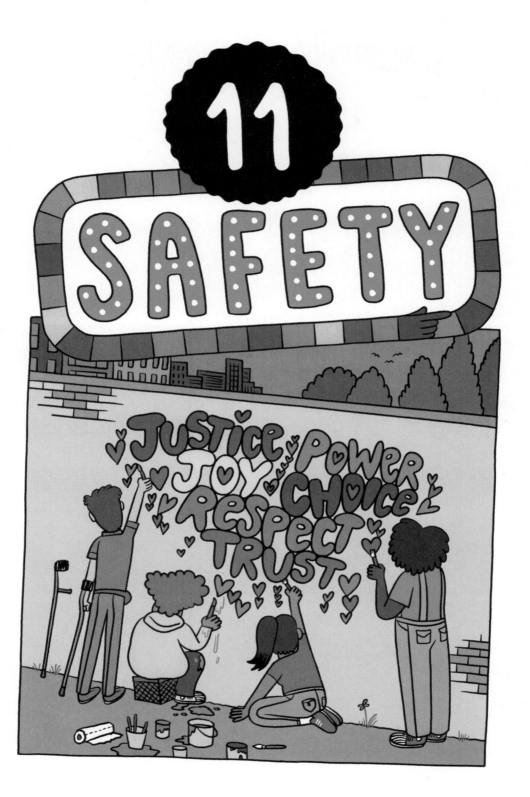

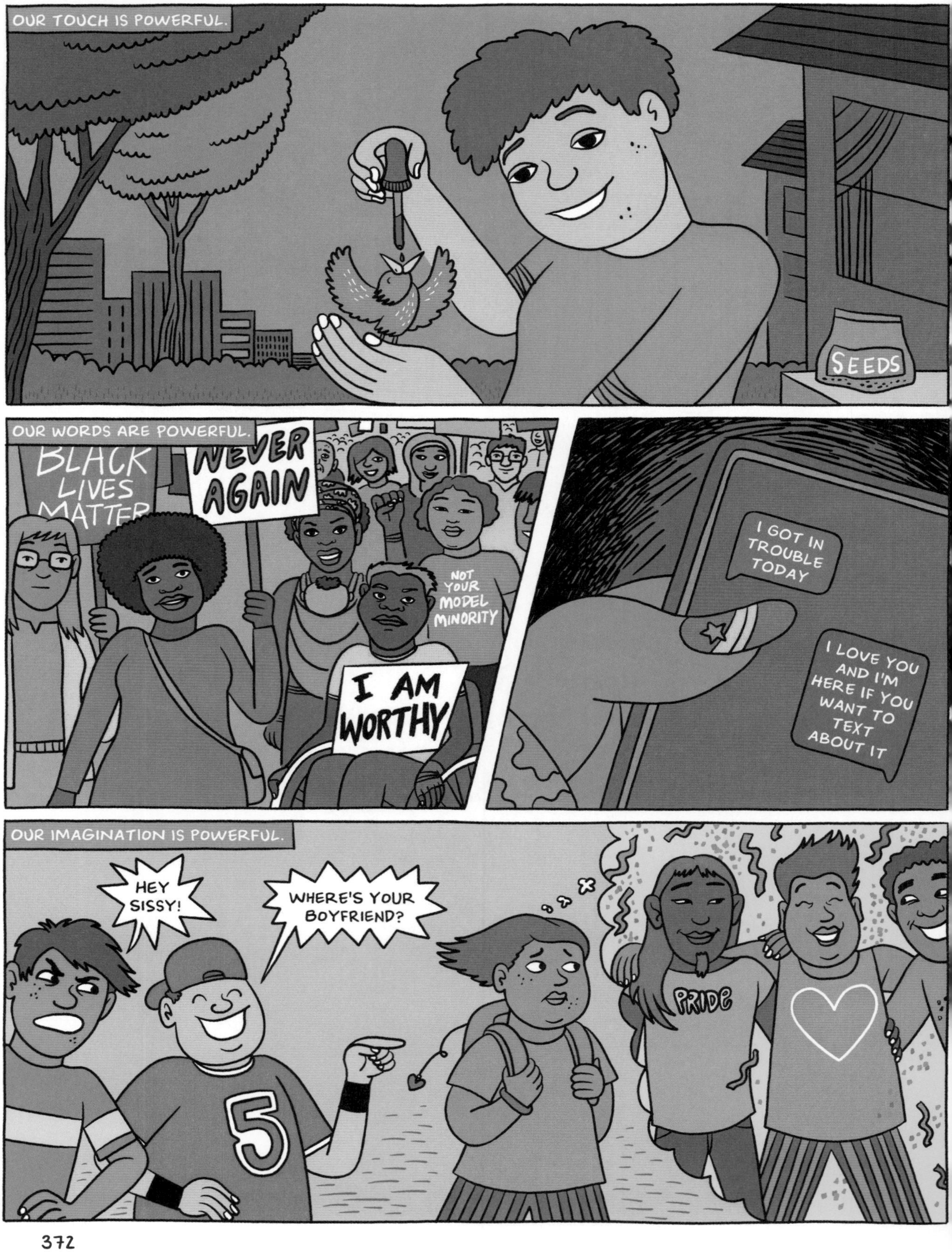
OUR TOUCH IS POWERFUL.
SEEDS
OUR WORDS ARE POWERFUL.
BLACK LIVES MATTER
NEVER AGAIN
NOT YOUR MODEL MINORITY
I AM WORTHY
I GOT IN TROUBLE TODAY
I LOVE YOU AND I'M HERE IF YOU WANT TO TEXT ABOUT IT
OUR IMAGINATION IS POWERFUL.
HEY SISSY!
WHERE'S YOUR BOYFRIEND?
PRIDE
5

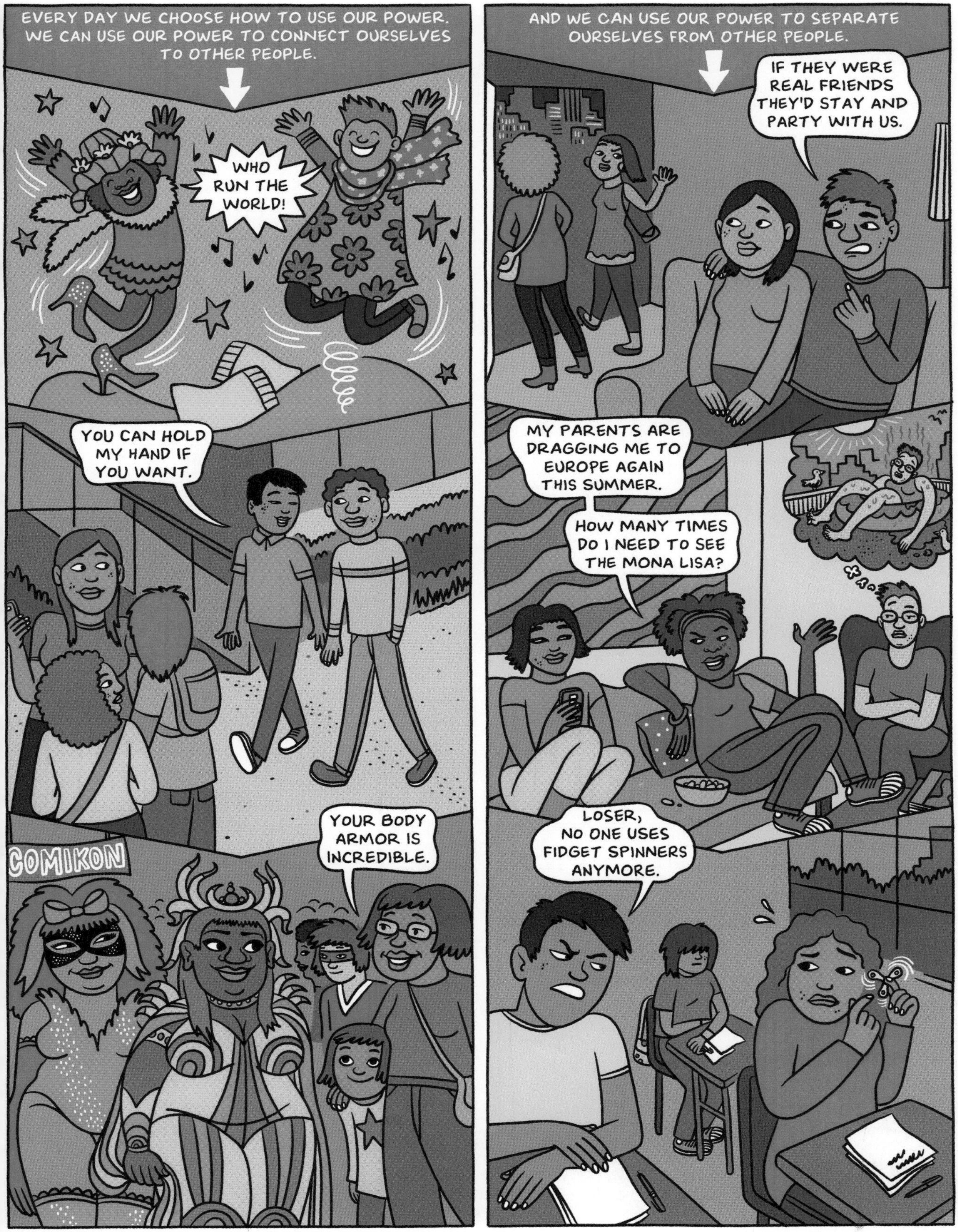
EVERY DAY WE CHOOSE HOW TO USE OUR POWER. WE CAN USE OUR POWER TO CONNECT OURSELVES TO OTHER PEOPLE.
WHO RUN THE WORLD!
YOU CAN HOLD MY HAND IF YOU WANT.
COMIKON
YOUR BODY ARMOR IS INCREDIBLE.
AND WE CAN USE OUR POWER TO SEPARATE OURSELVES FROM OTHER PEOPLE.
IF THEY WERE REAL FRIENDS THEY'D STAY AND PARTY WITH US.
MY PARENTS ARE DRAGGING ME TO EUROPE AGAIN THIS SUMMER.
HOW MANY TIMES DO I NEED TO SEE THE MONA LISA?
LOSER, NO ONE USES FIDGET SPINNERS ANYMORE.

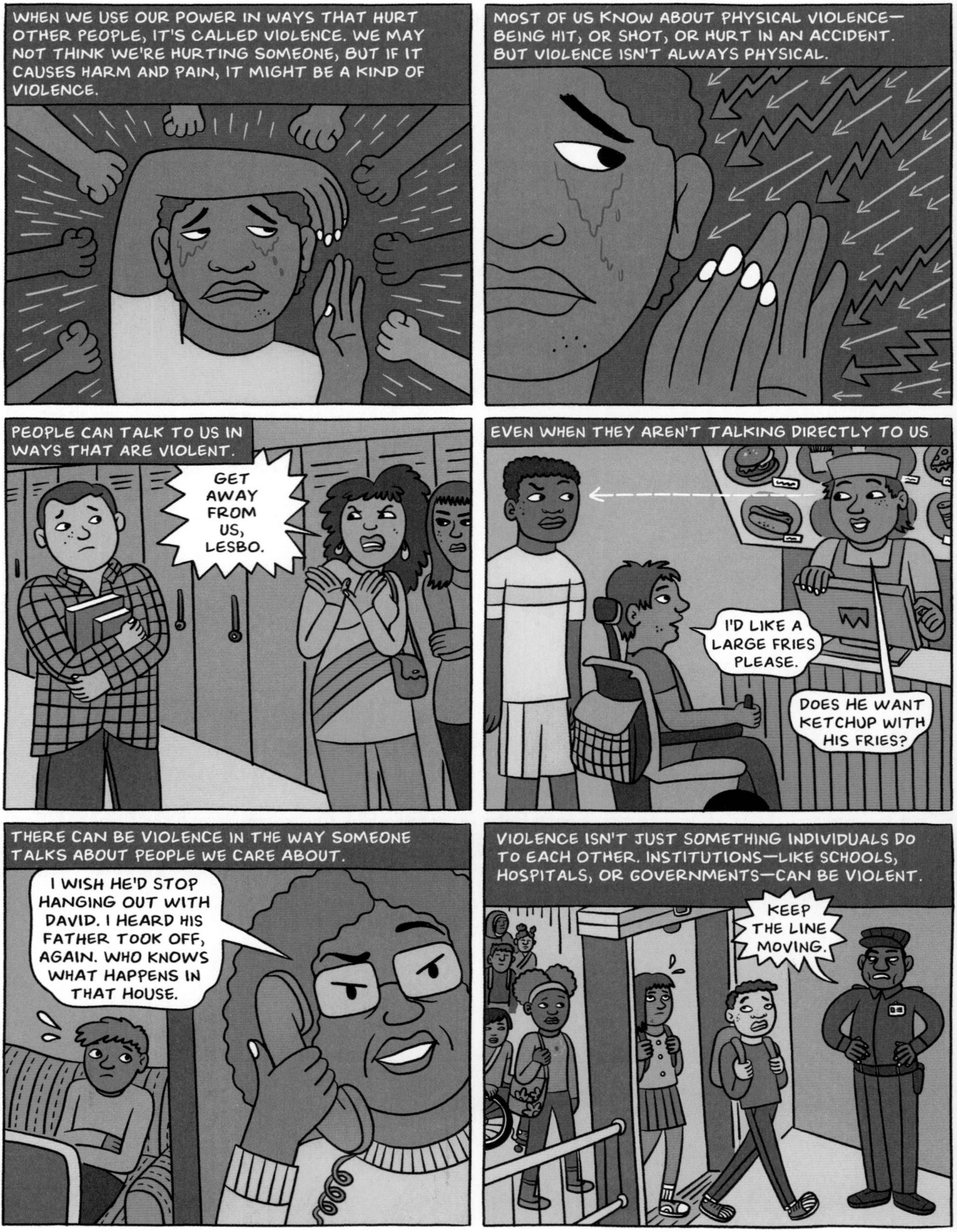
WHEN WE USE OUR POWER IN WAYS THAT HURT OTHER PEOPLE, IT'S CALLED VIOLENCE. WE MAY NOT THINK WE'RE HURTING SOMEONE, BUT IF IT CAUSES HARM AND PAIN, IT MIGHT BE A KIND OF VIOLENCE.
MOST OF US KNOW ABOUT PHYSICAL VIOLENCE—BEING HIT, OR SHOT, OR HURT IN AN ACCIDENT. BUT VIOLENCE ISN'T ALWAYS PHYSICAL.
PEOPLE CAN TALK TO US IN WAYS THAT ARE VIOLENT.
GET AWAY FROM US, LESBO.
EVEN WHEN THEY AREN'T TALKING DIRECTLY TO US.
I'D LIKE A LARGE FRIES PLEASE.
DOES HE WANT KETCHUP WITH HIS FRIES?
THERE CAN BE VIOLENCE IN THE WAY SOMEONE TALKS ABOUT PEOPLE WE CARE ABOUT.
I WISH HE'D STOP HANGING OUT WITH DAVID. I HEARD HIS FATHER TOOK OFF, AGAIN. WHO KNOWS WHAT HAPPENS IN THAT HOUSE.
VIOLENCE ISN'T JUST SOMETHING INDIVIDUALS DO TO EACH OTHER. INSTITUTIONS—LIKE SCHOOLS, HOSPITALS, OR GOVERNMENTS—CAN BE VIOLENT.
KEEP THE LINE MOVING.

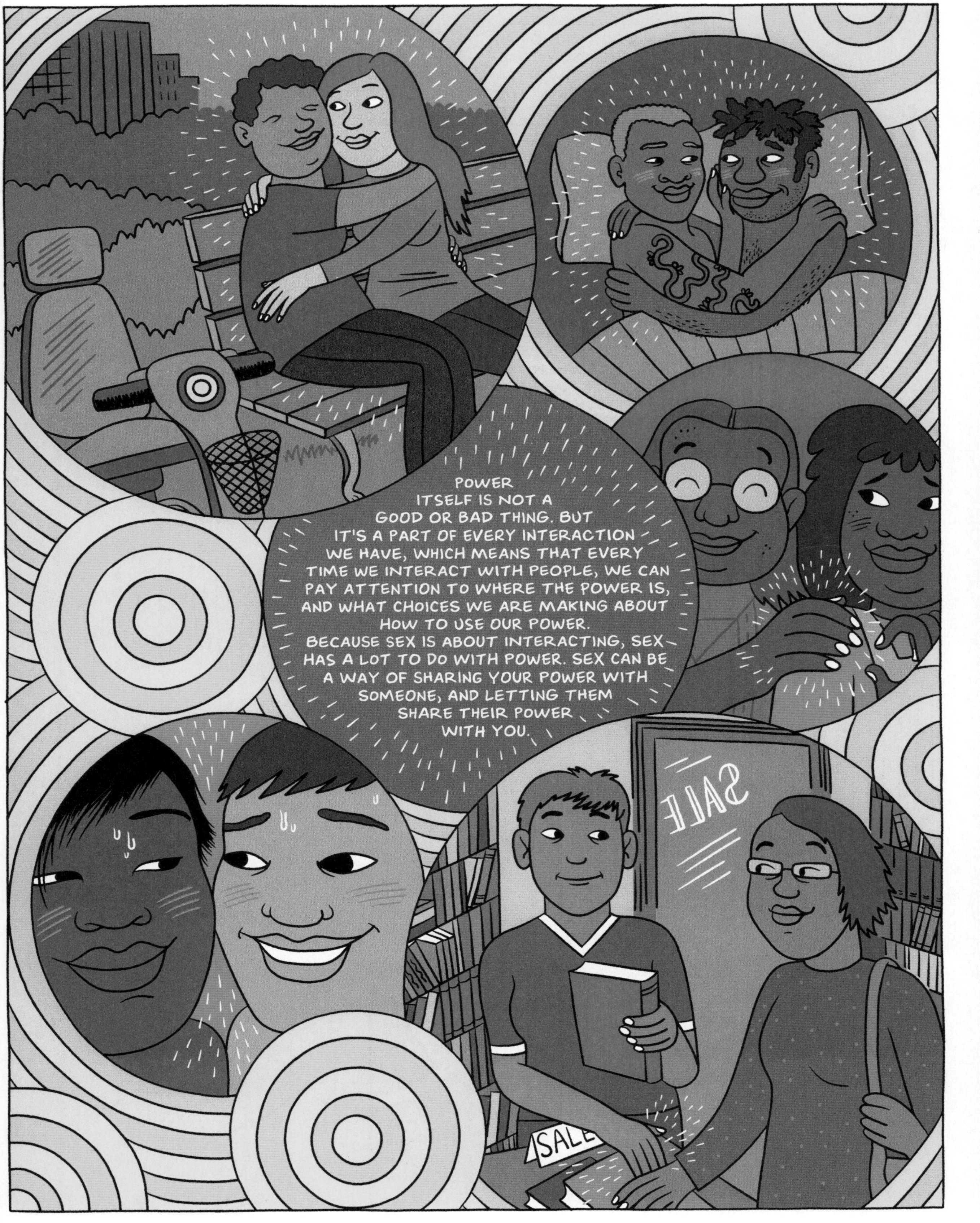
POWER ITSELF IS NOT A GOOD OR BAD THING. BUT IT'S A PART OF EVERY INTERACTION WE HAVE, WHICH MEANS THAT EVERY TIME WE INTERACT WITH PEOPLE, WE CAN PAY ATTENTION TO WHERE THE POWER IS, AND WHAT CHOICES WE ARE MAKING ABOUT HOW TO USE OUR POWER.
BECAUSE SEX IS ABOUT INTERACTING, SEX HAS A LOT TO DO WITH POWER. SEX CAN BE A WAY OF SHARING YOUR POWER WITH SOMEONE, AND LETTING THEM SHARE THEIR POWER WITH YOU.
SALE
SALE

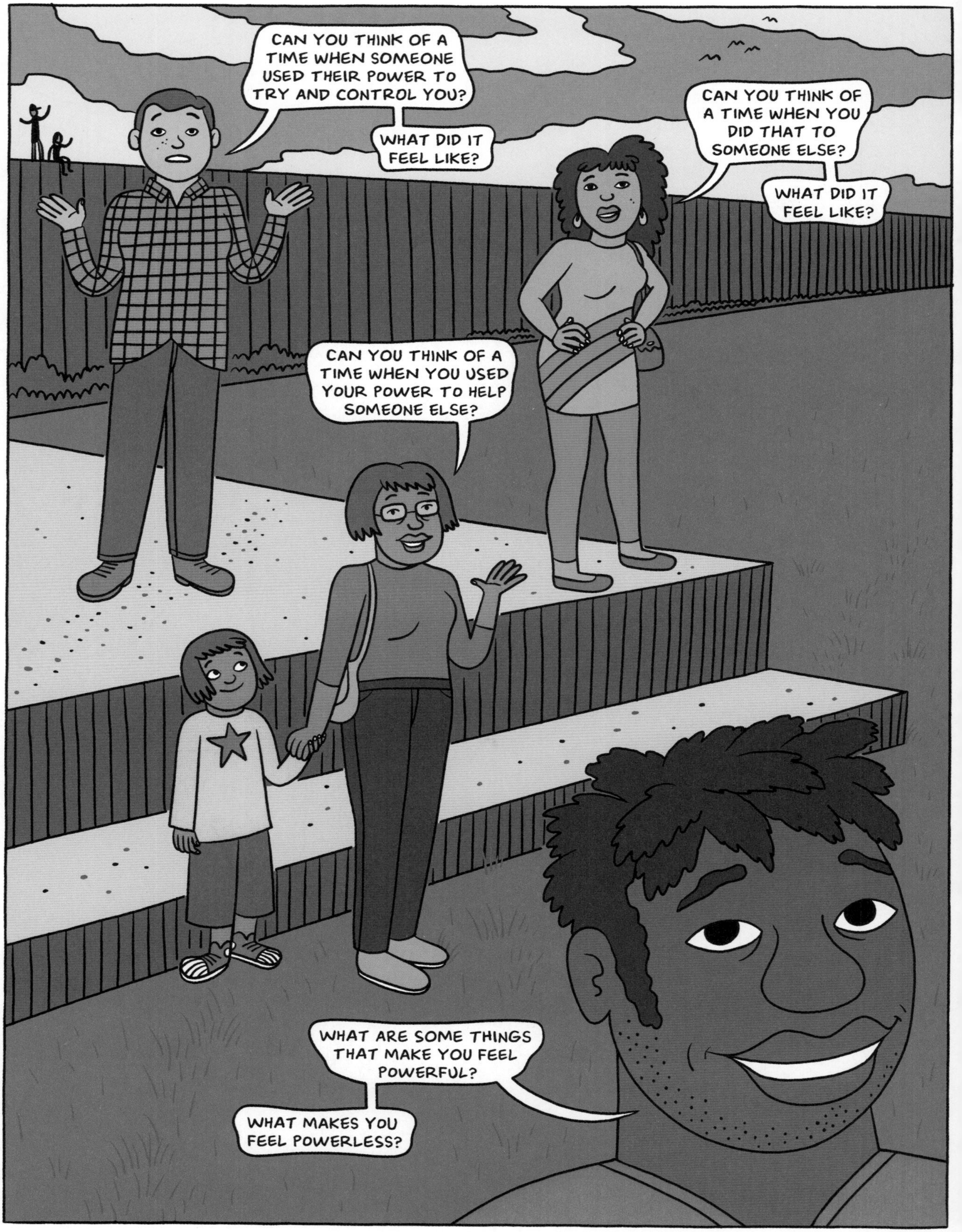
CAN YOU THINK OF A TIME WHEN SOMEONE USED THEIR POWER TO TRY AND CONTROL YOU?
WHAT DID IT FEEL LIKE?
CAN YOU THINK OF A TIME WHEN YOU DID THAT TO SOMEONE ELSE?
WHAT DID IT FEEL LIKE?
CAN YOU THINK OF A TIME WHEN YOU USED YOUR POWER TO HELP SOMEONE ELSE?
WHAT ARE SOME THINGS THAT MAKE YOU FEEL POWERFUL?
WHAT MAKES YOU FEEL POWERLESS?

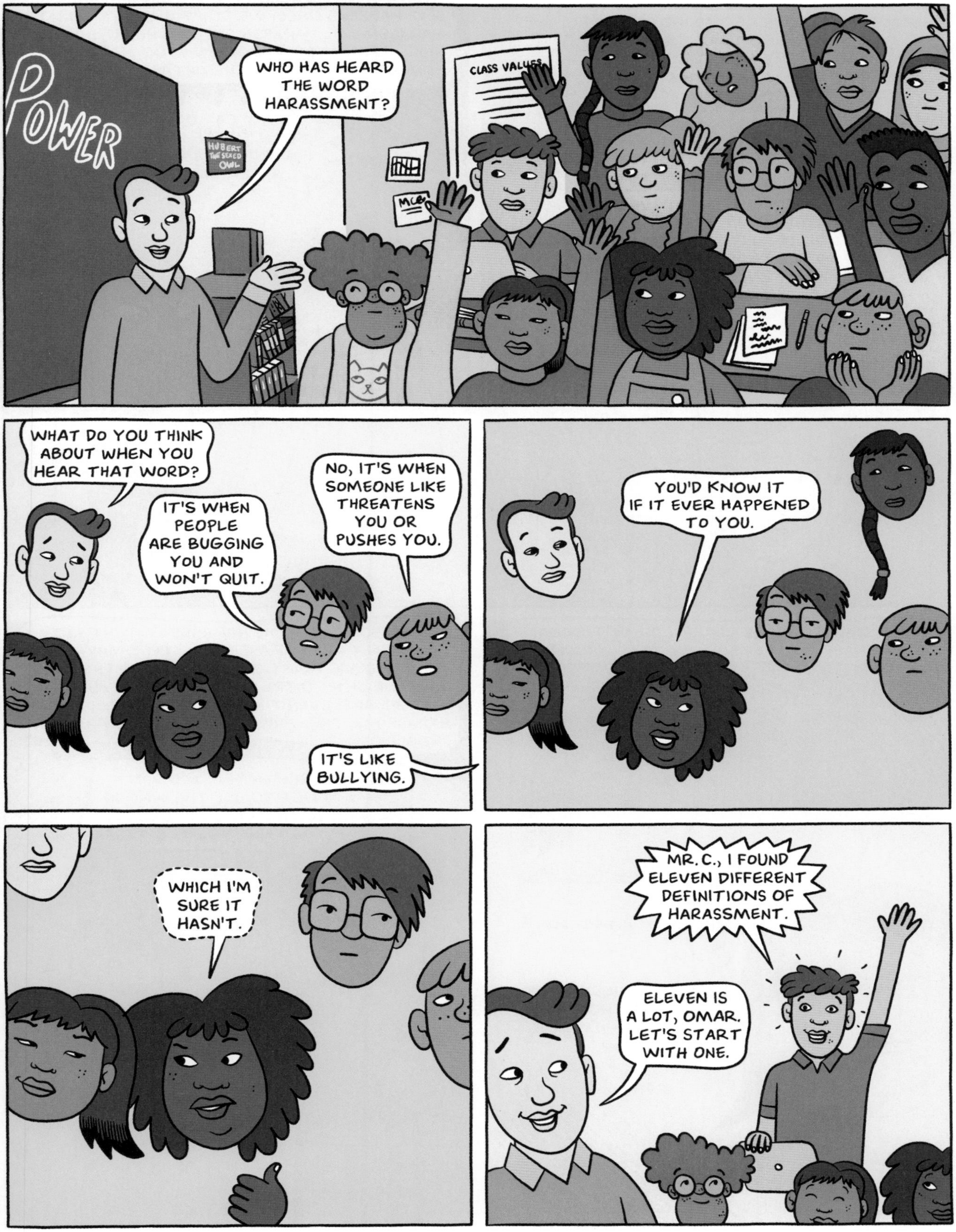
POWER
HUBERT THE SEXED OWL
CLASS VALUES
MCG
WHO HAS HEARD THE WORD HARASSMENT?
WHAT DO YOU THINK ABOUT WHEN YOU HEAR THAT WORD?
IT'S WHEN PEOPLE ARE BUGGING YOU AND WON'T QUIT.
NO, IT'S WHEN SOMEONE LIKE THREATENS YOU OR PUSHES YOU.
IT'S LIKE BULLYING.
YOU'D KNOW IT IF IT EVER HAPPENED TO YOU.
WHICH I'M SURE IT HASN'T.
MR. C., I FOUND ELEVEN DIFFERENT DEFINITIONS OF HARASSMENT.
ELEVEN IS A LOT, OMAR. LET'S START WITH ONE.

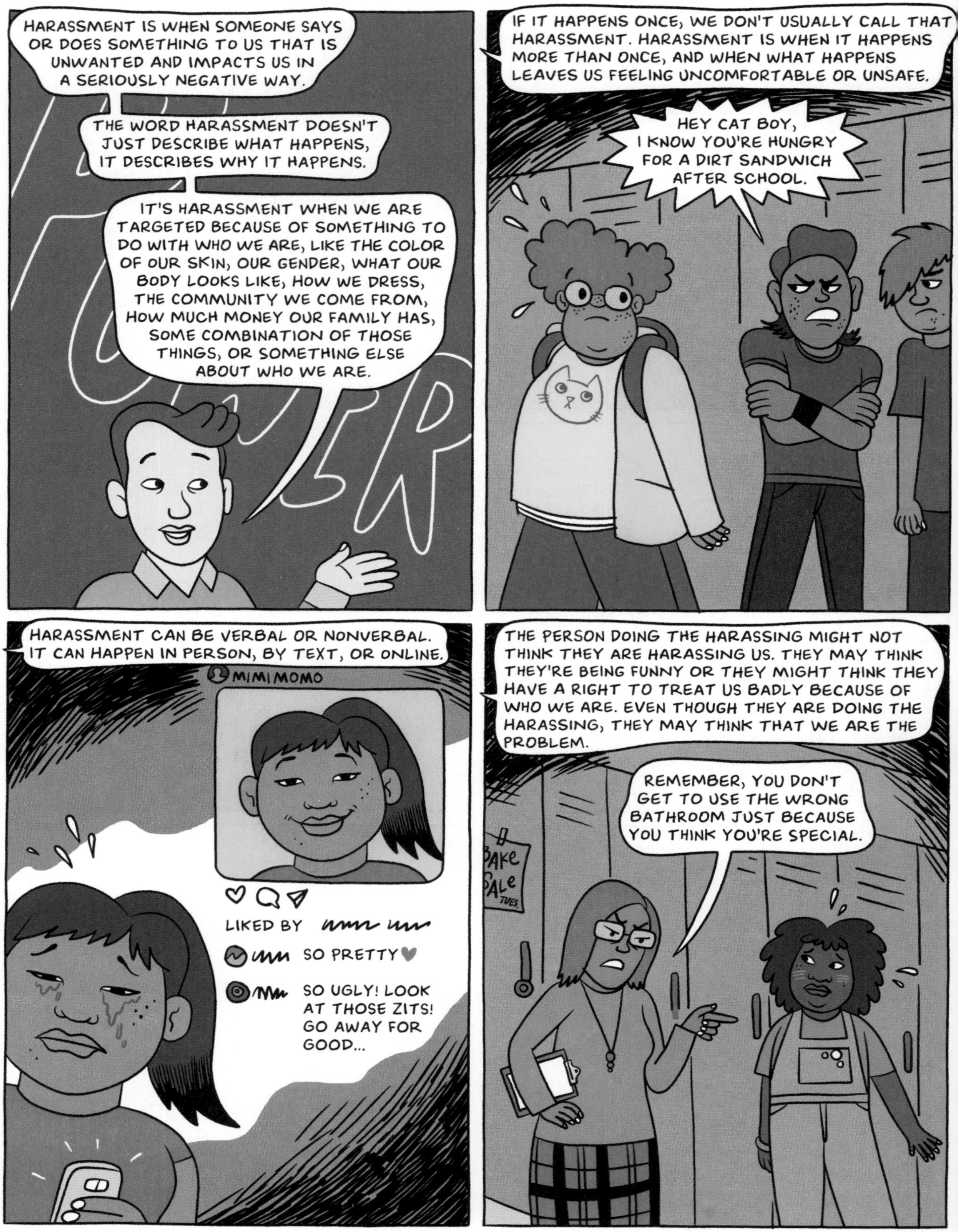
HARASSMENT IS WHEN SOMEONE SAYS OR DOES SOMETHING TO US THAT IS UNWANTED AND IMPACTS US IN A SERIOUSLY NEGATIVE WAY.
THE WORD HARASSMENT DOESN'T JUST DESCRIBE WHAT HAPPENS, IT DESCRIBES WHY IT HAPPENS.
IT'S HARASSMENT WHEN WE ARE TARGETED BECAUSE OF SOMETHING TO DO WITH WHO WE ARE, LIKE THE COLOR OF OUR SKIN, OUR GENDER, WHAT OUR BODY LOOKS LIKE, HOW WE DRESS, THE COMMUNITY WE COME FROM, HOW MUCH MONEY OUR FAMILY HAS, SOME COMBINATION OF THOSE THINGS, OR SOMETHING ELSE ABOUT WHO WE ARE.
IF IT HAPPENS ONCE, WE DON'T USUALLY CALL THAT HARASSMENT. HARASSMENT IS WHEN IT HAPPENS MORE THAN ONCE, AND WHEN WHAT HAPPENS LEAVES US FEELING UNCOMFORTABLE OR UNSAFE.
HEY CAT BOY, I KNOW YOU'RE HUNGRY FOR A DIRT SANDWICH AFTER SCHOOL.
HARASSMENT CAN BE VERBAL OR NONVERBAL. IT CAN HAPPEN IN PERSON, BY TEXT, OR ONLINE.
MIMIMOMO
LIKED BY
SO PRETTY
SO UGLY! LOOK AT THOSE ZITS! GO AWAY FOR GOOD...
THE PERSON DOING THE HARASSING MIGHT NOT THINK THEY ARE HARASSING US. THEY MAY THINK THEY'RE BEING FUNNY OR THEY MIGHT THINK THEY HAVE A RIGHT TO TREAT US BADLY BECAUSE OF WHO WE ARE. EVEN THOUGH THEY ARE DOING THE HARASSING, THEY MAY THINK THAT WE ARE THE PROBLEM.
REMEMBER, YOU DON'T GET TO USE THE WRONG BATHROOM JUST BECAUSE YOU THINK YOU'RE SPECIAL.
BAKE SALE TUES.

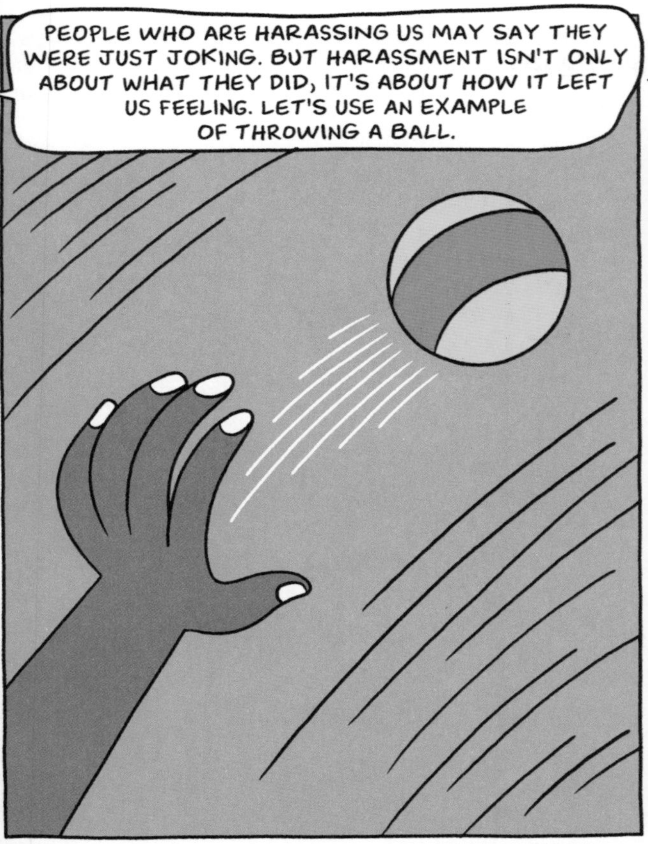
PEOPLE WHO ARE HARASSING US MAY SAY THEY WERE JUST JOKING. BUT HARASSMENT ISN'T ONLY ABOUT WHAT THEY DID, IT'S ABOUT HOW IT LEFT US FEELING. LET'S USE AN EXAMPLE OF THROWING A BALL.

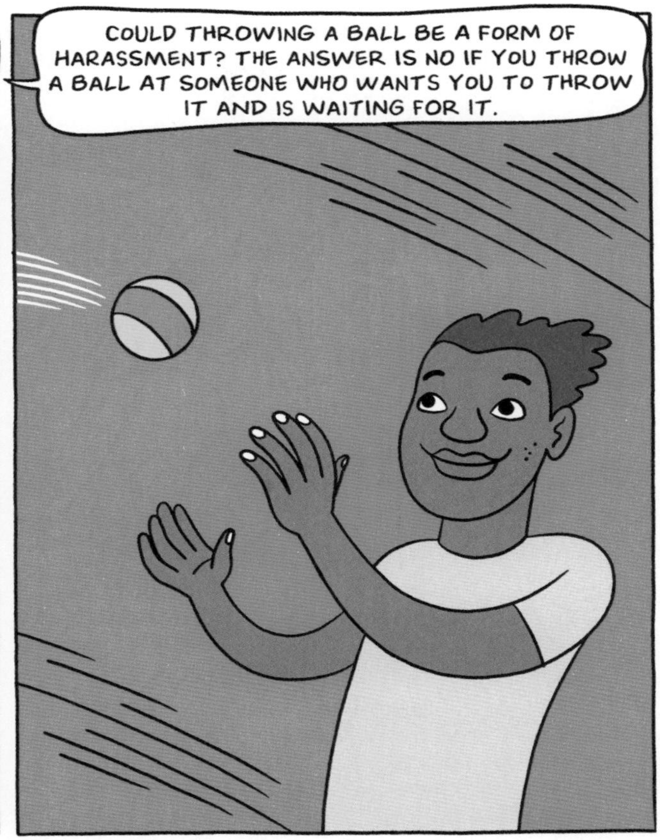
COULD THROWING A BALL BE A FORM OF HARASSMENT? THE ANSWER IS NO IF YOU THROW A BALL AT SOMEONE WHO WANTS YOU TO THROW IT AND IS WAITING FOR IT.

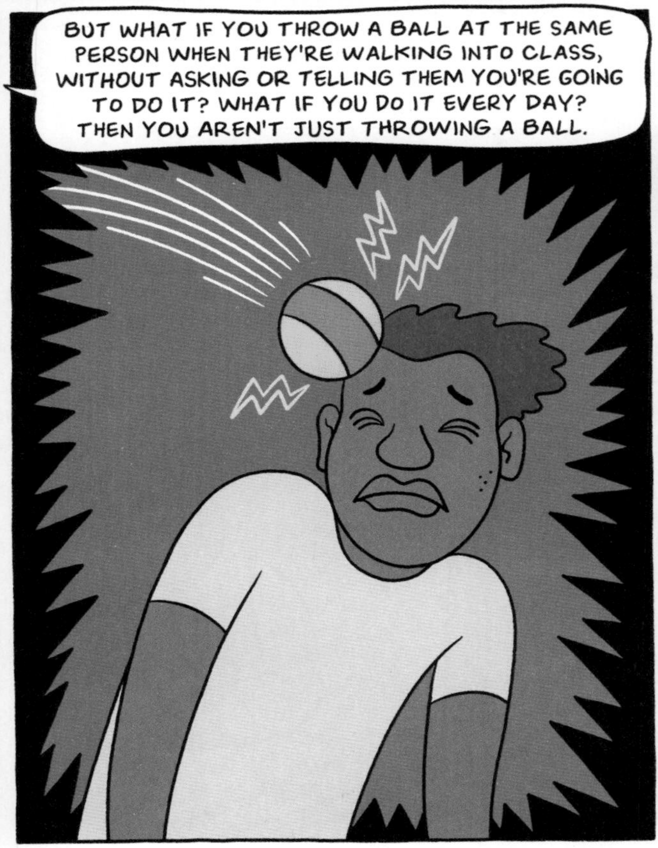
BUT WHAT IF YOU THROW A BALL AT THE SAME PERSON WHEN THEY'RE WALKING INTO CLASS, WITHOUT ASKING OR TELLING THEM YOU'RE GOING TO DO IT? WHAT IF YOU DO IT EVERY DAY? THEN YOU AREN'T JUST THROWING A BALL.

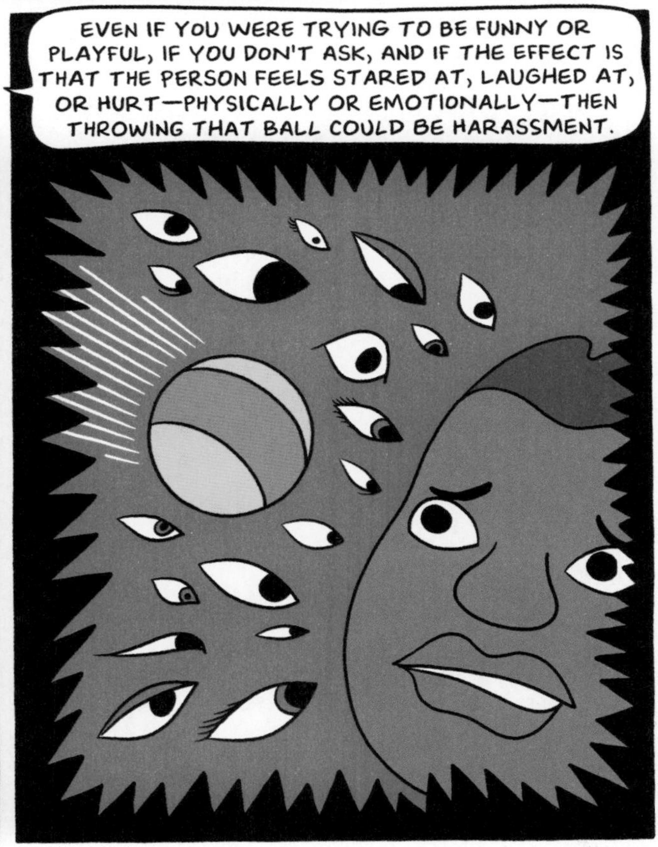
EVEN IF YOU WERE TRYING TO BE FUNNY OR PLAYFUL, IF YOU DON'T ASK, AND IF THE EFFECT IS THAT THE PERSON FEELS STARED AT, LAUGHED AT, OR HURT—PHYSICALLY OR EMOTIONALLY—THEN THROWING THAT BALL COULD BE HARASSMENT.

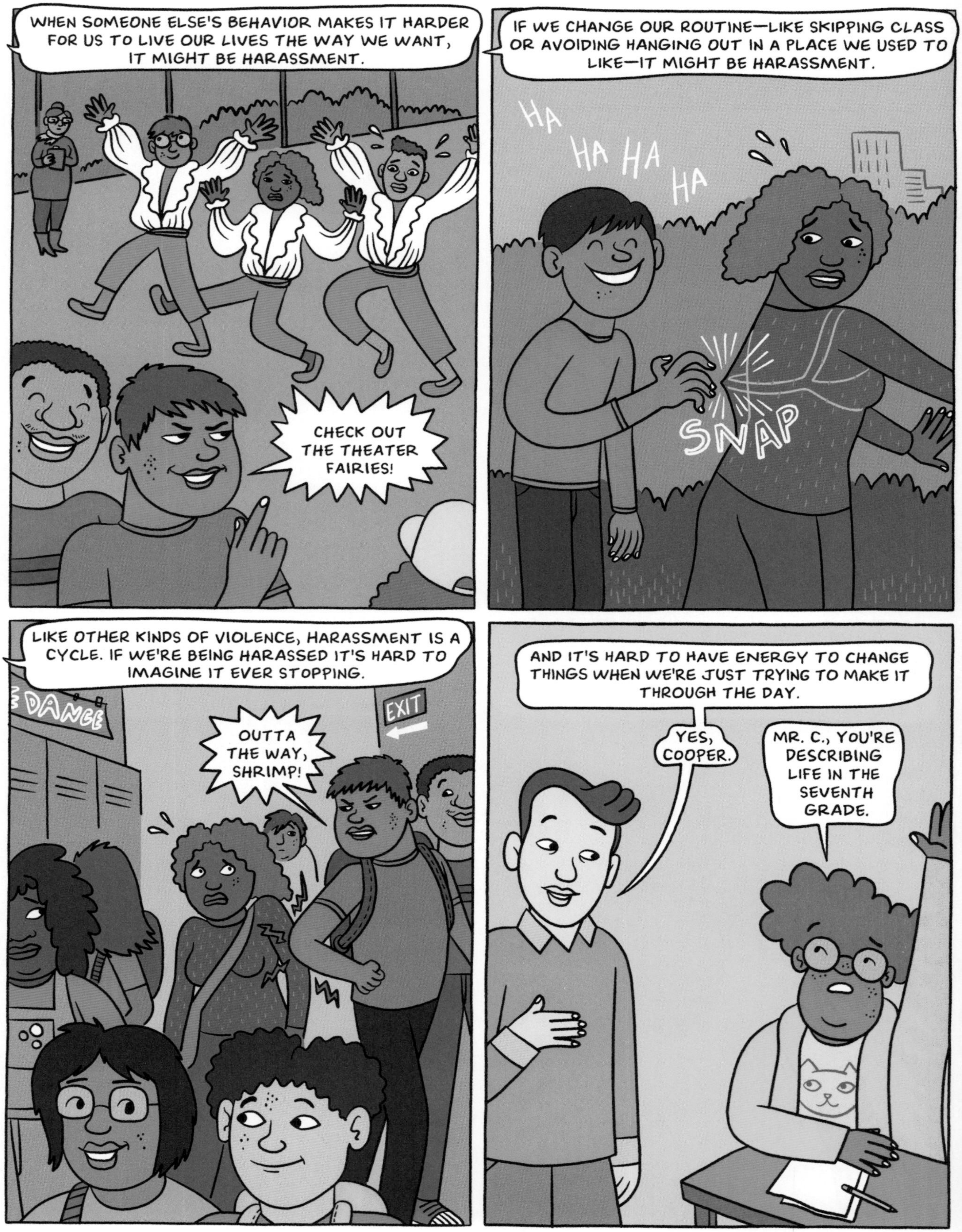
WHEN SOMEONE ELSE'S BEHAVIOR MAKES IT HARDER FOR US TO LIVE OUR LIVES THE WAY WE WANT, IT MIGHT BE HARASSMENT.
CHECK OUT THE THEATER FAIRIES!
IF WE CHANGE OUR ROUTINE—LIKE SKIPPING CLASS OR AVOIDING HANGING OUT IN A PLACE WE USED TO LIKE—IT MIGHT BE HARASSMENT.
HA HA HA HA
SNAP
LIKE OTHER KINDS OF VIOLENCE, HARASSMENT IS A CYCLE. IF WE'RE BEING HARASSED IT'S HARD TO IMAGINE IT EVER STOPPING.
DANCE
EXIT
OUTTA THE WAY, SHRIMP!
AND IT'S HARD TO HAVE ENERGY TO CHANGE THINGS WHEN WE'RE JUST TRYING TO MAKE IT THROUGH THE DAY.
YES, COOPER.
MR. C., YOU'RE DESCRIBING LIFE IN THE SEVENTH GRADE.

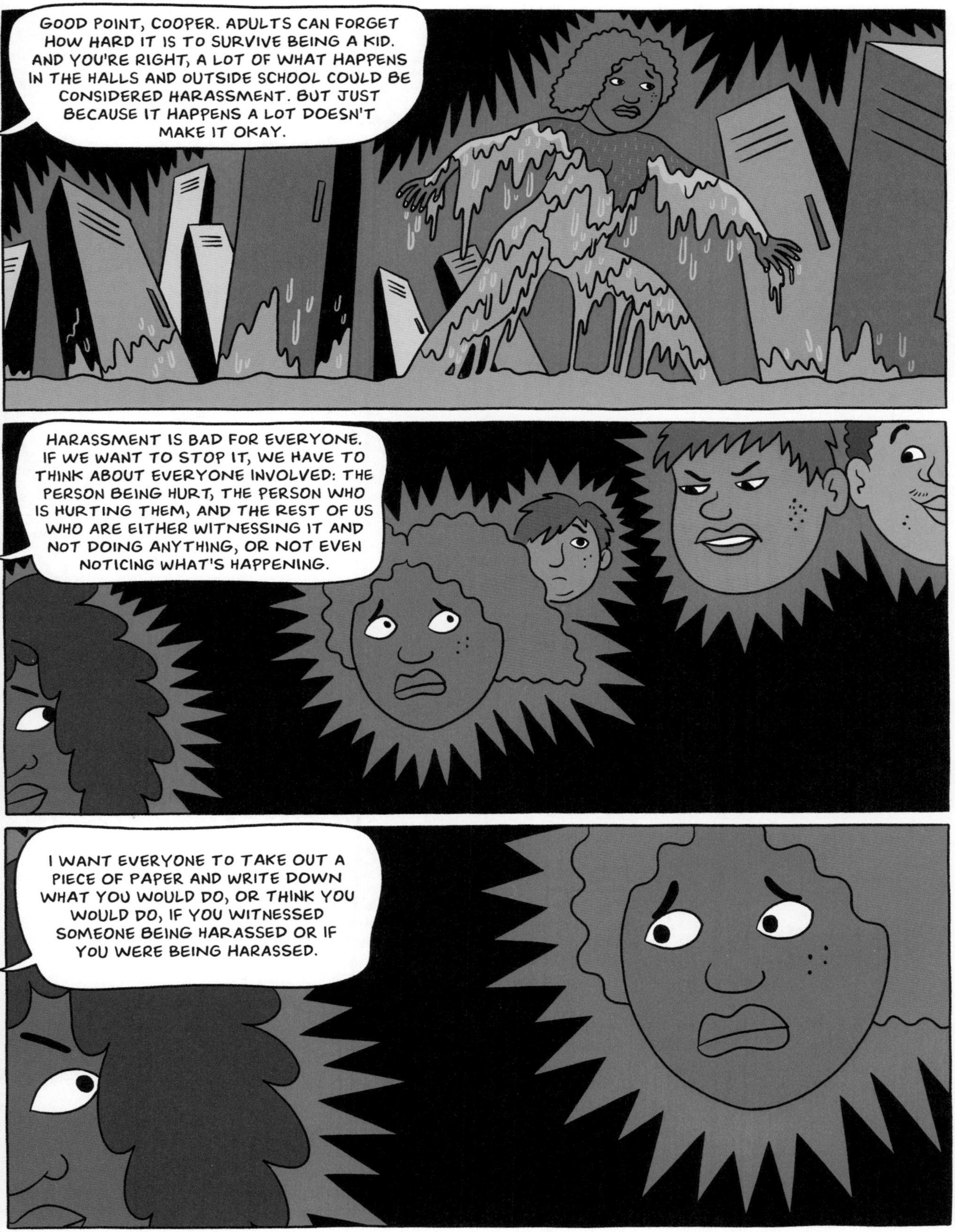
GOOD POINT, COOPER. ADULTS CAN FORGET HOW HARD IT IS TO SURVIVE BEING A KID. AND YOU'RE RIGHT, A LOT OF WHAT HAPPENS IN THE HALLS AND OUTSIDE SCHOOL COULD BE CONSIDERED HARASSMENT. BUT JUST BECAUSE IT HAPPENS A LOT DOESN'T MAKE IT OKAY.
HARASSMENT IS BAD FOR EVERYONE. IF WE WANT TO STOP IT, WE HAVE TO THINK ABOUT EVERYONE INVOLVED: THE PERSON BEING HURT, THE PERSON WHO IS HURTING THEM, AND THE REST OF US WHO ARE EITHER WITNESSING IT AND NOT DOING ANYTHING, OR NOT EVEN NOTICING WHAT'S HAPPENING.
I WANT EVERYONE TO TAKE OUT A PIECE OF PAPER AND WRITE DOWN WHAT YOU WOULD DO, OR THINK YOU WOULD DO, IF YOU WITNESSED SOMEONE BEING HARASSED OR IF YOU WERE BEING HARASSED.

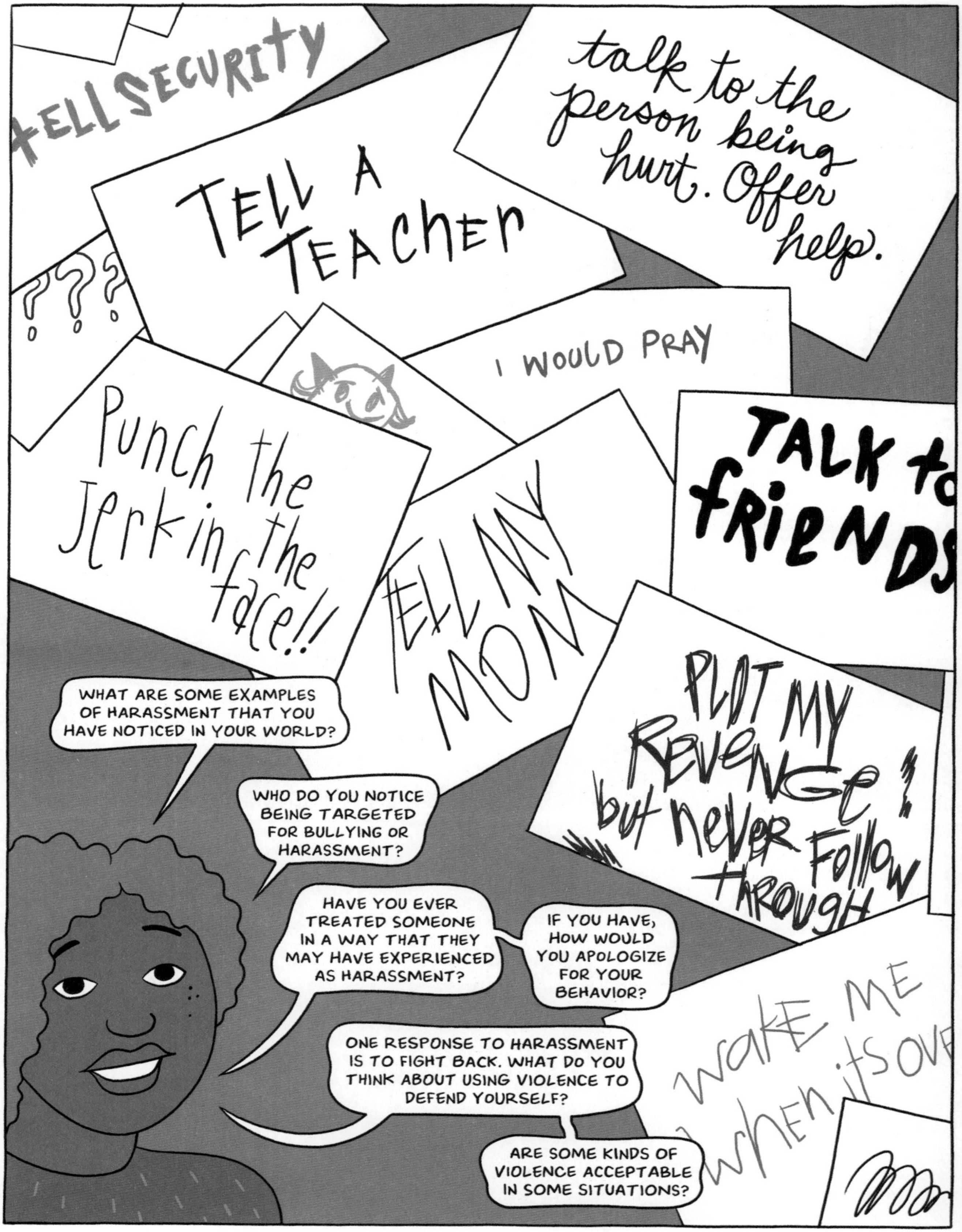
TELL SECURITY
talk to the person being hurt. Offer help.
TELL A TEACHER
???
I WOULD PRAY
Punch the Jerk in the face!!
TALK TO FRIENDS
TELL MY MOM
PLOT MY REVENGE but never follow through
wake me when it's ove
WHAT ARE SOME EXAMPLES OF HARASSMENT THAT YOU HAVE NOTICED IN YOUR WORLD?
WHO DO YOU NOTICE BEING TARGETED FOR BULLYING OR HARASSMENT?
HAVE YOU EVER TREATED SOMEONE IN A WAY THAT THEY MAY HAVE EXPERIENCED AS HARASSMENT?
IF YOU HAVE, HOW WOULD YOU APOLOGIZE FOR YOUR BEHAVIOR?
ONE RESPONSE TO HARASSMENT IS TO FIGHT BACK. WHAT DO YOU THINK ABOUT USING VIOLENCE TO DEFEND YOURSELF?
ARE SOME KINDS OF VIOLENCE ACCEPTABLE IN SOME SITUATIONS?

NERD ALERT WHAT DOES IT MEAN TO BE ACCOUNTABLE?

BEING ACCOUNTABLE MEANS TAKING RESPONSIBILITY FOR OUR BEHAVIOR AND DOING SOMETHING ABOUT IT WHEN WE HAVE CAUSED HARM. IT CAN BE HARD TO ADMIT THAT WE'VE HURT SOMEONE, BUT WE ALL DO IT AT SOME POINT. ACTING LIKE IT DIDN'T HAPPEN OR HOPING NO ONE TALKS ABOUT IT ONLY MAKES IT WORSE.

IN ORDER FOR US TO TAKE RESPONSIBILITY FOR OUR ACTIONS—INCLUDING OUR WORDS—WE NEED TO KNOW THE IMPACT OF OUR ACTIONS. THIS MEANS LISTENING TO THOSE WE HAVE HURT AND TRYING TO UNDERSTAND HOW OUR ACTIONS IMPACTED THEM.

AND IT MEANS WANTING TO WORK WITH THE PEOPLE WE HARM TO CHANGE THINGS FOR ALL OF US. WORKING TOGETHER TO MAKE THINGS BETTER FOR EVERYONE IS ONE WAY TO HEAL SOME OF THE HARM.

HOW TO APOLOGIZE

BIANCA I LAUREANO IS A SEX EDUCATOR (AND PRETTY COOL PERSON) WHO WRITES AND TALKS A LOT ABOUT JUSTICE AND ACCOUNTABILITY. SHE REMINDS US THAT EVERYONE MESSES UP AND HURTS SOMEONE AT SOME POINT. SO, A BIG PART OF ACCOUNTABILITY IS KNOWING HOW TO APOLOGIZE.

BIANCA SAYS THERE ARE THREE PARTS TO A MEANINGFUL APOLOGY:

1. START BY ACKNOWLEDGING WHAT YOU DID THAT YOU NOW KNOW CAUSED HARM. DON'T MAKE EXCUSES, JUST SAY WHAT HAPPENED.
2. ACKNOWLEDGE THE WAY YOUR WORDS OR ACTIONS IMPACTED OTHERS. SHOW THAT YOU UNDERSTAND THE POWER OF WHAT YOU DID, EVEN IF YOU DIDN'T MEAN TO DO IT. DON'T FOCUS ON WHAT YOU MEANT (YOUR INTENT), FOCUS ON HOW IT IMPACTED OTHERS.
3. BE CLEAR ABOUT WHAT YOU WILL DO TO CHANGE YOUR BEHAVIOR. THIS IS THE ACCOUNTABILITY PART. SHARE WHAT YOU LEARNED, HOW YOU WILL TRY TO DO IT DIFFERENTLY NEXT TIME, AND WHAT ELSE YOU CAN OFFER TO MAKE CHANGE.

ACCOUNTABILITY IS A WAY OF CARING FOR OTHERS AND OURSELVES.

JIMI THE JOKER
HEY BEANSTALK! WHERE'S JACK?
HA HA
?
HEY SHRIMP! WHERE'S THE BARBIE?
HA HA
HEY MEATBALL! WHERE'S THE SPAGHETTI?
HA HA
UGH
POOL
HEY JELLY! WHERE'S THE ROLL?
LIZ, YOU GOT A FAT BUTT!
HA HA
JIMI, WHY DO YOU TRY SO HARD TO BE MEAN?
I'M JUST KIDDING AROUND LIZ!
EVERY DAY, ALL DAY YOU BODY SHAME EVERYBODY!
I'M SORRY I UPSET YOU, LIZ.
THANKS FOR CORRECTING ME. YOU'RE A GOOD FRIEND.
NO MORE BODY JOKES FROM NOW ON.
EVERY BODY IS DIFFERENT, EVERY BODY HAS BEAUTY IN IT, RIGHT?
YUP, AND DON'T YOU FORGET IT!
CHECK OUT MY BUBBLE BUTT! IT'S BIGGER THAN YOURS!
CUTE, HUH?
THE BEST!

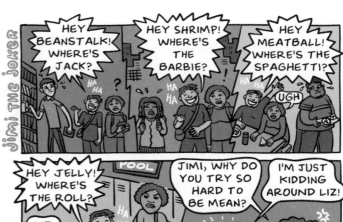

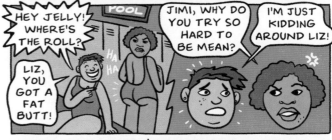

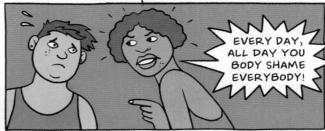

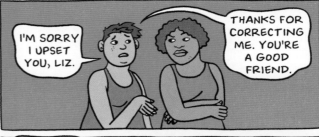

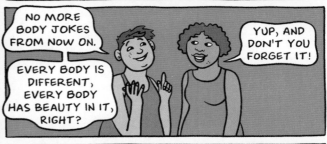

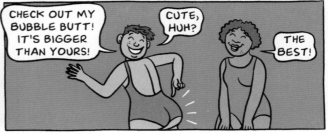

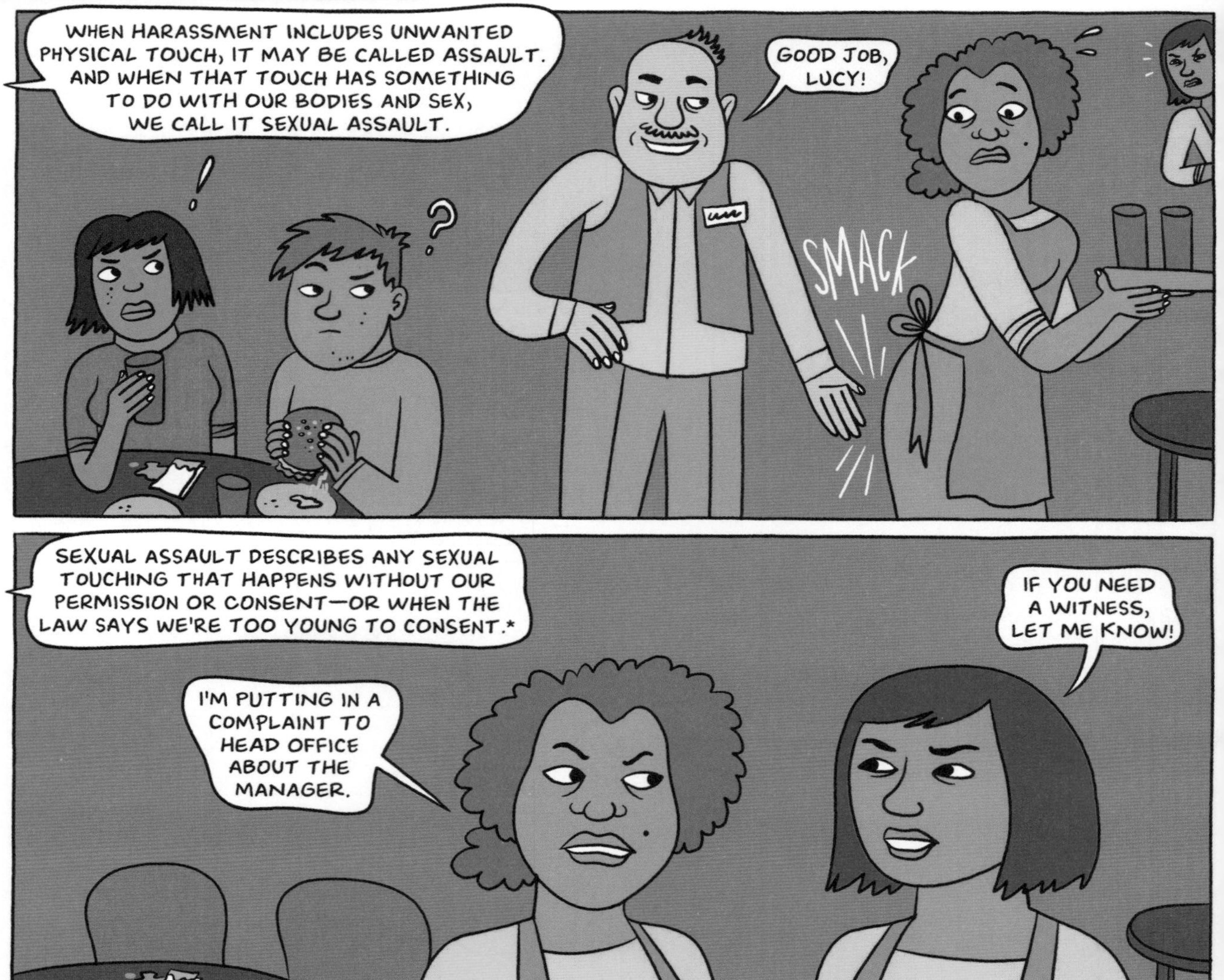
WHEN HARASSMENT INCLUDES UNWANTED PHYSICAL TOUCH, IT MAY BE CALLED ASSAULT. AND WHEN THAT TOUCH HAS SOMETHING TO DO WITH OUR BODIES AND SEX, WE CALL IT SEXUAL ASSAULT.
GOOD JOB, LUCY!
SMACK
SEXUAL ASSAULT DESCRIBES ANY SEXUAL TOUCHING THAT HAPPENS WITHOUT OUR PERMISSION OR CONSENT—OR WHEN THE LAW SAYS WE'RE TOO YOUNG TO CONSENT.*
I'M PUTTING IN A COMPLAINT TO HEAD OFFICE ABOUT THE MANAGER.
IF YOU NEED A WITNESS, LET ME KNOW!
SEXUAL ASSAULT CAN INCLUDE GRABBING OR KISSING OR MORE. IT CAN INCLUDE PHYSICAL FORCE OR USING WORDS—LIKE THREATS OR ATTEMPTS TO MAKE SOMEONE FEEL GUILTY—TO PRESSURE SOMEONE SO THEY FEEL THEY DON'T HAVE A CHOICE.
IT DOESN'T MATTER IF THE PERSON DOING THE ASSAULT FOLLOWS THROUGH ON THREATS OF VIOLENCE—IF THEY USE A THREAT AND THEN THERE IS TOUCH WITHOUT PERMISSION OR CONSENT, IT MIGHT BE SEXUAL ASSAULT.
ALCOHOL AND OTHER DRUGS CAN ALSO AFFECT THINGS: SOMETIMES THEY ARE USED INTENTIONALLY IN SEXUAL ASSAULTS. OTHER TIMES, WE MAY USE THEM VOLUNTARILY, BUT THEY MAY MAKE US LESS ABLE TO PROTECT OURSELVES FROM SEXUAL ASSAULT.

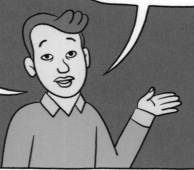

* IF YOU SKIPPED IT, YOU CAN READ ABOUT THE AGE OF CONSENT ON P. 233

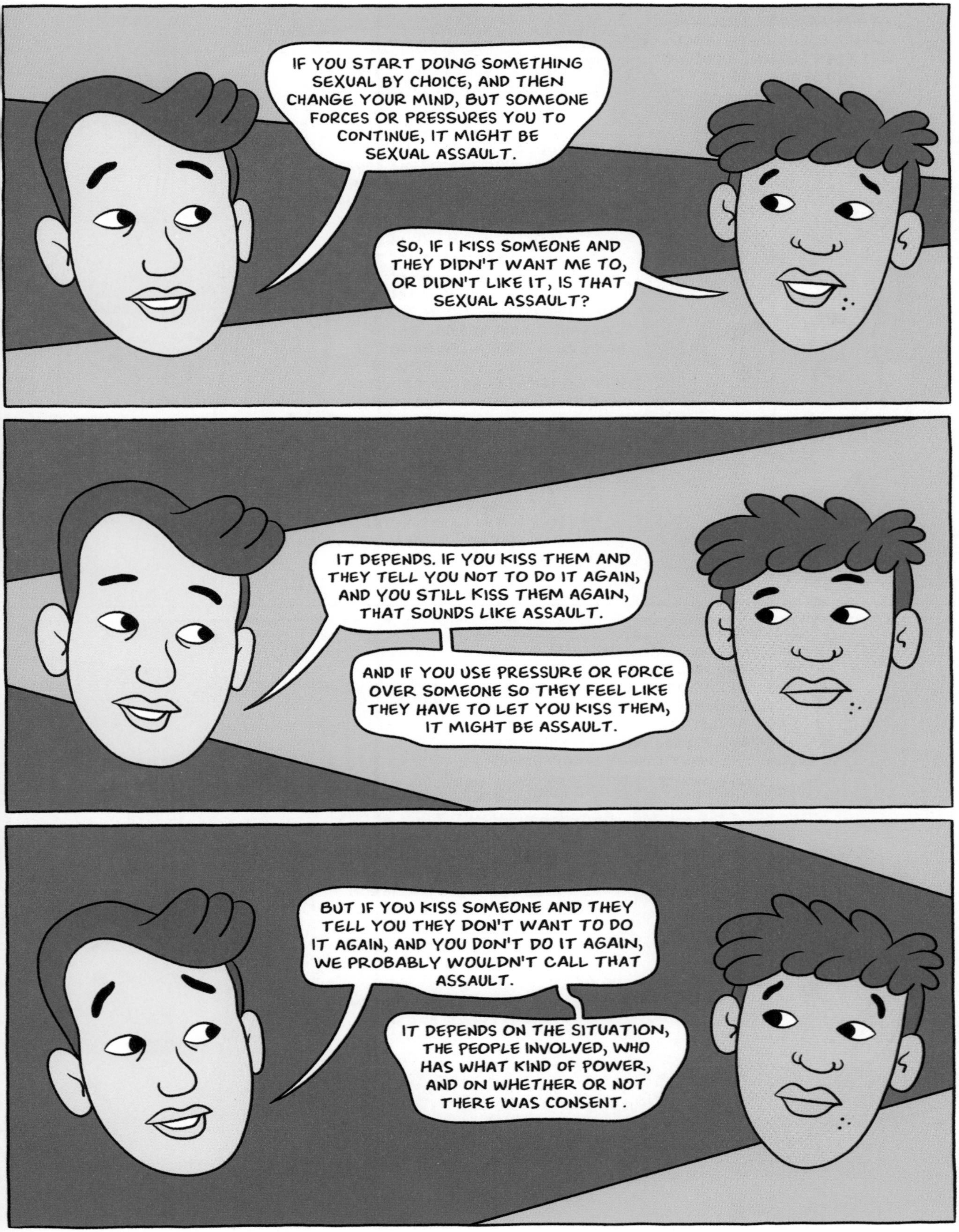
IF YOU START DOING SOMETHING SEXUAL BY CHOICE, AND THEN CHANGE YOUR MIND, BUT SOMEONE FORCES OR PRESSURES YOU TO CONTINUE, IT MIGHT BE SEXUAL ASSAULT.
SO, IF I KISS SOMEONE AND THEY DIDN'T WANT ME TO, OR DIDN'T LIKE IT, IS THAT SEXUAL ASSAULT?
IT DEPENDS. IF YOU KISS THEM AND THEY TELL YOU NOT TO DO IT AGAIN, AND YOU STILL KISS THEM AGAIN, THAT SOUNDS LIKE ASSAULT.
AND IF YOU USE PRESSURE OR FORCE OVER SOMEONE SO THEY FEEL LIKE THEY HAVE TO LET YOU KISS THEM, IT MIGHT BE ASSAULT.
BUT IF YOU KISS SOMEONE AND THEY TELL YOU THEY DON'T WANT TO DO IT AGAIN, AND YOU DON'T DO IT AGAIN, WE PROBABLY WOULDN'T CALL THAT ASSAULT.
IT DEPENDS ON THE SITUATION, THE PEOPLE INVOLVED, WHO HAS WHAT KIND OF POWER, AND ON WHETHER OR NOT THERE WAS CONSENT.

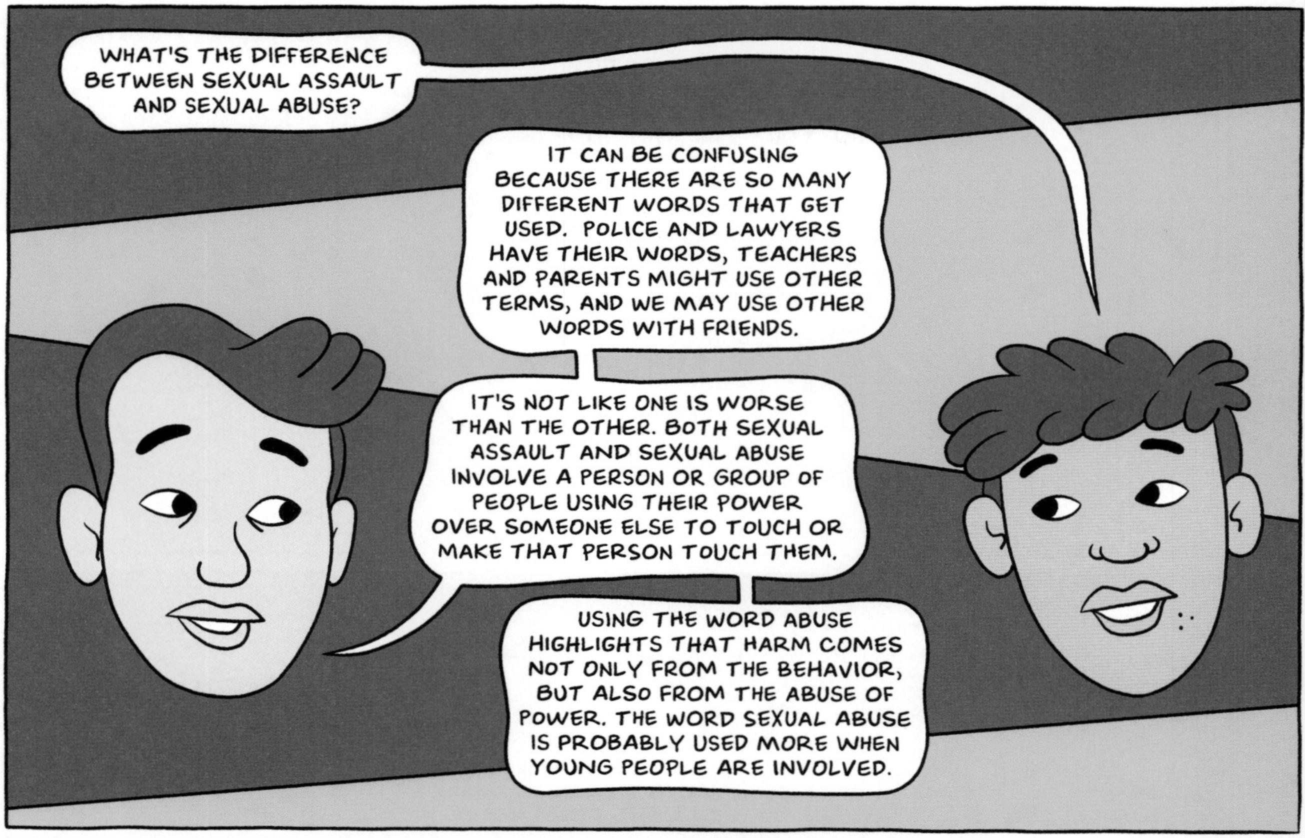
WHAT'S THE DIFFERENCE BETWEEN SEXUAL ASSAULT AND SEXUAL ABUSE?
IT CAN BE CONFUSING BECAUSE THERE ARE SO MANY DIFFERENT WORDS THAT GET USED. POLICE AND LAWYERS HAVE THEIR WORDS, TEACHERS AND PARENTS MIGHT USE OTHER TERMS, AND WE MAY USE OTHER WORDS WITH FRIENDS.
IT'S NOT LIKE ONE IS WORSE THAN THE OTHER. BOTH SEXUAL ASSAULT AND SEXUAL ABUSE INVOLVE A PERSON OR GROUP OF PEOPLE USING THEIR POWER OVER SOMEONE ELSE TO TOUCH OR MAKE THAT PERSON TOUCH THEM.
USING THE WORD ABUSE HIGHLIGHTS THAT HARM COMES NOT ONLY FROM THE BEHAVIOR, BUT ALSO FROM THE ABUSE OF POWER. THE WORD SEXUAL ABUSE IS PROBABLY USED MORE WHEN YOUNG PEOPLE ARE INVOLVED.

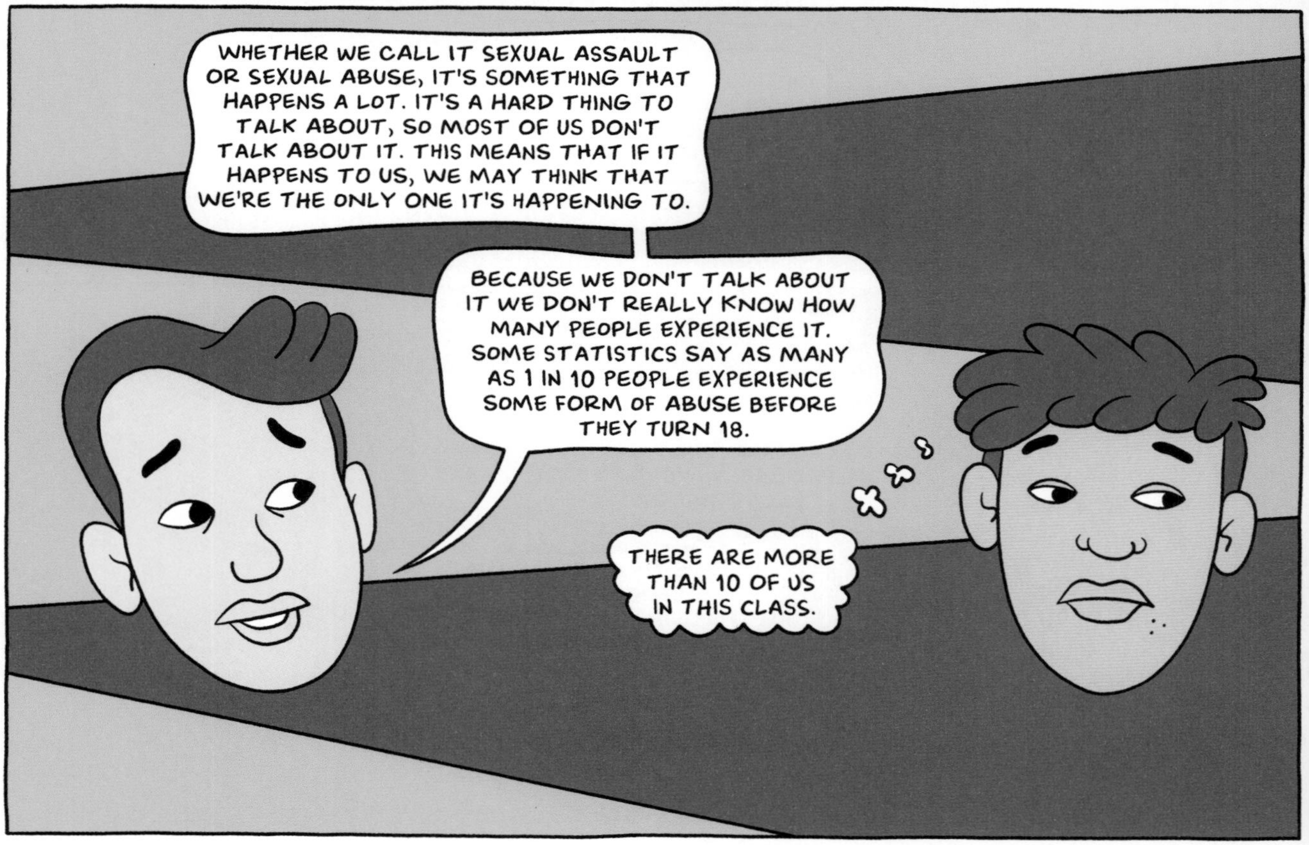
WHETHER WE CALL IT SEXUAL ASSAULT OR SEXUAL ABUSE, IT'S SOMETHING THAT HAPPENS A LOT. IT'S A HARD THING TO TALK ABOUT, SO MOST OF US DON'T TALK ABOUT IT. THIS MEANS THAT IF IT HAPPENS TO US, WE MAY THINK THAT WE'RE THE ONLY ONE IT'S HAPPENING TO.
BECAUSE WE DON'T TALK ABOUT IT WE DON'T REALLY KNOW HOW MANY PEOPLE EXPERIENCE IT. SOME STATISTICS SAY AS MANY AS 1 IN 10 PEOPLE EXPERIENCE SOME FORM OF ABUSE BEFORE THEY TURN 18.
THERE ARE MORE THAN 10 OF US IN THIS CLASS.

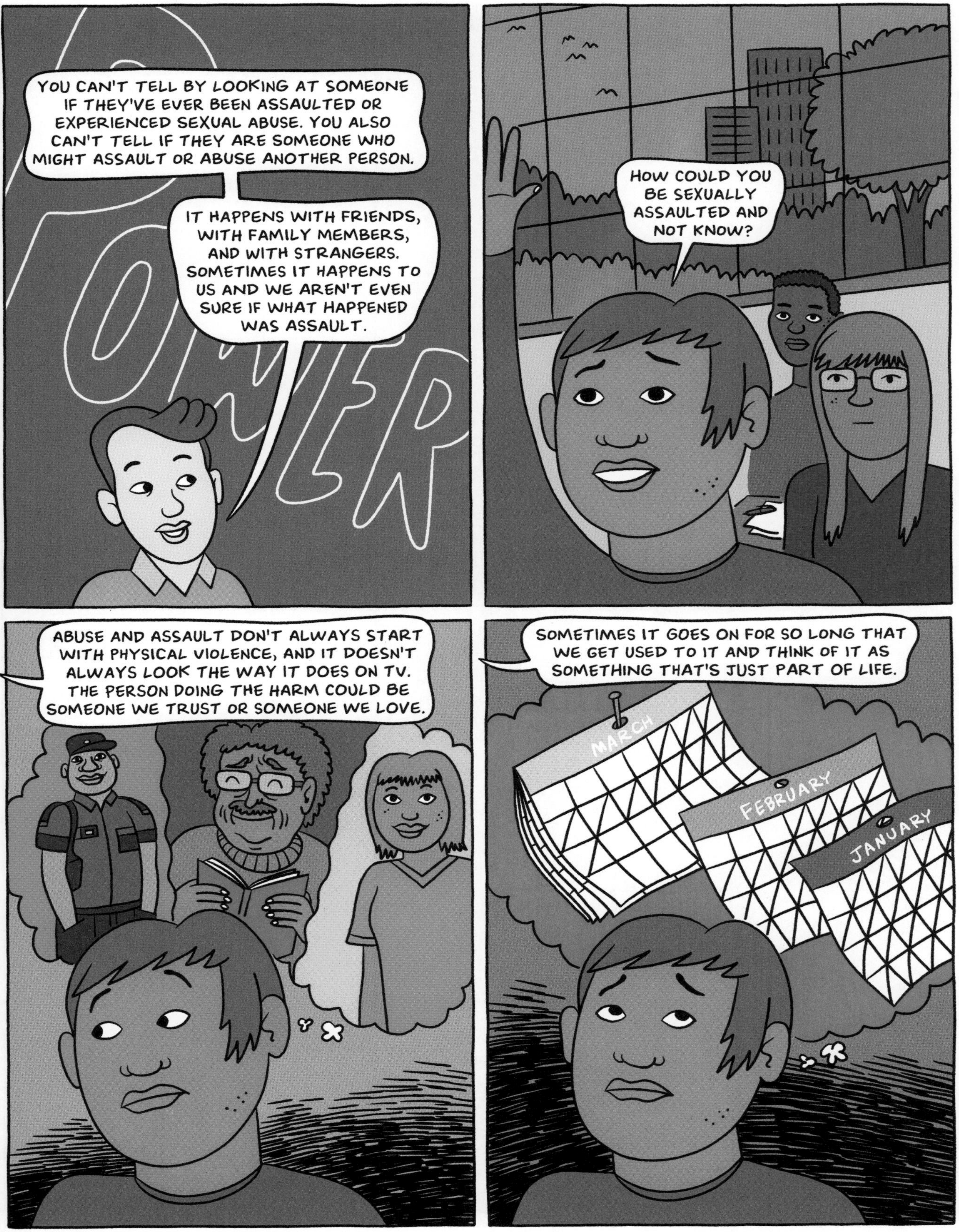
YOU CAN'T TELL BY LOOKING AT SOMEONE IF THEY'VE EVER BEEN ASSAULTED OR EXPERIENCED SEXUAL ABUSE. YOU ALSO CAN'T TELL IF THEY ARE SOMEONE WHO MIGHT ASSAULT OR ABUSE ANOTHER PERSON.
IT HAPPENS WITH FRIENDS, WITH FAMILY MEMBERS, AND WITH STRANGERS. SOMETIMES IT HAPPENS TO US AND WE AREN'T EVEN SURE IF WHAT HAPPENED WAS ASSAULT.
POWER
HOW COULD YOU BE SEXUALLY ASSAULTED AND NOT KNOW?
ABUSE AND ASSAULT DON'T ALWAYS START WITH PHYSICAL VIOLENCE, AND IT DOESN'T ALWAYS LOOK THE WAY IT DOES ON TV. THE PERSON DOING THE HARM COULD BE SOMEONE WE TRUST OR SOMEONE WE LOVE.
SOMETIMES IT GOES ON FOR SO LONG THAT WE GET USED TO IT AND THINK OF IT AS SOMETHING THAT'S JUST PART OF LIFE.
MARCH
FEBRUARY
JANUARY

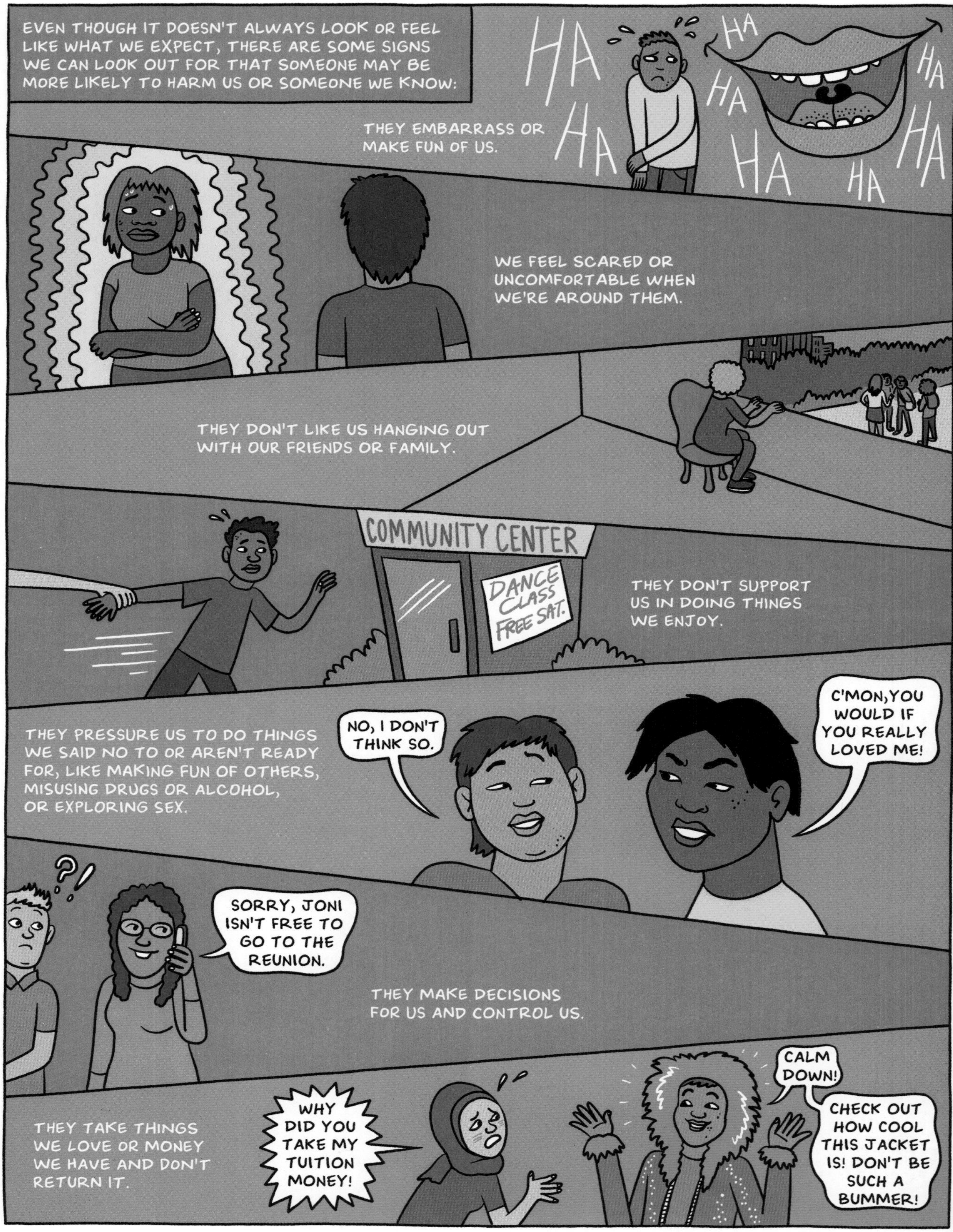
EVEN THOUGH IT DOESN'T ALWAYS LOOK OR FEEL LIKE WHAT WE EXPECT, THERE ARE SOME SIGNS WE CAN LOOK OUT FOR THAT SOMEONE MAY BE MORE LIKELY TO HARM US OR SOMEONE WE KNOW:
THEY EMBARRASS OR MAKE FUN OF US.
HA HA HA HA HA HA HA HA HA
WE FEEL SCARED OR UNCOMFORTABLE WHEN WE'RE AROUND THEM.
THEY DON'T LIKE US HANGING OUT WITH OUR FRIENDS OR FAMILY.
COMMUNITY CENTER
DANCE CLASS FREE SAT.
THEY DON'T SUPPORT US IN DOING THINGS WE ENJOY.
THEY PRESSURE US TO DO THINGS WE SAID NO TO OR AREN'T READY FOR, LIKE MAKING FUN OF OTHERS, MISUSING DRUGS OR ALCOHOL, OR EXPLORING SEX.
NO, I DON'T THINK SO.
C'MON, YOU WOULD IF YOU REALLY LOVED ME!
?!
SORRY, JONI ISN'T FREE TO GO TO THE REUNION.
THEY MAKE DECISIONS FOR US AND CONTROL US.
THEY TAKE THINGS WE LOVE OR MONEY WE HAVE AND DON'T RETURN IT.
WHY DID YOU TAKE MY TUITION MONEY!
CALM DOWN!
CHECK OUT HOW COOL THIS JACKET IS! DON'T BE SUCH A BUMMER!

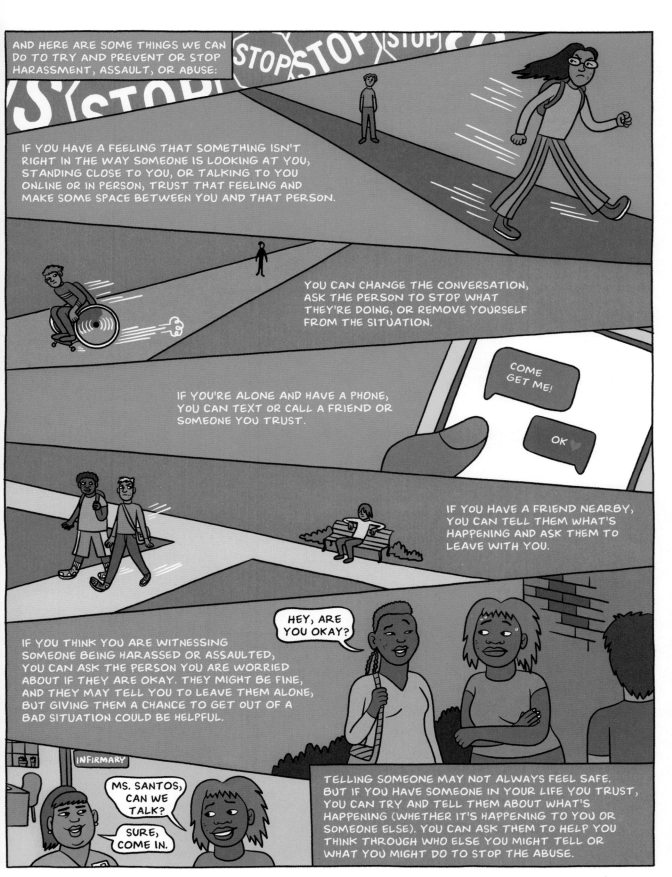

AND HERE ARE SOME THINGS WE CAN DO TO TRY AND PREVENT OR STOP HARASSMENT, ASSAULT, OR ABUSE:

IF YOU HAVE A FEELING THAT SOMETHING ISN'T RIGHT IN THE WAY SOMEONE IS LOOKING AT YOU, STANDING CLOSE TO YOU, OR TALKING TO YOU ONLINE OR IN PERSON, TRUST THAT FEELING AND MAKE SOME SPACE BETWEEN YOU AND THAT PERSON.

YOU CAN CHANGE THE CONVERSATION, ASK THE PERSON TO STOP WHAT THEY'RE DOING, OR REMOVE YOURSELF FROM THE SITUATION.

IF YOU'RE ALONE AND HAVE A PHONE, YOU CAN TEXT OR CALL A FRIEND OR SOMEONE YOU TRUST.

COME GET ME!

OK ♥

IF YOU HAVE A FRIEND NEARBY, YOU CAN TELL THEM WHAT'S HAPPENING AND ASK THEM TO LEAVE WITH YOU.

IF YOU THINK YOU ARE WITNESSING SOMEONE BEING HARASSED OR ASSAULTED, YOU CAN ASK THE PERSON YOU ARE WORRIED ABOUT IF THEY ARE OKAY. THEY MIGHT BE FINE, AND THEY MAY TELL YOU TO LEAVE THEM ALONE, BUT GIVING THEM A CHANCE TO GET OUT OF A BAD SITUATION COULD BE HELPFUL.

HEY, ARE YOU OKAY?

INFIRMARY

MS. SANTOS, CAN WE TALK?

SURE, COME IN.

TELLING SOMEONE MAY NOT ALWAYS FEEL SAFE. BUT IF YOU HAVE SOMEONE IN YOUR LIFE YOU TRUST, YOU CAN TRY AND TELL THEM ABOUT WHAT'S HAPPENING (WHETHER IT'S HAPPENING TO YOU OR SOMEONE ELSE). YOU CAN ASK THEM TO HELP YOU THINK THROUGH WHO ELSE YOU MIGHT TELL OR WHAT YOU MIGHT DO TO STOP THE ABUSE.

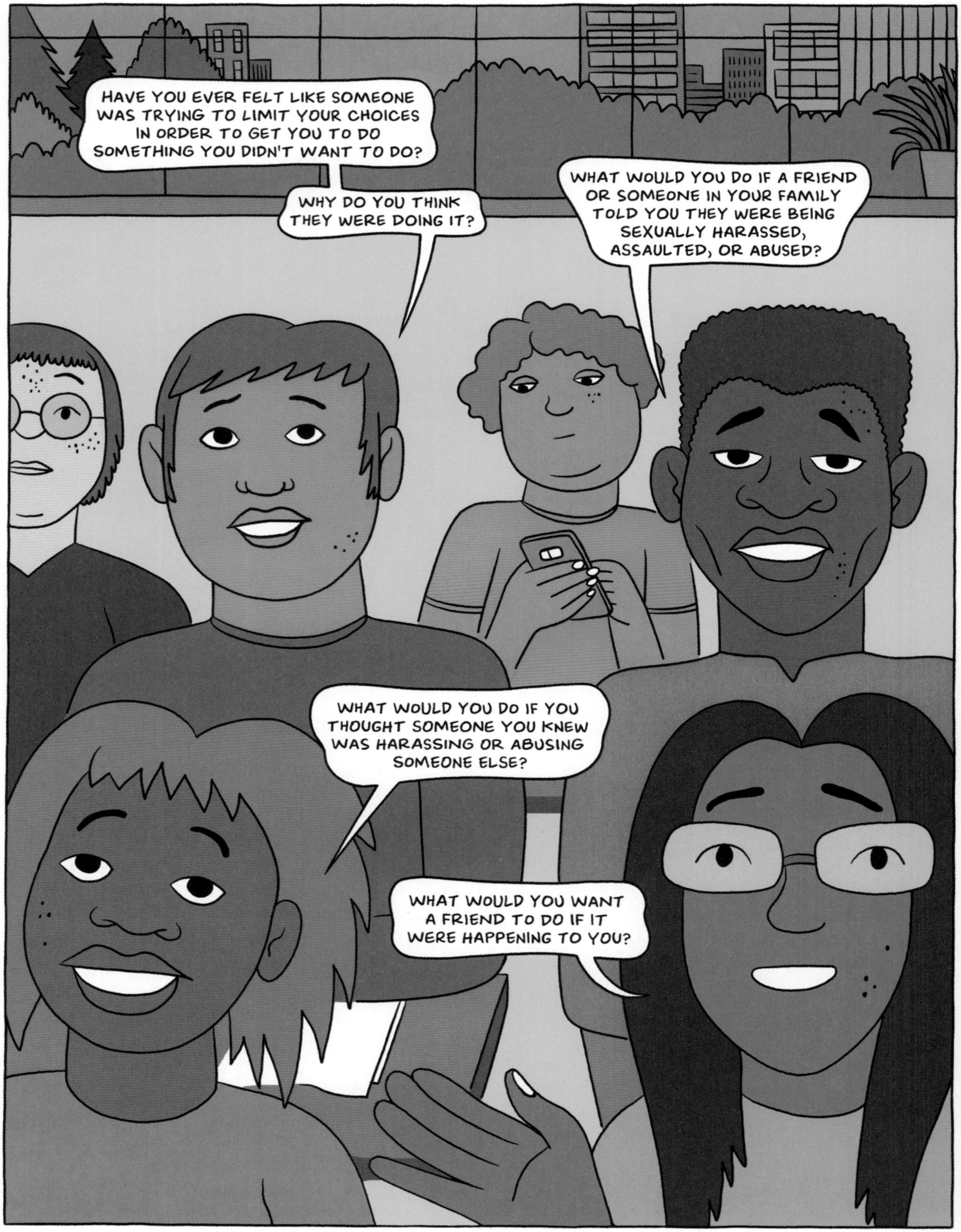
HAVE YOU EVER FELT LIKE SOMEONE WAS TRYING TO LIMIT YOUR CHOICES IN ORDER TO GET YOU TO DO SOMETHING YOU DIDN'T WANT TO DO?
WHY DO YOU THINK THEY WERE DOING IT?
WHAT WOULD YOU DO IF A FRIEND OR SOMEONE IN YOUR FAMILY TOLD YOU THEY WERE BEING SEXUALLY HARASSED, ASSAULTED, OR ABUSED?
WHAT WOULD YOU DO IF YOU THOUGHT SOMEONE YOU KNEW WAS HARASSING OR ABUSING SOMEONE ELSE?
WHAT WOULD YOU WANT A FRIEND TO DO IF IT WERE HAPPENING TO YOU?

THE NEXT CHAPTER DESCRIBES ONE KIND OF ABUSE OF POWER—
SEXUAL ABUSE THAT CAN HAPPEN WHEN WE ARE YOUNGER.

JAN HINDMAN WAS A THERAPIST WHO WORKED WITH YOUNG
PEOPLE EXPERIENCING SEXUAL ABUSE AND WITH PEOPLE WHO
SEXUALLY ABUSED YOUNG PEOPLE. JAN CAME UP WITH HER
OWN TERM FOR SEXUAL ABUSE WHEN IT HAPPENS TO US WHEN
WE'RE YOUNGER. SHE CALLED IT "SECRET TOUCH."

IT'S IMPORTANT TO KNOW THIS HAPPENS, AND TO KNOW WE
CAN TALK ABOUT IT. BUT IT CAN BE A LOT TO TAKE IN. IF YOU
START TO READ THIS SECTION AND IT FEELS LIKE TOO MUCH,
TAKE A BREAK. IF YOU HAVE SOMEONE IN YOUR LIFE YOU
TRUST, YOU MIGHT WANT TO READ IT WITH THEM OR ASK
THEM TO READ IT ON THEIR OWN, AND THEN YOU CAN BOTH
TALK ABOUT IT.

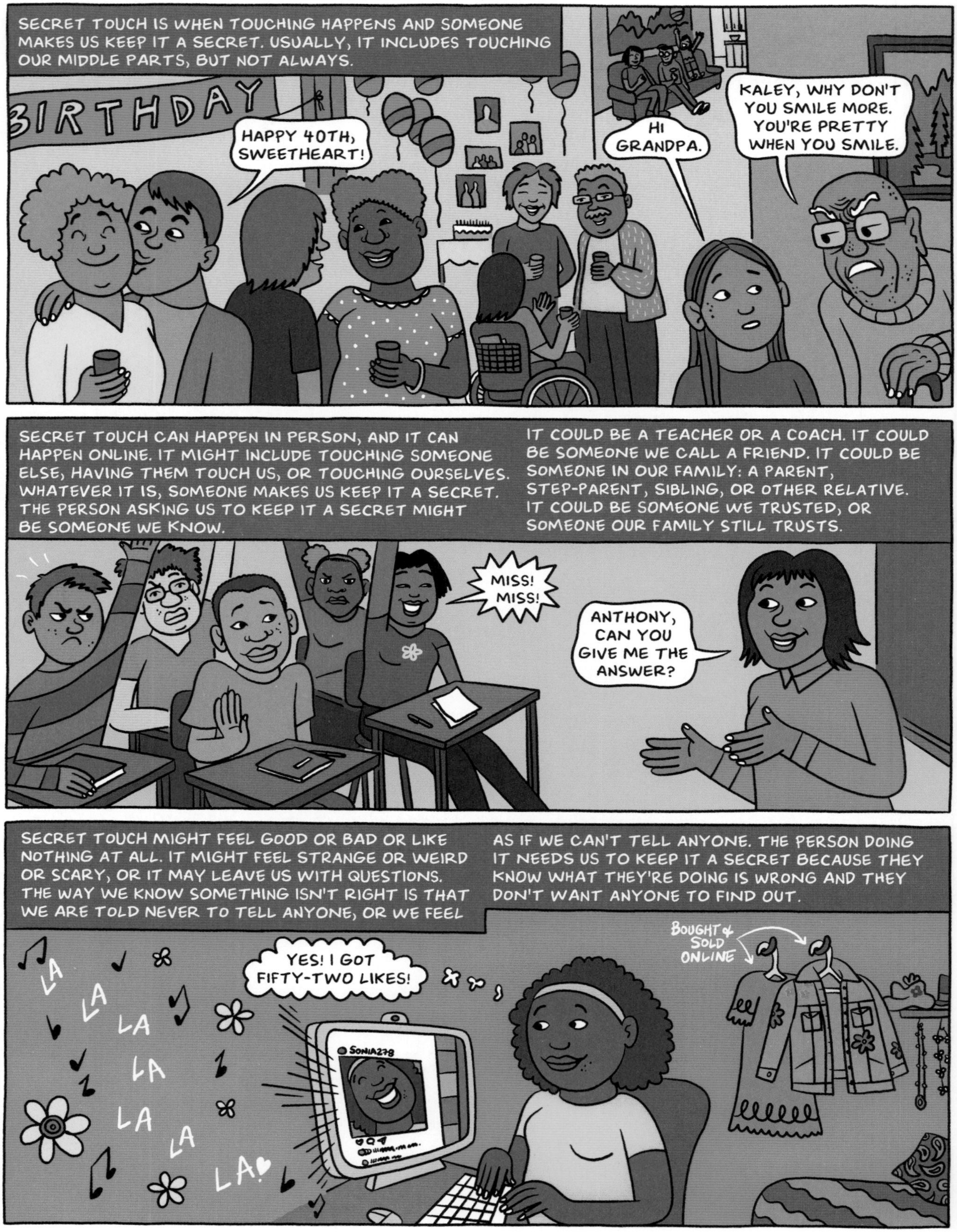
SECRET TOUCH IS WHEN TOUCHING HAPPENS AND SOMEONE MAKES US KEEP IT A SECRET. USUALLY, IT INCLUDES TOUCHING OUR MIDDLE PARTS, BUT NOT ALWAYS.
BIRTHDAY
HAPPY 40TH, SWEETHEART!
HI GRANDPA.
KALEY, WHY DON'T YOU SMILE MORE. YOU'RE PRETTY WHEN YOU SMILE.
SECRET TOUCH CAN HAPPEN IN PERSON, AND IT CAN HAPPEN ONLINE. IT MIGHT INCLUDE TOUCHING SOMEONE ELSE, HAVING THEM TOUCH US, OR TOUCHING OURSELVES. WHATEVER IT IS, SOMEONE MAKES US KEEP IT A SECRET. THE PERSON ASKING US TO KEEP IT A SECRET MIGHT BE SOMEONE WE KNOW.
IT COULD BE A TEACHER OR A COACH. IT COULD BE SOMEONE WE CALL A FRIEND. IT COULD BE SOMEONE IN OUR FAMILY: A PARENT, STEP-PARENT, SIBLING, OR OTHER RELATIVE. IT COULD BE SOMEONE WE TRUSTED, OR SOMEONE OUR FAMILY STILL TRUSTS.
MISS! MISS!
ANTHONY, CAN YOU GIVE ME THE ANSWER?
SECRET TOUCH MIGHT FEEL GOOD OR BAD OR LIKE NOTHING AT ALL. IT MIGHT FEEL STRANGE OR WEIRD OR SCARY, OR IT MAY LEAVE US WITH QUESTIONS. THE WAY WE KNOW SOMETHING ISN'T RIGHT IS THAT WE ARE TOLD NEVER TO TELL ANYONE, OR WE FEEL AS IF WE CAN'T TELL ANYONE. THE PERSON DOING IT NEEDS US TO KEEP IT A SECRET BECAUSE THEY KNOW WHAT THEY'RE DOING IS WRONG AND THEY DON'T WANT ANYONE TO FIND OUT.
LA LA LA LA LA LA LA!
YES! I GOT FIFTY-TWO LIKES!
SONIA278
BOUGHT & SOLD ONLINE

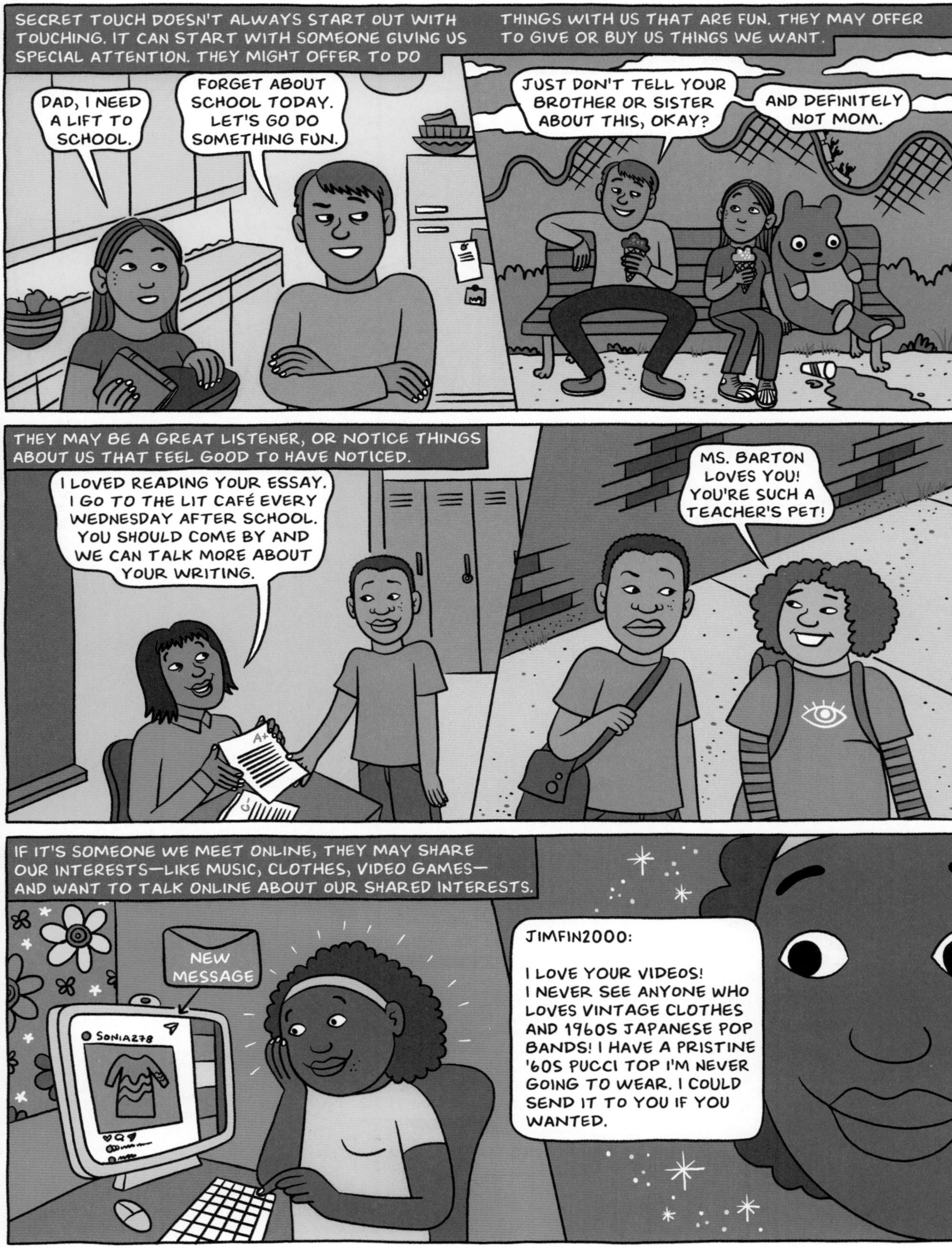
SECRET TOUCH DOESN'T ALWAYS START OUT WITH TOUCHING. IT CAN START WITH SOMEONE GIVING US SPECIAL ATTENTION. THEY MIGHT OFFER TO DO THINGS WITH US THAT ARE FUN. THEY MAY OFFER TO GIVE OR BUY US THINGS WE WANT.
DAD, I NEED A LIFT TO SCHOOL.
FORGET ABOUT SCHOOL TODAY. LET'S GO DO SOMETHING FUN.
JUST DON'T TELL YOUR BROTHER OR SISTER ABOUT THIS, OKAY?
AND DEFINITELY NOT MOM.
THEY MAY BE A GREAT LISTENER, OR NOTICE THINGS ABOUT US THAT FEEL GOOD TO HAVE NOTICED.
I LOVED READING YOUR ESSAY. I GO TO THE LIT CAFÉ EVERY WEDNESDAY AFTER SCHOOL. YOU SHOULD COME BY AND WE CAN TALK MORE ABOUT YOUR WRITING.
MS. BARTON LOVES YOU! YOU'RE SUCH A TEACHER'S PET!
IF IT'S SOMEONE WE MEET ONLINE, THEY MAY SHARE OUR INTERESTS—LIKE MUSIC, CLOTHES, VIDEO GAMES—AND WANT TO TALK ONLINE ABOUT OUR SHARED INTERESTS.
NEW MESSAGE
SONIA278
JIMFIN2000:
I LOVE YOUR VIDEOS! I NEVER SEE ANYONE WHO LOVES VINTAGE CLOTHES AND 1960S JAPANESE POP BANDS! I HAVE A PRISTINE '60S PUCCI TOP I'M NEVER GOING TO WEAR. I COULD SEND IT TO YOU IF YOU WANTED.

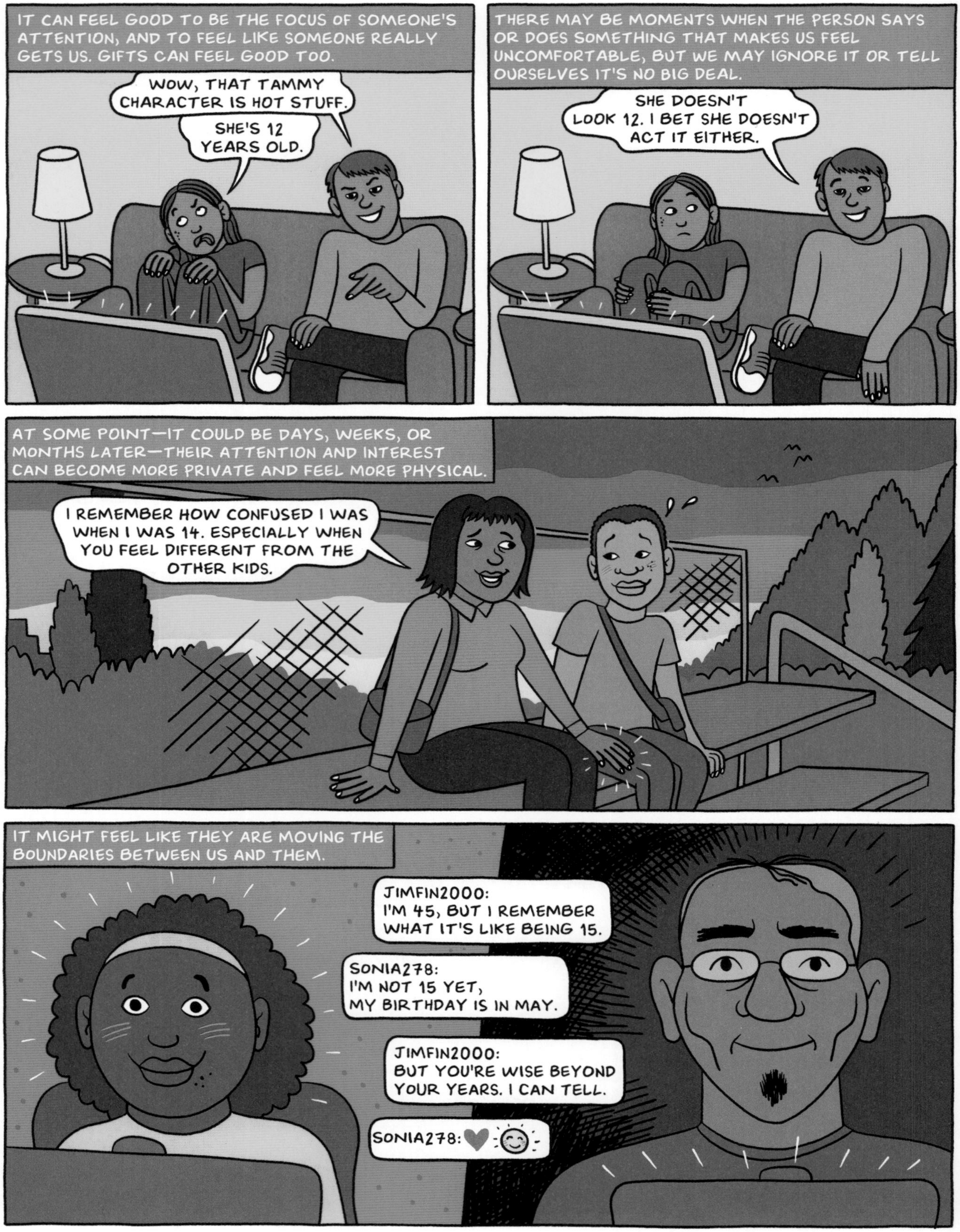
IT CAN FEEL GOOD TO BE THE FOCUS OF SOMEONE'S ATTENTION, AND TO FEEL LIKE SOMEONE REALLY GETS US. GIFTS CAN FEEL GOOD TOO.
WOW, THAT TAMMY CHARACTER IS HOT STUFF.
SHE'S 12 YEARS OLD.
THERE MAY BE MOMENTS WHEN THE PERSON SAYS OR DOES SOMETHING THAT MAKES US FEEL UNCOMFORTABLE, BUT WE MAY IGNORE IT OR TELL OURSELVES IT'S NO BIG DEAL.
SHE DOESN'T LOOK 12. I BET SHE DOESN'T ACT IT EITHER.
AT SOME POINT—IT COULD BE DAYS, WEEKS, OR MONTHS LATER—THEIR ATTENTION AND INTEREST CAN BECOME MORE PRIVATE AND FEEL MORE PHYSICAL.
I REMEMBER HOW CONFUSED I WAS WHEN I WAS 14. ESPECIALLY WHEN YOU FEEL DIFFERENT FROM THE OTHER KIDS.
IT MIGHT FEEL LIKE THEY ARE MOVING THE BOUNDARIES BETWEEN US AND THEM.
JIMFIN2000: I'M 45, BUT I REMEMBER WHAT IT'S LIKE BEING 15.
SONIA278: I'M NOT 15 YET, MY BIRTHDAY IS IN MAY.
JIMFIN2000: BUT YOU'RE WISE BEYOND YOUR YEARS. I CAN TELL.
SONIA278:

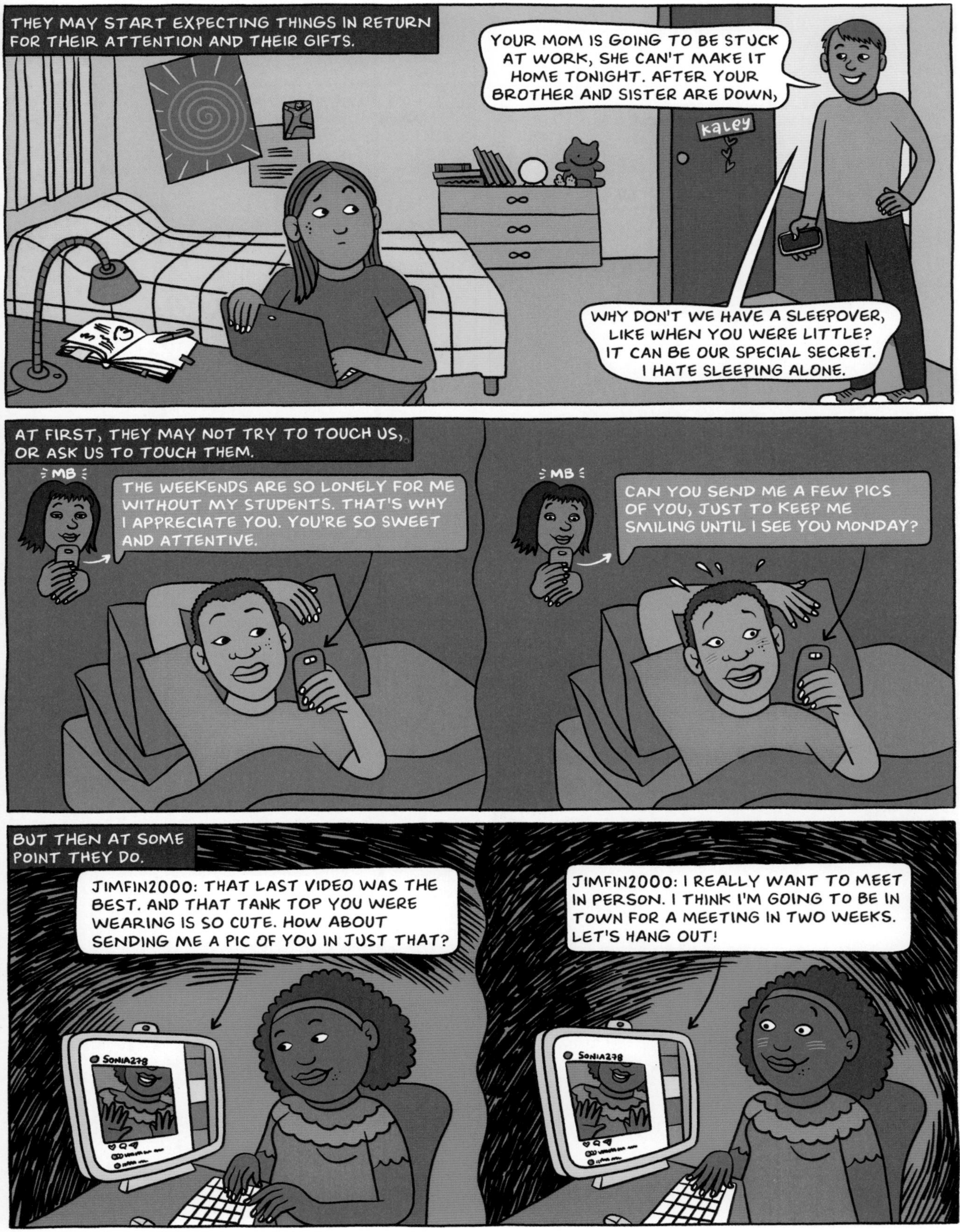
THEY MAY START EXPECTING THINGS IN RETURN FOR THEIR ATTENTION AND THEIR GIFTS.
YOUR MOM IS GOING TO BE STUCK AT WORK, SHE CAN'T MAKE IT HOME TONIGHT. AFTER YOUR BROTHER AND SISTER ARE DOWN,
kaley
WHY DON'T WE HAVE A SLEEPOVER, LIKE WHEN YOU WERE LITTLE? IT CAN BE OUR SPECIAL SECRET. I HATE SLEEPING ALONE.
AT FIRST, THEY MAY NOT TRY TO TOUCH US, OR ASK US TO TOUCH THEM.
MB
THE WEEKENDS ARE SO LONELY FOR ME WITHOUT MY STUDENTS. THAT'S WHY I APPRECIATE YOU. YOU'RE SO SWEET AND ATTENTIVE.
MB
CAN YOU SEND ME A FEW PICS OF YOU, JUST TO KEEP ME SMILING UNTIL I SEE YOU MONDAY?
BUT THEN AT SOME POINT THEY DO.
JIMFIN2000: THAT LAST VIDEO WAS THE BEST. AND THAT TANK TOP YOU WERE WEARING IS SO CUTE. HOW ABOUT SENDING ME A PIC OF YOU IN JUST THAT?
SONIA278
JIMFIN2000: I REALLY WANT TO MEET IN PERSON. I THINK I'M GOING TO BE IN TOWN FOR A MEETING IN TWO WEEKS. LET'S HANG OUT!
SONIA278

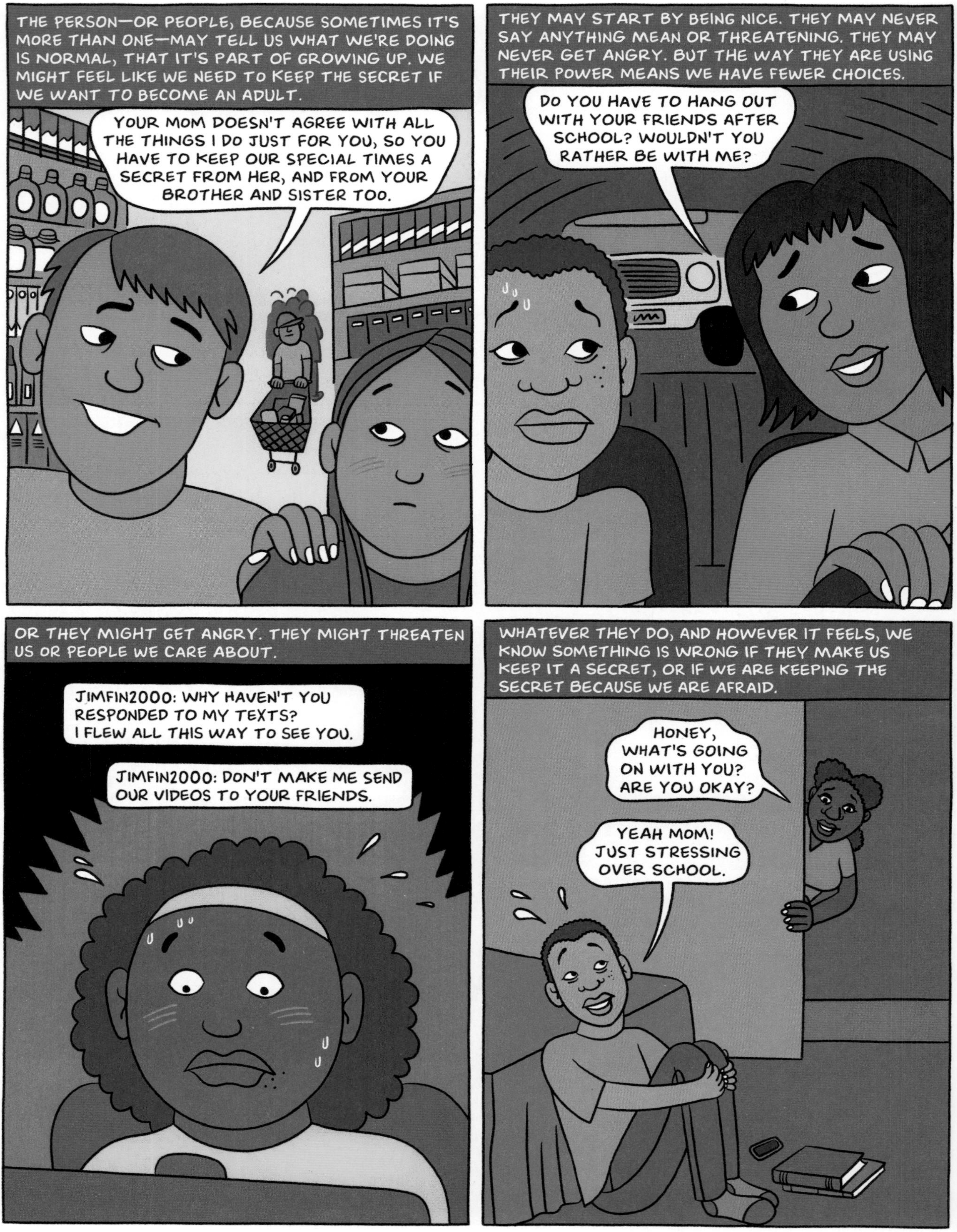
THE PERSON—OR PEOPLE, BECAUSE SOMETIMES IT'S MORE THAN ONE—MAY TELL US WHAT WE'RE DOING IS NORMAL, THAT IT'S PART OF GROWING UP. WE MIGHT FEEL LIKE WE NEED TO KEEP THE SECRET IF WE WANT TO BECOME AN ADULT.
YOUR MOM DOESN'T AGREE WITH ALL THE THINGS I DO JUST FOR YOU, SO YOU HAVE TO KEEP OUR SPECIAL TIMES A SECRET FROM HER, AND FROM YOUR BROTHER AND SISTER TOO.
THEY MAY START BY BEING NICE. THEY MAY NEVER SAY ANYTHING MEAN OR THREATENING. THEY MAY NEVER GET ANGRY. BUT THE WAY THEY ARE USING THEIR POWER MEANS WE HAVE FEWER CHOICES.
DO YOU HAVE TO HANG OUT WITH YOUR FRIENDS AFTER SCHOOL? WOULDN'T YOU RATHER BE WITH ME?
OR THEY MIGHT GET ANGRY. THEY MIGHT THREATEN US OR PEOPLE WE CARE ABOUT.
JIMFIN2000: WHY HAVEN'T YOU RESPONDED TO MY TEXTS? I FLEW ALL THIS WAY TO SEE YOU.
JIMFIN2000: DON'T MAKE ME SEND OUR VIDEOS TO YOUR FRIENDS.
WHATEVER THEY DO, AND HOWEVER IT FEELS, WE KNOW SOMETHING IS WRONG IF THEY MAKE US KEEP IT A SECRET, OR IF WE ARE KEEPING THE SECRET BECAUSE WE ARE AFRAID.
HONEY, WHAT'S GOING ON WITH YOU? ARE YOU OKAY?
YEAH MOM! JUST STRESSING OVER SCHOOL.

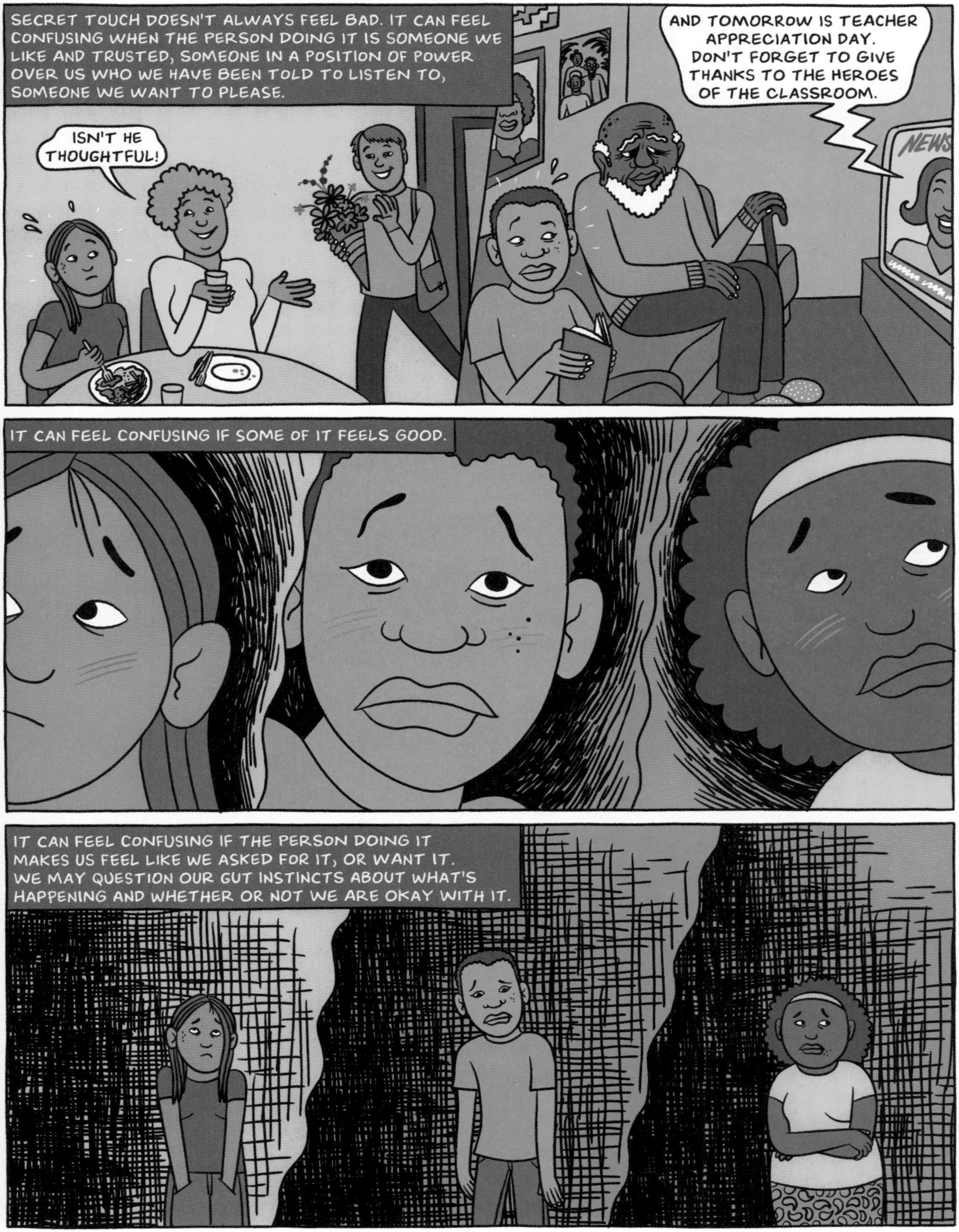
SECRET TOUCH DOESN'T ALWAYS FEEL BAD. IT CAN FEEL CONFUSING WHEN THE PERSON DOING IT IS SOMEONE WE LIKE AND TRUSTED, SOMEONE IN A POSITION OF POWER OVER US WHO WE HAVE BEEN TOLD TO LISTEN TO, SOMEONE WE WANT TO PLEASE.
ISN'T HE THOUGHTFUL!
AND TOMORROW IS TEACHER APPRECIATION DAY. DON'T FORGET TO GIVE THANKS TO THE HEROES OF THE CLASSROOM.
NEWS
IT CAN FEEL CONFUSING IF SOME OF IT FEELS GOOD.
IT CAN FEEL CONFUSING IF THE PERSON DOING IT MAKES US FEEL LIKE WE ASKED FOR IT, OR WANT IT. WE MAY QUESTION OUR GUT INSTINCTS ABOUT WHAT'S HAPPENING AND WHETHER OR NOT WE ARE OKAY WITH IT.

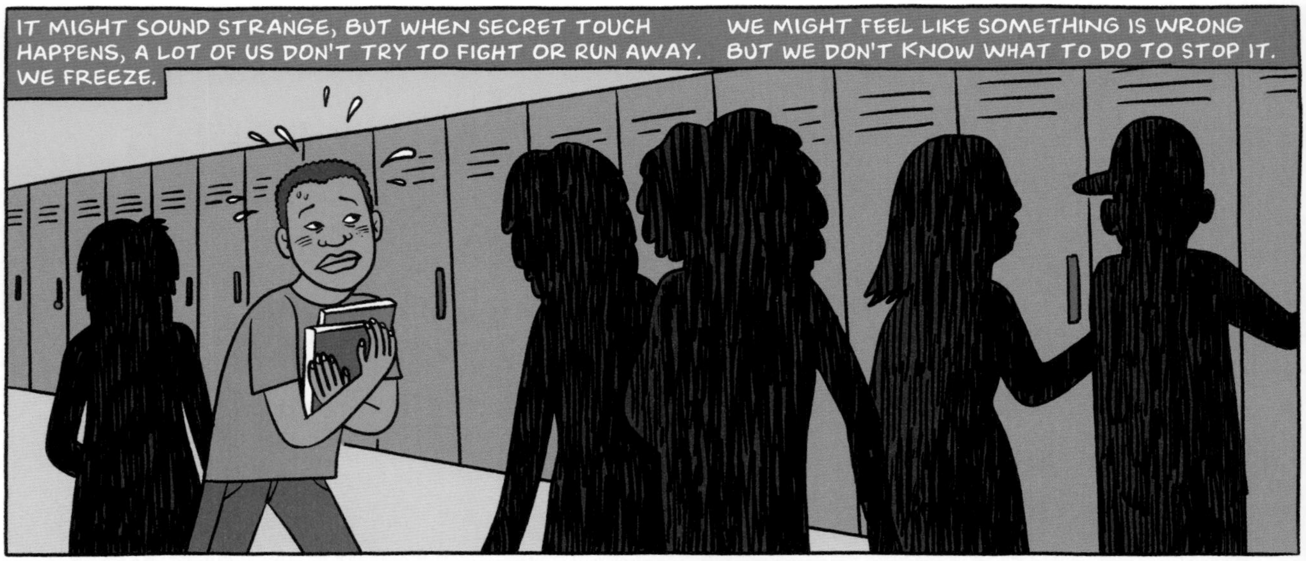
IT MIGHT SOUND STRANGE, BUT WHEN SECRET TOUCH HAPPENS, A LOT OF US DON'T TRY TO FIGHT OR RUN AWAY. WE FREEZE.
WE MIGHT FEEL LIKE SOMETHING IS WRONG BUT WE DON'T KNOW WHAT TO DO TO STOP IT.

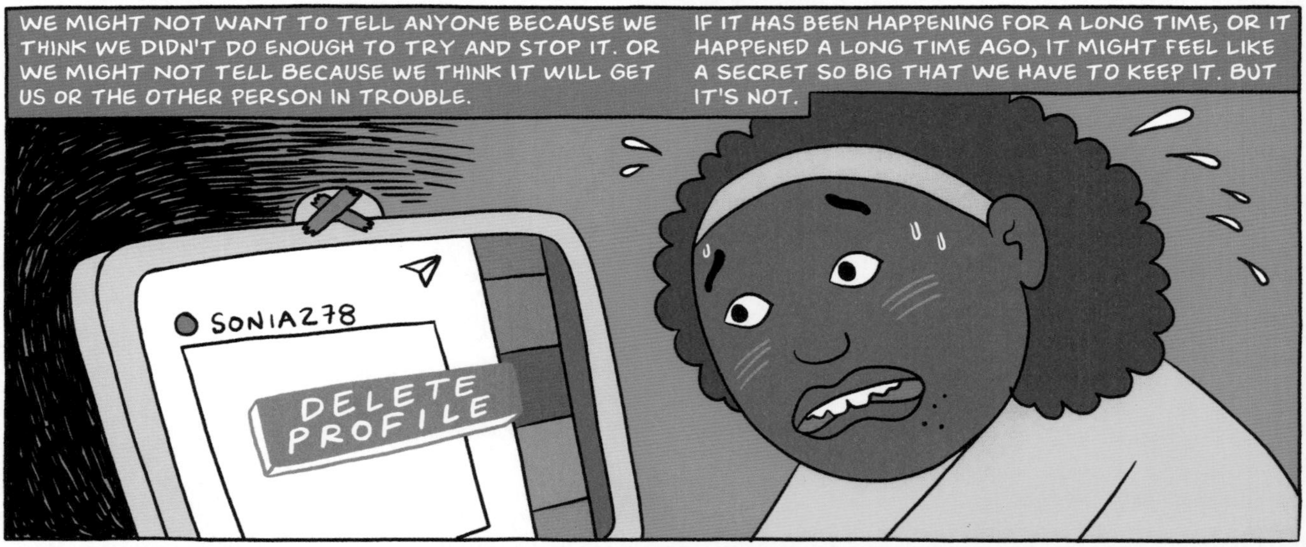
WE MIGHT NOT WANT TO TELL ANYONE BECAUSE WE THINK WE DIDN'T DO ENOUGH TO TRY AND STOP IT. OR WE MIGHT NOT TELL BECAUSE WE THINK IT WILL GET US OR THE OTHER PERSON IN TROUBLE.
IF IT HAS BEEN HAPPENING FOR A LONG TIME, OR IT HAPPENED A LONG TIME AGO, IT MIGHT FEEL LIKE A SECRET SO BIG THAT WE HAVE TO KEEP IT. BUT IT'S NOT.
SONIA278
DELETE PROFILE

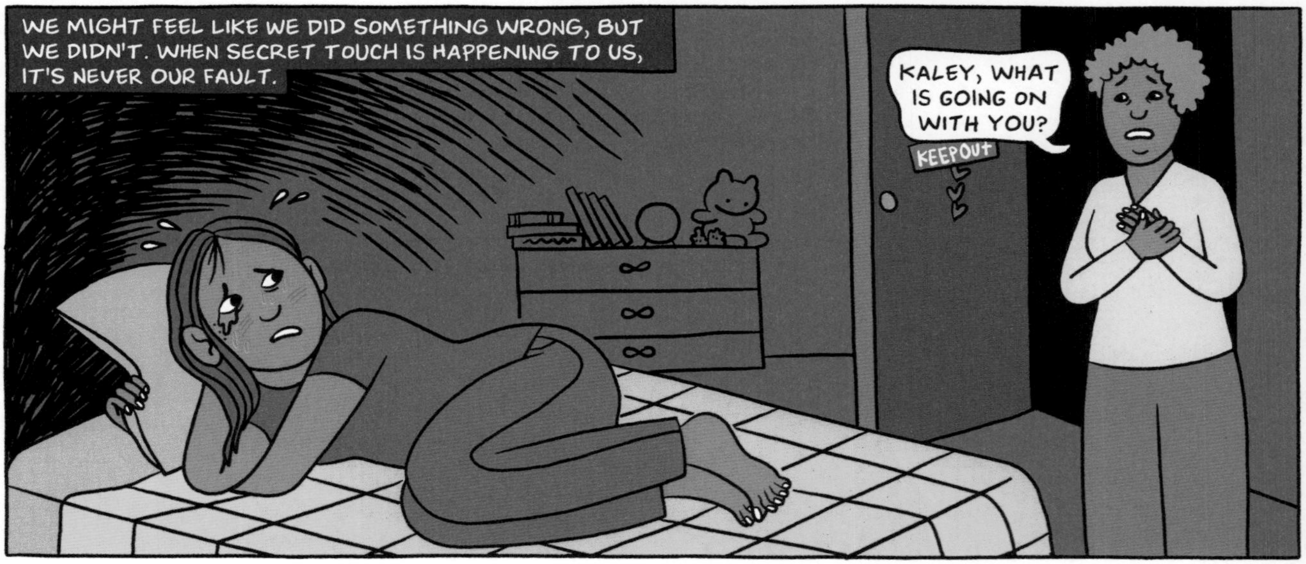
WE MIGHT FEEL LIKE WE DID SOMETHING WRONG, BUT WE DIDN'T. WHEN SECRET TOUCH IS HAPPENING TO US, IT'S NEVER OUR FAULT.
KALEY, WHAT IS GOING ON WITH YOU?
KEEPOUT

WHAT WE CAN DO

TELLING SOMEONE ISN'T EASY. IF WE DIDN'T TELL SOMEONE WHEN IT STARTED HAPPENING, WE MIGHT THINK IT'S TOO LATE TO TELL NOW.

THAT IS NOT TRUE. IT'S NEVER TOO LATE TO TALK TO SOMEONE ABOUT WHAT HAPPENED, OR WHAT IS STILL HAPPENING.

THE FIRST PERSON WE TELL MIGHT NOT KNOW WHAT TO DO, OR MIGHT NOT BELIEVE US. IF THAT HAPPENS, WE CAN TRY TO FIND ANOTHER PERSON WE FEEL SAFE AND COMFORTABLE WITH AND TELL THEM.

IF IT'S HAPPENING TO YOU, YOU CAN TRY TO TALK ABOUT WHAT HAPPENED, OR WHERE IT HAPPENED, OR WHO IT HAPPENED WITH. IF IT'S STILL HAPPENING, YOU CAN TRY TO FIND A SAFER PLACE TO BE. YOU CAN TRY TO AVOID BEING ALONE WITH THE PERSON.

IF IT'S HAPPENING TO SOMEONE YOU KNOW, THERE ARE ALSO WAYS TO TRY AND HELP.

YOU CAN TALK TO THE PERSON AND ASK THEM WHAT THEY NEED. THEY MIGHT WANT SOMEONE THEY CAN TALK TO. THEY MIGHT WANT HELP FIGURING OUT HOW TO MAKE IT STOP AND WHERE TO GO FOR HELP. THEY MIGHT WANT HELP TELLING SOMEONE ELSE IN THEIR LIFE.

IF YOU DON'T FEEL LIKE YOU CAN TELL ANYONE YOU KNOW, THERE ARE PLACES YOU CAN CALL OR TEXT TO GET SUPPORT WITHOUT GIVING YOUR NAME. YOU CAN FIND THOSE IN THE BACK OF THE BOOK.

IF YOU HAVE A FRIEND WHO IS TELLING YOU IT'S HAPPENING TO THEM, IT CAN BE HARD FOR YOU TOO AND YOU DESERVE TO BE SUPPORTED. IF YOU DON'T KNOW WHO TO ASK, YOU CAN ALSO CONTACT A SUPPORT LINE.

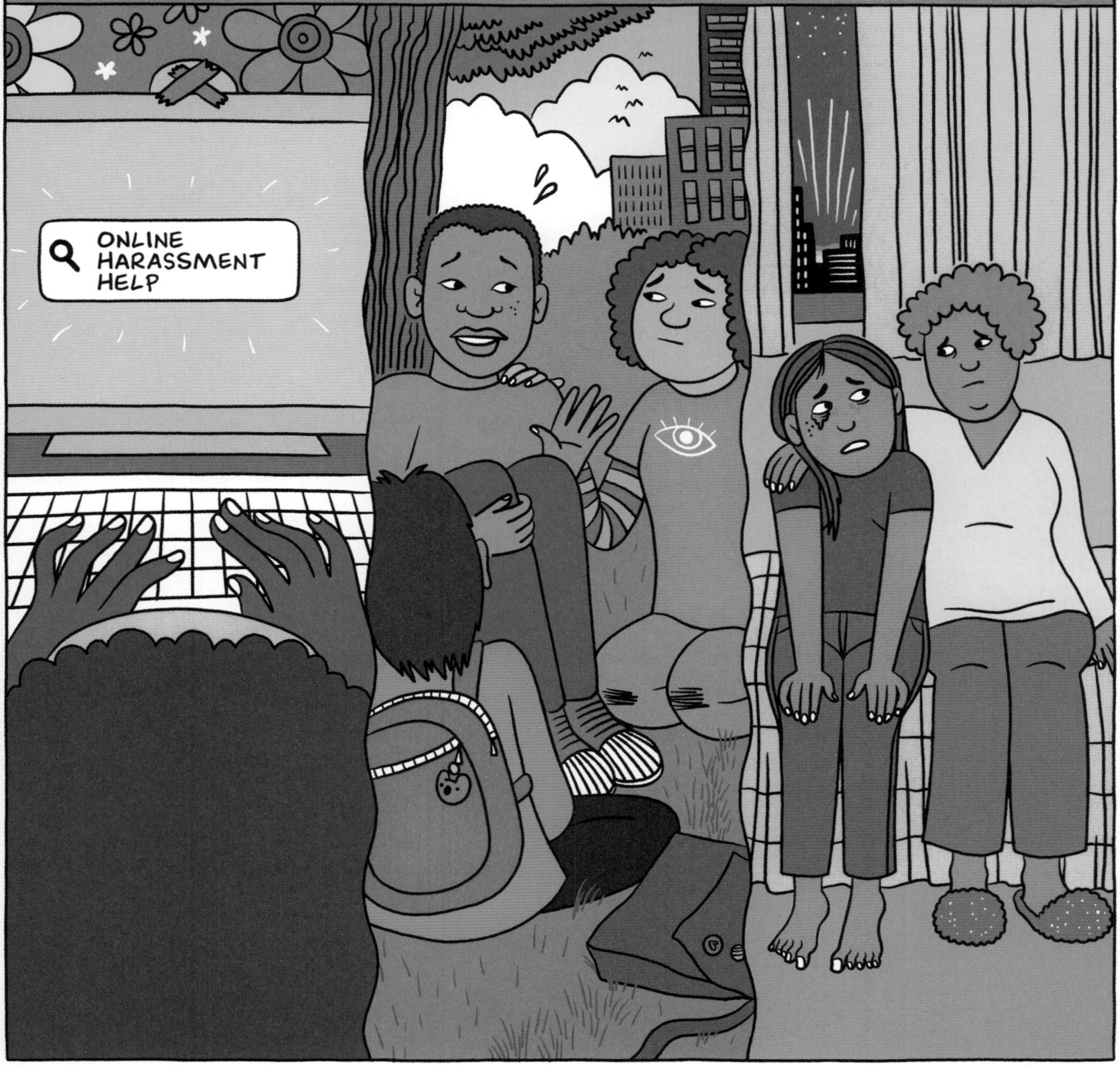
ONLINE HARASSMENT HELP

NERD ALERT WILL POLICE BE INVOLVED?

IF YOU THINK THAT YOU OR SOMEONE YOU KNOW IS EXPERIENCING ABUSE, INCLUDING SECRET TOUCH, YOU MIGHT WONDER IF TELLING SOMEONE MEANS THE POLICE WILL GET INVOLVED. DEPENDING ON WHO YOU TELL, THIS MAY HAPPEN.

IF SOMEONE IS HURTING YOU OR SOMEONE ELSE, THEY SHOULD BE STOPPED. POLICE AREN'T THE ONLY OPTION.

- YOU CAN TRY TO FIND A FRIEND OR FAMILY MEMBER YOU TRUST.
- YOU CAN CONTACT THE SUPPORT LINES IN THE BACK OF THE BOOK.
- IF THERE IS A TEACHER OR COUNSELOR YOU TRUST, YOU CAN TALK TO THEM WITHOUT NAMING THE PEOPLE INVOLVED. THEY MAY BE REQUIRED TO CONTACT AUTHORITIES, WHICH COULD INCLUDE THE POLICE, BUT YOU ARE NOT REQUIRED TO GIVE ANY MORE INFORMATION.

ONE OF THE HARDEST THINGS ABOUT SECRET TOUCH IS THE WAY IT MAKES US FEEL ALONE. BUT WE AREN'T ALONE. THIS HAPPENS TO SO MANY OF US AND THERE ARE PEOPLE WHO WANT TO HELP US STOP WHAT'S HAPPENING.

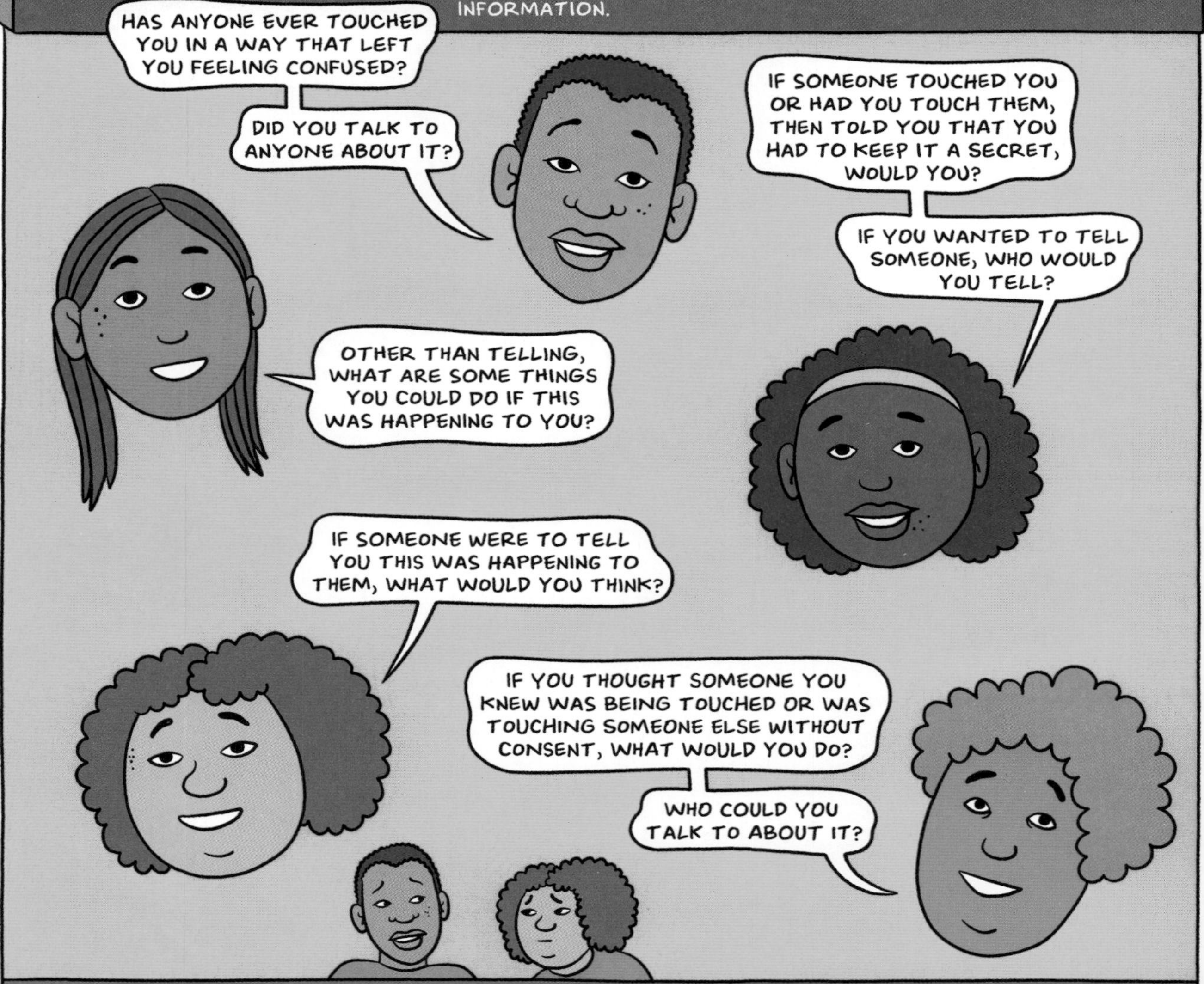
HAS ANYONE EVER TOUCHED YOU IN A WAY THAT LEFT YOU FEELING CONFUSED?
DID YOU TALK TO ANYONE ABOUT IT?
IF SOMEONE TOUCHED YOU OR HAD YOU TOUCH THEM, THEN TOLD YOU THAT YOU HAD TO KEEP IT A SECRET, WOULD YOU?
IF YOU WANTED TO TELL SOMEONE, WHO WOULD YOU TELL?
OTHER THAN TELLING, WHAT ARE SOME THINGS YOU COULD DO IF THIS WAS HAPPENING TO YOU?
IF SOMEONE WERE TO TELL YOU THIS WAS HAPPENING TO THEM, WHAT WOULD YOU THINK?
IF YOU THOUGHT SOMEONE YOU KNEW WAS BEING TOUCHED OR WAS TOUCHING SOMEONE ELSE WITHOUT CONSENT, WHAT WOULD YOU DO?
WHO COULD YOU TALK TO ABOUT IT?

BEING A SUPPORT: IF SOMEONE TELLS YOU ABOUT ABUSE THEY HAVE EXPERIENCED, THERE ISN'T ONE RIGHT THING TO SAY OR ONE RIGHT WAY TO RESPOND. YOU CAN LISTEN, YOU CAN ASK WHAT THE PERSON NEEDS AND WANTS, AND THEN YOU CAN TRY TO SUPPORT THEM.

TELLING THEM WHAT THEY SHOULD DO, OR DOING THINGS FOR THEM WITHOUT THEIR PERMISSION, ISN'T ALWAYS AS HELPFUL AS WE IMAGINE IT IS. BODY AUTONOMY MEANS WE ALL GET TO MAKE OUR OWN DECISIONS ABOUT HOW TO DEAL WITH ABUSE. RESPECTING BODY AUTONOMY MEANS LISTENING AND HELPING WHEN THAT HELP IS REQUESTED.

TRAUMA IS A WORD PEOPLE USE TO DESCRIBE THE WAY OUR BODIES AND MINDS RESPOND WHEN WE EXPERIENCE SOMETHING SIGNIFICANT THAT ISN'T OKAY, LIKE HARASSMENT, ASSAULT, AND SECRET TOUCH.

THE WORD TRAUMA ORIGINALLY MEANT "WOUND." WHEN WE CALL SOMETHING "TRAUMATIC," THAT MEANS IT HAS WOUNDED US IN A DEEP, DISTURBING, AND LASTING WAY. TRAUMA SOUNDS LIKE A BAD THING, BUT IT'S ONE WAY WE TRY TO PROTECT OURSELVES WHEN SOMETHING OVERWHELMING HAPPENS.

EVERYONE RESPONDS DIFFERENTLY WHEN THEY EXPERIENCE SOMETHING TRAUMATIC. SOME PEOPLE CAN'T STOP THINKING ABOUT WHAT HAPPENED AND MAY BE FLOODED WITH FEELINGS. OTHERS MAY NOT BE ABLE TO REMEMBER WHAT HAPPENED AT ALL, AND MAY FEEL NOTHING.

EVERY RESPONSE TO SOMETHING TRAUMATIC IS VALID AND REAL, WHETHER IT'S BIG OR SMALL. IF SOMETHING WE EXPERIENCED STAYS WITH US AND BOTHERS US, OUR FEELINGS ABOUT IT ARE IMPORTANT, AND IT'S OKAY TO ASK FOR HELP.

WHETHER WE THINK IT'S A BIG DEAL OR A SMALL THING, WE ALL DESERVE TO HAVE PEOPLE LISTEN AND HELP US.

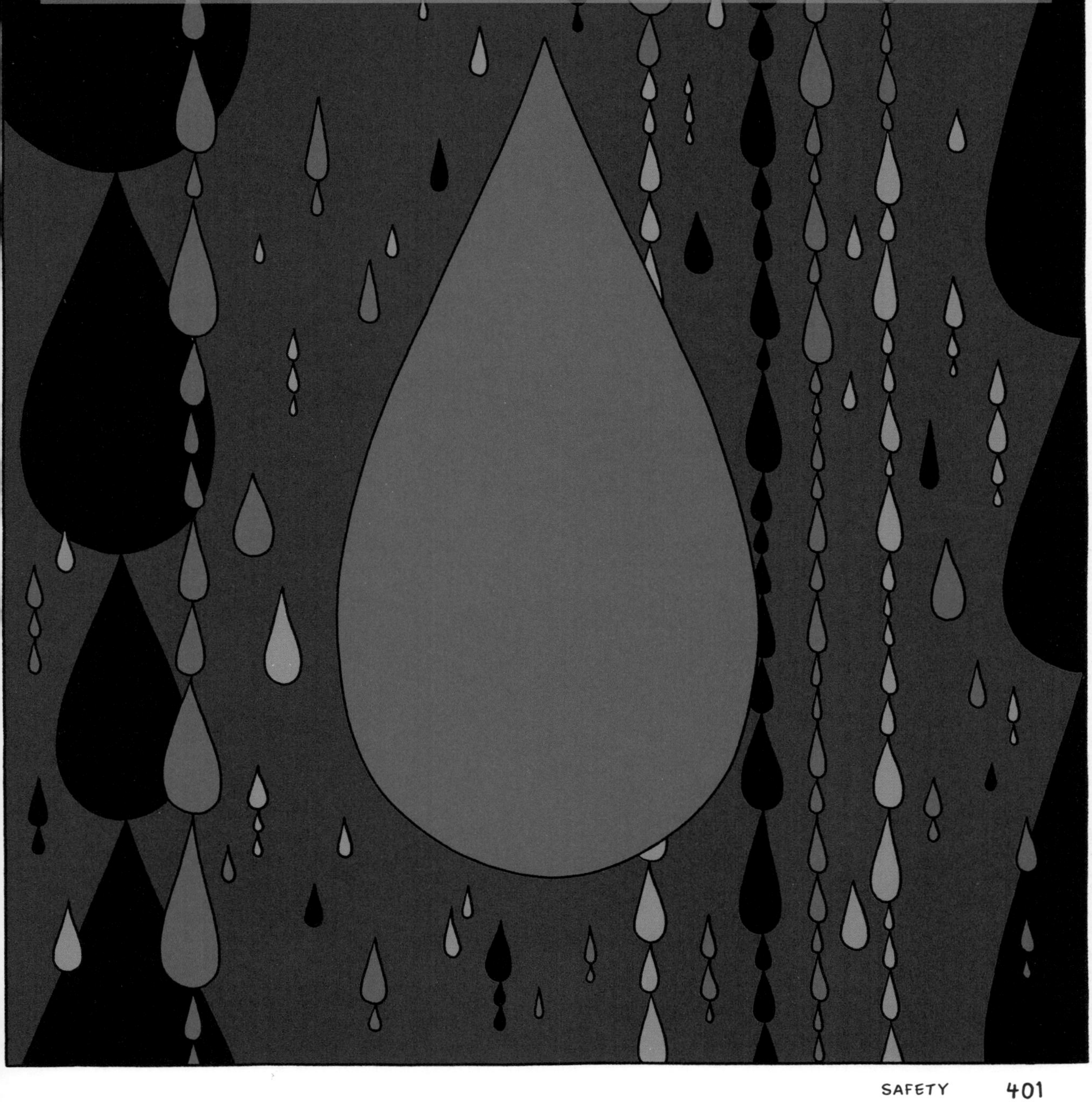

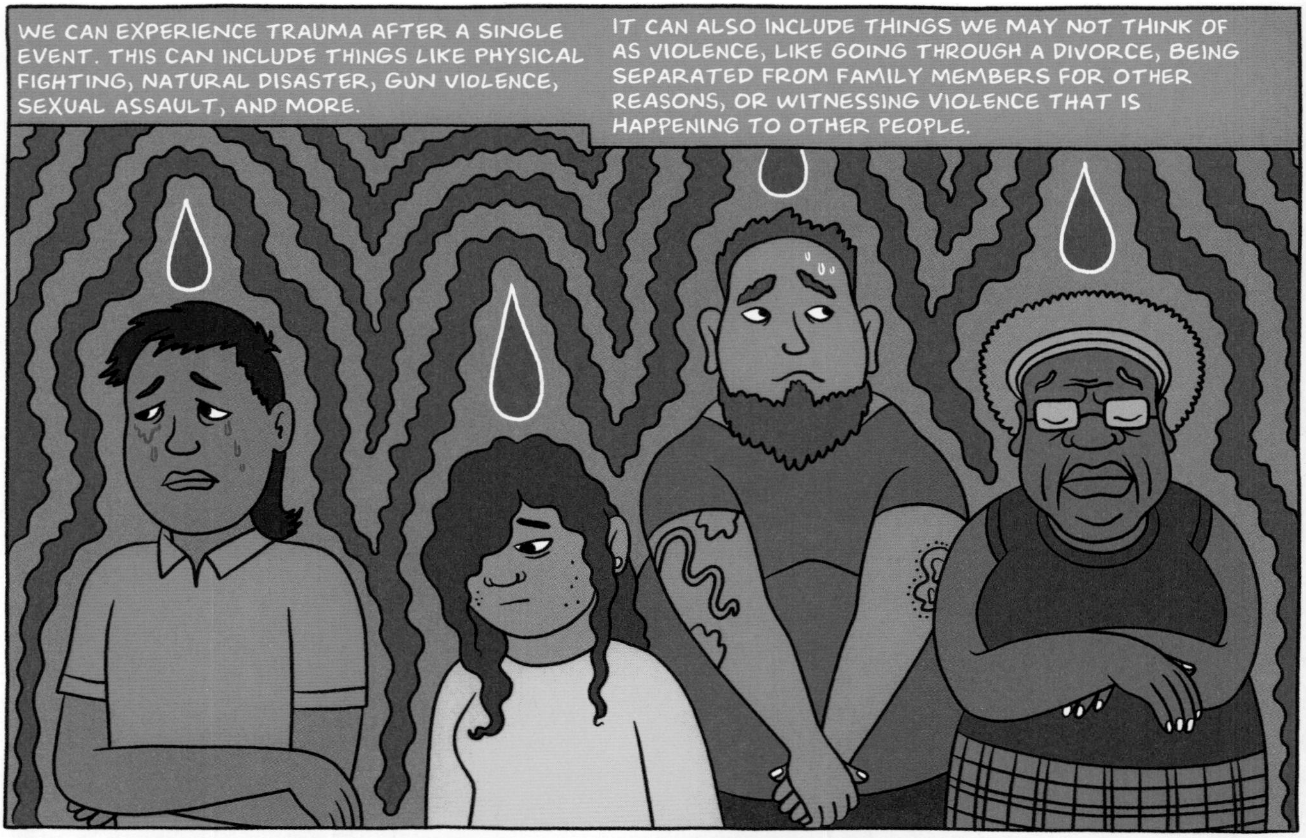
WE CAN EXPERIENCE TRAUMA AFTER A SINGLE EVENT. THIS CAN INCLUDE THINGS LIKE PHYSICAL FIGHTING, NATURAL DISASTER, GUN VIOLENCE, SEXUAL ASSAULT, AND MORE.
IT CAN ALSO INCLUDE THINGS WE MAY NOT THINK OF AS VIOLENCE, LIKE GOING THROUGH A DIVORCE, BEING SEPARATED FROM FAMILY MEMBERS FOR OTHER REASONS, OR WITNESSING VIOLENCE THAT IS HAPPENING TO OTHER PEOPLE.

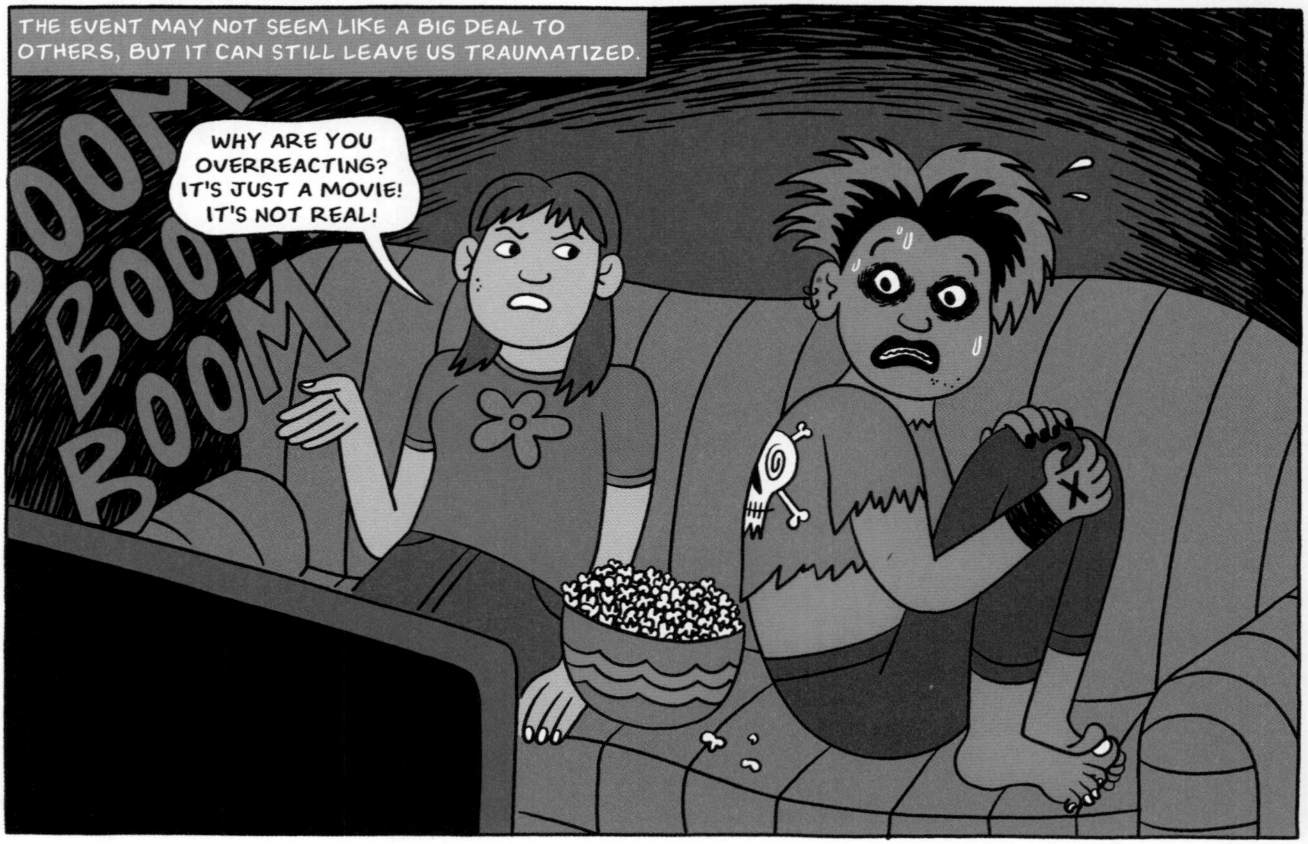
THE EVENT MAY NOT SEEM LIKE A BIG DEAL TO OTHERS, BUT IT CAN STILL LEAVE US TRAUMATIZED.
BOOM BOOM BOOM
WHY ARE YOU OVERREACTING? IT'S JUST A MOVIE! IT'S NOT REAL!

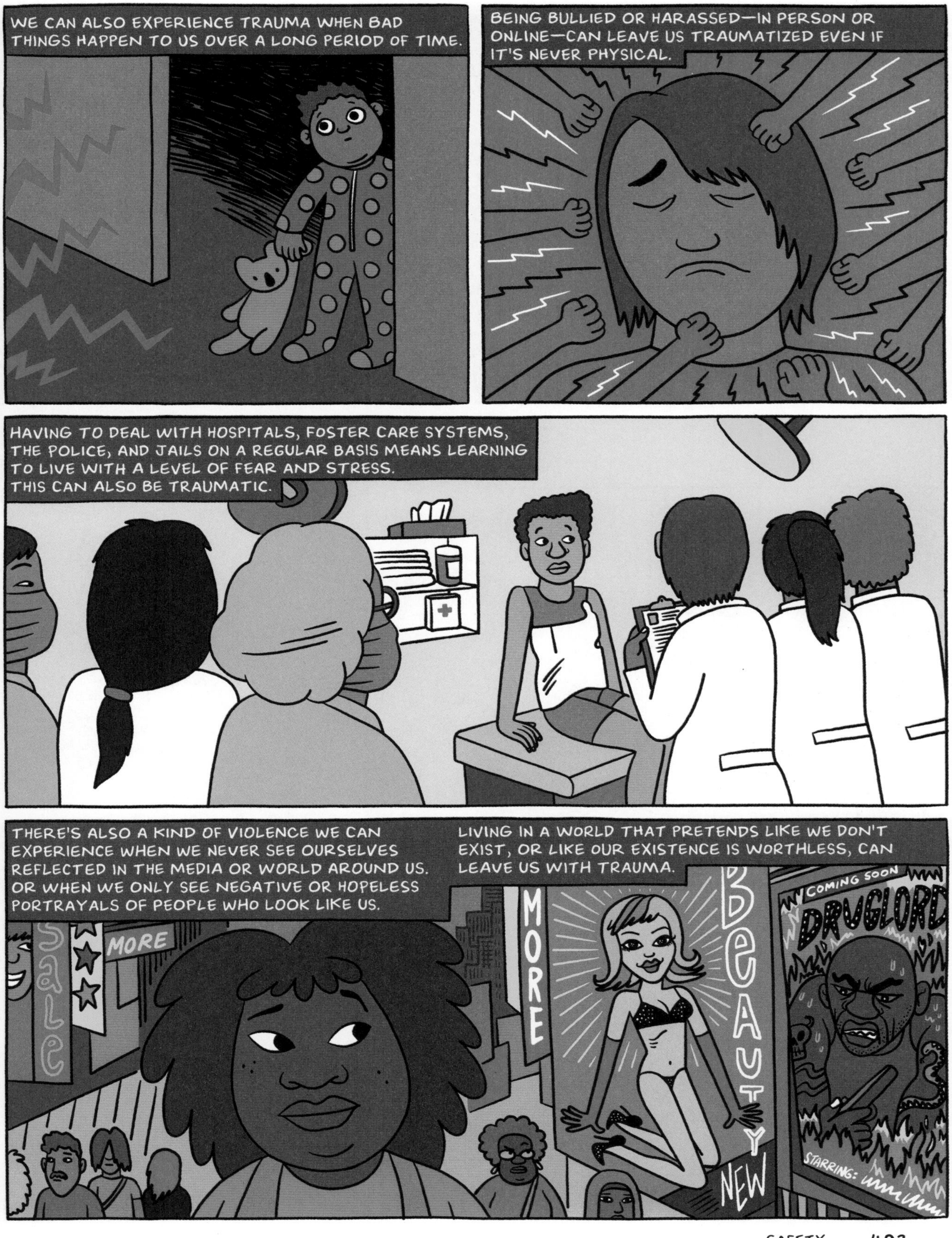
WE CAN ALSO EXPERIENCE TRAUMA WHEN BAD THINGS HAPPEN TO US OVER A LONG PERIOD OF TIME.
BEING BULLIED OR HARASSED—IN PERSON OR ONLINE—CAN LEAVE US TRAUMATIZED EVEN IF IT'S NEVER PHYSICAL.
HAVING TO DEAL WITH HOSPITALS, FOSTER CARE SYSTEMS, THE POLICE, AND JAILS ON A REGULAR BASIS MEANS LEARNING TO LIVE WITH A LEVEL OF FEAR AND STRESS. THIS CAN ALSO BE TRAUMATIC.
THERE'S ALSO A KIND OF VIOLENCE WE CAN EXPERIENCE WHEN WE NEVER SEE OURSELVES REFLECTED IN THE MEDIA OR WORLD AROUND US. OR WHEN WE ONLY SEE NEGATIVE OR HOPELESS PORTRAYALS OF PEOPLE WHO LOOK LIKE US.
LIVING IN A WORLD THAT PRETENDS LIKE WE DON'T EXIST, OR LIKE OUR EXISTENCE IS WORTHLESS, CAN LEAVE US WITH TRAUMA.
Sale
MORE
MORE
Beauty
BEAUTY
NEW
COMING SOON
DRUGLORD
STARRING:

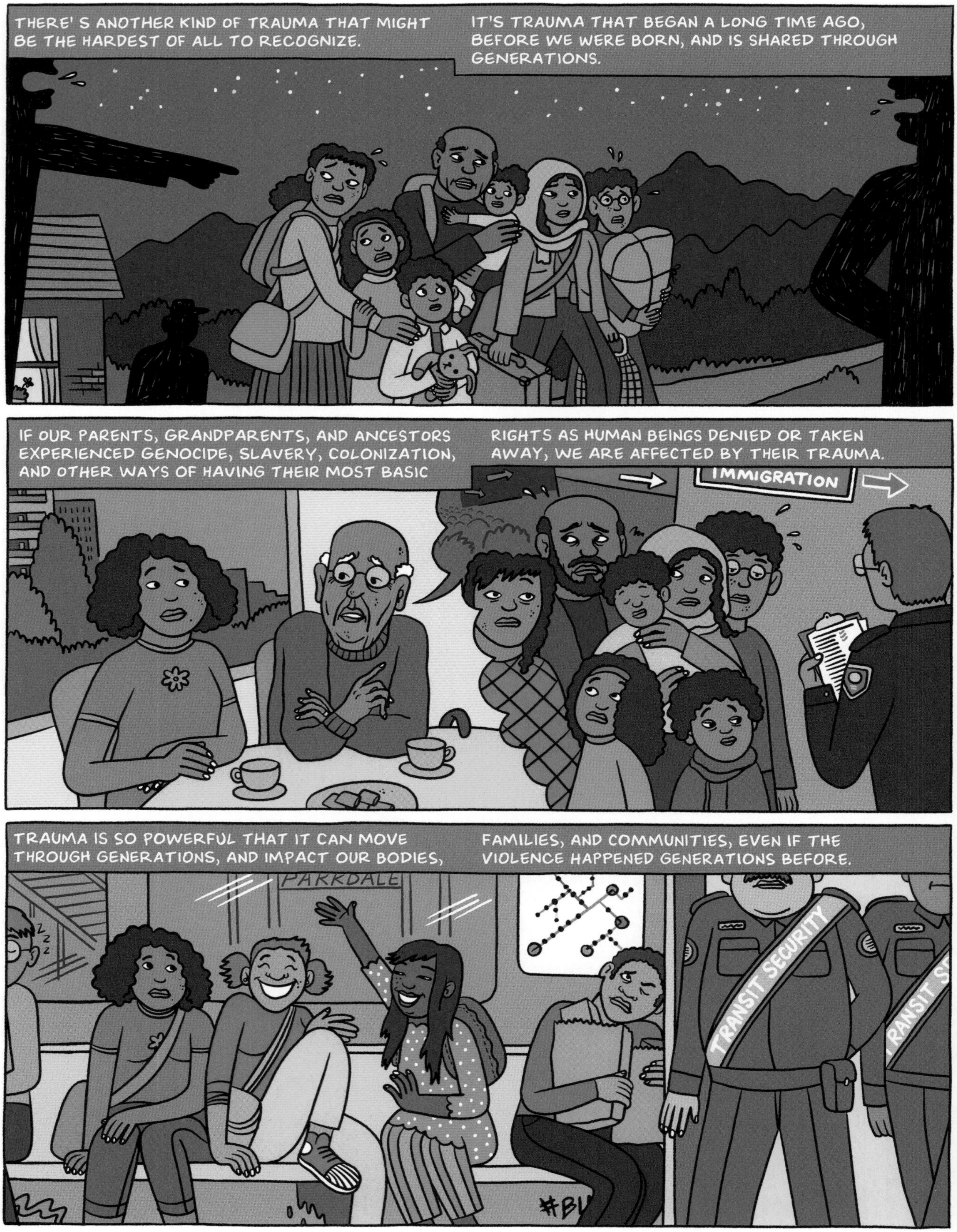
THERE'S ANOTHER KIND OF TRAUMA THAT MIGHT BE THE HARDEST OF ALL TO RECOGNIZE.
IT'S TRAUMA THAT BEGAN A LONG TIME AGO, BEFORE WE WERE BORN, AND IS SHARED THROUGH GENERATIONS.
IF OUR PARENTS, GRANDPARENTS, AND ANCESTORS EXPERIENCED GENOCIDE, SLAVERY, COLONIZATION, AND OTHER WAYS OF HAVING THEIR MOST BASIC
RIGHTS AS HUMAN BEINGS DENIED OR TAKEN AWAY, WE ARE AFFECTED BY THEIR TRAUMA.
IMMIGRATION
TRAUMA IS SO POWERFUL THAT IT CAN MOVE THROUGH GENERATIONS, AND IMPACT OUR BODIES,
FAMILIES, AND COMMUNITIES, EVEN IF THE VIOLENCE HAPPENED GENERATIONS BEFORE.
PARKDALE
TRANSIT SECURITY

TRAUMA CAN SCRAMBLE US UP, MAKING IT DIFFICULT TO THINK CLEARLY AND KNOW OUR OWN FEELINGS, OR HOW TO BE WITH THE PEOPLE AROUND US. IT CAN MAKE US FEEL LIKE WE'RE BOTH HERE AND NOT HERE.

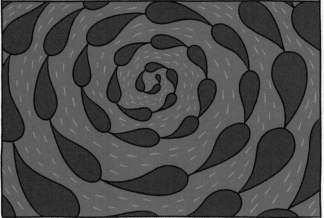

LIVING WITH TRAUMA CAN MAKE IT HARDER TO DO THINGS THAT OTHERS TAKE FOR GRANTED. LIKE LEARNING—IN AND OUT OF SCHOOL—MAKING AND KEEPING FRIENDS, AND LISTENING TO OUR INNER VOICE OR GUT INSTINCTS ABOUT WHAT WE WANT AND NEED.

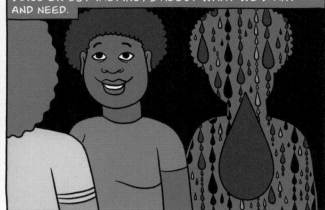

SOMETIMES TRAUMA MEANS EVERYTHING FEELS EXTRA. JUST MAKING IT THROUGH THE DAY CAN FEEL LIKE AN IMPOSSIBLE TASK.

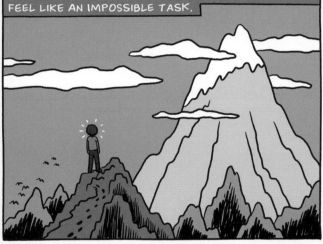

SOMETIMES TRAUMA MEANS EVERYTHING FEELS LESS. LIKE WE ARE MOVING THROUGH LIFE WITHOUT REALLY LIVING IT.

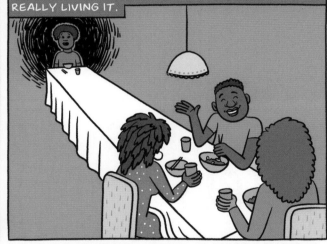

WHEN IT COMES TO SEX AND SEXY FEELINGS, TRAUMA CAN MEAN SOME OF US ARE VERY INTERESTED IN SEX AND SOME OF US HAVE NO INTEREST AT ALL OR ARE FEARFUL OF SEX.

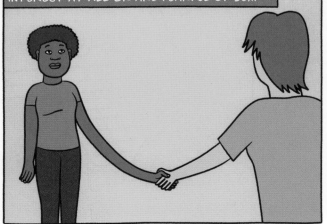

BECAUSE TRAUMA IS SOMETHING WE EXPERIENCE IN OUR BODIES AND MINDS, IT CAN CHANGE THE WAY WE FEEL IN OUR BODIES. EVEN IF WE ARE WITH SOMEONE WE LIKE, WHO WE WANT TO BE WITH, WE MAY STILL FEEL LIKE WE'RE OUTSIDE OUR BODY, OR WE MAY FEEL NOTHING AT ALL.

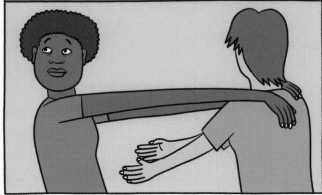

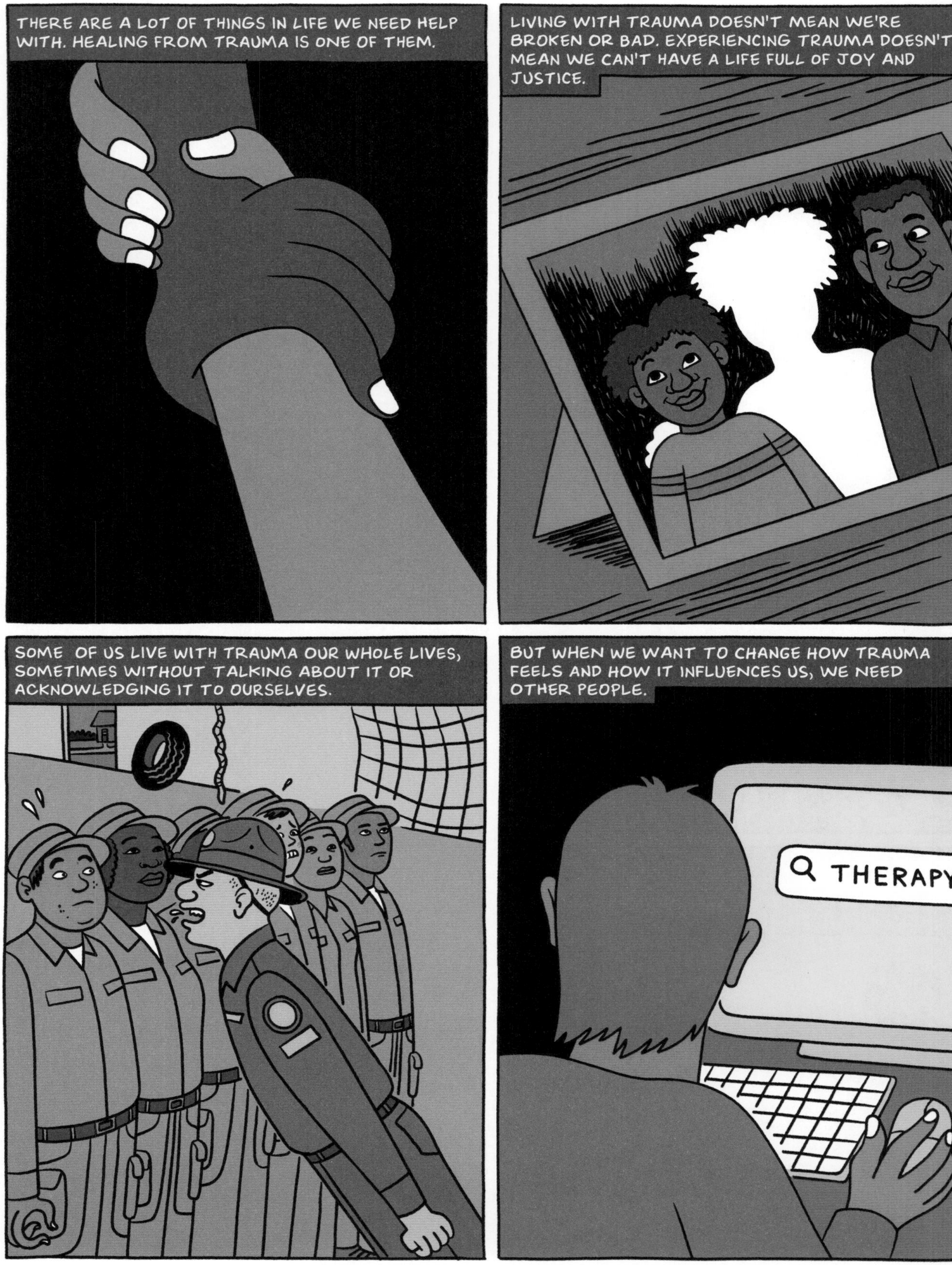

THERE ARE A LOT OF THINGS IN LIFE WE NEED HELP WITH. HEALING FROM TRAUMA IS ONE OF THEM.
LIVING WITH TRAUMA DOESN'T MEAN WE'RE BROKEN OR BAD. EXPERIENCING TRAUMA DOESN'T MEAN WE CAN'T HAVE A LIFE FULL OF JOY AND JUSTICE.
SOME OF US LIVE WITH TRAUMA OUR WHOLE LIVES, SOMETIMES WITHOUT TALKING ABOUT IT OR ACKNOWLEDGING IT TO OURSELVES.
BUT WHEN WE WANT TO CHANGE HOW TRAUMA FEELS AND HOW IT INFLUENCES US, WE NEED OTHER PEOPLE.
THERAPY

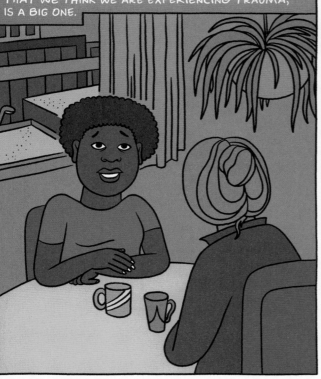

THE CHOICE TO TELL SOMEONE ABOUT VIOLENCE WE HAVE EXPERIENCED, OR TO TELL SOMEONE THAT WE THINK WE ARE EXPERIENCING TRAUMA, IS A BIG ONE.

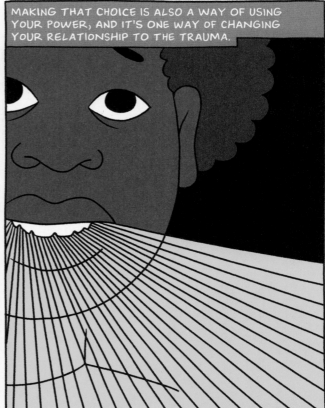

MAKING THAT CHOICE IS ALSO A WAY OF USING YOUR POWER, AND IT'S ONE WAY OF CHANGING YOUR RELATIONSHIP TO THE TRAUMA.

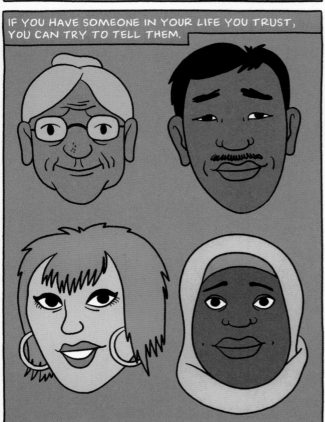

IF YOU HAVE SOMEONE IN YOUR LIFE YOU TRUST, YOU CAN TRY TO TELL THEM.

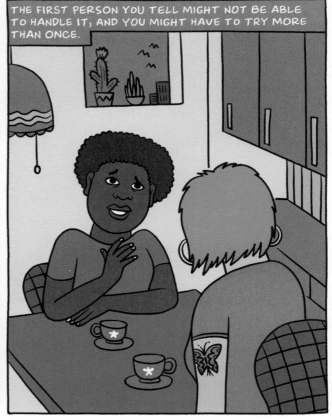

THE FIRST PERSON YOU TELL MIGHT NOT BE ABLE TO HANDLE IT, AND YOU MIGHT HAVE TO TRY MORE THAN ONCE.

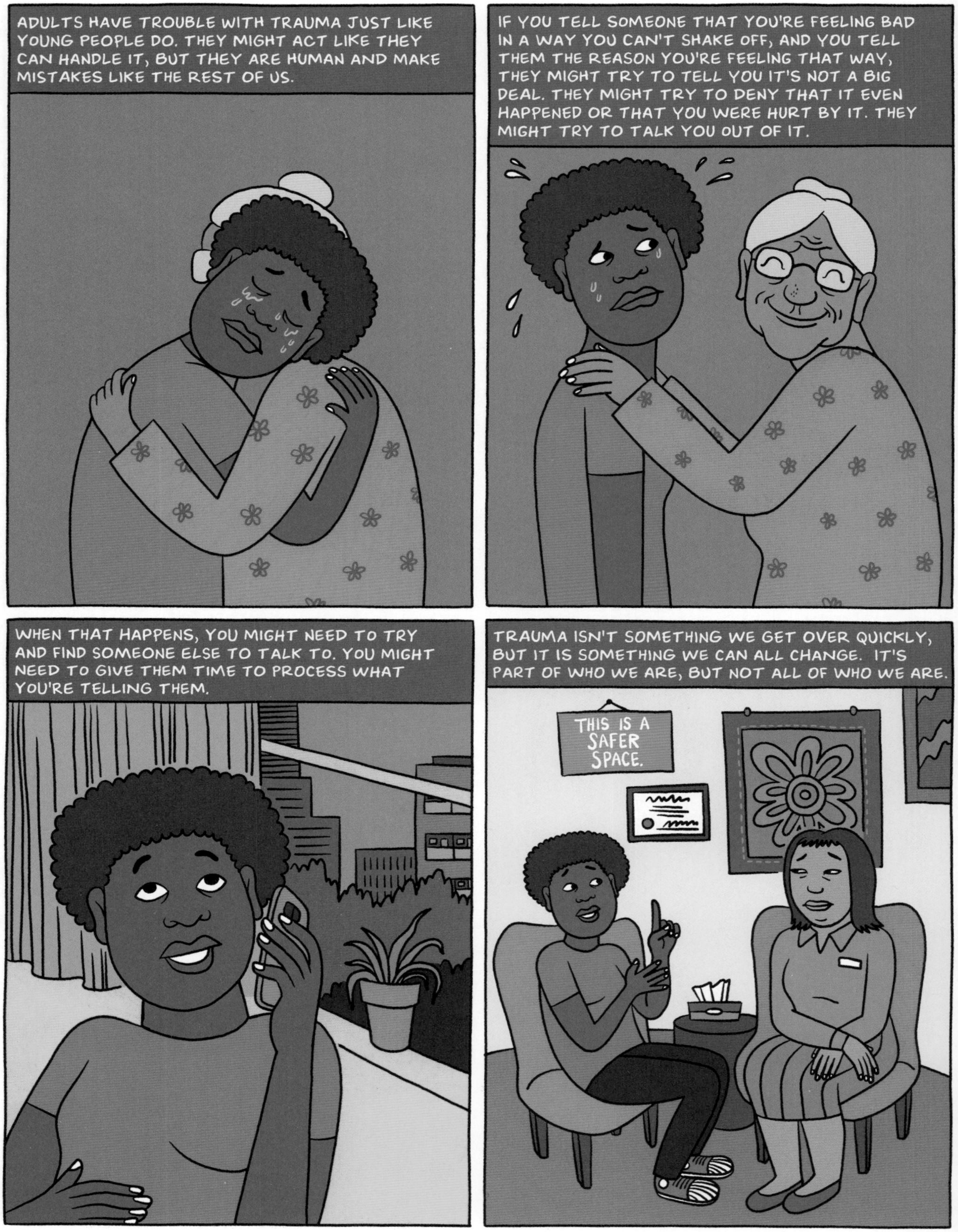
ADULTS HAVE TROUBLE WITH TRAUMA JUST LIKE YOUNG PEOPLE DO. THEY MIGHT ACT LIKE THEY CAN HANDLE IT, BUT THEY ARE HUMAN AND MAKE MISTAKES LIKE THE REST OF US.
IF YOU TELL SOMEONE THAT YOU'RE FEELING BAD IN A WAY YOU CAN'T SHAKE OFF, AND YOU TELL THEM THE REASON YOU'RE FEELING THAT WAY, THEY MIGHT TRY TO TELL YOU IT'S NOT A BIG DEAL. THEY MIGHT TRY TO DENY THAT IT EVEN HAPPENED OR THAT YOU WERE HURT BY IT. THEY MIGHT TRY TO TALK YOU OUT OF IT.
WHEN THAT HAPPENS, YOU MIGHT NEED TO TRY AND FIND SOMEONE ELSE TO TALK TO. YOU MIGHT NEED TO GIVE THEM TIME TO PROCESS WHAT YOU'RE TELLING THEM.
TRAUMA ISN'T SOMETHING WE GET OVER QUICKLY, BUT IT IS SOMETHING WE CAN ALL CHANGE. IT'S PART OF WHO WE ARE, BUT NOT ALL OF WHO WE ARE.
THIS IS A SAFER SPACE.

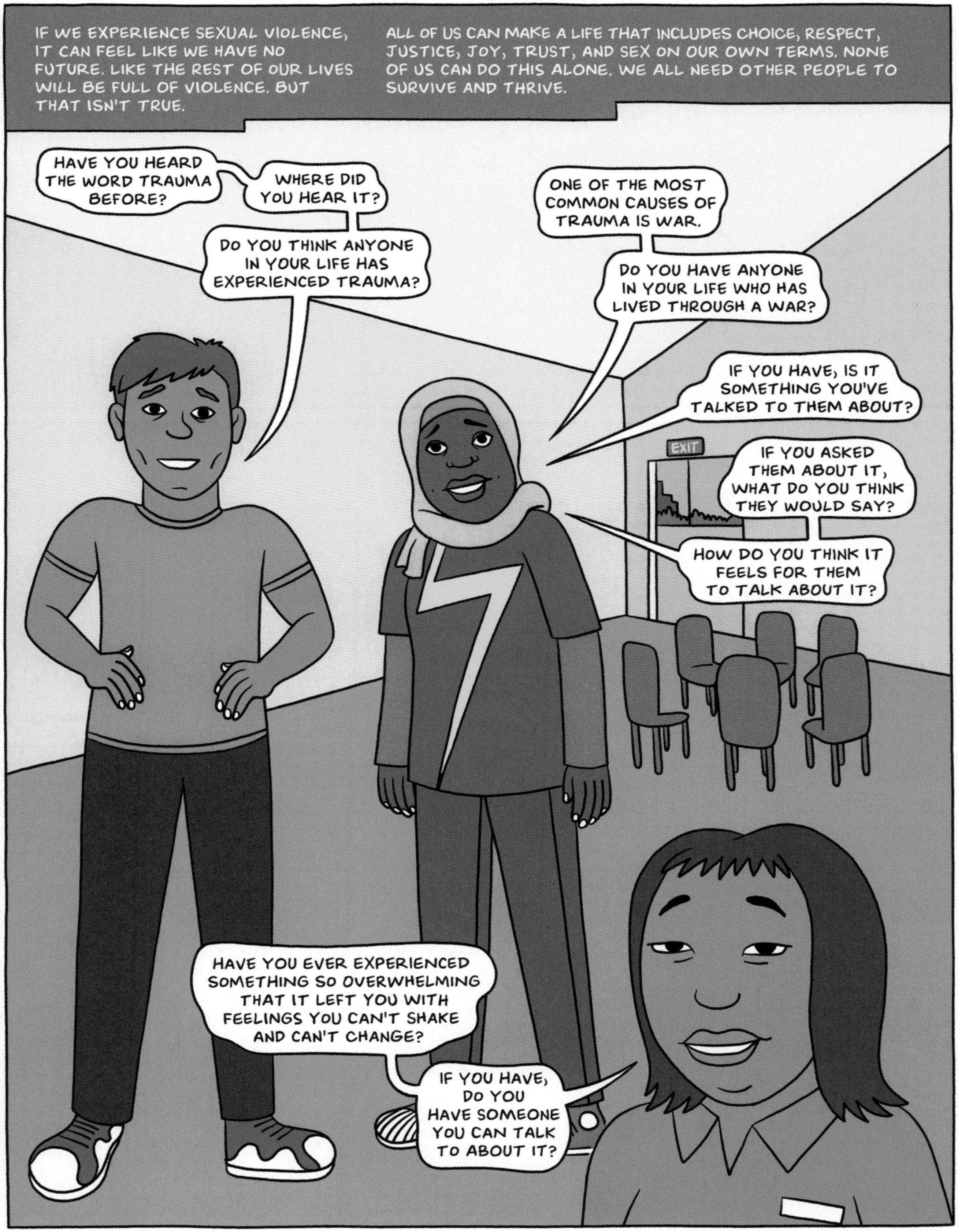
IF WE EXPERIENCE SEXUAL VIOLENCE, IT CAN FEEL LIKE WE HAVE NO FUTURE. LIKE THE REST OF OUR LIVES WILL BE FULL OF VIOLENCE. BUT THAT ISN'T TRUE.
ALL OF US CAN MAKE A LIFE THAT INCLUDES CHOICE, RESPECT, JUSTICE, JOY, TRUST, AND SEX ON OUR OWN TERMS. NONE OF US CAN DO THIS ALONE. WE ALL NEED OTHER PEOPLE TO SURVIVE AND THRIVE.
HAVE YOU HEARD THE WORD TRAUMA BEFORE?
WHERE DID YOU HEAR IT?
DO YOU THINK ANYONE IN YOUR LIFE HAS EXPERIENCED TRAUMA?
ONE OF THE MOST COMMON CAUSES OF TRAUMA IS WAR.
DO YOU HAVE ANYONE IN YOUR LIFE WHO HAS LIVED THROUGH A WAR?
IF YOU HAVE, IS IT SOMETHING YOU'VE TALKED TO THEM ABOUT?
EXIT
IF YOU ASKED THEM ABOUT IT, WHAT DO YOU THINK THEY WOULD SAY?
HOW DO YOU THINK IT FEELS FOR THEM TO TALK ABOUT IT?
HAVE YOU EVER EXPERIENCED SOMETHING SO OVERWHELMING THAT IT LEFT YOU WITH FEELINGS YOU CAN'T SHAKE AND CAN'T CHANGE?
IF YOU HAVE, DO YOU HAVE SOMEONE YOU CAN TALK TO ABOUT IT?

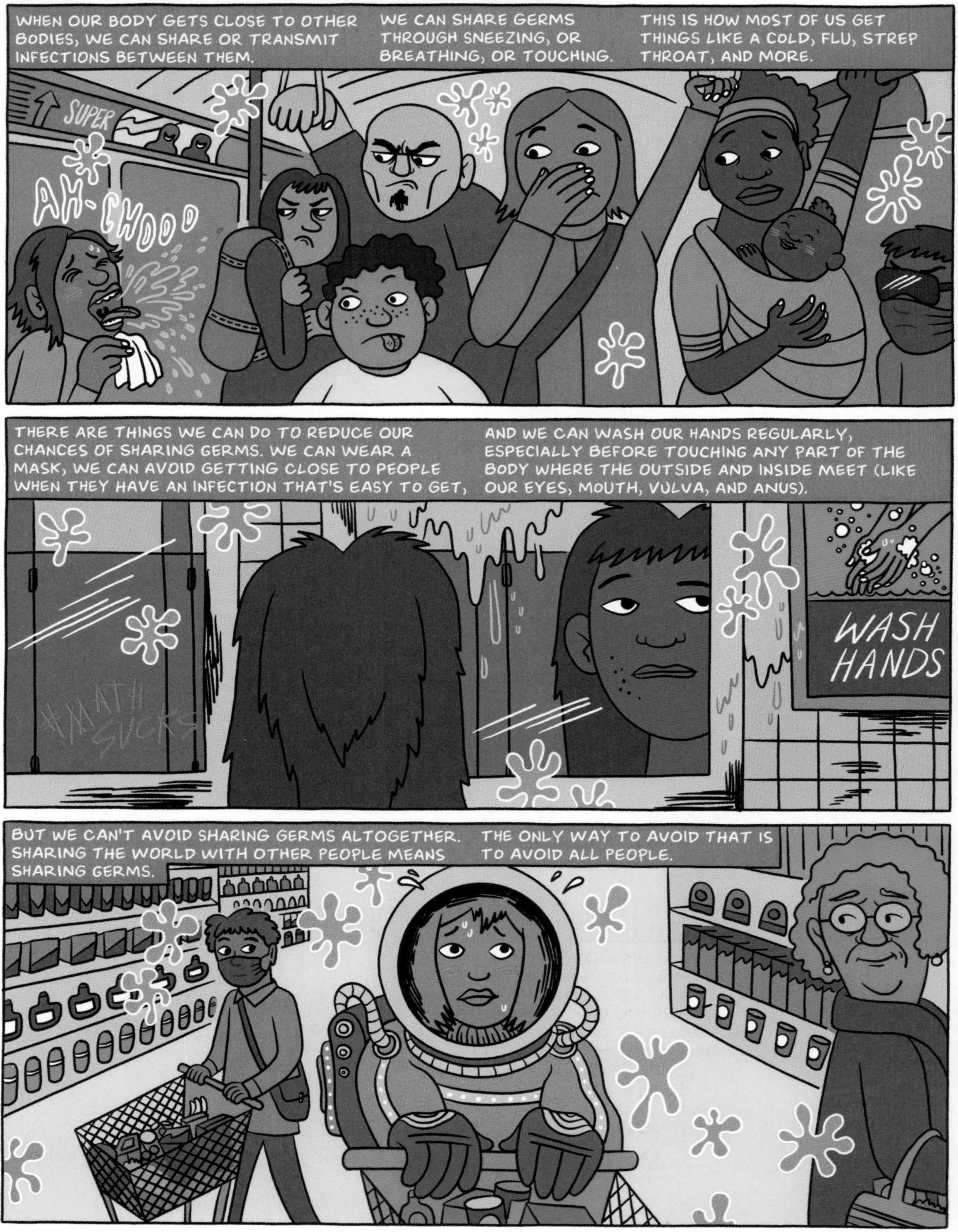
WHEN OUR BODY GETS CLOSE TO OTHER BODIES, WE CAN SHARE OR TRANSMIT INFECTIONS BETWEEN THEM.
WE CAN SHARE GERMS THROUGH SNEEZING, OR BREATHING, OR TOUCHING.
THIS IS HOW MOST OF US GET THINGS LIKE A COLD, FLU, STREP THROAT, AND MORE.
SUPER
AH-CHOOO
THERE ARE THINGS WE CAN DO TO REDUCE OUR CHANCES OF SHARING GERMS. WE CAN WEAR A MASK, WE CAN AVOID GETTING CLOSE TO PEOPLE WHEN THEY HAVE AN INFECTION THAT'S EASY TO GET,
AND WE CAN WASH OUR HANDS REGULARLY, ESPECIALLY BEFORE TOUCHING ANY PART OF THE BODY WHERE THE OUTSIDE AND INSIDE MEET (LIKE OUR EYES, MOUTH, VULVA, AND ANUS).
#MATH SUCKS
WASH HANDS
BUT WE CAN'T AVOID SHARING GERMS ALTOGETHER. SHARING THE WORLD WITH OTHER PEOPLE MEANS SHARING GERMS.
THE ONLY WAY TO AVOID THAT IS TO AVOID ALL PEOPLE.

WHEN WE SHARE AN INFECTION DURING SEX IT'S CALLED A SEXUALLY TRANSMITTED INFECTION, OR STI FOR SHORT.

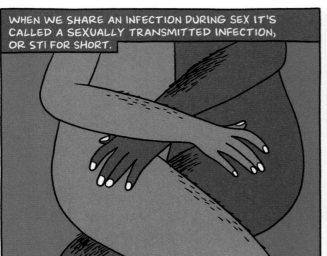

STIS AREN'T BETTER OR WORSE THAN INFECTIONS SHARED THROUGH OTHER ACTIVITIES. INFECTIONS CAN MAKE US VERY SICK IF THEY AREN'T TREATED. BUT MANY INFECTIONS—INCLUDING THE ONES WE CAN SHARE DURING SEX—CAN BE EASILY TREATED AND GOTTEN RID OF ENTIRELY.

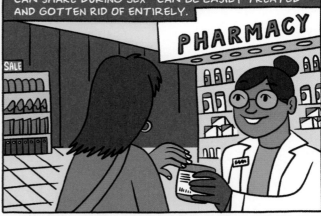

STIS ARE THOUGHT OF AS WORSE AND SCARIER— NOT BECAUSE OF WHAT THEY DO TO OUR BODIES, BUT BECAUSE OF STIGMA.*

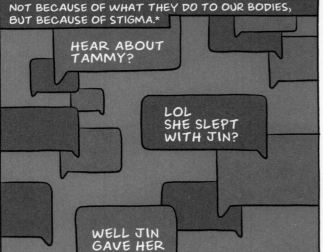

HEAR ABOUT TAMMY?

LOL SHE SLEPT WITH JIN?

WELL JIN GAVE HER

WHEN SOMEONE SAYS THEY HAVE A COLD, PEOPLE MIGHT AVOID BEING CLOSE TO THEM FOR A WHILE. BUT THEY DON'T USUALLY ACT LIKE THERE'S SOMETHING WRONG WITH THE PERSON.

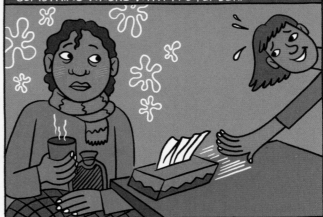

BUT IF SOMEONE SAYS THEY HAVE AN STI, OR IF OTHER PEOPLE THINK THEY HAVE AN STI, THAT PERSON IS OFTEN TREATED NOT JUST AS IF THEY HAVE AN INFECTION, BUT AS IF THEY ARE AN INFECTION.

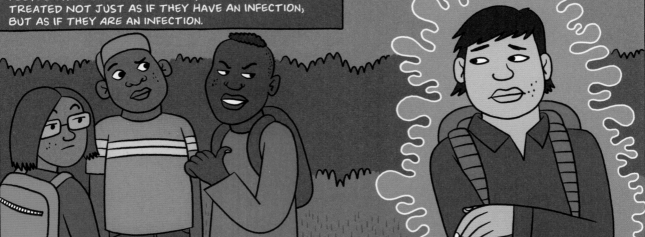

* READ MORE ABOUT STIGMA ON P. 243

STIS ARE VERY COMMON. MANY PEOPLE GET ONE, OR MORE THAN ONE, IN THEIR LIFETIME. WHEN YOU TALK TO PEOPLE WHO HAVE HAD AN STI, MANY WILL SAY THAT IT'S THE STIGMA—THE WAY THEY ARE TREATED—THAT HURTS MORE THAN THE STI ITSELF.

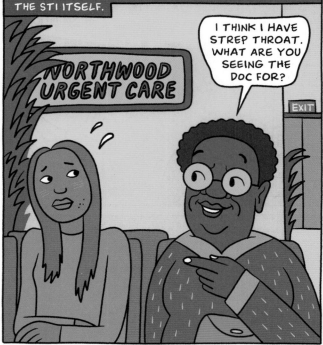

NORTHWOOD URGENT CARE

EXIT

I THINK I HAVE STREP THROAT. WHAT ARE YOU SEEING THE DOC FOR?

BEFORE YOU START EXPLORING SEX WITH ANOTHER PERSON, IT'S IMPORTANT TO KNOW ABOUT STIS, WHAT TO DO IF YOU THINK YOU HAVE ONE, AND WHAT YOU CAN DO TO REDUCE YOUR CHANCES OF GETTING OR SHARING ONE.

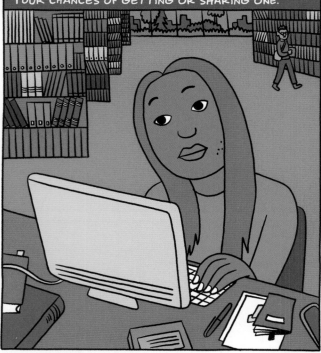

THAT'S THE INFORMATION MOST SEX EDUCATION FOCUSES ON. AND YOU CAN FIND THE NAMES OF RELIABLE SOURCES FOR STI INFORMATION IN THE BACK OF THE BOOK.

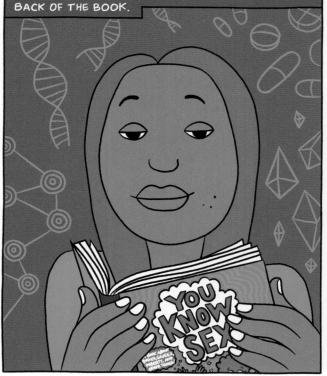

YOU KNOW SEX

WE DECIDED NOT TO INCLUDE THAT INFORMATION HERE. INSTEAD, WE WANTED TO SHARE A FEW THINGS ABOUT STIS WE HAVEN'T SEEN IN MANY SEX EDUCATION BOOKS—PLUS TWO ACTIVITIES FOR ANYONE WHO WANTS TO LEARN MORE.

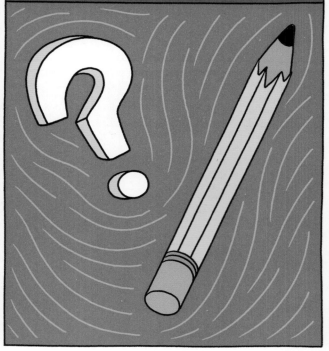

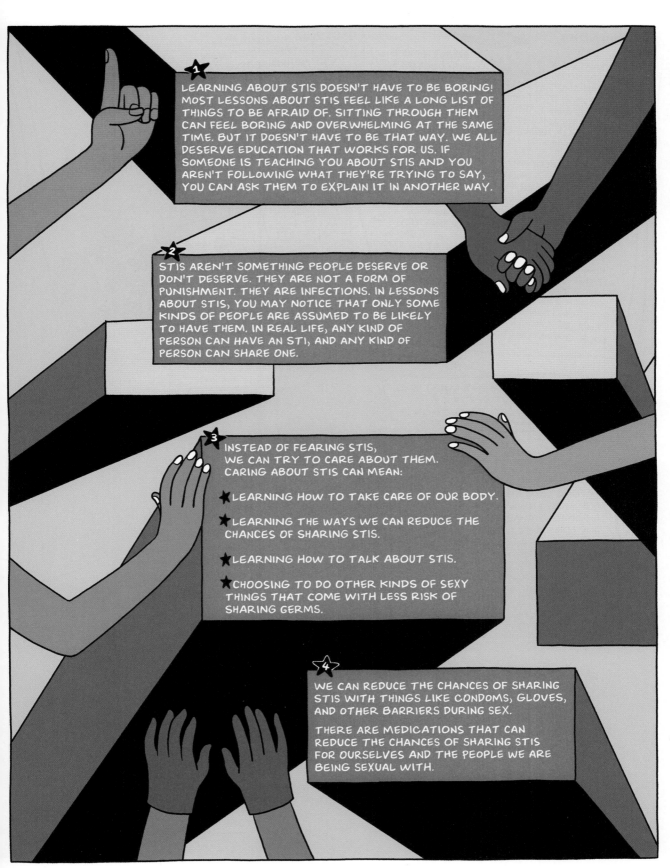

1 LEARNING ABOUT STIS DOESN'T HAVE TO BE BORING! MOST LESSONS ABOUT STIS FEEL LIKE A LONG LIST OF THINGS TO BE AFRAID OF. SITTING THROUGH THEM CAN FEEL BORING AND OVERWHELMING AT THE SAME TIME. BUT IT DOESN'T HAVE TO BE THAT WAY. WE ALL DESERVE EDUCATION THAT WORKS FOR US. IF SOMEONE IS TEACHING YOU ABOUT STIS AND YOU AREN'T FOLLOWING WHAT THEY'RE TRYING TO SAY, YOU CAN ASK THEM TO EXPLAIN IT IN ANOTHER WAY.

2 STIS AREN'T SOMETHING PEOPLE DESERVE OR DON'T DESERVE. THEY ARE NOT A FORM OF PUNISHMENT. THEY ARE INFECTIONS. IN LESSONS ABOUT STIS, YOU MAY NOTICE THAT ONLY SOME KINDS OF PEOPLE ARE ASSUMED TO BE LIKELY TO HAVE THEM. IN REAL LIFE, ANY KIND OF PERSON CAN HAVE AN STI, AND ANY KIND OF PERSON CAN SHARE ONE.

3 INSTEAD OF FEARING STIS, WE CAN TRY TO CARE ABOUT THEM. CARING ABOUT STIS CAN MEAN:

★ LEARNING HOW TO TAKE CARE OF OUR BODY.

★ LEARNING THE WAYS WE CAN REDUCE THE CHANCES OF SHARING STIS.

★ LEARNING HOW TO TALK ABOUT STIS.

★ CHOOSING TO DO OTHER KINDS OF SEXY THINGS THAT COME WITH LESS RISK OF SHARING GERMS.

4 WE CAN REDUCE THE CHANCES OF SHARING STIS WITH THINGS LIKE CONDOMS, GLOVES, AND OTHER BARRIERS DURING SEX.

THERE ARE MEDICATIONS THAT CAN REDUCE THE CHANCES OF SHARING STIS FOR OURSELVES AND THE PEOPLE WE ARE BEING SEXUAL WITH.

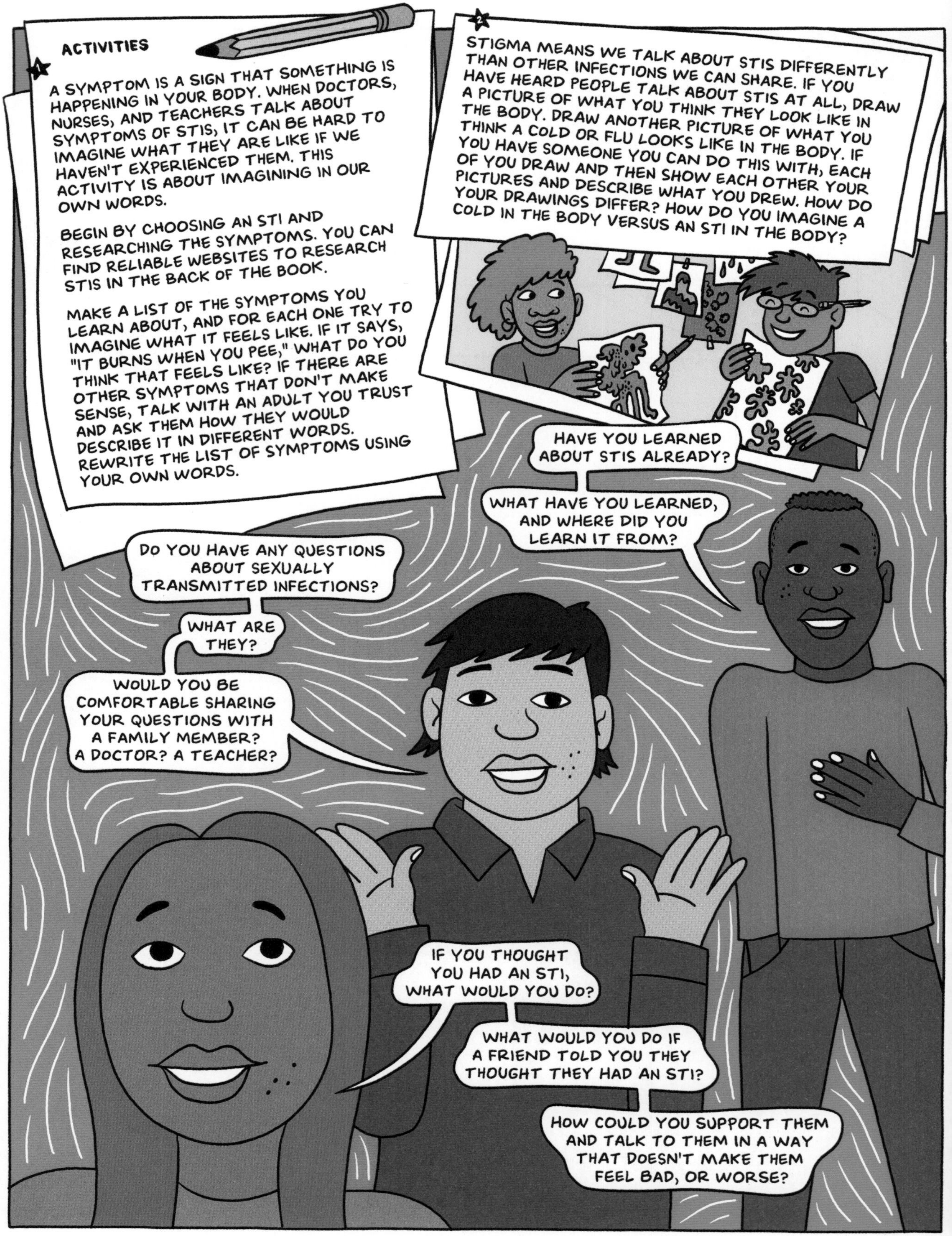
ACTIVITIES
1
A SYMPTOM IS A SIGN THAT SOMETHING IS HAPPENING IN YOUR BODY. WHEN DOCTORS, NURSES, AND TEACHERS TALK ABOUT SYMPTOMS OF STIS, IT CAN BE HARD TO IMAGINE WHAT THEY ARE LIKE IF WE HAVEN'T EXPERIENCED THEM. THIS ACTIVITY IS ABOUT IMAGINING IN OUR OWN WORDS.
BEGIN BY CHOOSING AN STI AND RESEARCHING THE SYMPTOMS. YOU CAN FIND RELIABLE WEBSITES TO RESEARCH STIS IN THE BACK OF THE BOOK.
MAKE A LIST OF THE SYMPTOMS YOU LEARN ABOUT, AND FOR EACH ONE TRY TO IMAGINE WHAT IT FEELS LIKE. IF IT SAYS, "IT BURNS WHEN YOU PEE," WHAT DO YOU THINK THAT FEELS LIKE? IF THERE ARE OTHER SYMPTOMS THAT DON'T MAKE SENSE, TALK WITH AN ADULT YOU TRUST AND ASK THEM HOW THEY WOULD DESCRIBE IT IN DIFFERENT WORDS. REWRITE THE LIST OF SYMPTOMS USING YOUR OWN WORDS.
2
STIGMA MEANS WE TALK ABOUT STIS DIFFERENTLY THAN OTHER INFECTIONS WE CAN SHARE. IF YOU HAVE HEARD PEOPLE TALK ABOUT STIS AT ALL, DRAW A PICTURE OF WHAT YOU THINK THEY LOOK LIKE IN THE BODY. DRAW ANOTHER PICTURE OF WHAT YOU THINK A COLD OR FLU LOOKS LIKE IN THE BODY. IF YOU HAVE SOMEONE YOU CAN DO THIS WITH, EACH OF YOU DRAW AND THEN SHOW EACH OTHER YOUR PICTURES AND DESCRIBE WHAT YOU DREW. HOW DO YOUR DRAWINGS DIFFER? HOW DO YOU IMAGINE A COLD IN THE BODY VERSUS AN STI IN THE BODY?
HAVE YOU LEARNED ABOUT STIS ALREADY?
WHAT HAVE YOU LEARNED, AND WHERE DID YOU LEARN IT FROM?
DO YOU HAVE ANY QUESTIONS ABOUT SEXUALLY TRANSMITTED INFECTIONS?
WHAT ARE THEY?
WOULD YOU BE COMFORTABLE SHARING YOUR QUESTIONS WITH A FAMILY MEMBER? A DOCTOR? A TEACHER?
IF YOU THOUGHT YOU HAD AN STI, WHAT WOULD YOU DO?
WHAT WOULD YOU DO IF A FRIEND TOLD YOU THEY THOUGHT THEY HAD AN STI?
HOW COULD YOU SUPPORT THEM AND TALK TO THEM IN A WAY THAT DOESN'T MAKE THEM FEEL BAD, OR WORSE?

SINCE TODAY IS OUR LAST CLASS, I'M WONDERING IF THERE ARE ANY QUESTIONS WE HAVEN'T COVERED?
HUBERT THE SEX ED OWL
CLASS VALUES

WHY HAS PUBERTY STARTED FOR EVERYONE BUT ME?
HOW CAN I GET SOMEONE TO STOP LIKING ME?
HOW CAN I GET SOMEONE TO LIKE ME?
WHEN WILL I HAVE MY FIRST KISS?
WHY DO PEOPLE THINK SEX JOKES ARE FUNNY?
HOW CAN I AVOID MY FIRST KISS?
HOW CAN I TALK TO MY PARENTS ABOUT ANY OF THIS?
I T NORMAL TO HINK ABOUT EX A LOT?
I T NORMAL IF I EVER REALLY TH K ABOUT SEX?
BOTH PEOPLE KE SEX THE AMOUNT?
HAT IF I DON'T T NK I'LL EVER LI E SOMEONE L E THAT?
IF I HAVE BODY AUTONOMY, HOW COME I HAVE TO GO TO SCHOOL?
I DON'T HAVE A Q ESTION NOW BUT KNO I WILL LATER. WHA DO I DO THEN?
HOW DO YOU KNOW YOU'RE READY FOR SEX?
IS IT OKAY TO LOOK UP SEX STUFF ONLINE?
CLASS VALUES
!

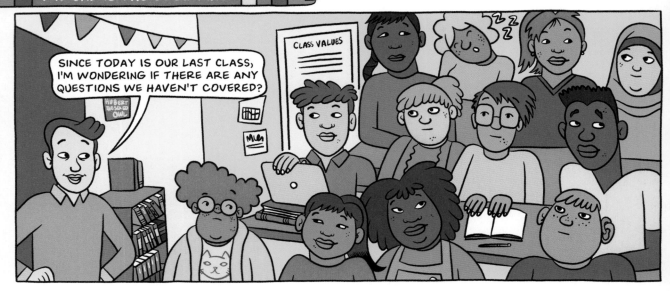

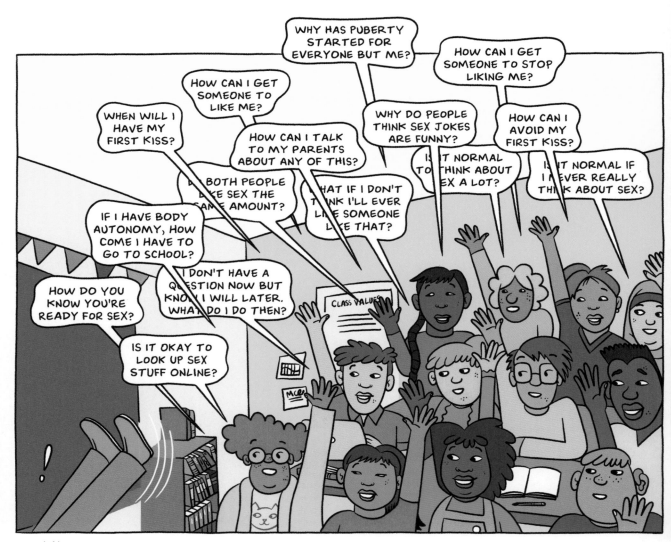

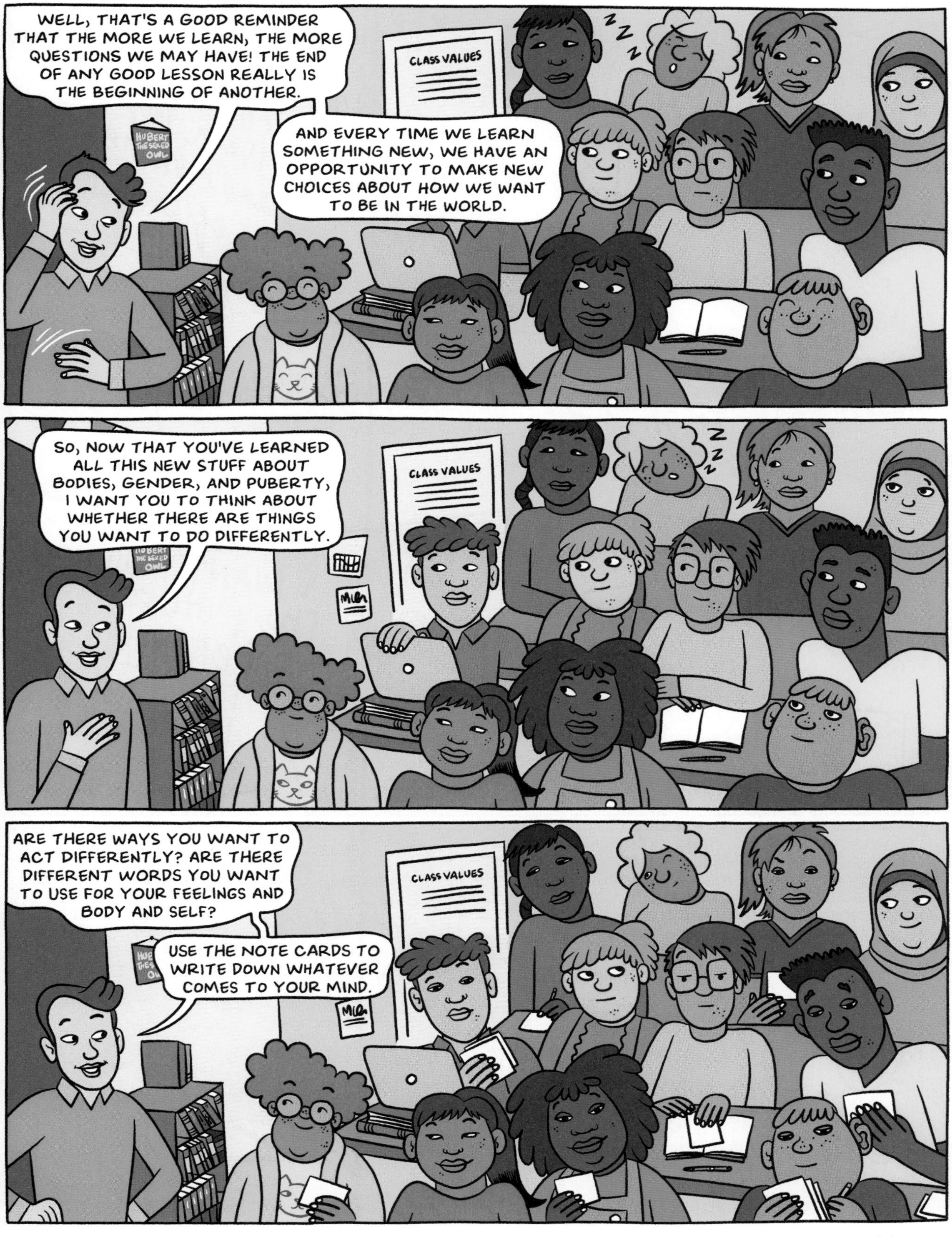
WELL, THAT'S A GOOD REMINDER THAT THE MORE WE LEARN, THE MORE QUESTIONS WE MAY HAVE! THE END OF ANY GOOD LESSON REALLY IS THE BEGINNING OF ANOTHER.
AND EVERY TIME WE LEARN SOMETHING NEW, WE HAVE AN OPPORTUNITY TO MAKE NEW CHOICES ABOUT HOW WE WANT TO BE IN THE WORLD.
CLASS VALUES
HUBERT THE SEXED OWL
Z Z Z
SO, NOW THAT YOU'VE LEARNED ALL THIS NEW STUFF ABOUT BODIES, GENDER, AND PUBERTY, I WANT YOU TO THINK ABOUT WHETHER THERE ARE THINGS YOU WANT TO DO DIFFERENTLY.
ARE THERE WAYS YOU WANT TO ACT DIFFERENTLY? ARE THERE DIFFERENT WORDS YOU WANT TO USE FOR YOUR FEELINGS AND BODY AND SELF?
USE THE NOTE CARDS TO WRITE DOWN WHATEVER COMES TO YOUR MIND.

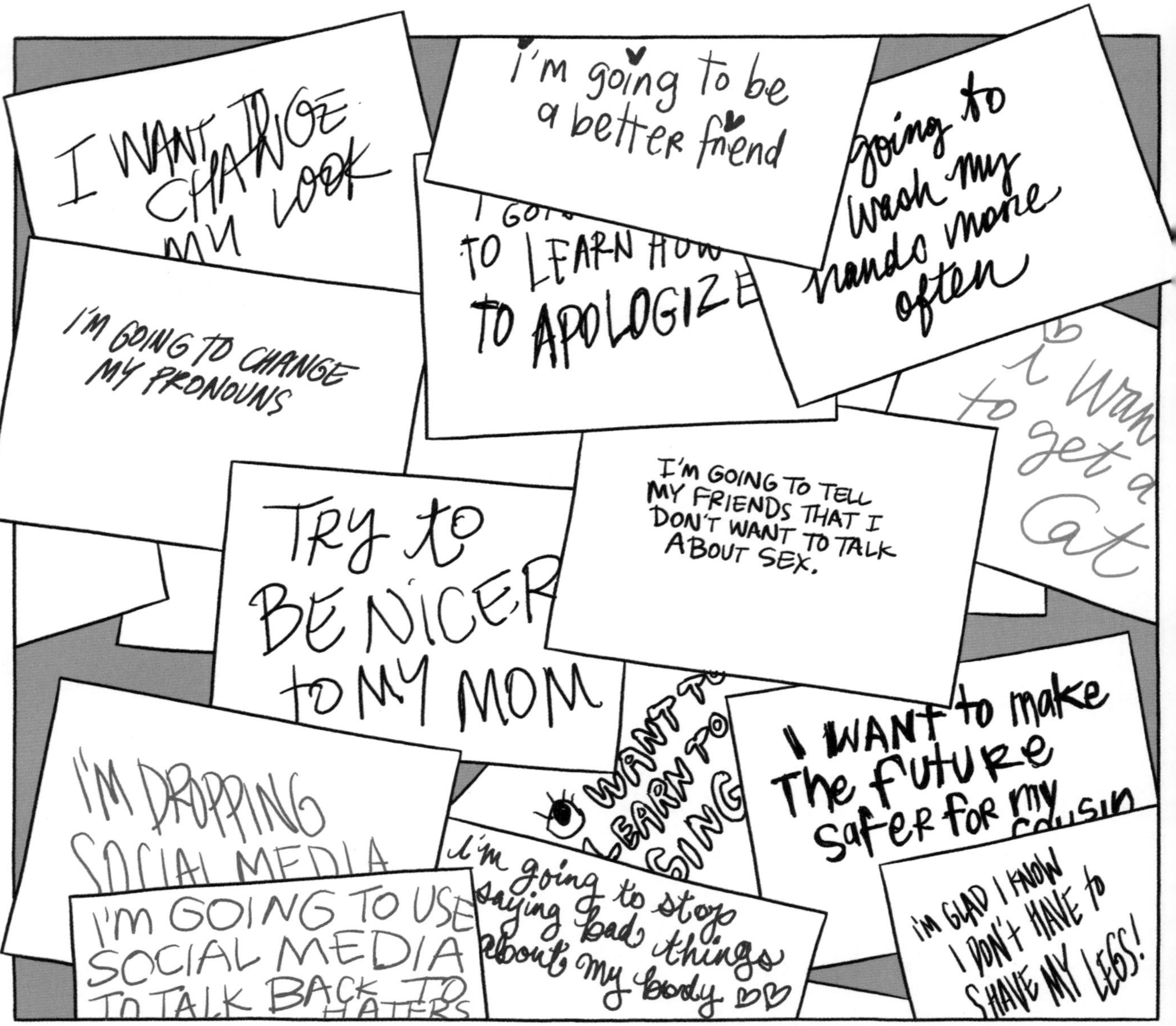
I WANT TO CHANGE MY LOOK
i'm going to be a better friend
going to wash my hands more often
I'M GOING TO CHANGE MY PRONOUNS
TO LEARN HOW TO APOLOGIZE
I WANT TO GET A CAT
TRY TO BE NICER TO MY MOM
I'M GOING TO TELL MY FRIENDS THAT I DON'T WANT TO TALK ABOUT SEX.
I'M DROPPING SOCIAL MEDIA
I WANT TO LEARN TO SING
I WANT to make The future safer for my cousin
I'M GOING TO USE SOCIAL MEDIA TO TALK BACK TO HATERS
i'm going to stop saying bad things about my body
I'M GLAD I KNOW I DON'T HAVE TO SHAVE MY LEGS!

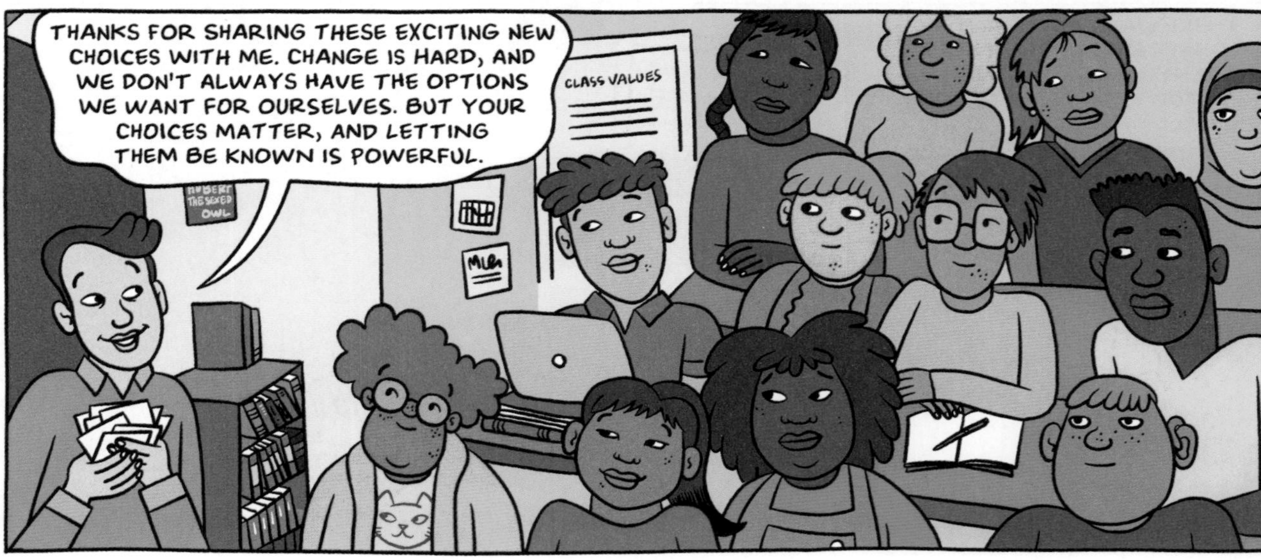
THANKS FOR SHARING THESE EXCITING NEW CHOICES WITH ME. CHANGE IS HARD, AND WE DON'T ALWAYS HAVE THE OPTIONS WE WANT FOR OURSELVES. BUT YOUR CHOICES MATTER, AND LETTING THEM BE KNOWN IS POWERFUL.
CLASS VALUES
ROBERT THE SEXED OWL

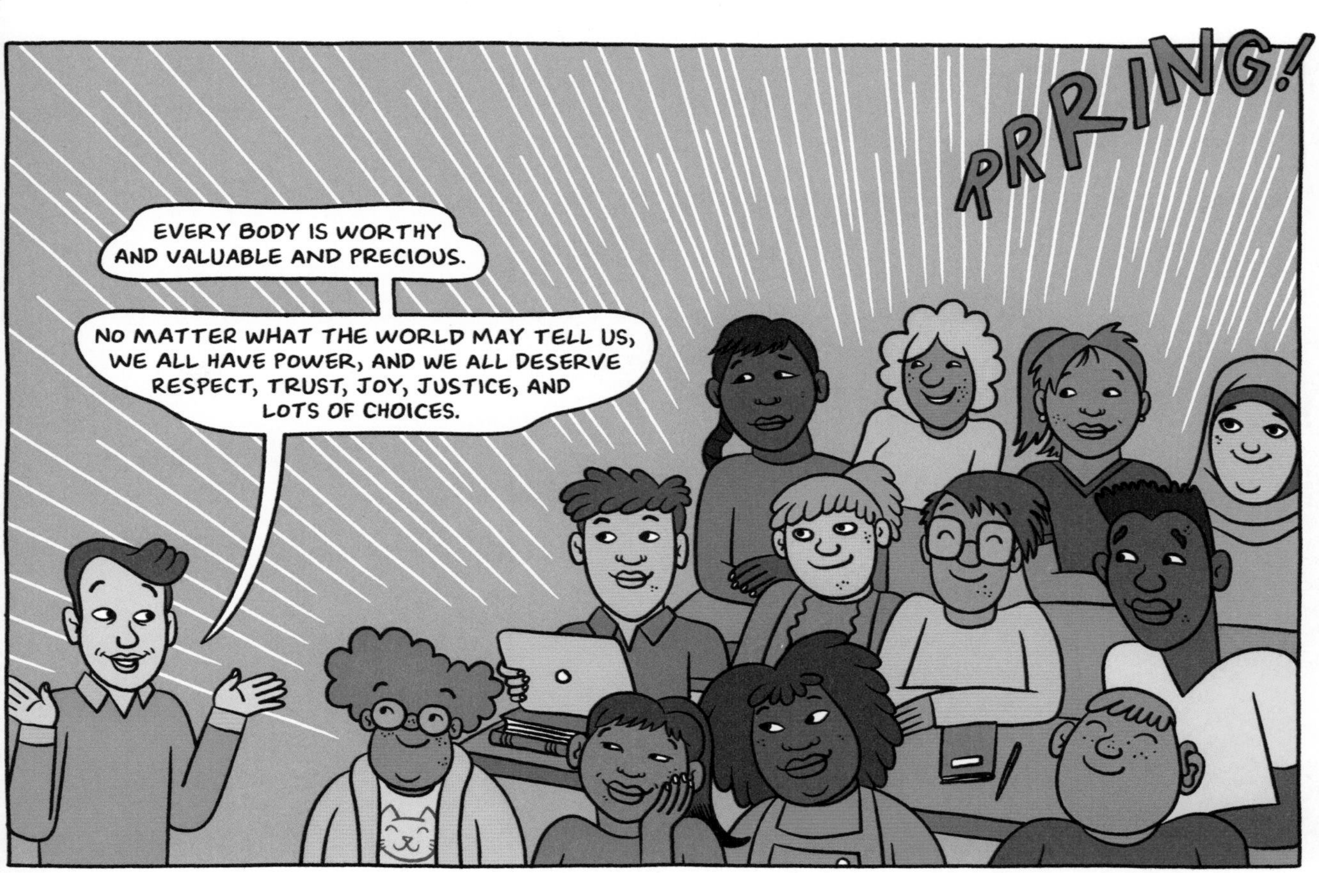
RRRING!
EVERY BODY IS WORTHY AND VALUABLE AND PRECIOUS.
NO MATTER WHAT THE WORLD MAY TELL US, WE ALL HAVE POWER, AND WE ALL DESERVE RESPECT, TRUST, JOY, JUSTICE, AND LOTS OF CHOICES.

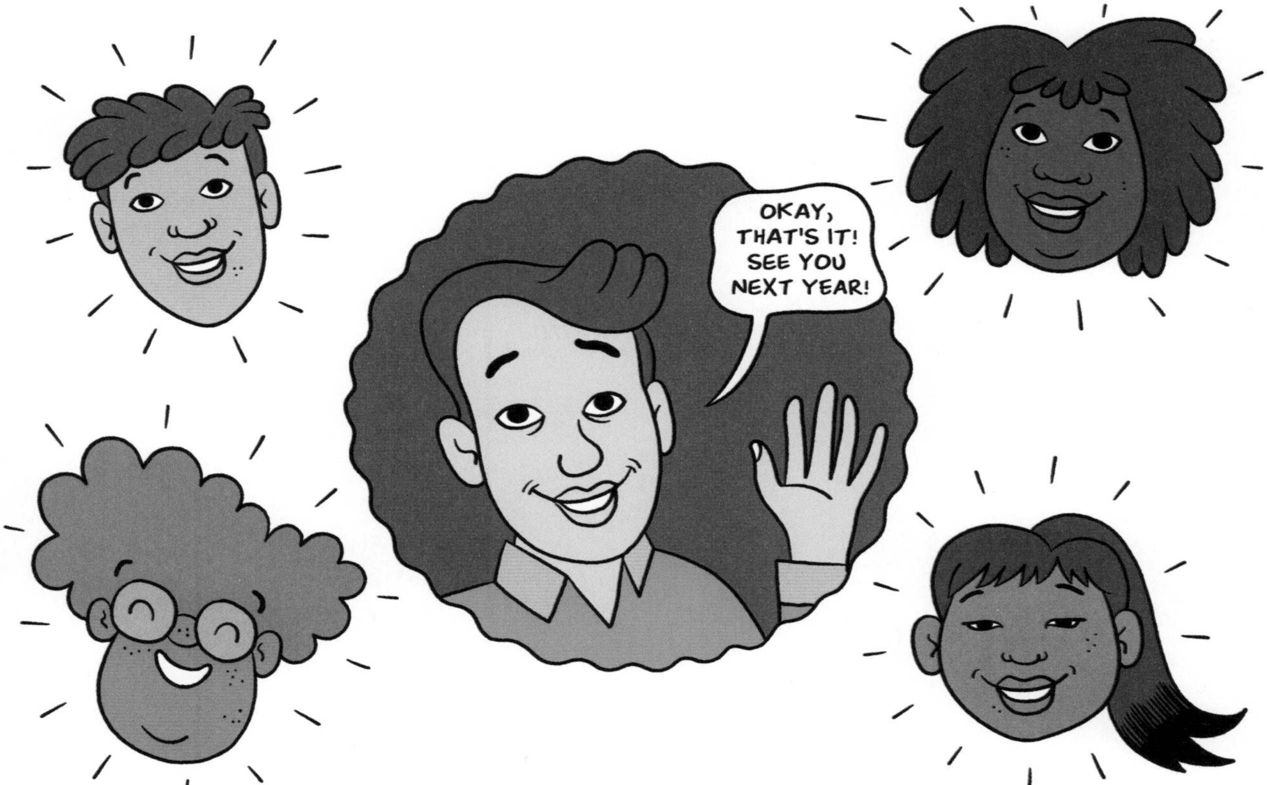
OKAY, THAT'S IT! SEE YOU NEXT YEAR!

GLOSSARY

THE MEANING OF A WORD CAN CHANGE DEPENDING ON WHERE AND WHEN IT'S USED. ONE WAY THAT PEOPLE TRY TO USE POWER OVER OTHERS IS BY CLAIMING THAT *THEIR* DEFINITION OF A WORD IS THE ONLY CORRECT DEFINITION. YOUNG PEOPLE HAVE OFTEN RESPONDED BY USING THEIR POWER WITH EACH OTHER TO EXPAND THE POSSIBILITIES OF WHAT WORDS MEAN, MAKING MORE ROOM IN A WORD FOR PEOPLE TO FIND THEMSELVES, AND WHEN THEY CAN'T, MAKING NEW WORDS.

THE DEFINITIONS THAT FOLLOW ARE NOT PERFECT OR THE BEST. THEY ARE A PLACE TO START.

ABLEISM IS DISCRIMINATION BASED ON THE BELIEF THAT THERE IS ONE RIGHT WAY TO HAVE A BODY/MIND. ABLEISM INCLUDES THINGS WE DO, WAYS WE THINK ABOUT OURSELVES AND OTHERS, POLICIES, AND SYSTEMS THAT PEOPLE ENGAGE IN THAT DEHUMANIZE AND ISOLATE PEOPLE CONSIDERED DISABLED—WHETHER THEY THINK ABOUT THEMSELVES AS DISABLED OR NOT. ABLEISM IS CONNECTED TO OTHER KINDS OF DISCRIMINATION INCLUDING RACISM, SEXISM, CLASSISM, AND MORE. BECAUSE ABLEISM FOCUSES ON BODIES, AND INCLUDES RULES ABOUT WHAT MAKES A "NORMAL" OR WORTHY BODY, ABLEISM IS SOMETHING THAT HURTS EVERYONE WHO HAS A BODY (WHICH IS TO SAY, ANYONE WHO IS ALIVE).

ADOPTING/ADOPTION IS ONE WAY A BABY OR CHILD BECOMES PART OF A FAMILY. WHEN IT'S USED LEGALLY, ADOPTING REFERS TO AN ADULT BECOMING THE LEGAL GUARDIAN OF A CHILD. LEGAL ADOPTION IS A PROCESS CONTROLLED BY GOVERNMENTS, AND WHEN IT HAPPENS IT MEANS THAT THE ADULT HAS ALL THE RIGHTS AND RESPONSIBILITIES OF A BIRTH PARENT. SOME PEOPLE USE THIS TERM TO DESCRIBE BECOMING A PARENT EVEN IF THERE ISN'T A LEGAL ADOPTION.

AMENORRHEA IS A MEDICAL TERM THAT DESCRIBES WHEN SOMEONE WITH OVARIES AND A UTERUS, WHO HAS STARTED MENSTRUATING, MISSES AT LEAST THREE PERIODS IN A ROW. AMENORRHEA OCCURS DURING PREGNANCY, BUT CAN HAPPEN BECAUSE OF MEDICATIONS, CHANGES IN HORMONES, AND MORE. READ MORE ABOUT MENSTRUATION ON P. 172.

AROUSAL—WHAT WE CALL "SEXY FEELINGS" IN THIS BOOK—MEANS FEELING SEXUALLY EXCITED. AROUSAL IS SOMETHING WE CAN FEEL, AND IS ALSO SOMETHING WE CAN OBSERVE IN AND ON A BODY (BLUSHING, SWEATING, HEAVY BREATHING, ERECTIONS, AND MORE). READ MORE ON P. 194.

BIPOC IS AN ACRONYM THAT STANDS FOR BLACK, INDIGENOUS, AND PEOPLE OF COLOR.

BLACK GIRL MAGIC ON PAGE 19 ZAI HAS A POSTER THAT SAYS "BLACK GIRL MAGIC." THE PHRASE "BLACK GIRLS ARE MAGIC" WAS COINED BY CASHAWN THOMPSON, AN EARLY CHILDCARE DEVELOPMENT EXPERT AND TRAINED DOULA WHO IS A THIRD GENERATION RESIDENT OF WASHINGTON, D.C. ABOUT THE PHRASE, CASHAWN HAS SAID:

"WHEN I SAY BLACK GIRLS ARE MAGIC, I AM TALKING ABOUT THE BLACK GIRL WITH DISABILITIES, I AM TALKING ABOUT THE LESBIAN BLACK WOMAN, I AM TALKING THE TRANS BLACK WOMAN, I AM DEFINITELY TALKING THE

POOR BLACK WOMEN AND GIRLS. NOBODY GETS LEFT BEHIND. BECAUSE WHO ARE WE WITHOUT ALL OF US?"

LEARN MORE ABOUT CASHAWN AT HTTP://CASHAWN.COM

CISGENDER IS A TERM USED TO DESCRIBE PEOPLE WHOSE GENDER IDENTITY FITS WITH THEIR SEX ASSIGNMENT AT BIRTH. IT CAN BE HELPFUL AS A WAY OF POINTING OUT HOW MOST PEOPLE ASSUME THAT OUR GENDER MATCHES OUR SEX ASSIGNED AT BIRTH. BUT CISGENDER HAS ITS OWN PROBLEMS. CISGENDER RELIES ON A BINARY, WHICH MEANS THAT THERE ARE ONLY TWO OPTIONS: EITHER YOUR GENDER MATCHES YOUR SEX ASSIGNMENT OR IT DOESN'T. AS WELL, SOME PEOPLE WHO HAVE BEEN LABELED AND/ OR IDENTIFY AS INTERSEX HAVE POINTED OUT THAT IT ERASES THE VIOLENCE THEY EXPERIENCED. OTHERS POINT OUT THAT FITTING OR NOT FITTING INTO YOUR SEX OR GENDER ASSIGNED AT BIRTH IS MORE COMPLICATED THAN A BINARY ALLOWS. READ MORE ABOUT GENDER IDENTITIES ON P. 114.

COERCION IS ANOTHER WORD TO DESCRIBE FORCING SOMEONE TO DO SOMETHING. COERCION CAN HAPPEN THROUGH PHYSICAL FORCE, OR THROUGH EMOTIONAL AND MENTAL PRESSURE AND MANIPULATION. READ MORE ON P. 377.

COLONIZATION IS A TERM THAT DESCRIBES THE ONGOING PROCESS DURING WHICH ONE GROUP OF PEOPLE TAKES CONTROL OF ANOTHER GROUP OF PEOPLE. COLONIZATION INCLUDES THE THEFT AND CONTROL OF LAND, BODIES, AND/OR PERSONAL PROPERTY AS WELL AS THE THEFT OF IDEAS, ART, AND CULTURE. COLONIZATION IS SOMETHING THAT HAPPENED AND IS HAPPENING AROUND THE WORLD. IT LOOKS AND WORKS DIFFERENTLY IN DIFFERENT PLACES. IN NORTH AMERICA, COLONIZATION IS DEEPLY TIED TO WHITE SUPREMACY.

CRIMINALIZATION IS WHEN A PERSON IS TURNED INTO A CRIMINAL BY MAKING THE THINGS THEY DO (OFTEN THINGS THEY NEED TO DO TO SURVIVE) ILLEGAL. FOR EXAMPLE, LAWS THAT MAKE IT ILLEGAL TO SLEEP OUTSIDE ON PUBLIC PROPERTY CRIMINALIZE THOSE OF US WITH NO SAFE PLACE TO LIVE. CRIMINALIZATION DOESN'T ONLY TARGET WHAT PEOPLE DO, IT TARGETS GROUPS OF PEOPLE AS A WAY OF CONTROLLING THEM AND REDUCING THEIR OPTIONS AND OPPORTUNITIES. YOU CAN FIND AN EXAMPLE OF CRIMINALIZATION ON P. 77.

DEAF GAIN IS A TERM DEVELOPED BY DEAF COMMUNITIES TO REFRAME THE IDEA THAT NOT BEING ABLE TO HEAR IS ONLY A LOSS. INSTEAD OF "HEARING LOSS"— WHICH FOCUSES ON WHAT SOMEONE IS MISSING—DEAF GAIN HIGHLIGHTS THE BEAUTY, JOY, AND MANY BENEFITS THAT COME WITH NOT HEARING THROUGH YOUR EARS.

DEPRESSION IS A WORD PEOPLE USE TO DESCRIBE WHEN THEY FEEL DOWN, SAD, HOPELESS, AND MORE. IT'S ALSO A WORD THAT MENTAL HEALTH PROFESSIONALS USE AS A DIAGNOSIS, OR LABEL. LIKE ALL LABELS, IT MAY BE HELPFUL, BECAUSE IT MAKES IT EASIER FOR US TO ACCESS COUNSELING, THERAPY, AND OTHER KINDS OF HELP. AND IT MAY BE HARMFUL WHEN IT IS USED TO MAKE US FEEL AS IF WE HAVE FEWER OPTIONS OR IS USED TO EXCLUDE US FROM PARTICIPATING IN LIFE. FIND MENTAL HEALTH RESOURCES ON P. 428.

DESIRE IS AN EXPERIENCE OF DEEP WANTING. WHEN WE SAY WE DESIRE SOMETHING IT USUALLY MEANS IT'S SOMETHING WE FEEL A SIGNIFICANT WANT FOR. WE EXPERIENCE DESIRE IN OUR BODY AND MIND, BUT WE ALL EXPERIENCE IT DIFFERENTLY. WE MAY DESIRE SOMETHING AND CHOOSE NOT TO PURSUE THAT THING, AND WE MAY DESIRE SOMETHING AND GET THE THING WE WANT, THEN FIND THAT IT ISN'T WHAT WE THOUGHT IT WOULD BE.

DOUCHE OR **DOUCHING** REFERS TO INSERTING WATER, AND SOMETIMES OTHER CHEMICALS, INTO THE VAGINA OR ANUS. VAGINAL DOUCHES ARE MARKETED AS "CLEANING" THE VAGINA. BUT HEALTH PROFESSIONALS DO NOT RECOMMEND THEM BECAUSE THE VAGINA IS SELF-LUBRICATING AND SELF-CLEANING, AND SO DOUCHING CAN CREATE PROBLEMS WITH NO REAL BENEFIT. COMPANIES THAT MAKE DOUCHES MAKE PEOPLE FEEL EMBARRASSED OR ASHAMED OF THEIR BODIES IN ORDER TO SELL A PRODUCT.

DYSMENORRHEA IS A MEDICAL TERM THAT DESCRIBES THE VERY COMMON EXPERIENCE OF PAINFUL PERIODS AND MENSTRUAL CRAMPS. READ MORE ABOUT MENSTRUATION ON P. 172.

FEMME IS A QUEER GENDER IDENTITY, OR A PART OF SOME PEOPLE'S GENDER IDENTITY THAT HAS TO DO WITH QUEERING IDEAS AND EXPRESSIONS OF FEMININITY. THERE'S NO ONE WAY TO IDENTIFY AS FEMME, BUT ALL FEMMES ARE MAKING THE TRADITIONAL, HETERO-NORMATIVE UNDERSTANDING OF FEMININITY MORE COMPLICATED (AND COOL). SEARCH FOR FEMMES WRITING ABOUT FEMMES. CHECK OUT AUTOSTRADDLE'S "WHAT WE MEAN WHEN WE SAY 'FEMME': A ROUNDTABLE." READ MORE ABOUT GENDER IDENTITIES ON P. 114.

FOSTERING / FOSTER FAMILY
DESCRIBES WHEN A CHILD IS
LIVING WITH AND LOOKED
AFTER BY A FAMILY THAT IS NOT
CONSIDERED THEIR PERMANENT
FAMILY. SOME FAMILIES CHOOSE
TO FOSTER SO THAT THEY CAN
EVENTUALLY ADOPT AND BRING
THE CHILD INTO THEIR FAMILY
FOREVER. SOME FAMILIES
ACT AS TEMPORARY FOSTER
HOMES AND DO NOT HAVE
THE INTENTION OF BECOMING
PARENTS TO THE CHILDREN OVER
THE COURSE OF THEIR LIVES.

GENOCIDE DESCRIBES THE
INTENTIONAL KILLING OF A
LARGE GROUP OF PEOPLE,
BASED ON THEIR ETHNICITY,
RELIGION, POLITICAL
AFFILIATION, OR WHERE THEY
ARE LIVING. THE INTENTION
OF GENOCIDE IS TO ERASE AN
ENTIRE GROUP OF PEOPLE
FROM THE PLANET.

HETERONORMATIVE DESCRIBES
THE WAY PEOPLE WHO
ARE HETEROSEXUAL (OR
STRAIGHT) ARE ASSUMED TO
BE NORMAL, AND EVERYONE
ELSE IS TREATED AS OUTSIDE
THAT NORM. IT DESCRIBES
THE WAY THE WORLD IS SET
UP TO BE EASIER TO MOVE
THROUGH FOR PEOPLE WHO
IDENTIFY THEMSELVES AS, OR
PRESENT THEMSELVES TO
BE, HETEROSEXUAL. BECAUSE
HETERONORMATIVITY
REQUIRES STRAIGHT PEOPLE
TO CONFORM TO CERTAIN
ROLES AND STANDARDS, IT
DOESN'T ONLY HARM GAY AND
QUEER PEOPLE, IT HARMS
STRAIGHT PEOPLE TOO.

HIV, WHICH IS SHORT FOR
HUMAN IMMUNODEFICIENCY
VIRUS, IS NOT THE MOST
COMMON SEXUALLY
TRANSMITTED INFECTION,
BUT IT'S ONE WE HEAR
ABOUT A LOT. WHEN IT
FIRST APPEARED, A LOT OF
PEOPLE DIED FROM DISEASES
RELATED TO HIV. IF LEFT
UNTREATED, HIV LEADS TO AIDS
(ACQUIRED IMMUNODEFICIENCY
SYNDROME), WHICH LEAVES
OUR BODIES OPEN TO DISEASES
IT CANNOT FIGHT. BUT TODAY,
IF SOMEONE HAS ACCESS TO
TREATMENT, THAT DOESN'T
HAPPEN. BECAUSE WE DON'T
ALL HAVE EQUAL ACCESS TO
TREATMENT, HIV CAN ALSO
BE A LOT MORE THAN AN
INCONVENIENCE. IN SOME WAYS,
HIV IS ABOUT MORE THAN A
VIRUS. BECAUSE PEOPLE LIVE
THEIR WHOLE LIVES WITH
HIV, THEY MAKE FAMILY AND
COMMUNITY, ART AND CULTURE,
ALL AROUND HIV. PEOPLE WITH
HIV STILL GET DISCRIMINATED
AGAINST BY INDIVIDUALS AND
SYSTEMS LIKE SCHOOLS AND
GOVERNMENTS, SO WE NEED
TO TALK ABOUT THAT TOO.
WORKING FOR JUSTICE MEANS
WORKING TO REDUCE STIGMA
ABOUT HIV. READ MORE ABOUT
HIV AND STIGMA ON P. 243.

HOMOPHOBIA IS A TERM
USED TO DESCRIBE NEGATIVE,
HATEFUL, AND SOMETIMES
VIOLENT BELIEFS AND ACTIONS
DIRECTED TOWARD GAYS
AND LESBIANS. WHILE IT IS
WIDELY USED, THE WORD
"PHOBIA" HAS BEEN CRITICIZED
BY PEOPLE WHO EXPERIENCE
PHOBIAS, WHICH ARE REAL AND
DEBILITATING IRRATIONAL
FEARS OF EVERYTHING FROM
SNAKES TO BIG OPEN SPACES.
FOR THAT REASON, WE CHOSE
NOT TO USE THE TERM IN
THIS BOOK, AND INSTEAD
JUST DESCRIBE WHAT IT IS:
PREJUDICE, VIOLENCE, AND
OPPRESSION BASED ON SEXUAL
ORIENTATION. READ MORE
ABOUT SEXUAL ORIENTATION
ON P. 198.

HPV, WHICH IS SHORT FOR
HUMAN PAPILLOMAVIRUS, IS
ONE OF THE MOST COMMON
SEXUALLY TRANSMITTED
INFECTIONS (STIS). YOU MAY
HAVE HEARD OF IT BECAUSE
THERE'S A VACCINE FOR YOUNG
PEOPLE THAT REDUCES THE
CHANCES OF GETTING SOME
KINDS OF HPV. NOT EVERYONE
GETS THE VACCINE. IT'S A
CHOICE THAT YOUR PARENTS
USUALLY MAKE FOR YOU. IF YOU
ARE LOOKING FOR RELIABLE
INFORMATION ABOUT HPV AND
OTHER STIS, CHECK OUT THE
RESOURCE SECTION ON P. 410.

INDIGENOUS IS A TERM
THAT IS USED BY PEOPLE
WHOSE ANCESTORS WERE THE
FIRST PEOPLES TO LIVE ON
PARTICULAR LANDS. THE TERM
ACKNOWLEDGES THAT THEIR
WAYS OF BEING ARE VALUABLE
AND ARE NOT THE SAME AS
THE SETTLER OR COLONIAL
SOCIETIES THAT OCCUPY THEIR
LAND. INDIGENOUS PEOPLE
IDENTIFY THEMSELVES AS
BELONGING TO A SPECIFIC
PEOPLE, SO IT'S BEST TO LEARN
THE SPECIFIC COMMUNITY A
PERSON IDENTIFIES AS BEING
PART OF.

LATINX IS A GOOD EXAMPLE
OF HOW LANGUAGE CHANGES.
IT'S A RELATIVELY NEW TERM
USED BY SOME PEOPLE WHO
TRACE THEIR ANCESTRY TO THE
PART OF THE WORLD CALLED
CENTRAL AND SOUTH AMERICA.
IT IS A GENDER-INCLUSIVE
EXPANSION OF THE TERMS
LATINA AND LATINO, WHICH
ARE STILL MORE COMMON.
LATINX IS PREFERRED BY SOME
AS IT INCLUDES PEOPLE OF
ALL GENDERS. BUT OTHERS,
INCLUDING FOLKS WHO ARE
GENDER EXPANSIVE, DON'T USE
IT AND FIND OTHER WAYS OF
NAMING THEMSELVES.

MISOGYNY DESCRIBES HATRED
AND PREJUDICE DIRECTED
TOWARD GIRLS AND WOMEN.
IT IS A MORE VIOLENT
EXPRESSION OF SEXISM, WHICH
IS DISCRIMINATION BASED
ON GENDER. ACTING IN A WAY
THAT DISCRIMINATES AGAINST
WOMEN—LIKE EXCLUDING THEM
FROM A GROUP ACTIVITY
BECAUSE THEY ARE WOMEN—IS
SEXISM. SPEAKING OR ACTING
WITH ANGER AND VIOLENCE
TOWARD GIRLS AND WOMEN—
SNAPPING BRA STRAPS,
THREATENING TO BEAT UP A
GIRL BECAUSE YOU DISAGREE
WITH SOMETHING SHE SAID OR
DID—IS MISOGYNY. MISOGYNY,
LIKE SEXISM, ISN'T JUST IN THE
THINGS WE SAY AND DO, IT CAN
BE FOUND IN THE WAY SCHOOLS,
GOVERNMENTS, AND THE MEDIA
ARE ORGANIZED AND RUN.

MISOGYNOIR IS A WORD THAT WAS FIRST USED BY QUEER BLACK FEMINIST MOYA BAILEY TO DESCRIBE THE WAY THAT RACISM AND MISOGYNY INTERACT TO HARM BLACK WOMEN IN WAYS THAT ARE DIFFERENT THAN THE EXPERIENCES OF RACISM OR MISOGYNY ALONE. MISOGYNOIR IS AN IMPORTANT WORD BECAUSE IT DESCRIBES VERY REAL HARM THAT WAS MADE INVISIBLE FOR A LONG TIME.

ORGY IS A TERM USED TO DESCRIBE A GROUP OF PEOPLE HAVING SEX IN THE SAME PLACE AT THE SAME TIME. ORGIES DO HAPPEN, BUT PROBABLY NOT AS MUCH AS PEOPLE TALK ABOUT THEM HAPPENING. YOU MAY COME ACROSS THIS WORD IN POP-UP ADVERTISING AND FREE PORN.

RACISM IS A WORD THAT PEOPLE USE IN DIFFERENT WAYS. A LOT OF PEOPLE THINK RACISM IS SAYING THE "N WORD" OR BEING MEAN TO BLACK OR BROWN PEOPLE. THOSE MAY BE EXAMPLES OF RACISM, BUT RACISM IS MORE THAN ONLY ATTITUDES OR BELIEFS. RACISM IS A MISUSE OF POWER, BY INDIVIDUALS, GOVERNMENTS, AND SOCIETIES, THAT IS GROUNDED IN AND GUIDED BY WHITE SUPREMACY. RACISM DESCRIBES THE WAY PEOPLE WITH DARKER SKIN ARE DENIED ACCESS TO BASIC THINGS LIKE GETTING A JOB, FINDING A PLACE TO LIVE, BEING ABLE TO FIND AND AFFORD FOOD, GETTING MEDICAL CARE, AND BEING SAFE IN THEIR HOME AND ON THE STREETS BASED SOLELY ON RACE. PEOPLE USE DIFFERENT TERMS FOR RACISM TO POINT OUT ALL THE WAYS IT SHOWS UP IN OUR LIVES AND OUR WORLD, INCLUDING INSTITUTIONAL RACISM, SYSTEMIC RACISM, INTERNALIZED RACISM, AND MORE. WHAT RACISM LOOKS LIKE AND HOW IT WORKS IS DIFFERENT FROM ONE COUNTRY TO ANOTHER.

RAPE IS A TERM PEOPLE USE FOR SEXUAL ASSAULT THAT INVOLVED PENETRATION. READ MORE ABOUT SEXUAL ASSAULT ON P. 384.

SEX CHARACTERISTICS ARE PHYSICAL TRAITS THAT DOCTORS AND RESEARCHERS USE TO CATEGORIZE BODIES AS EITHER MALE OR FEMALE. THEY DISTINGUISH BETWEEN PRIMARY SEX CHARACTERISTICS (INCLUDING THE GONADS AND THE GENITALS) AND SECONDARY SEX CHARACTERISTICS THAT DEVELOP AS WE GROW (INCLUDING THINGS LIKE GROWTH OF BODY HAIR, DEVELOPMENT OF BREASTS, LOWERING OF VOICE, AND MORE). BECAUSE HUMAN BODIES DON'T ACTUALLY FIT WELL INTO A BINARY MODEL, SEX CHARACTERISTICS DO NOT ALWAYS ALL MATCH. WE MAY HAVE GONADS, GENITALS, AND SECONDARY SEX CHARACTERISTICS THAT ARE A BLEND OF WHAT IS TYPICALLY THOUGHT OF AS MALE OR FEMALE. THE TERM VARIATION OF SEX CHARACTERISTICS (VSC) DESCRIBES THIS REALITY. EVEN THOUGH OUR BODIES HAVE ALWAYS BEEN DIVERSE AND BEAUTIFUL, THE TERM VSC IS RELATIVELY NEW.

SEX TOYS ARE TOYS THAT MAY BE USED AS PART OF SEX. THEY ARE CALLED TOYS BECAUSE THEY HELP ADULTS EXPLORE USING THEIR IMAGINATIONS AND CREATE SENSORY EXPERIENCES THAT CAN BE FUN. RULES DIFFER FROM COUNTRY TO COUNTRY ABOUT HOW OLD YOU HAVE TO BE BEFORE YOU CAN BUY A SEX TOY, BUT LIKE PORNOGRAPHY, THEY ARE MADE WITH ADULTS AS THEIR INTENDED AUDIENCE.

SEXUALITY IS A WORD THAT INCLUDES ALL THE ASPECTS OF SEX DESCRIBED IN THIS BOOK, AND MORE. OUR SEXUALITY INCLUDES OUR IDENTITIES AND ORIENTATIONS, THE ACTIVITIES WE CHOOSE TO ENGAGE IN AND THE ONES WE CHOOSE NOT TO ENGAGE IN, OUR SEXUAL FEELINGS AND THOUGHTS, AND ALL THE WAYS WE ARE IMPACTED BY SEXUAL MESSAGES IN THE WORLD AROUND US.

SEXUALIZATION IS A WORD THAT DESCRIBES WHEN WE ARE TREATED AS IF OUR VALUE IS ONLY CONNECTED TO BEING A SEXUAL OBJECT, HAVING A BODY THAT OTHER PEOPLE FIND SEXUALLY ATTRACTIVE. SEXUALIZATION HAPPENS THROUGH WORDS AND ACTIONS. WE ARE NOT ALL SEXUALIZED IN THE SAME WAY OR THE SAME AMOUNT, AND THIS FORM OF OPPRESSION AND DISCRIMINATION CONNECTS WITH OTHERS INCLUDING RACISM, ABLEISM, SEXISM, CLASSISM, AND MORE.

SEX WORK IS A TERM USED TO DESCRIBE ANY KIND OF WORK THAT INVOLVES PROVIDING SEXUAL SERVICES IN EXCHANGE FOR COMPENSATION—USUALLY MONEY. SEX WORK MIGHT INCLUDE NUDE DANCING, GIVING EROTIC MASSAGES, OR HAVING ANY KIND OF SEX WITH SOMEONE WHERE THE PRIMARY MOTIVATION IS COMPENSATION. SEX WORK HAS HAPPENED FOR AS LONG AS HUMANS HAVE RECORDED HISTORY, BUT THE TERM IS CREDITED TO SEX WORKER AND ACTIVIST CAROL LEIGH, WHO WANTED TO EMPHASIZE THE FACT THAT FOR SEX WORKERS, IT IS PRIMARILY A JOB.

SLAVERY IS A WORD THAT DESCRIBES THE SYSTEM OF FORCING PEOPLE TO DO LABOR AND HOLDING THEM AGAINST THEIR WILL. PEOPLE WHO ARE ENSLAVED ARE DENIED BASIC RIGHTS AND FREEDOMS AND ARE USUALLY CONSIDERED PROPERTY, NOT HUMAN BEINGS. SLAVERY HAS EXISTED ALL OVER THE WORLD, AND CONTINUES TO EXIST IN MANY PARTS OF THE WORLD TODAY. THE LEGACY OF SLAVERY —AND ITS CURRENT WORKINGS—LOOK AND FEEL DIFFERENT IN EACH COUNTRY.

STERILIZATION IS A FORM OF PERMANENT BIRTH CONTROL THAT PREVENTS SOMEONE FROM BEING ABLE TO MAKE A BABY. THERE ARE DIFFERENT METHODS FOR STERILIZING SOMEONE WITH A PENIS AND SCROTUM AND SOMEONE WITH OVARIES AND A UTERUS. STERILIZATION DOES NOT PROVIDE PROTECTION FROM STIS. WHILE IT SHOULD BE AN AVAILABLE OPTION THAT PEOPLE CAN CHOOSE, HISTORICALLY STERILIZATION HAS BEEN USED WITHOUT CONSENT, AS A FORM OF EUGENICS, TARGETING INDIGENOUS PEOPLE, PEOPLE OF COLOR, DISABLED PEOPLE, AND PEOPLE WITH LESS MONEY. READ MORE ABOUT BIRTH CONTROL ON P. 326.

TOXIC SHOCK SYNDROME (TSS) IS A VERY RARE BUT LIFE-THREATENING COMPLICATION OF CERTAIN KINDS OF INFECTIONS. EVEN THOUGH IT'S RARE, IT IS STILL MENTIONED IN SEX EDUCATION MATERIALS ABOUT WEARING TAMPONS, MENSTRUAL CUPS, AND SOME KINDS OF CONTRACEPTION (INCLUDING THE SPONGE AND DIAPHRAGMS). IF YOU USE TAMPONS, YOU MAY HAVE READ INSTRUCTIONS THAT SAY TO USE THE LOWEST ABSORBENCY YOU NEED, AND TO CHANGE YOUR TAMPON EVERY 4 TO 8 HOURS (SOME PLACES SAY DIFFERENT TIMES). THE REASON FOR THIS IS THAT KEEPING A TAMPON IN FOR EXTENDED PERIODS CAN INCREASE THE RISK OF TSS. READ MORE ABOUT MENSTRUATION ON P. 172.

TRANSITIONING IS A WORD SOME PEOPLE USE TO DESCRIBE THEIR PROCESS OF CHANGING SOME OR ALL ASPECTS OF THEIR GENDER AND/OR SEX IDENTITY. JUST LIKE THERE ISN'T ONE WAY TO EXPRESS YOUR GENDER, THERE ISN'T ONE WAY TO TRANSITION. THE TERM "SOCIAL TRANSITION" REFERS TO CHANGING THINGS LIKE NAME, PRONOUNS, AND HOW SOMEONE PRESENTS THEMSELVES IN PUBLIC. THE TERM "MEDICAL TRANSITION" MAY INCLUDE TAKING HORMONES TO PAUSE CHANGES THAT HAPPEN DURING PUBERTY OR TO CHANGE THE SHAPE AND FEEL OF ONE'S BODY, AND IT MAY ALSO INCLUDE SURGERY. THERE ARE MANY DIFFERENT WAYS TO TRANSITION, AND IT CAN TAKE PLACE OVER ANY LENGTH OF TIME. TRANSITIONING CAN BE A USEFUL WORD FOR THINKING ABOUT HOW YOU WANT TO BE SEEN—AND HOW TO HAVE PEOPLE INTERACT WITH AND TALK TO YOU IN WAYS THAT FEEL MORE LIKE THEY SEE YOU AS YOU WANT TO BE SEEN. READ MORE ABOUT GENDER ON P. 101.

TRANSMISOGYNY IS A TERM THAT DESCRIBES THE WAYS THAT TRANSPHOBIA AND MISOGYNY CONNECT AND COMBINE TO PRODUCE A PARTICULAR KIND OF HATE, VIOLENCE, AND DISCRIMINATION AGAINST TRANS WOMEN AND ANYONE WHO IS TRANS AND AT ALL FEMININE PRESENTING. IT WAS COINED BY TRANS WRITER AND ACTIVIST JULIA SERANO IN HER BOOK *WHIPPING GIRL*.

TRANSPHOBIA IS A TERM USED TO DESCRIBE NEGATIVE, HATEFUL, AND SOMETIMES VIOLENT BELIEFS AND ACTIONS DIRECTED TOWARD TRANSGENDER PEOPLE. WHILE IT IS WIDELY USED, THE WORD "PHOBIA" HAS BEEN CRITICIZED BY PEOPLE WHO EXPERIENCE PHOBIAS, WHICH ARE REAL AND DEBILITATING IRRATIONAL FEARS OF EVERYTHING FROM SNAKES TO BIG OPEN SPACES. FOR THAT REASON, WE CHOSE NOT TO USE THE TERM IN THIS BOOK, AND INSTEAD JUST DESCRIBE WHAT IT IS: PREJUDICE, VIOLENCE, AND OPPRESSION BASED ON A FEAR AND HATRED OF TRANS PEOPLE AND TRANS BODIES.

WHITE SUPREMACY DESCRIBES THE SYSTEM THAT IS FOUNDATIONAL IN MANY PARTS OF THE WORLD THAT GIVES WHITE PEOPLE AND WHITENESS POWER AND BENEFITS OVER PEOPLE WHO ARE NOT DEFINED AS WHITE. EDUCATOR AND WRITER HILARY NORTH-ELLASANTE DESCRIBES WHITE SUPREMACY THIS WAY:

"AN IDEOLOGY, OR SET OF IDEAS THAT CONSIDERS PEOPLE WITH A 'WHITE' RACIAL IDENTITY, OFTEN LIGHTER-SKINNED PEOPLE OF EUROPEAN DESCENT, AS SUPERIOR TO DARKER-SKINNED 'PEOPLE OF COLOR,' WHO ARE INDIGENOUS, OF AFRICAN, ASIAN, AND/OR LATINX DESCENT. SYSTEMS ROOTED IN WHITE SUPREMACY ARE ORGANIZED SO THAT LAWS, JOBS, AND OPPORTUNITIES BENEFIT WHITE PEOPLE AND DISADVANTAGE PEOPLE OF COLOR. THE UNITED STATES IS ONE EXAMPLE OF A COUNTRY THAT WAS ESTABLISHED TO BENEFIT WHITE PEOPLE, AND WHITE SUPREMACY HAS PLAYED AN IMPORTANT ROLE IN THE CREATION OF ALL LAWS AND SYSTEMS IN THE U.S."

INDEX

RESOURCES

SUPPORT LINES

IF YOU'RE FEELING STUCK AND DON'T HAVE SOMEONE TO TALK TO, THERE ARE LOTS OF PLACES WHERE YOU CAN TEXT OR CALL TO COMMUNICATE WITH SOMEONE ANONYMOUSLY ABOUT WHAT'S GOING ON. EVEN THOUGH THEY ARE SOMETIMES CALLED "CRISIS" LINES, YOU MAY CONTACT THESE LINES IF YOU AREN'T SURE WHAT TO DO NEXT.

IF YOU CALL OR TEXT A SUPPORT LINE AND HAVE A BAD EXPERIENCE, YOU CAN TRY AGAIN. THE PEOPLE WHO WORK ON SUPPORT LINES ARE TRAINED, BUT THEY ARE STILL PEOPLE, AFTER ALL, AND YOU MAY NOT CONNECT WELL TO THE FIRST PERSON YOU TEXT OR TALK WITH.

MOST OF THESE SERVICES ARE AVAILABLE 24 HOURS A DAY, 7 DAYS A WEEK.

LOVE IS RESPECT
DATING AND RELATIONSHIP SUPPORT: TEXT **LOVEIS** TO 22522, OR PHONE 1-866-331-9474

KIDS HELP PHONE
(CANADA) TEXT **CONNECT** TO 686868, OR PHONE 1-800-668-6868 (FRENCH/ENGLISH)

CRISIS TEXT LINE
TEXT **HOME** TO 741741

THE TREVOR PROJECT (LGBTQ)
TEXT **START** TO 678-678, OR PHONE 1-866-488-7386

STRONGHEARTS NATIVE HELPLINE
CHAT THROUGH STRONGHEARTSHELPLINE.ORG, OR PHONE 1-844-762-8483

TRANS LIFELINE
PHONE 877-330-6366 (CANADA), OR 877-565-8860 (US; SPANISH/ENGLISH)

NATIONAL SUICIDE PREVENTION LIFELINE
(US) PHONE 1-800-273-8255 (SPANISH, ENGLISH, WITH CHAT AND TEXT SERVICES FOR DEAF/HARD OF HEARING)

CANADA SUICIDE PREVENTION SERVICE
TEXT 45645, OR PHONE 1-833-456-4566 (ENGLISH), OR 1-866-277-3553 (FRENCH)

TIPS FOR LEARNING MORE

WE ALL LEARN DIFFERENTLY. SOME OF US LEARN BEST THROUGH READING AND RESEARCH, SOME OF US LEARN BEST IN CONVERSATION WITH OTHERS. LEARNING FROM PEOPLE WHO SHARE PARTS OF OUR EXPERIENCE OR IDENTITIES CAN FEEL DIFFERENT THAN LEARNING FROM PEOPLE WHO HAVE VERY DIFFERENT BACKGROUNDS AND EXPERIENCES FROM US.

THERE IS SO MUCH KNOWLEDGE AND EXPERIENCE ONLINE, AND IN BOOKS, VIDEOS, PODCASTS, AND MORE, THAT WE DON'T THINK WE CAN TELL YOU WHAT THE BEST RESOURCE IS FOR YOU. SO INSTEAD OF SHARING A LONG LIST OF SPECIFIC RESOURCES, WE'LL SHARE SOME PLACES TO START A SEARCH FOR MORE INFORMATION.

WE ALL DESERVE SUPPORT AND INFORMATION THAT SPEAKS TO OUR LIVES. WE SHOULDN'T HAVE TO IGNORE PARTS OF WHO WE ARE, OR PRETEND WE'RE SOMEONE WE'RE NOT, IN ORDER TO GET HELP. A GOOD STARTING PLACE FOR INFORMATION CAN BE TO ASK SOMEONE WHO YOU HAVE THINGS IN COMMON WITH.

WHEN SEARCHING ONLINE, REMEMBER THAT YOU CAN ADD IDENTITY TERMS TO YOUR SEARCH WORDS. FOR EXAMPLE, IF YOU WANT TO KNOW MORE ABOUT HAIR AND PUBERTY, YOU CAN SEARCH FOR THOSE TERMS, BUT YOU COULD ALSO ADD "QUEER," "JEWISH," "BLACK," OR OTHER WORDS THAT CONNECT TO WHO YOU ARE. IT WON'T ALWAYS WORK, BUT IT MAY LEAD YOU TO INFORMATION THAT FEELS MORE LIKE PARTS OF YOU.

NO RESOURCE (BOOK, WEBSITE, INSTAGRAM FEED) CAN PROVIDE ALL THE ANSWERS OR CONNECT TO EVERY PART OF WHO WE ARE. AND ALL RESOURCES LEAVE SOME OF US OUT. A RESOURCE MAY CONNECT TO SOME PARTS OF YOU BUT IGNORE OR HARM OTHER PARTS. IT DEPENDS A LOT ON WHO PEOPLE ARE PAYING ATTENTION TO AND LEARNING FROM. FOR EXAMPLE, THERE'S A GREAT VIDEO ON YOUTUBE CALLED "SELF-CARE IN MIDDLE SCHOOL" (SERIOUSLY, YOU SHOULD CHECK IT OUT). BUT AFTER WATCHING IT, WE NOTICED THAT THE ORGANIZATION THAT CREATED IT SUPPORTS "TREATMENTS" THAT MANY PEOPLE CALL ABLEIST AND HARMFUL.

WITH ANY RESOURCE— INCLUDING THE ONES BELOW— THERE ARE SOME QUESTIONS YOU CAN ASK YOURSELF:

★ WHOSE VOICE IS TELLING THE STORY?

★ WHO IS MISSING?

★ HOW WOULD OTHER PEOPLE THINK ABOUT THIS?

★ WHO IS BEING HELD UP HERE, AND WHO IS BEING IGNORED OR TALKED ABOUT POORLY?

★ WHAT ASSUMPTIONS ARE BEING MADE BY THE PEOPLE SHARING THE INFORMATION? WHAT ARE THEY ASSUMING ABOUT YOU, YOUR FRIENDS, AND YOUR COMMUNITY?

HERE ARE IDEAS ON WHERE TO SEARCH FOR MORE INFORMATION BASED ON TOPICS WE COVERED IN *YOU KNOW, SEX.*

ASL / DEAF LANGUAGE AND CULTURE

ON PAGE 115 ZAI MEETS (AND IMMEDIATELY CRUSHES OUT ON) LISA, A DEAF STUDENT WHO GOES TO THE SCHOOL WHERE ZAI'S MOM WORKS. YOU CAN LEARN MORE ABOUT DEAF ART, LANGUAGE, AND CULTURE FROM THE MANY YOUNG DEAF FOLKS SHARING, ESPECIALLY ON SOCIAL MEDIA. HERE ARE A FEW OTHER RESOURCES TO CHECK OUT:

★ DEAF QUEER RESOURCE CENTER IS AN ONLINE HUB.

★ GALLAUDET UNIVERSITY, A DEAF UNIVERSITY IN THE US, OFFERS FREE LESSONS FOR AMERICAN SIGN LANGUAGE.

★ SEARCH FOR, AND LEARN ABOUT, BLACK AMERICAN SIGN LANGUAGE (BASL).

BINDERS / BINDING

BINDERS SHOW UP ON SEVERAL PAGES IN THE BOOK. BINDERS ARE UNDERGARMENTS DESIGNED TO COMPRESS A PART OF THE BODY TO MAKE IT LOOK FLATTER AND SMOOTHER, OFTEN AS PART OF EXPLORING GENDER EXPRESSION OR GENDER TRANSITION. SAFETY WISE: DON'T USE DUCT TAPE, SARAN WRAP, OR ACE BANDAGES FOR BINDING. DON'T WEAR THEM OVERNIGHT, DO TAKE DAYS OFF FROM WEARING A BINDER, AND DO WEAR ONE THAT FITS WELL. CHECK OUT:

* DO A SEARCH FOR "SAFE CHEST BINDING."

* POINT OF PRIDE'S CHEST BINDER PROGRAM IS ONE OF MANY PROGRAMS WHERE PEOPLE CAN ACCESS LOW-COST/ FREE BINDERS.

BIRTH CONTROL

HAVING ACCESS TO SAFE AND RELATIVELY AFFORDABLE BIRTH CONTROL HAS CHANGED MANY PEOPLE'S LIVES FOR THE BETTER. BUT MANY BIRTH CONTROL METHODS WERE DEVELOPED AND TESTED ON WOMEN OF COLOR AND INDIGENOUS WOMEN IN WAYS THAT HARMED THEM AND THAT ARE RARELY TALKED ABOUT.

* LEARN ABOUT THE HISTORY OF BIRTH CONTROL BY SEARCHING FOR "REPRODUCTIVE JUSTICE TIMELINE."

* LEARN ABOUT DIFFERENT KINDS OF BIRTH CONTROL, HOW THEY WORK, AND HOW TO ACCESS THEM FROM THESE ORGANIZATIONS:

* PLANNEDPARENTHOOD.ORG (AVAILABLE IN ENGLISH / SPANISH)

* SCARLETEEN.COM

* SEXANDU.CA (AVAILABLE IN ENGLISH / FRENCH)

BODY ACCEPTANCE/ BODY LOVE

IN OUR BOOK YOU SEE ALL SORTS OF BODIES LOOKING BEAUTIFUL. WE LIVE IN A WORLD THAT TELLS US OTHERWISE, BUT THERE IS NO RIGHT OR WRONG WAY TO HAVE A BODY, AND ALL OUR BODIES HAVE BEAUTY IN THEM. THERE ARE PEOPLE AND MOVEMENTS THAT ARE RESISTING THE INCORRECT IDEA THAT WHAT'S BEAUTIFUL IS SKINNY, LIGHT SKINNED, ATHLETIC. CHECK OUT:

* SEARCH: "FAT ACCEPTANCE" / "FAT LIBERATION" / "#NOBODYISDISPOSIBLE"

* SONYA RENEE TAYLOR

DISABILITY / DISABILITY JUSTICE

DISABILITY IS MORE THAN A DESCRIPTION OF A BODY: FOR MANY PEOPLE IT'S AN IDENTITY, TIED TO A PROUD HISTORY AND CULTURE. CHECK OUT:

* AUTISTIC SELF ADVOCACY NETWORK

* AUTISTIC WOMEN & NON-BINARY NETWORK

* BLACK DISABLED ART HISTORY 101 BY LEROY MOORE

* THE HARRIET TUBMAN COLLECTIVE

* KRIP-HOP NATION

* YOUTUBE VIDEO SERIES: "SEX ED FOR PEOPLE WITH I/DD"

GENDER

IF YOU WANT TO FIND OUT MORE ABOUT GENDER IDENTITIES OR THE WAYS PEOPLE ARE EXPLORING AND SHIFTING THEIR GENDER (INCLUDING USING HORMONES) THERE ARE MANY SUPPORTIVE ORGANIZATIONS, AND YOU MAY BE ABLE TO FIND ONE CLOSE(ISH) TO WHERE YOU LIVE. SEARCHING TERMS LIKE "GENDER AFFIRMATIVE" OR "GENDER SUPPORTIVE"—PLUS OTHER TERMS THAT FIT FOR YOU—IS A GOOD PLACE TO START.

AS YOU SEEK INFORMATION, YOU MAY ALSO COME ACROSS INDIVIDUALS AND GROUPS THAT WANT TO DENY YOUNG PEOPLE'S BODY AUTONOMY AND

STOP THEM FROM EXPRESSING GENDER IN WAYS BEYOND THE BINARY. CHECK OUT:

* GENDERCREATIVEKIDS.CA (AVAILABLE IN FRENCH / ENGLISH)

* GENDERWHEEL.COM BY MAYA GONZALEZ

* OURTRANSTRUTH.ORG, YOUTH-LED STORYTELLING PROJECT

* TRANSFAMILIES.ORG

INTERSEX

AROUND THE WORLD INTERSEX EDUCATORS AND ACTIVISTS ARE CREATING ORGANIZATIONS TO STOP NONCONSENSUAL SURGERIES. CHECK OUT:

* INTERACT: ADVOCATES FOR INTERSEX YOUTH

* INTERSEX JUSTICE PROJECT

* OII INTERSEX NETWORK

MENSTRUATION / PERIODS

MENSTRUATION ISN'T JUST A BIG DEAL FOR THE BODIES THAT EXPERIENCE IT, IT'S ALSO BIG BUSINESS FOR COMPANIES THAT MAKE PRODUCTS RELATED TO IT. IF YOU WANT TO LEARN MORE ABOUT THE POLITICS OF PERIODS, YOU CAN SEARCH FOR TERMS LIKE "SUSTAINABLE MENSTRUAL PRODUCTS" OR "MENSTRUAL EQUITY."

FOR INFORMATION, CHECK OUT THESE RELIABLE ORGANIZATIONS:

* PLANNEDPARENTHOOD.ORG (AVAILABLE IN ENGLISH / SPANISH)

* SCARLETEEN.COM

* SEXANDU.CA (AVAILABLE IN ENGLISH / FRENCH)

SEX / GENDER ACTIVISM / JUSTICE

THERE IS A LOT OF INJUSTICE IN THE WORLD—BUT THERE ARE ALSO A LOT OF PEOPLE AROUND THE WORLD WORKING TOGETHER TO CHANGE THAT.

IF YOU THINK YOU WANT TO BE PART OF THAT CHANGE, YOU CAN CONNECT WITH OTHER ACTIVISTS IN YOUR COMMUNITY AND ONLINE AROUND THE WORLD. CHECK OUT:

* ACTION CANADA FOR SEXUAL HEALTH AND RIGHTS

* ADVOCATES FOR YOUTH

* BLACK AND PINK

* NATIVE YOUTH SEXUAL HEALTH NETWORK

* RADICAL MONARCHS

* REFLECTION PRESS: WRITE NOW MAKE BOOKS

TRAUMA

IF YOU WANT TO LEARN MORE ABOUT TRAUMA, AND YOU HAVE SOMEONE TRUSTWORTHY TO TALK TO, THEY MAY BE THE BEST PLACE TO START. IF YOU DON'T, YOU CAN USE ANY OF THE HELP/SUPPORT LINES LISTED AT THE BEGINNING OF THIS SECTION. MOST RESOURCES THAT USE THE WORD "TRAUMA" ARE GEARED TO OLDER PEOPLE, SO YOU MAY WANT TO SEARCH USING OTHER TERMS, LIKE "VIOLENCE," "BULLYING," "SELF-CARE," OR "TAKING CARE OF MYSELF."

ACKNOWLEDGEMENTS

WE MAKE BOOKS SLOWLY, AND WITH COMMUNITY. PEOPLE SHARED THEIR TIME AND EXPERIENCE WITH US THROUGH CONVERSATIONS AND BY READING DRAFTS OVER A PERIOD OF MANY YEARS. WHILE WE ARE RESPONSIBLE FOR ANY ERRORS, OMISSIONS, AND BAD PUNS, MUCH OF THE RICHNESS, INSIGHT, AND WISDOM IN THIS BOOK CAME FROM THE CONTRIBUTIONS OF THE FOLLOWING PEOPLE:

ALANNA GAIL KIBBE, ALEJANDRA OSPINA, ALISON HOWELL, AMINA SAM-O, ANNA-LOUISE CRAGO, ANOOSH JORJORIAN, ANDY TANK, ANYA, LINDA & ROBERT J. PECHÉ, BEC SOKHA KEO, BETHANY GEHMAN, BETTY TANK, CAITLIN MACINTYRE, CATHERINE FITZPATRICK, COLIN SILVERBERG, CORAL MALONEY, CYNTHIA LOYST, DANIEL SILVERBERG, DEESHA NARICHANIA, ELI ABRAHAM, ELINOR WHIDDEN (AKA THE ARCHDUKE), ELIZABETH BOSKEY, ELLEN FRIEDRICHS, EMMA KLEIMAN, ESTHER IGNAGNI, FRANCES GRIMSTAD MD,MS, HAZEL LIVINGSTON, HEATHER JAMIESON, HILARY NORTH-ELLASANTE, IAN KHARA ELLASANTE, JAKE PYNE, JANEEN MODDEJONGE, JASMIN TECSON, JENNIFER LUU, JESS ABRAHAM, JIZ LEE, JONATHAN S. BRAJTBORD, MD, DR. JUDITH PERRY, JUDITH TAYLOR, KARI PERRY & LIANA HARTEL, KARLEEN PENDLETON JIMÉNEZ, KATRINA PEDDLE, KOOMAH, LAIA M. BAGUÉS, JARE & ELIAN ITZAZELAIA, LAN LI, LOREE ERICKSON, LORI SELKE WITH SIMONE AND BRUCE, MAY CHAZAN & ZOE HODSON, MICHELE CHAI, MICHELLE BOURGEOIS, MICHELLE DEMOLE, MICHELLE MANTIONE, MICHELLE MURPHY, MICHELLE NAGY, MIRIAM KAUFMAN, MORÉNIKE GIWA ONAIWU, M. MORGAN LEFAY HOLMES, NAUSHABA PATEL, NIKI PARKER, OI YEE AGNES HO, LMSW, PATRICIA BERNE, RAYNA RAPP, REBECCA PICHERACK, SUZANNE & GEOFF SISKIND WITH MOSES & CHARLIE, THEODORE (TED) KERR, TRACEY BROWN, TYLER COHEN, VENITA RAY, VIVIANA CORNEJO, XAVIER NORTH.

SPECIAL THANKS (AND SONGWRITING CO-CREDIT) TO KIA CORTHRON, MARIKO TAMAKI, AND TARA-MICHELLE ZINIUK FOR HELP WITH THE SONG LYRICS ON PAGE 87. AND TO LISA ROSS-RIZIKOV FOR HER GROUNDBREAKING '90S ZINE *DIS-CHARGE*, WHICH INSPIRED OUR PAGE ON THE TOPIC!

THANKS TO OUR TYPOGRAPHER AND BOOK DESIGNER ZAB HOBART FOR 10 YEARS OF COLLABORATING WITH US AND MAKING OUR WORK READABLE AND BEAUTIFUL. THANKS ALSO TO OUR EDITOR VERONICA LIU, THE METICULOUS LAUREN HOOKER, AND THE TEAM AT SEVEN STORIES PRESS FOR PATIENCE, PERSEVERANCE, AND LETTING US MAKE THE BOOKS WE WANT TO MAKE.

CORY WANTS TO THANK BIANCA I LAUREANO AND ZOË WOOL FOR READING AND REREADING PARTS OF THIS MANUSCRIPT MORE TIMES THAN REASONABLE HUMANS SHOULD BE ASKED TO, FOR LAUGHING AT AND WITH HIM DURING DIALOGUE CONSULTATIONS, AND GENERALLY MAKING LIFE BETTER. AND SADIE FOR MAKING IT IMPOSSIBLE TO WORK TOO HARD OR TAKE HIMSELF TOO SERIOUSLY.

FIONA WANTS TO THANK CRAIG DANIELS FOR SUPPORT AND CHEERLEADING THROUGH MANY MANY DAYS OF CREATING AND DRAWING. SHE THANKS SHEILA SMYTH, JEAN SMYTH, AND MARGARET POWELL FOR ROOTING HER ON NEAR THE FINISH LINE. AND GRATITUDE FOR THE MANY SUPPORTERS AND READERS OF OUR PREVIOUS BOOKS, ESPECIALLY THE ONES WHO HAVE GROWN UP TO MEET THIS NEW BOOK.

THIS BOOK WAS WRITTEN AND CREATED ON INDIGENOUS LAND. IT WAS CONCEIVED BY TWO WHITE SETTLERS LIVING IN *TKARONTO*. WE ARE GRATEFUL TO THOSE WHO CARE FOR THE LAND WE LIVE ON, WHO INVITE US TO DO THE SAME, AND WHO REMIND US TO CHERISH THE BEAUTY IN THIS WORLD WHILE WE FIGHT THE INJUSTICES IN IT.